Geriatrics Medicine and Gerontology

Geriatrics Medicine and Gerontology

Editor: Roger Simpson

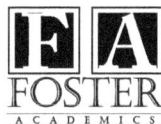

FA
FOSTER
A C A D E M I C S

www.fosteracademics.com

www.fosteracademics.com

FA FOSTER
ACADEMICS

Cataloging-in-Publication Data

Geriatrics medicine and gerontology / edited by Roger Simpson.
    p. cm.
Includes bibliographical references and index.
ISBN 978-1-63242-493-8
1. Geriatrics. 2. Older people--Health and hygiene. 3. Older people--Diseases. 4. Gerontology.
5. Aging. I. Simpson, Roger.
RC952 .G47 2017
618.97--dc23

Foster Academics,
118-35 Queens Blvd., Suite 400,
Forest Hills, NY 11375, USA

ISBN 978-1-63242-493-8 (Hardback)

Contents

Preface

Geriatrics is a branch of medicine that focuses on healthcare of elderly people. This field of medicine is also known as gerontology. This book provides significant information of this discipline to help develop a good understanding of geriatrics and related fields. It aims to put forward the various sub-fields of this discipline so as to get a holistic understanding of geriatrics. It picks up individual branches and explains their need and contribution in the field of geriatrics. For all readers who are interested in the study of care of old people, this book will serve as excellent guide to develop a comprehensive knowledge in a lucid manner.

Significant researches are present in this book. Intensive efforts have been employed by authors to make this book an outstanding discourse. This book contains the enlightening chapters which have been written on the basis of significant researches done by the experts.

Finally, I would also like to thank all the members involved in this book for being a team and meeting all the deadlines for the submission of their respective works. I would also like to thank my friends and family for being supportive in my efforts.

Editor

Associations between Multiple Accelerometry-Assessed Physical Activity Parameters and Selected Health Outcomes in Elderly People – Results from the KORA-Age Study

Sandra Ortlieb[1,2], Lukas Gorzelniak[2], Dennis Nowak[3,4], Ralf Strobl[5,6], Eva Grill[5,6], Barbara Thorand[7], Annette Peters[7], Klaus A. Kuhn[2], Stefan Karrasch[1,8,9], Alexander Horsch[2,10,11¶], Holger Schulz[1*¶]

1 Institute of Epidemiology I, Helmholtz Zentrum München, German Research Center for Environmental Health, Neuherberg, Germany, 2 Institute of Medical Statistics and Epidemiology, Technische Universität München, Munich, Germany, 3 Institute and Outpatient Clinic for Occupational, Social and Environmental Medicine, Ludwig-Maximilians-Universität, Munich, Germany, 4 Comprehensive Pneumology Center Munich (CPC-M), Member of the German Center for Lung Research, Munich, Germany, 5 Institute for Medical Information Processing, Biometrics and Epidemiology, Ludwig-Maximilians-Universität München, Munich, Germany, 6 German Center for Vertigo and Balance Disorders, Ludwig-Maximilians-Universität München, Munich, Germany, 7 Institute of Epidemiology II, Helmholtz Zentrum München, German Research Center for Environmental Health, Neuherberg, Germany, 8 Institute and Outpatient Clinic for Occupational, Social and Environmental Medicine, Ludwig-Maximilians-Universität, Munich, Germany, 9 Institute of General Practice, University Hospital Klinikum rechts der Isar, Technische Universität München, Munich, Germany, 10 Department of Computer Science, University of Tromsø, Tromsø, Norway, 11 Department of Clinical Medicine, University of Tromsø, Tromsø, Norway

Abstract

Introduction: Accelerometry is an important method for extending our knowledge about intensity, duration, frequency and patterns of physical activity needed to promote health. This study has used accelerometry to detect associations between intensity levels and related activity patterns with multimorbidity and disability. Moreover, the proportion of people meeting the physical activity recommendations for older people was assessed.

Methods: Physical activity was measured in 168 subjects (78 males; 65–89 years of age), using triaxial GT3X accelerometers for ten consecutive days. The associations between physical activity parameters and multimorbidity or disability was examined using multiple logistic regression models, which were adjusted for gender, age, education, smoking, alcohol consumption, lung function, nutrition and multimorbidity or disability.

Results: 35.7% of the participants met the physical activity recommendations of at least 150 minutes of moderate to vigorous activity per week. Only 11.9% reached these 150 minutes, when only bouts of at least 10 minutes were counted. Differences in moderate to vigorous activity between people with and without multimorbidity or disability were more obvious when shorter bouts instead of only longer bouts were included. Univariate analyses showed an inverse relationship between physical activity and multimorbidity or disability for light and moderate to vigorous physical activity. A higher proportion of long activity bouts spent sedentarily was associated with higher risk for multimorbidity, whereas a high proportion of long bouts in light activity seemed to prevent disability. After adjustment for covariates, there were no significant associations, anymore.

Conclusions: The accumulated time in moderate to vigorous physical activity seems to have a stronger relationship with health and functioning when shorter activity bouts and not only longer bouts were counted. We could not detect an association of the intensity levels or activity patterns with multimorbidity or disability in elderly people after adjustment for covariates.

Editor: Nuria Garatachea, University of Zaragoza, Spain

Funding: The KORA research platform (KORA, Cooperative Health Research in the Region of Augsburg) was initiated and financed by the Helmholtz Zentrum München, German Research Center for Environmental Health (formerly GSF, National Research Center for Environment and Health), which is funded by the German Federal Ministry of Education and Research and by the State of Bavaria. KORA Age was financed by the German Federal Ministry of Education and Research (BMBF FKZ 01ET0713). Further support was provided by the BMBF funded Competence Network ASCONET, subnetwork COSYCONET (FKZ 01GI0882). The research was supported by the Graduate School of Information Science in Health (GSISH) and the Technische Universität München Graduate School. Lukas Gorzelniak received university grant monies as a PhD scholarship from 3/1/2009 to 6/30/2012. The funders had no role in study design, data collection and analysis, decision to publish, or preparation of the manuscript.

Competing Interests: The authors have declared that no competing interests exist.

* Email: schulz@helmholtz-muenchen.de

¶ These authors shared last authorship.

Introduction

Population aging will be a substantial societal phenomenon in the next half century. Due to the increase in life expectancy and the associated increase in the number of individuals at risk for chronic diseases and injuries, the aging of the population will produce crucial societal challenges [1]. Physical activity (PA) is a fundamental component targeted at preventing diseases and maintaining functional independence as well as in therapeutic intervention and rehabilitation programs for older adults.

Many studies have shown significant associations between PA and certain chronic diseases, including coexistence of selected diseases with high prevalence (e.g. cardiovascular diseases and diabetes) [2,3]. In contrast, studies about the associations of multimorbidity (the coexistence of multiple chronic diseases) and PA are rare. Only one article about this subject was included in the review by Marengoni et al. [4] in 2011, who examined occurrence, causes, and consequences of multimorbidity. Hudon et al. [5] did not identify an association between multimorbidity and PA. Recently, two further studies were published which showed an inverse association between PA and multimorbidity [6,7]. The relationship between PA and functional limitations or disability has been better investigated: two reviews dealt with this topic and reported consistent results demonstrating a positive influence of PA on the relationship of aging and disability [8,9]. However, all studies on the associations between disability or multimorbidity and PA used self-reports to assess PA.

Although moderate to vigorous physical activity (MVPA) has been shown to provide beneficial effects to the health and functioning of older people [10,11], little is known about the impact of light PA and the activity patterns needed to promote health in elderly people. The global recommendations on PA from the World Health Organization (WHO) [11] suggest that adults, including older adults, should perform a minimum of 150 min of at least moderate intensity PA per week for beneficial health effects. Moreover, the activity should be performed in bouts of at least 10 min duration. Moderate PA is defined as considerable increases in heart rate and breathing, such as brisk walking, and vigorous PA is even more exhausting [12]. The proportion of elderly people who meet the recommended PA guidelines diminishes from 47% −63%, found through questionnaires, to 6% −26%, when assessed by use of accelerometers [13].

Due to low costs and high feasibility, PA was usually measured by means of questionnaires in large epidemiological studies. The instrument requires a thorough and objective consideration of the questions addressed but it often comes along with recall bias, socially desirable responses, and the influence of mood, depression, anxiety, cognition, and disability on responses [14]. Accelerometers resolve some of the limitations of self-report instruments: they are not affected by random and systematic errors introduced by respondents and interviewers, and they provide valid and reliable estimates about basic characteristics (frequency, duration and intensity of PA) as well as of PA patterns [15,16]. Moreover, accelerometers have improved the ability to examine the relationship between PA and different health outcomes and thus present supportive statistics for public health planning and intervention [17].

Recently, sedentary PA, as characterized by activities involving mainly sitting, has been proposed as a risk factor for all-cause disease that is independent of MVPA [18]. The role of light PA (e.g. self-care, cooking, casual walking or shopping), measured by accelerometers, with regard to health effects has been less studied [19,20]. This might be of particular interest for older people who

are limited in their exercise capacity due to age-related physical or mental restrictions [21]. In this respect, the patterns of PA have been proposed as a new group of PA outcomes that may offer additional information beyond reports of activity counts and activity type recognition [22].

In our study, we will examine the associations between the volume of PA (divided into sedentary PA: ≤ 100 counts per min (cpm), light PA: 101–1951 cpm, and MVPA: ≥ 1952 cpm) as well as PA patterns (with the so called GINI-Index [22,23] as quantification) measured by accelerometers and specific health outcomes (disability and multimorbidity). Each health outcome is a clinically distinct entity with different prognosis and health care implications [24] and should therefore be observed individually. In this context, we will answer the following research questions: 1) Is there an association between the volume of sedentary or light PA and the two health outcomes, independent of MVPA? 2) Is there an association between PA patterns and the two health outcomes? 3) Are there differences and similarities regarding the relationship of PA with disability and multimorbidity? The answers to these questions will allow us to present novel information about the associations between sedentary PA, light PA as well as PA patterns and different health outcomes. Furthermore, we will assess the proportion of people fulfilling the current global recommendations of PA for older people under different methodical conditions, i.e. assess the impact of different bout lengths varying between 1 and the WHO recommended 10 min in subjects with and without disability or multimorbidity, and translate our results into advice for the prevention of chronic diseases and disability in elderly people.

Methods

The KORA-Age study was approved by the Ethical Committee of the Bavarian medical association (Ethik-Kommission Nr. 08064), written informed consent has been obtained from the participants and all investigations have been conducted according to the principles expressed in the Declaration of Helsinki.

Study population

Data from the present study derived from the KORA (Cooperative Health Research in the Region of Augsburg)-Age cohort. The KORA-Age study investigates the determinants and consequences of health status changes of older adults in a representative population based sample over a period of 3 years. Details have been described previously [25]. Since lung function is an important predictor of morbidity and mortality [26], 200 eligible individuals with extreme lung function values within the normal range had been selected from the first and fourth quartiles of the study population and grouped into a 'better' and a 'worse' lung function group. Activity counts from the non-dominant side of the hip were measured in 191 subjects at a rate of 30 Hz and stored at an epoch length of 2 sec by means of a GT3X (ActiGraph, Pensacola, FL, USA) accelerometers during daily living. Data filtering was set to default ('normal') as recommended by ActiGraph. PA was recorded up to 10 days, starting from the day at the study center where the accelerometers were handed out, until the eleventh day, which was the day the subjects were instructed to return the devices. PA data from the first recorded day as well as any other day with a wear time of less than ten hours were excluded. To be included in the study, subjects had to have a minimum of four valid days. After exclusion of subjects with insufficient days of recordings (n = 19) or accelerometer malfunctions (n = 4), the final study sample comprised 78 men and 90 women. Participants had 8.1±1.5 (mean ± SD) days of valid accelerometer data. The mean wear time was 740±114 min per day.

Details about the study design, participants and other methodic procedures have been described previously [22].

Measures

Independent variables. The independent variables included: gender; age (65–69, 70–74, 75–79, >79); BMI (under-weight if <18.5 kg/m^2, normal weight if 18.5–24.9 kg/m^2, overweight if 25.0–29.9 kg/m^2 and obesity if ≥30.0 kg/m^2); education (≤10 years vs. >10 years); smoking habits (never, formerly smoked vs. currently smokes); alcohol consumption (teetotalism vs. no teetotalism); lung function ('better' vs. 'worse' lung function group) and risk of malnutrition measured by the Geriatric Nutritional Risk Index (GNRI) (major risk if <82, moderate risk if ≥82 and < 92), low risk if >92 and ≤98, and no risk if >98) [27]. No person was at major risk and only 4 people were on moderate risk. Therefore we merged moderate and low risk.

Physical activity: To represent the characteristics of PA, multiple variables were obtained from uniaxial accelerometer data. As an overall measure of PA average counts per minute (cpm) were calculated for each subject. Times in different intensity levels were calculated by the most commonly used PA cut points applied for adults: *sedentary PA* was defined as ≤100 cpm [14] and the cut points by Freedson et al. [28] were used for *light* (101– 1951 cpm), *moderate* (1952–5724 cpm), and *vigorous PA* (5725–9498 cpm). *PA patterns:* In the present study, a *bout* is defined as consecutive min spent in a specific intensity level, i.e. sedentary PA, light PA or MVPA, without interruption. To determine the time participants spent in the MVPA level and the portion of people fulfilling the current PA recommendations of ≥ 150 min of MVPA per week [11], we applied different cut offs for the bout lengths, ranging from 1 min to 10 min: i.e. the recommended ≥150 min of MVPA per week had to be performed in bouts of at least 1 min up to at least 10 min. We averaged MVPA over all valid days of recordings and multiplied it by seven, in order to test if a person met the PA recommendations of ≥ 150 min per week.

Activity patterns are characterized by the distribution of frequency of bouts of different duration. This information is combined by the so-called *GINI-index (G)*, introduced by Chastin and colleagues [23]. The index expresses how the PA time in a specific intensity level is accumulated with respect to the bout lengths. The index value *G* ranges from 0 to 1 and has to be interpreted as follows: *High G values*: large difference between minimal and maximal bout lengths and relatively high proportion of few long bouts in relation to the overall time. *Low G values*: small difference between minimal and maximal bout length, i.e. the activity pattern is characterized by a lot of relatively short bouts of similar length. A G value of 0 would result if all the bouts were the same length. Note that this does not depend on the length of these bouts, but only on their relationship to each other.

Dependent variables. *Multimorbidity* was defined as the presence of ≥2 *chronic diseases* out of a list of 13 chronic diseases: hypertension, eye disease, heart disease, diabetes mellitus, joint disease, lung disease, gastrointestinal disease, mental disease, stroke, cancer, kidney disease, neurological disease, liver disease. Chronic health conditions were determined through a self-administered questionnaire and a standardized telephone interview adapted from the self-report-generated Charlson Comorbidity Index [29].

Disability was quantified using the Health Assessment Questionnaire Disability Index (HAQ-DI) [30] during a telephone interview. The instrument consists of 20 questions in eight domains (dressing and grooming, hygiene, arising, reach, eating, grip, walking, and common daily activities), which can be answered on a scale from 0 (no difficulty), 1 (some difficulty), 2 (much difficulty) to 3 (unable to perform). The HAQ-DI score is the mean of the eight domains. In line with the literature [31], disability was defined as HAQ-DI >0. The HAQ had shown high validity, a good test-retest reliability, and internal consistency, and can be applied very well to elderly people [31]. For more detailed information regarding disability within the KORA-Age framework see Strobl et al. [32].

Statistical analyses

Some of the metric variables were not normally distributed. Thus, the Wilcoxon two-sample test was used for metric variables to test for differences between people with and without a diagnosis of multimorbidity or disability, and Chi^2-test for categorical variables. For the multiple logistic regression models, we used the interquartile range (IQR) of each PA variable as scaling distance. The IQR is defined as the distance between the 25th and 75th percentiles and thus describes values of the predictor that are relatively well-represented in the sample [33]. The association between the six PA parameters (sedentary PA, light PA, MVPA, G for sedentary PA (G$_{sedentary}$), G for light PA (G$_{light}$) or G for MVPA (G$_{MVPA}$)) and multimorbidity as well as disability was examined using multiple logistic regression models. Statistical models were adjusted for gender, age, BMI, education, smoking, alcohol consumption, lung function group, nutrition, and one of the health outcomes (multimorbidity, disability), as appropriate. Results are presented as odds ratios (OR) and 95% confidence intervals. Statistically significant differences were assumed at a significance level of p<0.05. Statistical analyses were conducted using SAS version 9.2 (SAS institute Cary, NC).

Results

Descriptive characteristics

Table 1 presents the characteristics of the study sample: 168 people (46.4% male, 53.6% female) were included in the study with a median (5%, 95%) age of 73 (65, 86) years and a median BMI of 27 (23, 35) kg/m^2. More than half of the study sample (51.8%) was multimorbid and 41.7% of the participants were disabled. 29.7% of all participants were both disabled and multimorbid (results not shown in the table). More detailed information about the subject characteristics and clinical parameters stratified by multimorbidity and disability are presented in table 1 (median values) and table S1 (mean values).

PA and bout length. Overall, most of the time in MVPA (55%) was performed in bouts of one min (Figure 1). 47.6% of the participants did not achieve at least one 10-min bout. 35.7% of the participants met the current PA recommendations [11] of performing ≥150 min of MVPA, regardless of bout length, and 11.9% reached this in bouts of at least 10 min (Figure 2A). Differences in terms of MVPA between people with and without a diagnosis of disability or multimorbidity were stronger under consideration of short bouts instead of only using longer bouts, and more obvious with regard to disablity compared to multimorbidity. Furthermore, there was little difference between disabled individuals and people which were both disabled and multimorbid (Figure 2A and 2B). In addition, mean values are presented in Figure S1.

Table 2 shows the PA variables stratified by presence of disability and presence of multimorbidity. The median (5%/ 95%) activity per day was 221 (67/487) cpm. Lower values were

Table 1. Characteristics of the participants, stratified by multimorbidity and disability. Median (5%, 95%).

	all	multimorbidity		disability	
	n = 168	no	yes	no	yes
		n = 81	n = 87	n = 98	n = 70
Age (years)	73 (65/86)	**69 (65/84)**	**77 (67/87)**	**71 (65/84)**	**76 (67/87)**
BMI (kg/m^2)	27 (23/35)	27 (21/35)	27 (23/37)	**27 (21/34)**	**28 (23/38)**
Gender, m (n, (%))	78 (46.4)	40 (49.4)	38 (43.7)	**56 (57.1)**	**22 (31.4)**
Education ≤10 years (n (%))	110 (65.5)	56 (69.1)	54 (62.1)	59 (60.2)	51 (72.9)
Alcohol abstinence, yes (n (%))	23 (13.7)	8 (9.9)	15 (17.2)	**9 (9.2)**	**14 (20.0)**
Smoker or ex-smoker (n (%))	97 (57.7)	46 (56.8)	51 (58.6)	56 (57.1)	41 (58.6)
GNRI	109 (96/124)	108 (97/123)	109 (95/126)	108 (96/122)	110 (96/129)
Health outcomes					
Lung group, better (n (%))	92 (54.7)	47 (58.0)	45 (51.7)	58 (59.2)	34 (48.6)
Disability, yes (n (%))	70 (41.7)	**20 (24.7)**	**50 (57.5)**	–	–
Multimorbidity, yes (n (%))	87 (51.8)	–	–	**37 (37.8)**	**50 (71.4)**

Significant differences are written in bold, p≤0.05. Wilcoxon-test was used for metric variables and Chi^2-test for categorical variables; GNRI = Geriatric Nutritional Risk Index.

observed in subjects with multimorbidity (181 (62/455) cpm) and disability (174 (57 439) cpm) while subjects without multimorbidity or disability showed significantly higher values. Overall, the participants passed a median time of 65% being sedentary, 32% in light activity and 2% in MVPA. Values of G tended to increase with decreasing intensity level: $G_{sedentary} = 0.63$, $G_{light} = 0.48$, and $G_{MVPA} = 0.43$ (see Table S2 for mean values). According to this, the accumulated PA time in the sedentary level was composed of a higher proportion of long bouts compared to the light or MVPA level. Multimorbid participants were generally less active. They spent 4% more of their time in the sedentary level (p<0.01), 2% less in the light level (p = 0.02) and 1% less in the MVPA level (p< 0.01) compared to people who were not multimorbid. Moreover, $G_{sedentary}$ was significantly higher in multimorbid people (p<0.01).

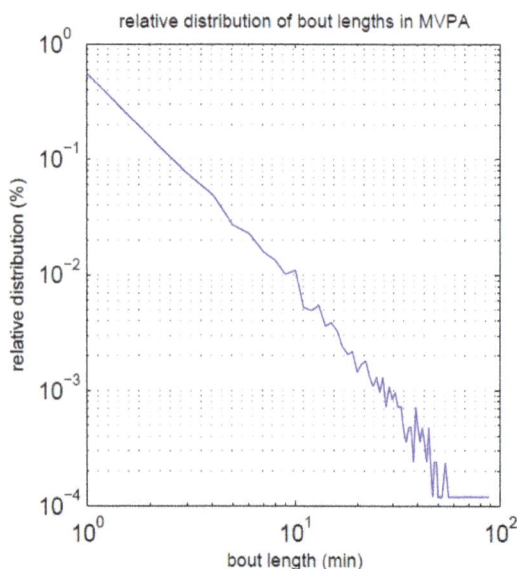

Figure 1. Distribution of PA bouts of moderate to vigorous physical activity.

The results for disability were similar with regard to the intensity levels, but not in terms of the PA patterns: G_{light} and G_{MVPA} were significantly lower in disabled people compared to people without diagnosis of disability (p = 0.04 and p<0.01).

Table 3 presents associations between the six PA variables and the prevalence of multimorbidity or disability, respectively. For the multiple regression models, each PA variable was scaled by its interquartile range (IQR). The resulting regression coefficient from IQR compares a person in the middle of the upper half of the predictor distribution to a person in the middle of the lower half of the distribution.

PA and multimorbidity. The risk of multimorbidity seemed to be 1.7 times higher for an elderly person with a typical 'high' (75th percentile) value on sedentary PA compared to a person with a typically 'low' (25th percentile) value (model 1). In contrast, high values of light PA and MVPA showed a protective effect (OR = 0.88, p = 0.02 and OR = 0.99, p<0.01). Since the participants spent little time in MVPA and the variance of MVPA was very low, even an OR of 0.99 emerged as a statistically significant risk. High $G_{sedentary}$ values appeared to increase the risk of multimorbidity by the factor 1.5 compared to low values. After adjustment for age and sex (model 2) all results tended into the same direction, however they were not significant, anymore. The same applied to model 3 (also adjusted for BMI, smoking, education, alcohol consumption, nutrition, lung function, and disability). Instead, higher age and presence of disability were significant predictors for multimorbidity, no matter which of the PA variables was included in the model.

PA and disability. The risk of disability appeared to be twice as high for participants with a typical 'high' value on sedentary PA compared to people with a typically 'low' value. In contrast, high values of light PA and MVPA showed a significant protective effect (OR = 0.84, p<0.01 and OR = 0.99, p<0.01). Due to the low variance of MVPA, even an OR of 0.99 emerged as a significant result. High G_{light} values reduced the risk of multimorbidity by 21% compared to low values. Significant associations between the three intensity levels and disability persisted, even after adjustment for age and sex (model 2). However, there were no significant relations, anymore, after controlling for further covariates (model

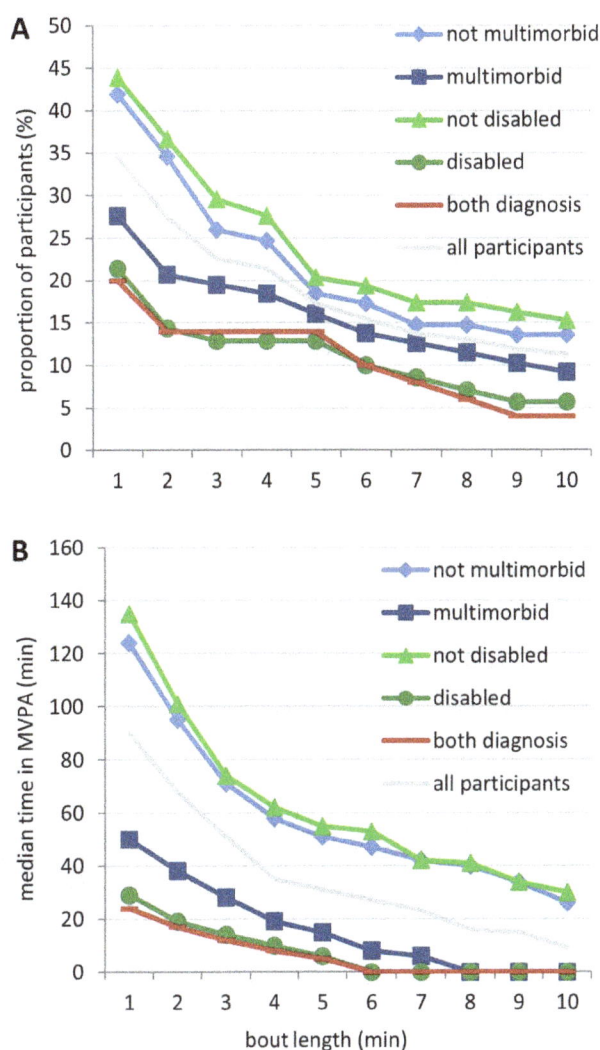

Figure 2. Moderate to vigorous physical activity (MVPA) in relation to different minimal bout lengths. A) Proportion of participants (%) fulfilling ≥150 min of MVPA/week vs. minimal bout length. B) Median time in MVPA per week (min). Each bout length refers to the minimal number of consecutive min in MVPA required for inclusion in the calculation of accumulated time in MVPA, i.e. if bout length is 3 then bouts of length 1 and 2 are excluded.

3). Instead, female gender and presence of multimorbidity emerged as significant risk factors for disability, no matter which of the PA variables was included in the model.

When comparing the models of the two health outcomes multimorbidity and disability, all results point in the same direction. According to model 2, the relationship between disability and PA seemed to be stronger than the relationship between multimorbidity and PA. The more variables were included in the model, the weaker became the associations between PA variables and health outcomes.

Discussion

To the best of our knowledge, this is the first study examining the association between PA patterns and multimorbidity or disability on a sample of elderly people using accelerometry.

One striking finding was that shorter bouts (e.g. 1-min bouts) of MVPA seem to provide more distinct evidence about the positive effect of MVPA with multimorbidity and disability than longer bouts (e.g. 10-min bouts). An explanation for this may be the relatively short overall time that elderly people spend in this level and especially the low proportion of long bouts. This finding is in contrast to the current PA recommendations [11] which request that PA is performed in bouts of at least 10 min (in the following called '10-min bout rule') for beneficial health effects.

The majority of older adults (61.3%) failed to meet the PA recommendations [11] of 150 min of MVPA per week. When the 10-min bout rule was applied, only 11.9% fulfilled the recommendations. Differences in terms of MVPA between people with and without disability or multimorbidity were more obvious in connection with disability than with multimorbidity. Furthermore, disability seemed to be the limiting factor with regard to MVPA in people which were both disabled and multimorbid. Troiano et al. [34] reported that 7.6% of people ≥60 years met the recommendations of at least 150 min MVPA per week and according to MVPA performed in 10-min bouts only 2.4%. According to Tucker et al. [13] 8.5% of people aged 60–69 and 6.3% of people ≥70 years met the recommendations taking into account the 10-min bout rule. An explanation for the somewhat higher rates of people achieving the recommendations in our study might be that the participants had to attend the KORA study center and thus seemed to have better general health as compared to other studies: The prevalence of multimorbidity (defined as 2+ concurrent diseases) of older people widely varied (55−98%) across studies [4]. A large epidemiological study by van den Bussche et al. [35] determined a multimorbidity prevalence of 62% in Germany among people aged 65 or above and a comparable study about disability observed a prevalence of 63.6% [36] while we observed lower prevalence values, 52% of elderly people in our population were multimorbid and 42% were disabled.

There were differences between participants with and without a diagnosis of multimorbidity in terms of all intensity levels (sedentary PA, light PA, MVPA). The more time people spent actively, the lower was the risk of multimorbidity, regardless intensity of the movement. PA patterns of elderly people with and without multimorbidity only differed with regard to the PA level: people without a diagnosis seemed to get up more often. The associations were lost after adjusting for BMI, smoking, education, alcohol consumption, nutrition, lung function, and disability. Only higher age and disability showed significant associations with multimorbidity. Few large population-based health studies also investigated the relationship between PA and multimorbidity or the number of chronic diseases and reached inconsistent results: Hudon et al. [5] examined people aged 45–68 and found no relationship between multimorbidity and PA levels when age, education, income, employment, long-term limitations on activity, self-rated general health, and psychological distress were controlled for. In contrast, a study about Brazilian women aged 40 to 65 determined an increased likelihood of having two or more morbid conditions for inactive women after adjustment for sociodemographic, behavioral, clinical, and reproductive factors [6]. Likewise, two other studies reported an associations between multimorbidity and the frequency of PA (15 min, ≥12 times per month for positive effects) [37] or a mean PA score [7] in people aged ≥65 years of age after adjusting for predictor variables. However, comparisons between these studies and our results are limited because they used questionnaires to assess PA. Furthermore, the studies used different covariates, different definitions of PA (e.g. 'active' and 'inactive' vs. continuous), different definitions of multimorbidity (e.g. 'multimorbid' vs. 'not multimorbid' vs.

Table 2. PA variables by mulitmorbidity and disability. Median (5%/95%).

PA variables	all	n	not multimorbid	n	multimorbid	n
Average PA (cpm)	221 (67/487)	**168**	**250 (120/487)**	81	**181 (62/455)**	**87**
Sedentary PA time (%)	0.65 (0.48/0.82)	168	**0.63 (0.46/0.79)**	81	**0.67 (0.51/0.84)**	87
Light PA time (%)	0.32 (0.18/0.48)	168	**0.33 (0.20/0.51)**	81	**0.31 (0.16/0.48)**	87
MVPA time (%)	0.02 (0.00/0.08)	168	**0.02 (0.00/0.08)**	81	**0.01 (0.00/0.07)**	87
$G_{sedentary}$	0.63 (0.57/0.68)	168	**0.62 (0.57/0.68)**	81	**0.64 (0.58/0.68)**	87
G_{light}	0.48 (0.37/0.55)	168	0.48 (0.38/0.55)	81	0.47 (0.37/0.55)	87
G_{MVPA}	0.43 (0.00/0.66)	156	0.45 (0.00/0.67)	77	0.40 (0.00/0.65)	79
	all	n	not disabled	n	disabled	n
Average PA (cpm)	221 (67/487)	**168**	**269 (119/542)**	98	**174 (57/439)**	**70**
Sedentary PA time (%)	0.65 (0.48/0.82)	168	**0.64 (0.46/0.77)**	98	**0.68 (0.54/0.84)**	70
Light PA time (%)	0.32 (0.18/0.48)	168	**0.32 (0.21/0.51)**	98	**0.31 (0.16/0.45)**	70
MVPA time (%)	0.02 (0.00/0.08)	168	**0.02 (0.00/0.09)**	98	**0.01 (0.00/0.07)**	70
$G_{sedentary}$	0.63 (0.57/0.68)	168	0.63 (0.57/0.68)	98	0.63 (0.57/0.70)	70
G_{light}	0.48 (0.37/0.55)	168	**0.48 (0.40/0.55)**	98	**0.47 (0.35/0.55)**	70
G_{MVPA}	0.43 (0.00/0.66)	156	**0.46 (0.13/0.68)**	96	**0.37 (0.00/0.62)**	60

Results emerged from Wilcoxon-test. Significant differences are written in bold, $p \le 0.05$; cpm = counts per minute; G = GINI-Index; high G = mainly few long bouts are responsible for the activity pattern; low G = mainly short bouts of similar length contribute to the activity pattern.

number of chronic conditions) and they partially included other age groups. Nonetheless, the present study supports the findings by Hudon et al. [5] that there is no association between multimorbidity and PA after controlling for covariates, based on objective assessment of PA.

According to the univariate results, PA was associated with disability. The risk for disability was twice as high in people with a high proportion of time spent sedentarily compared to people with less time in this level, whereas high levels of light PA and MVPA seemed protective (OR = 0.84 and OR = 0.99). Since the participants spent little time in MVPA and the variance of MVPA was very low, the OR of 0.99 emerged as significant risk. PA patterns of elderly people with and without disability only differed in terms of light PA. A high proportion of long bouts in light activity appeared protective against disability (OR = 0.8). After adjustment of the predictor variables, there were no significant associations,

Table 3. OR and 95% CI describing the associations between PA variables and prevalent diseases.

	Model 1[a]	p	Model 2[b]	p	Model 3[c]	p
Multimorbidity						
Sedentary PA, IQR	**1.66 (1.14, 2.40)**	**<.01**	1.32 (0.88, 2.00)	0.18	1.11 (0.70, 1.76)	0.67
Light PA, IQR	**0.88 (0.78, 0.98)**	**0.02**	0.93 (0.82, 1.06)	0.28	0.99 (0.86, 1.14)	0.86
MVPA, IQR	**0.99 (0.99, 1.00)**	**<.01**	1.00 (0.99, 1.00)	0.15	1.00 (0.99, 1.00)	0.30
$G_{sedentary}$, IQR	**1.48 (1.12, 1.97)**	**<.01**	1.33 (0.97, 1.82)	0.07	1.46 (1.03, 2.06)	0.03
G_{light}, IQR	0.90 (0.75, 1.08)	0.25	1.00 (0.81, 1.23)	0.98	1.13 (0.88, 1.46)	0.33
G_{MVPA}, IQR	1.02 (0.86, 1.21)	0.79	1.03 (0.86, 1.25)	0.73	1.07 (0.86, 1.33)	0.55
Disability						
Sedentary PA, IQR	**1.99 (1.33, 2.98)**	**<.01**	**1.74 (1.10, 2.75)**	**0.02**	1.52 (0.91, 2.53)	0.11
Light PA, IQR	**0.84 (0.75, 0.94)**	**<.01**	**0.86 (0.76, 0.99)**	**0.03**	0.89 (0.76, 1.03)	0.11
MVPA, IQR	**0.99 (0.98, 1.00)**	**<.01**	**0.99 (0.99, 1.00)**	**0.02**	1.00 (0.99, 1.00)	0.31
$G_{sedentary}$, IQR	1.19 (0.90, 1.58)	0.21	1.01 (0.74, 1.38)	0.94	0.89 (0.63, 1.25)	0.50
G_{light}, IQR	**0.79 (0.65, 0.95)**	**0.02**	0.85 (0.68, 1.06)	0.14	0.84 (0.65, 1.09)	0.18
G_{MVPA}, IQR	0.99 (0.83, 1.18)	0.88	0.96 (0.80, 1.16)	0.68	0.96 (0.79, 1.17)	0.70

Significant estimates are written in bold, $p \le 0.05$. P-values result from multiple logistic regression models.
[a]unadjusted.
[b]adjusted for age and sex.
[c]also adjusted for BMI, smoking, education, alcohol consumption, nutrition, lung function, and multimorbidity or disability.
G = GINI-Index; high G = mainly few long bouts are responsible for the activity pattern; low G = mainly short bouts of similar length contribute to the activity pattern;

anymore. Even if PA parameters do not appear to be related to disability, it is related to other variables such as gender and multimorbidity. Strong evidence from questionnaire-based literature indicates that older adults who participate in regular PA have a reduced risk of functional limitations [32,38]. Significant results were shown for MVPA after controlling for potential predictors, whereas findings for light PA are inconsistent [39]. We found two other accelerometer-based studies which researched the relationship between PA and disability. They showed a significant association between daily PA and disability after controlling for other predictors [40,41]. However, they did not provide information about the exact intensity levels they applied.

Neither of the mentioned studies used a disability or multimorbidity index that accounted for the severity of the functional limitation or of any disease. A previous study showed that chronic diseases were only associated with another health outcome when the severity of the disease was considered [42].

To our knowledge, the present study is the first one that examined the association between accelerometry-assessed PA levels and multimorbidity in elderly people and the only one that presents information about the relationship of PA patterns with disability and multimorbidity. Due to the objective measurement, our results are not affected by recall biases associated with self-report in older people at risk for cognitive decline.

However, since our participants had to visit the study center, a selection bias is possible which may be responsible for somewhat lower rates of multimorbid and disabled people and slightly increased MVPA. As our study was cross-sectional, we cannot assure causality for any of the associations. For greater understanding of the associations, longitudinal or intervention studies are required. Another limitation of this study is the limited validity of the cut-points applied to classify activities into intensity levels [43] in elderly people [44]. We chose the algorithm by Freedson et al. [28] because it had the highest potential to provide comparable data [14,19,45]. More information on this issue can be found elsewhere [22]. Furthermore, the GT3X accelerometer used in this study is likely to underestimate activities due to its inability to measure water-related activities (e.g. swimming) and to detect the types of activities performed (e.g. cycling, gymnastics, or strength trainings) [16]. Other characteristics, such as self-rated health status or psychological distress level, may have been included in the model [5]. However, we wanted this study to be focused on the relationship of PA with multimorbidity and disability and decided not to include further covariates in the analysis.

Conclusion

In elderly people, MVPA seems to have a stronger relationship with multimorbidity and disability when shorter bouts and not only longer bouts were counted. In older people who are both disabled and multimorbid, disability seems to be the limiting factor for the performance of MVPA. From the univariate analysis presented, the following conclusions can be drawn: multimorbid people should interrupt their periods of inactivity more frequently, whereas disabled people should increase the proportion of long bouts in light activities. Again, associations between disability and PA were stronger than those between multimorbidity and PA. These conclusions should be treated with caution and are limited in their validity, since the findings were not significant after adjustment for covariates. According to multiple logistic regression analyses other variables emerged as significant predictors: higher age and disability were associated with higher risk of multimorbidity; female gender and multimorbidity were associated with higher risk of disability. Studies which take into account the severity of the disease of functional limitation could contribute to a greater understanding of the associations.

Supporting Information

Figure S1 Moderate to vigorous physical activity (MVPA) in relation to different minimal bout lengths. Mean (SD) time in MVPA per week (min). Each bout length refers to the minimal number of consecutive min in MVPA required for inclusion in the calculation of accumulated time in MVPA, i.e. if bout length is 3 then bouts of length 1 and 2 are excluded.

Table S1 Characteristics of the participants, stratified by multimorbidity and disability. Mean (SD). GNRI = Geriatric Nutritional Risk Index.

Table S2 PA variables by mulitmorbidity and disability. Mean (SD). cpm = counts per minute; G = GINI-Index; high G = mainly few long bouts are responsible for the activity pattern; low G = mainly short bouts of similar length contribute to the activity pattern.

Acknowledgments

Thanks to the subjects for their agreement to participate in the KORA-Age study and also to wear the accelerometers. Thanks to Claudia Flexeder (HMGU) for the statistical support.

Author Contributions

Conceived and designed the experiments: LG DN SK AP BT EG RS KAK HS AH. Performed the experiments: LG DN SK AP BT EG RS KAK HS AH. Analyzed the data: SO AH HS. Contributed reagents/materials/analysis tools: AH HS LG SK SO. Wrote the paper: SO. Manuscript revision and final approval of the version to be published: SO LG DN RS EG BT AP KAK SK AH HS.

References

1. Sidall C, Kjaeserud G, Dziworski W, Przywara B, Xavier A (2007) Healthy Ageing: Keystone for a Sustainable Europe. EU Health Policy in the Context of Demographic Change: Discussion Paper of the Services of DG SANCO, DG ECFIN.

2. Tanasescu M, Leitzmann M, Rimm E, Willett W, Stampfer M, et al. (2002) Exercise type and intensity in relation to coronary heart disease in men. JAMA 288: 1994–2000.

3. Knowler W, Barrett-Connor E, Fowler S, Hamman R, Lachin J, et al. (2002) Reduction in the incidence of type 2 diabetes with lifestyle intervention or metformin. NEnglJMed 346: 393–403.

4. Marengoni A, Angleman S, Melis R, Mangialasche F, Karp A, et al. (2011) Aging with multimorbidity: A systematic review of the literature. Ageing Research Reviews 10: 430–439.

5. Hudon C, Soubhi H, Fortin M (2008) Relationship between multimorbidity and physical activity: Secondary analysis from the Quebec health survey. BMC Public Health 8: 304.

6. de Souza Santos Machado V, Valadares A, da Costa-Paiva L, Moraes S, Pinto-Neto A (2012) Multimorbidity and associated factors in Brazilian women aged 40 to 65 years: a population-based study [Abstract]. Menopause 19: 569–575.

7. Autenrieth C, Kirchberger I, Heier M, Zimmermann A, Peters A, et al. (2013) Physical activity is inversely associated with multimorbidity in elderly men: Results from the KORA-Age Augsburg Study. Prev Med 57: 17–19.

8. Paterson D, Warburton D (2010) Physical activity and functional limitations in older adults: a systematic review related to Canada's Physical Activity Guidelines. Int J Behav Nutr Phys Act 7: 38.

9. Tak E, Kuiper R, Chorus A, Hopman-Rock M (2013) Prevention of onset and progression of basic ADL disability by physical activity in community dwelling older adults: A meta-analysis. Ageing Res Rev 12: 329–338.

10. Nelson ME, Rejeski WJ, Blair SN, Duncan PW, Judge JO, et al. (2007) Physical activity and public health in older adults: recommendation from the American College of Sports Medicine and the American Heart Association. Med Sci Sports Exerc 39: 1435–1445.

11. WHO (2010) Global Recommendations on Physical Activity for Health. Geneva: World Health Organization.

12. Haskell WL, Lee IM, Pate RR, Powell KE, Blair SN, et al. (2007) Physical activity and public health: updated recommendation for adults from the American College of Sports Medicine and the American Heart Association. Med Sci Sports Exerc 39: 1423–1434.

13. Tucker JM, Welk GJ, Beyler NK (2011) Physical activity in U.S.: adults compliance with the Physical Activity Guidelines for Americans. Am J Prev Med 40: 454–461.

14. Gorman E, Hanson H, Yang P, Khan K, Liu-Ambrose T, et al. (2014) Accelerometry analysis of physical activity and sedentary behavior in older adults: a systematic review and data analysis. Eur Rev Aging Phys Act 11: 35–49.

15. Troiano RP (2005) A Timely Meeting: Objective Measurement of Physical Activity. Med Sci Sports Exerc 37: S487–489.

16. Matthews CE, Hagströmer M, Pober DM, Bowles HR (2012) Best Practices for Using Physical Activity Monitors in Population Based Research - review. Med Sci Sports Exerc 44: 68–76.

17. Strath S, Pfeiffer K, Whitt-Glover M (2012) Accelerometer Use with Children, Older Adults, and Adults with Functional Limitations. Med Sci Sports Exerc 44: 77–85.

18. Bankoski A, Harris TB, McClain JJ, Brychta RJ, Caserotti P, et al. (2011) Sedentary Activity Associated With Metabolic Syndrome Independent of Physical Activity. Diabetes Care 34: 497–503.

19. Bento (2012) Use of accelerometry to measure physical activity in adults and the elderly. Rev Saúde Pública 46: 561–570.

20. Withall J, Stathi A, Davis M, Coulson J, Thompson J, et al. (2014) Objective indicators of physical activity and sedentary time and associations with subjective well-being in adults aged 70 and over. Int J Environ Res Public Health 11: 643–656.

21. Tudor-Locke C, Myers A (2001) Challenges and Opportunities for Measuring Physical Activity in Sedentary Adults. Sports Med 31: 91–100.

22. Ortlieb S, Dias A, Gorzelniak L, Nowak D, Karrasch S, et al. (2014) Exploring Patterns of Accelerometry-assessed Physical Activity in Elderly People. Int J Behav Nutr Phys Act 11: 28.

23. Chastin SFM, Granat MH (2010) Methods for objective measure, quantification and analysis of sedentary behaviour and inactivity. Gait & Posture 31: 82–86.

24. Fried L, Ferrucci L, Darer J, Williamson J, Anderson G (2004) Untangling the Concepts of Disability, Frailty, and Comorbidity: Implications for Improved Targeting and Care. Journal of Gerontology 59: 255–263.

25. Peters A, Döring A, Ladwig KH, Meisinger C, Linkohr B, et al. (2011) Multimorbidity and successful aging: the population-based KORA-Age study. Z Gerontol Geriatr 44: 41–54.

26. Mannino D, Buist A, Petty T, Enright P, Redd S (2003) Lung function and mortality in the United States: data from the First National Health and Nutrition Examination Survey follow up study. Thorax 58: 388–393.

27. Bouillanne O, Morineau G, Dupont C, Coulombel I, Vincent J-P, et al. (2005) Geriatric Nutritional Risk Index: a new index for evaluating at-risk elderly medical patients. Am J Clin Nutr 82: 777–783.

28. Freedson PS, Melanson E, Sirard J (1998) Calibration of the Computer Science and Applications, Inc. accelerometer. Med Sci Sports Exerc 30: 777–781.

29. Chaudhry S, Jin L, Meltzer D (2005) Use of a self-report-generated Charlson Comorbidity Index for predicting mortality. Med Care 43: 607–615.

30. Fries J, Spitz P, Young D (1982) The dimensions of health outcomes: the health assessment questionnaire, disability and pain scales. J Rheumatol 9: 789–793.

31. Krishnan E, Sokka T, Hakkinen A, Hubert H, Hannonen P (2004) Normative Values for the Health Assessment Questionnaire Disability Index. Arthritis Rheum 50: 953–960.

32. Strobl R, Müller M, Emeny R, Peters A, Grill E (2013) Distribution and determinants of functioning and disability in aged adults - results from the German KORA-Age study. BMC Public Health 13: 137.

33. Babyak M (2009) Statistical Tips from the Editors of Psychosomatic Medicine. Psychosom Med 24: 8.

34. Troiano RP, Berrigan D, Dodd KW, Masse LC, Tilert T, et al. (2008) Physical activity in the United States measured by accelerometer. Med Sci Sports Exerc 40: 181–188.

35. van den Bussche H, Schäfer I, Koller D, Hansen H, von Leitner E-C, et al. (2012) Multimorbidity in the German Elderly Population – Part 1: Prevalence in Ambulatory Medical Care. A Study Based on Statutory Health Insurance Data. Z Allg Med 88: 365–371.

36. Wilms H, Riedel-Heller S, Angermeyer M (2007) Limitations in activities of daily living and instrumental activities of daily living capacity in a representative sample: disentangling dementia- and mobility-related effects Compr Psychiatry 48: 95–101.

37. Kaplan M, Newsom J, McFarland B, Lu L (2001) Demographic and Psychosocial Correlates of Physical Activity in Late Life. Am J Prev Med 21: 306–312.

38. U.S. Department of Health and Human Services. Physical Activity Guidelines Advisory Committee Report, 2008. Available: http://www.health.gov/PAGuidelines/Report/. Accessed 2013 October 17.

39. He X, Baker D (2004) Body Mass Index, Physical Activity, and the Risk of Decline in Overall Health and Physical Functioning in Late Middle Age. Am J Public Health 94: 1567–1573.

40. Shah R, Buchman A, Leurgans S, Boyle P, Bennett D (2012) Association of total daily physical activity with disability in community-dwelling older persons: a prospective cohort study. BMC Geriatrics 12: 63.

41. Harris T, Owen C, Victor C, Adams R, Cook D (2009) What factors are associated with physical activity in older people, assessed objectively by accelerometry? Br J Sports Med 43: 442–450.

42. Fortin M, Bravo G, Hudon C, Lapointe L, Dubois M, et al. (2006) Psychological Distress and Multimorbidity in Primary Care. Ann Fam Med 4: 417–422.

43. Strath S, Bassett DJ, Swartz A (2003) Comparison of MTI accelerometer cut-points for predicting time spent in physical activity. Int J Sports Med 24: 298–303.

44. Santos-Lozano A, Santín-Medeiros F, Cardon G, Torres-Luque G, Bailón R, et al. (2013) Actigraph GT3X: Validation and Determination of Physical Activity Intensity Cut Points. Int J Sports Med 2013 34: 975–982.

45. Kaminsky L, Ozemek C (2012) A comparison of the Actigraph GT1M and GT3X accelerometers under standardized and free-living conditions. Physiol Meas 33: 1869–1876.

2

Weak Prediction Power of the Framingham Risk Score for Coronary Artery Disease in Nonagenarians

Josef Yayan*

Department of Internal Medicine, Division of Pulmonary, Allergy, and Sleep Medicine, Saarland University Medical Center, Homburg/Saar, Germany

Abstract

Background: Coronary artery disease (CAD) is caused by an acute myocardial infarction and is still feared as a life-threatening heart disease worldwide. In order to identify patients at high risk for CAD, previous studies have proposed various risk assessment scores for the prevention of CAD. The most commonly used risk assessment score for CAD worldwide is the Framingham Risk Score (FRS). The FRS is used for middle-aged people; hence, its appropriateness has not been demonstrated to predict the likelihood of CAD occurrence in very elderly people. This article examines the possible predictive value of FRS for CAD in very elderly people over 90 years of age.

Methods: Data on all patients over 90 years of age who received a cardiac catheter were collected from hospital charts from the Department of Internal Medicine, Saarland University Medical Center, and HELIOS Hospital Wuppertal, Witten/Herdecke University Medical Center, Germany, within a study period from 2004 to 2013. The FRSs and cardiovascular risk profiles of patients over 90 years of age with and without CAD after cardiac catheterization were compared.

Results: One hundred and seventy-five (91.15%, mean age 91.51 ± 1.80 years, 74 females [42.29%]; 95% confidence interval [CI], 0.87–0.95) of a total 192 of the very elderly patients were found to have CAD. Based on the results of our study, the FRS seems to provide weak predictive ability for CAD in very elderly people ($P = 0.3792$).

Conclusion: We found weak prediction power of FRS for CAD in nonagenarians.

Editor: Ralf Krahe, University of Texas MD Anderson Cancer Center, United States of America

Funding: The author has no funding or support to report.

* Email: josef.yayan@hotmail.com

Introduction

Coronary artery disease (CAD) is the most common heart disease and hides the high risk for the cause for the development of acute myocardial infarction [1]. Numerous studies and international and national clinical practice guidelines have proven that CAD is caused by the manifestation of atherosclerosis in coronary arteries [2–10]. According to data from epidemiological studies, CAD has an increasingly high mortality rate around the world [11]. For this reason, the prediction of CAD risk has gained significant attention in the medical science community worldwide. The identification of risk factors for CAD is a basic requirement for establishing possible targeted medical therapy for the primary and secondary prevention of CAD. Therefore, several national and international guidelines and recommendations for preventing CAD were previously published after identifying the risk factors for CAD [12–15]. There are still ongoing efforts and attempts to improve the risk assessment methods for the prediction of CAD. To achieve this goal, several risk prediction scores for CAD have been developed in recent years [16]. Five or 10 risk assessments for CAD have been assumed worldwide according to the recommendations of the guidelines [17–18]. Currently available CAD risk prediction scores are mostly based on multivariable regression analysis deduced from the Framingham Heart Study [19] in which the traditional risk factors for CAD are taken into consideration such as age, cholesterol levels, blood pressure, smoking, and body weight [20–21]. The Framingham Risk Score (FRS) provides an estimation of the probability of an individual developing CAD in 10 years to detect high-risk persons and to take preventive actions [22]. Based on data obtained through the FRS calculations, high-risk patients should be treated, according to the guidelines' recommendations, with lipid-lowering medication and aspirin in the primary prevention of CAD [23,24]. FRS and other presently common risk estimation scores are designed for people in middle age [20,25,26]. The mean age in the FRS was 49 years old and people younger than 30 years and older than 74 years of age were not considered [20,27]. Present risk prediction with the FRS might operate less effectively in elderly compared to middle-aged persons, and various traditional risk factors have a weak association with CAD risk in the elderly; for example, hypercholesterolemia is a strong cardiovascular risk factor in middle-aged individuals, but not in the elderly [27,28]. Thus, new questions arise as to whether the FRS could be used to estimate cardiovascular risk for very elderly people over 90 years of age. We conducted the present investigation to better understand the FRS as an eligible prediction system for CAD in very elderly people over 90 years of age. Therefore, we collected data on all patients of this age group with CAD according to the International Classification of Disease from the hospital database at the Department of Internal Medicine, Saarland University Medical Center, and HELIOS Hospital Wuppertal, Witten/Herdecke University Medical Center, Germany. We used a risk assessment tool based on information from the Framingham Heart Study to calculate the FRS after confirming the presence or absence of CAD by performing cardiac catheterization to examine the FRS as an eligible scoring system for very elderly people. The variety of calculated FRS for CAD in people over 90 years of age were age, gender, systolic blood pressure, total cholesterol, high density lipoproteins (HDL), tobacco smoking, and former smoking. CAD diagnosis was made only after cardiac catheterization. The FRS for CAD was compared in patients older than 90 years of age after excluding CAD by performing cardiac catheterization. Only once we have identified the cardiovascular risk factors of CAD can we develop appropriately tailored therapies for all patients to take precautions against CAD.

Materials and Methods

Ethics Statement

All patients' data were anonymized prior to analysis. Due to the retrospective nature of the study protocol, the Medical Association of Saarland's Institutional Review Board approved this study and waived the need for informed consent.

Patients

In this study, the FRS for CAD was retrospectively examined in patients over 90 years of age using hospital chart data at the Department of Internal Medicine, Saarland University Medical Center, and HELIOS Hospital Wuppertal, Witten/Herdecke University Medical Center, during the study period from 2004 to 2013.

The FRS for CAD in the last decade of a patient's life was considered theoretically, assuming that the average life expectancy would be 100 years of age. For the control group, the last highest decade of life was chosen to avoid any distortion in the data analysis due to age. The last highest decade of life refers to patients over 90 years old. Thus, the study population was composed of very elderly patients over 90 years of age diagnosed with CAD, and the control group was composed of elderly patients over 90 years of age without CAD, as determined after cardiac catheterization. All patients older than 90 years who were treated at the internal medicine emergency rooms or in one of the internal departments of the two hospitals were included after receiving a cardiac catheter in this study. Patients over 90 years who were treated in other departments or had no cardiac catheter were excluded from this study.

The FRS assessment tool from the National Heart, Lung, and Blood Institute (NHLBI) in Bethesda, Maryland [12,29] was used to calculate FRSs in very elderly people over 90 years of age after CAD was confirmed to be present or absent by cardiac catheterization. The study population received a point score based on the categorical values of age, total cholesterol, high-density lipoprotein cholesterol (HDL), blood pressure, diabetes, and smoking [30]. Former smokers were considered smokers when calculating the FRS in this study. All patients' 0–5 Risk Scores for CAD were determined, giving one point for existing cardiovascular risk factors. A score of 0 means no risk for CAD, 1 very low risk, 2 moderate risk, 3 increased risk, 4 high risk, and 5 very high risk for CAD. Once CAD was detected or excluded by cardiac catheterization, we calculated FRSs retrospectively using the data

from very elderly people over 90 years of age collected from the two hospital charts data, assuming that the examined cardiovascular risk factors in this study existing at the time of detection or exclusion of CAD would also have existed 10 years ago.

CAD has been defined as a chronic disease of the coronary arteries characterized by the manifestation of atherosclerosis with variable coronary artery stenosis, resulting in myocardial ischemia. CAD symptoms are classified as stable angina and ACS. ACS is a collective term for unstable angina, NSTEMI, and STEMI. The main symptom of coronary insufficiency is angina pectoris; it involves localized retrosternal pain triggered by physical and mental stress. Such chest pain may spread to the neck, lower jaw, shoulder, back, left arm to the fingertips, or the upper abdomen. Unstable angina refers to angina pectoris occurring for the first time, as well as a worsening of pain intensity and the duration of episodes.

NSTEMI was described for unstable angina and myocardial infarction with an increase in cardiac enzymes such as high-sensitivity cardiac troponin T without ST-segment elevation on an electrocardiogram. A 12-lead electrocardiogram was used at rest for the temporary recording of the sum of the heart's electrical activity to diagnose STEMI or cardiac arrhythmias in all patients. Typical ST-segmental change in the electrocardiogram for STEMI was considered ST-segment elevation>0.1 mV in at least one derivation. The diagnosis of CAD was made after cardiac catheterization. The quantitative determination of high-sensitivity troponin T in human plasma was measured after sample collection in lithium heparin SARSTEDT Monovette 4.7 ml (orange top) using a standard immunoturbidimetric assay on the COBAS INTEGRA system (the normal value is less than 14 pg/ml) after conservation from cardiac troponin T on September 2, 2010. A second measurement of high-sensitivity troponin T was carried out three hours after the first blood sample.

Prior to this, from January 1, 2004, to September 2, 2010, electrochemiluminescence immunoassay (ECLIA) was performed to determine cardiac troponin T (the normal value is less than 0.01 µg/l) on Elecsys 2010 and cobas e 411 immunoassay analyzers (Roche Diagnostics Ltd., Mannheim, Germany).

The classification of CAD was performed in each case according to the latest edition of the International Classification of Disease (ICD I25.11–I25.13) from 2004 to 2013. Coronary artery disease injuries were categorized as 1-, 2, or 3-vessel. Further, examiners visually estimated the degree of stenosis diameter as a percentage of the cardiac catheter, as per the stenosis morphology classification recommendations of the American College of Cardiology/American Heart Association [31].

We compared the cardiovascular risk factors in accordance with the guidelines of the International Atherosclerosis Society [32], such as arterial hypertension, diabetes mellitus, hypercholesterolemia, hyperlipidemia, obesity, tobacco smoking, and former smoking in very elderly patients over 90 years of age with and without CAD (ICD I25.0–I25.10) after completing cardiac catheterization.

Arterial hypertension was described as a condition in which the blood pressure of the arterial vascular system is chronically elevated. According to the World Health Organization (WHO) [33], hypertension can be diagnosed with a systolic blood pressure of at least 140 mmHg or a diastolic blood pressure of at least 90 mmHg (ICD I10.90). The manifestation of hypertension was described as a known history of hypertension where the patient has been treated with drugs. Blood pressure was measured by the indirect method following Riva-Rocci, 24-hour blood pressure measurement and blood pressure monitors DINAMAP (GE

Medical Systems Information Technologies Ltd., Freiburg, Germany).

Diabetes mellitus (ICD E14.90) was diagnosed as a chronic metabolic disease based on an absolute or relative lack of insulin with elevated blood glucose levels when fasting values were more than 126 mg/dl or when, occasionally, a measured value above 200 mg/dl was detected in the serum of the patients. Blood glucose was determined in the serum of all patients using the SARSTEDT serum Monovette 4.7 ml (brown top) blood collection system with a multifly blood collection needle.

As hypercholesterolemia (ICD E78.0) is considered a lipid metabolic disorder characterized by elevated blood cholesterol levels higher than 200 mg/dl, total cholesterol and HDL (reference range 35–65 mg/dl) were measured after 12 hours of fasting in all patients in the plasma after blood collection in lithium heparin SARSTEDT Monovette 4.7 ml (orange top) with a multifly blood collection needle as an enzymatic colorimetric test using Roche cobas c 701 systems (Roche Diagnostics Ltd., Mannheim, Germany). Hyperlipidemia (ICD E78.2–E78.3) is mainly diagnosed through elevated triglycerides in the blood plasma of patients. The reference range for hypertriglyceridemia has been specified as>200 mg/dl in blood plasma after 12 hours of fasting following blood collection in lithium heparin SARSTEDT Monovette 4.7 ml (orange top) with a multifly blood collection needle as an enzymatic colorimetric test using Roche cobas c 701 systems (Roche Diagnostics Ltd., Mannheim, Germany).

Obesity (ICD E66.99) was defined as the excessive growth of adipose tissue in the body. The transition from overweight to obese was achieved with a body mass index (BMI) of 30. The designation of obese was made by calculating the body weight in kilograms divided by height in meters squared. Nicotine abuse (ICD F17.1) was designated as the abusive consumption of products that contain nicotine, including cigarettes, cigars, and other tobacco products. The study population was categorized into smokers, former smokers, and non-smokers. The quantification of tobacco smoking by measuring packs per year was not considered in this study because the harmful effect of nicotine was not the focus of the research.

We analyzed acute and chronic comorbidities as predisposing factors for the development of CAD in elderly people. In addition, the length of the study and control groups' hospital stays was compared.

Statistical analysis

The data were expressed in proportion, mean, and standard deviation wherever appropriate. We calculated 95% confidence intervals (CIs) for the total number of patients with CAD. Odds ratios were calculated for the presence of cardiovascular risk factors for CAD, sex, and acute and chronic comorbidities. Gender difference was calculated using the chi-square test for two independent standard normal variables of two probabilities. A calculation of the chi-square test for four independent standard normal variables of two probabilities was used to compare the association between cardiovascular risk factors and stable angina, unstable angina, NSTEMI, or STEMI. Fisher's exact test for three variables of two probabilities was calculated for cardiovascular risk factors in different forms of CAD. One-way analysis of variance (ANOVA) for independent samples was performed to compare the duration of hospital stays, BMI, body height, body weight, cholesterol, HDL, and systolic blood pressure between the two groups. The survival rates for both groups were calculated using the Kaplan-Meier method. All tests were expressed as two-tailed, and a P value of <0.05 was considered statistically significant.

Results

In the two hospital databases, we found 126,931 patients who underwent cardiac catheterization at the Department of Internal Medicine, University Hospital of Saarland, and HELIOS Hospital Wuppertal, Witten/Herdecke University Medical Center, Germany, during the study period from 2004 to 2013. A total of 192 (0.15%, mean age 91.45±1.75 years, 97 females [50.52%]; 95% confidence interval [CI], 0.0013–0.0017) patients over 90 years of age with a cardiac catheter met the inclusion criteria for this trial. A total of 175 (91.15%, mean age 91.51±1.80 years, 74 females [42.29%]; 95% confidence interval [CI], 0.87–0.95) patients over 90 years of age had CAD (study group); in 17 patients (8.85%, mean age 90.77±0.88 years, 10 females [58.82%]; 95% CI, 0.05–0.13), CAD was excluded by means of cardiac catheter (control group). We found a higher prevalence of CAD in males, but without increased risk (1.4450 odds ratio; 95% CI, 0.5261–3.9687; P = 0.4752).

FRSs did not differ between very elderly people over 90 years of age compared with and without CAD (P = 0.3792, Table 1). The calculation of Risk Scores 0–5 including one point for each cardiovascular risk factor showed statistical difference only for risk score 3 with statistical difference (P = 0.0244) compared between both study groups (Table 1). A statistical difference was also found in systolic blood pressure with higher levels in the group without CAD with statistical difference (P = 0.465). The levels of cholesterol, HDL, and BMI were statistically no different between the two groups (Table 1). The duration of hospital stays showed no statistical significance between the two groups (Table 1).

Following the results of this study, we identified a five-fold higher cardiovascular risk of developing CAD in patients over 90 years of age with arterial hypertension (P = 0.0035, Table 2). Very elderly diabetics had a three-fold, those with hypercholesterolemia had a one-fold, and very elderly former smokers had a two-fold increased risk of developing CAD, but without a statistically significant difference (Table 2). Neither group was distinguished statistically according to the number of subjects of normal weight, although most of the patients in the study population were not overweight (Table 2).

The largest group in the study group had 3-vessel CAD, followed by 2-vessel CAD, and the small group 1-vessel CAD (Table 3). A comparison of the traditional cardiovascular risk factors with the number of coronary arteries that were afflicted with CAD showed no statistical difference (Table 3).

Only for hypertension did we find a statistically significant difference after comparing the tested traditional cardiovascular risk factors with the clinical manifestation of CAD, such as stable angina or ACS (P<0.0001, Table 4). We also found no statistically significant difference between risk factors and the acute comorbidities in the two groups (Table 5). Cases with a negative outcome were found numerically and exhibited a statistical difference in acute comorbidities such as syncope, falls, and attacks of gout (Table 5). These acute comorbidities showed no increased risk for CAD.

Chronic comorbidities exhibited no increased risk for CAD (Table 6). We found cases with negative outcomes with a statistically significant difference in terms of chronic lumbago and pacemakers. However, chronic lumbago and patients with pacemakers demonstrated no increased risk for CAD (Table 6).

There were six (3.43%, 4 [66.67%] females; 95% CI, 0.0073–0.0613) deaths in the study group and no deaths in the control group (P = 0.4379). Thus, the survival rate was 96.57% (95% CI, 0.94–0.99) in the study group and 100% in the control group.

Table 1. Comparison of demographic data, duration of hospital stay, cholesterol, high sensitivity lipoproteins, systolic blood pressure, Framingham Risk Score, and Risk Score between elderly people over 90 years of age with and without CAD.

	CAD (%)	Without CAD (%)	P value
Number of patients (N = 192)	175 (91.15)	17 (8.85)	
Male	88 (50.29)	7 (41.18)	0.4733
Female	87 (49.71)	10 (58.82)	0.4733
BMI (kg/m^2)	25.59±3.57	25.67±25.65	0.9205
Body height (cm)	166.31±8.85	163.13±8.36	0.1852
Body weight (kg)	70.38±10.61	68.27±11.58	0.4676
Duration of hospital stay (day)	6.02±8.03	6.29±6.21	0.8877
Framingham Score (%)	18.70±9.16	15±8.60	0.3792
Cholesterol (mg/dl)	168.89±42.21	196±27.40	0.1579
HDL (mg/dl)	52.96±20.86	59.6±13.48	0.4854
Systolic blood pressure (mmHg)	140.74±26.08	154.73±23.25	**0.0465**
Risk Score 0	16 (9.14)	3 (17.65)	0.2623
Risk Score 1	40 (22.86)	7 (41.18)	0.0935
Risk Score 2	60 (34.29)	3 (17.65)	0.163
Risk Score 3	41 (23.43)	0	**0.0244**
Risk Score 4	12 (6.86)	1 (5.88)	0.8786
Risk Score 5	6 (3.43)	0	0.4379

Abbreviations: CAD: coronary artery disease; BMI: body mass index; HDL: high sensitivity lipoproteins. **Notes:** Significant P values are shown in bold.

Discussion

Past researchers have assumed that the incidence of acute myocardial infarction increases with advancing aging [34,35]. According to the results of this study, after confirmation by cardiac catheterization, the FRS had an insufficient predictive value for CAD in very elderly people over 90 years of age with CAD. In this study, the assessment tool that was used to estimate 10-year risk after having a heart attack considered age, sex, total cholesterol, HDL, systolic blood pressure, smoking status, and whether patients were currently under medication for hypertension. However, age is in and of itself the strongest predictor of CAD.

For this reason, in one study, researchers examined the possibility of the prediction value of a risk factor on the prevalence of CAD to vary over a wide range of ages from middle age to old age [36]. The positive association between hypertension and CAD decreased considerably with age, primarily due to the significantly increased risk of CAD in elderly men without hypertension. The outcomes of total cholesterol on CAD also appeared to decrease with age, although variations were not statistically significant. In contrast, men with diabetes had a dependable two-fold additional risk of CAD transversely across all age groups, while a positive relationship with body mass index in younger men became negative in those who were the oldest. Due to the occasional smoking amongst the elderly, the relationship between smoking and CAD deteriorated with age. The results of this study suggest that changes in risk factor effects on the incidence of CAD with advancing age may require efficient approaches for CAD prevention as people age [35]. The influence of age on the incidence of CAD was not investigated in our study. Overall, the size of the study population in our study over the course of nearly 10 years was small. Therefore, we included the data of two

Table 2. Comparison of traditional risk factors for CAD in very elderly people over 90 years of age with and without CAD.

Risk factors	Elderly>90 years of age		Odds ratio	95% CI	P value
	CAD (n = 175) (%)	Without CAD (n = 17) (%)			
Hypertension	147 (84)	9 (52.94)	4.6667	1.6584–13.1318	**0.0035**
Diabetes	48 (27.43)	1 (5.88)	6.0472	0.7805–46.8540	0.0849
Hypercholesterolemia	17 (9.71)	1 (5.88)	1.7215	0.2148–13.7984	0.6090
Hyperlipidemia	47 (26.86)	3 (17.65)	1.7135	0.4712–6.2312	0.4136
Obesity	22 (12.57)	3 (17.65)	0.6710	0.1784–2.5236	0.5550
Smoker	6 (3.43)	0	1.3422	0.0725–24.8432	0.8433
Former smoker	14 (8)	0	3.1424	0.1796–54.9851	0.4330

Abbreviations: CAD: coronary artery disease; CI: confidence interval. **Notes:** Significant P values are shown in bold.

Table 3. Comparison of traditional cardiovascular risk factors in different forms of coronary artery disease.

| Risk factors | Coronary artery disease | | | |
	1-vessel (n = 26)(%)	2-vessel (n = 53)(%)	3-vessel (n = 96)(%)	P value
Hypertension	19 (73.08)	45 (84.91)	83 (86.46)	0.2433
Diabetes	4 (15.38)	12 (22.64)	32 (33.33)	0.1320
Hypercholesterolemia	4 (15.38)	5 (9.43)	8 (8.33)	0.5620
Hyperlipidemia	3 (11.54)	14 (26.42)	30 (31.25)	0.1290
Obesity	4 (15.38)	3 (5.66)	15 (15.63)	0.1748
Smoker	1 (3.85)	1 (1.89)	4 (4.17)	0.8601
Former smoker	0	3 (5.66)	11 (11.46)	0.1450

hospitals in this study. This may be due to the patients' biological age, because with increasing age, the population decreases. We found that for patients over 90 years of age, only those with hypertension had a high risk for CAD. Traditional cardiovascular risk factors such as progressing age, diabetes mellitus, hypertension, dyslipidemia, smoking, and obesity are known to have a relationship with CAD [36,37].

Veeranna et al. reported that age and male sex, but not hypertension or dyslipidemia, represented an increased risk for CAD. Only diabetes was an independent predictor of CAD, and smoking was associated with the occlusion of the left main trunk artery of the heart in their study [38]. This was quite different from our outcome, as we found a high risk of CAD in very elderly people with hypertension. Diabetes increased the risk of developing CAD, but without statistical significance, and smoking presented absolutely no increased risk for CAD in our analysis. While the number of male patients with CAD was slightly increased in our study, we could not find a statistically significant difference in sex regarding the risk for CAD.

In one study, researchers examined the influence of advancing age on clinical presentation and hospital reports in a large sample of patients with STEMI [39]. There was a significant converse relationship between age and the probability of presenting with STEMI. For each period of life, the probability of presenting with STEMI decreased. Noticeably fewer elderly patients were frequently treated by cardiologists, they were not examined as

thoroughly, and when presenting with STEMI, a smaller number were likely to be treated with cardiac catheterization. Hospital mortality was augmented in the elderly. Fewer elderly patients presented with STEMI but had considerable in-hospital mortality rates; however, they had obviously fewer intensive treatments and investigations [39]. The amount of STEMI was decreased in our study as well. We did not investigate whether the very elderly were treated less often with cardiac catheterization and by cardiologists.

Although several scoring systems have been recommended to compute cardiovascular risk factors, some information has been lacking on significant variables such as family history of CAD or LDL cholesterol. Based on acute coronary events happening within 10 years of follow-up after enrollment into the Prospective Cardiovascular Münster (PROCAM) study [26], the authors of the study developed a Cox proportional hazards model using the following eight independent risk factors for CAD, graded in order of importance: age, LDL cholesterol, smoking, HDL cholesterol, systolic blood pressure, family history of previous myocardial infarction, diabetes mellitus, and triglycerides. They then developed a point scoring system created on the beta-coefficients of this model. The exactness of this point scoring system was similar to coronary event prediction when the continuous variables themselves were used. The scoring system accurately predicted detected coronary events [26]. Similar to this model, we could detect a statistical difference only for risk score 3 in the predictive value of traditional risk factors for CAD for very elderly people in our study

Table 4. Comparison of cardiovascular risk factors with stable angina pectoris and acute coronary syndrome in very elderly people over 90 years of age with CAD.

| Risk factors | Coronary artery disease | | | | |
	Stable angina (n = 30)(%)	Unstable angina (n = 121)(%)	NSTEMI (n = 61)(%)	STEMI (n = 47)(%)	P value
Hypertension	30 (100)	99 (81.82)	52 (85.25)	24 (51.06)	**<0.0001**
Diabetes	8 (26.67)	31 (25.62)	17 (27.87)	5 (10.64)	0.1429
Hypercholesterolemia	3(10)	18 (14.88)	9 (14.75)	4 (8.51)	0.6594
Hyperlipidemia	8 (26.67)	30 (24.79)	18 (29.51)	6 (12.77)	0.2186
Obesity	3 (10)	16 (13.22)	9 (14.75)	3 (6.38)	0.5459
Smoker	2 (6.67)	3 (2.48)	2 (3.28)	0	0.3618
Former smoker	3 (10)	10 (8.26)	6 (9.84)	2 (4.26)	0.722

Abbreviations: NSTEMI: non-ST segment elevation myocardial infarction; STEMI: ST segment elevation myocardial infarction. **Notes:** Significant P values are shown in bold.

Table 5. Comparison of acute illnesses in patients with and without CAD.

Cardiovascular diseases	CAD (n = 175) (%)	Without CAD (n = 17) (%)	Odds ratio	95% CI	P value
Acute heart failure	103 (58.86)	9 (52.94)	1.2716	0.4683–3.4526	0.6373
Anemia	8 (4.57)	0	1.7761	0.0983–32.0995	0.6973
Cardiac arrhythmia	62 (35.42)	8 (47.06)	0.6173	0.2267–1.6804	0.3451
Cardiac decompensation	18 (10.29)	3 (17.65)	0.5350	0.1402–2.0412	0.3599
Circulatory collapse	1 (0.57)	0	0.0118	0.0118–7.6681	0.4672
Derailed blood pressure	8 (4.57)	0	1.7761	0.00983–32.0995	0.6973
Shock	4 (2.29)	0	0.9184	0.0475–17.7742	0.9551
Syncope	1 (0.57)	4 (23.53)	0.0187	0.0019–0.1795	**0.0006**
Pulmonary diseases					
Acute respiratory failure	2 (1.14)	1 (5.88)	0.1850	0.0159–2.1532	0.1778
Aspiration pneumonia	1 (0.57)	0	0.3009	0.0118–7.6681	0.4672
Bronchopulmonary infection	3 (1.71)	1 (7.14)	0.2791	0.0274–2.8411	0.2841
Pneumonia	2 (1.14)	0	0.5043	0.0233–10.9290	0.6627
Pulmonary edema	4 (2.89)	0	0.9184	0.0475–17.4442	0.9551
Gastrointestinal diseases					
Duodenal ulcer	1 (0.57)	0	0.3009	0.0118–7.6681	0.4672
Gastritis	2 (1.14)	0	0.5043	0.0233–10.9290	0.6627
Gastrointestinal bleeding	2 (1.14)	0	0.5043	0.0233–10.9290	0.4672
Hyperglycemia	1 (0.57)	0	0.3009	0.0118–7.6681	0.4672
Reflux esophagitis 2 (1.14)	0	0.5043	0.0233–10.9290	0.4672	
Kidney diseases					
Acute kidney injury	3 (1.71)	0	0.7101	0.0352–14.3174	0.8233
Acute urinary tract infection	10 (5.71)	1 (5.88)	0.3009	0.0118–7.6681	0.4672
Macrohematuria	3 (1.71)	0	0.7101	0.0352–14.3174	0.8233
Water-electrolyte imbalance	2 (1.14)	0	0.5043	0.0233–10.9290	0.4672
Thyroid diseases					
Hyperthyroidism	1 (0.57)	0	0.3009	0.0118–7.6681	0.4672
Hypothyroidism	5 (2.86)	0	1.1290	0.0599–21.2845	0.9354
Other conditions					
Acute stroke	1 (0.57)	0	0.3009	0.0118–7.6681	0.4672
Abscess	1 (0.57)	0	0.3009	0.0118–7.6681	0.4672
Dizziness	2 (1.14)	0	0.5043	0.0233–10.9290	0.4672
Fall	0	1 (5.88)	0.0313	0.0012–0.8004	**0.0362**
Attack of gout	0	1 (5.88)	0.0313	0.0012–0.8004	**0.0362**
Delirium	2 (1.14)	1 (5.88)	0.1850	0.0159–2.1532	0.1778

Abbreviations: CAD: coronary artery disease; CI: confidence interval. **Notes:** Significant P values are shown in bold.

when we calculated one point for each traditional risk factor, such as hypertension, diabetes, hypercholesterolemia, hyperlipidemia, obesity, and smoking. This risk assessment model was easy to calculate. Apparently, it makes no difference whether the exact numbers of serum lipids or their global viewpoint was used when calculating this risk factor. Because the risk factor of a family history of previous myocardial infarction cannot be influenced, we did not consider this established risk factor of family history for CAD when evaluating the very elderly in our study.

The question of the use of risk assessment for the primary prevention of CAD remains controversial. The validity of the FRS was assessed in a previous study [40]. Comparisons of prediction models and reality in tertiles were performed, and the individual

survival functions were calculated. The mean risk for men was increased. Cardiovascular disease events happened in the highest risk tertiles. The negative predictive values in both sexes were noteworthy, and the specificity in women and sensitivity in men were high when their risk for cardiovascular disease was high. This model overestimated the risk in older women and in middle-aged men. The cumulative probability of individual survival by tertiles was significant in both sexes [40]. The results of this study warrant the reclassification of FRS.

Rodondi et al. also reached the conclusion that the FRS miscalculates the risk for CAD in the elderly, mainly in women [27]. They proposed that traditional risk factors best predict CAD. We detected no sex differences in the mean study population in

Table 6. Comparison of chronic comorbidities in elderly people over 90 years of age with and without CAD.

Cardiovascular diseases	CAD (n = 175) (%)	Without CAD (n = 17) (%)	Odds ratio	95% CI	P value
Aneurysm	1 (0.57)	1 (5.88)	0.0920	0.0055–1.5408	0.0970
Cardiomyopathy	4 (2.29)	0	0.9184	0.0475–17.7742	0.9551
Carotid stenosis	3 (1.71)	1 (5.88)	0.2791	0.0274–2.8411	0.2810
Cor pulmonale	9 (5.14)	2 (11.76)	0.4066	0.0804–2.0563	0.2765
Hypertensive heart disease	29 (16.57)	4 (23.53)	0.6455	0.1965–2.1207	0.4708
Pacemaker	20 (11.43)	5 (29.41)	0.3097	0.0988–0.9707	**0.0443**
Peripheral arterial occlusive disease	17 (9.71)	0	3.8644	0.2226–67.0875	0.3533
State after syncope	3 (1.71)	0	0.7101	0.0352–14.3174	0.8233
Cardiac valvular defect	50 (28.57)	8 (47.06)	0.4500	0.1643–1.2322	0.1202
Chronic venous insufficiency	1 (0.57)	0	0.3009	0.0118–7.6681	0.4672
Varicose veins	2 (1.14)	0	0.5043	0.0233–10.9290	0.6627
State after bypass surgery	10 (5.71)	0	2.2205	0.1247–39.5395	0.5871
Pulmonary diseases					
Chronic obstructive pulmonary disease	12 (6.86)	2 (11.76)	0.5521	0.1129–2.7012	0.4639
Emphysema	2 (1.14)	0	0.5043	0.0233–10.9290	0.6627
Obstructive sleep apnea syndrome	1 (0.57)	0	0.3009	0.0118–7.6681	0.4672
State after tuberculosis	2 (1.14)	0	0.5043	0.0233–10.9290	0.6627
Gastrointestinal diseases					
Appendectomy	1 (0.57)	0	0.3009	0.0118–7.6681	0.4672
Cholecystectomy	16 (9.14)	1 (5.88)	1.6101	0.2002–12.9484	0.6543
Colonic diverticula	4 (2.29)	0	0.9184	0.0475–17.7742	0.9551
Gallbladder disease	1 (0.57)	0	0.3009	0.0118–7.6681	0.4672
Gastric carcinoma	6 (3.43)	0	1.3422	0.0725–24.8432	0.8433
Liver cysts	1 (0.57)	0	0.3009	0.0118–7.6681	0.4672
Pancreatic disease	1 (0.57)	0	0.3009	0.0118–7.6681	0.4672
Splenectomy	1 (0.57)	0	0.3009	0.0118–7.6681	0.4672
State after bowel surgery	3 (1.71)	0	0.7101	0.0352–14.3174	0.8233
State after hepatitis	3 (1.71)	0	0.7101	0.0352–14.3174	0.8233
State after hernia operation	4 (2.29)	0	0.9184	0.0475–17.7742	0.9551
State after gastric surgery	4 (2.29)	0	0.9184	0.0475–17.7742	0.9551
Kidney diseases					
Chronic renal failure	45 (25.71)	5 (29.41)	0.8308	0.2774–2.4883	0.7404
Contracted kidney	1 (0.57)	0	0.3009	0.0118–7.6681	0.4672
Diabetic nephropathy	3 (1.71)	0	0.7101	0.0352–14.3174	0.8233
Nephrectomy	3 (1.71)	0	0.7101	0.0352–14.3174	0.8233
Renal adenoma	2 (1.14)	0	0.5043	0.0233–10.9290	0.6627
Renal cysts	5 (2.86)	0	1.1290	0.0599–21.2845	0.9354
State after kidney stones	1 (0.57)	0	0.3009	0.0118–7.6681	0.4672
Diseases of the genitourinary system					
Benign prostate hyperplasia	4 (2.29)	1 (5.88)	0.3743	0.0394–3.5526	0.3920
Hysterectomy	4 (2.29)	0	0.9184	0.0475–17.7742	0.9551
Prostate cancer	3 (1.71)	1 (12.50)	0.2791	0.0274–2.8411	0.2810
Prostatectomy	3 (1.71)	0	0.7101	0.0352–14.3174	0.8233
State after bladder carcinoma	2 (1.14)	0	0.5043	0.0233–10.9290	0.6627
Thyroid diseases					
Struma	2 (1.14)	0	0.5043	0.0233–10.9290	0.6627
Strumectomy	2 (1.14)	1 (5.88)	0.1850	0.0159–2.1532	0.1778
Nervous system disorders					
Chronic lumbago	0	1 (5.88)	0.0313	0.0012–0.8004	**0.0362**

Table 6. Cont.

Cardiovascular diseases	CAD (n = 175) (%)	Without CAD (n = 17) (%)	Odds ratio	95% CI	P value
Disc herniation	2 (1.14)	0	0.5043	0.0233–10.9290	0.6627
Polyneuropathy	4 (2.29)	1 (5.88)	0.3743	0.0394–3.5526	0.3920
Parkinson disease	6 (3.43)	0	1.3422	0.0725–24.8432	0.8433
Restless legs syndrome	3 (1.71)	0	0.7101	0.0352–14.3174	0.8233
Spinal canal stenosis	2 (1.14)	1 (5.88)	0.1850	0.0159–2.1532	0.1778
Status after stroke	12 (6.86)	1 (5.88)	1.1779	0.1437–9.6544	0.8787
Orthopedic disorders					
Osteoarthritis	9 (5.14)	3 (17.65)	0.2530	0.0614–1.0425	0.0571
Osteoporosis	5 (2.86)	1 (5.88)	0.4706	0.0518–4.2786	0.5033
Rheumatism	2 (1.14)	0	0.5043	0.0233–10.9290	0.6627
Psychiatric disorders					
Alzheimer disease	1 (0.57)	0	0.3009	0.0118–7.6681	0.4672
Dementia	4 (2.29)	1 (5.88)	0.3743	0.0394–3.5526	0.3920
Depression	3 (1.71)	0	0.7101	0.0352–14.3174	0.8233
Ear, nose, and throat diseases					
Nasal polypectomy	1 (0.57)	0	0.3009	0.0118–7.6681	0.4672
Tonsillectomy	1 (0.57)	0	0.3009	0.0118–7.6681	0.4672
Skin disorders					
Allergy	1 (0.57)	0	0.3009	0.0118–7.6681	0.4672
Psoriasis	1 (0.57)	0	0.3009	0.0118–7.6681	0.4672
State post-herpes zoster	1 (0.57)	0	0.3009	0.0118–7.6681	0.4672
Ophthalmologic diseases	13 (7.43)	1 (5.88)	1.2840	0.1576–10.4623	0.8154
Gynecological disorders					
Status after breast cancer	3 (1.71)	0	0.7101	0.0352–14.3174	0.8233

Abbreviations: CAD: coronary artery disease; CI: confidence interval. **Notes:** Significant P values are shown in bold.

very elderly people over 90 years of age with and without CAD in our study.

In one study, classic risk factors' validity was examined with several new biomarkers in predicting cardiovascular mortality in the very elderly from the general population with no history of CAD [40]. All classic risk factors were comprised in the FRS as well as serum concentrations of the biomarkers homocysteine, folic acid, C reactive protein, and interleukin 6 [40]. Classic risk factors did not forecast cardiovascular mortality when used in the FRS. Of the novel biomarkers investigated, homocysteine had the greatest predictive value. The inclusion of some additional risk factors or a combination of factors into the homocysteine prediction model did not increase its discriminative value. In very elderly people with no history of CAD, only serum levels of homocysteine were able to precisely detect those at high risk of cardiovascular mortality, whereas classic risk factors incorporated into the FRS did not [40]. Further investigations are warranted to confirm these findings.

Other findings have suggested that the FRS and PROCAM should not be carried out to calculate the absolute CAD risk of middle-aged men without any CAD history because of a clear overestimation [41]. In our study, some FRSs overestimated the probability of CAD occurrence, mainly in the very elderly after excluding CAD by cardiac catheterization. In contrast, a small number very elderly people with CAD were underestimated after the calculation of FRSs in our study.

In previous studies, researchers found that risk factors could have supplementary predictive value outside of what the FRS can predict [42]. However, most of the results of the examined studies had mistakes in their design, methods, and descriptions that limit their reliability and validity [42]. While hypertension was treated by medication in the very elderly, our study showed that the risk for CAD was high. While diabetes has been found in nearly over one-quarter of elderly patients with CAD, about one-tenth had hypercholesterolemia in our study, without statistical significance. Neither hyperlipidemia nor obesity was an increased risk factor for CAD in the very elderly patients in our study population. The same result was reported by Kim et al. in relation to the elderly [43]. These results raise questions about the value of weight loss and diet for the prevention of CAD in the elderly.

The effects of smoking on mortality in the elderly population have been studied previously [44]. When comparing the mortality rates for older smokers, ex-smokers, and non-smokers, lower mortality was observed for non-smokers and former smokers than for older smokers [44]. We found more very elderly former smokers and smokers with CAD than non-smokers in our study, but this was not statistically significant.

However, it continues to be difficult to correlate CAD and atherosclerosis. Even when this was evaluated angiographically, the connection has not been well established, and previous studies have reported different and varying outcomes concerning the link between CAD and atherosclerosis [45–47]. The severity of CAD in the elderly seemed to correlate poorly with the prevalence of established traditional cardiovascular risk factors in our study.

There are probably reasons for the different risk profiles for CAD in very elderly people. The assessment and identification of cardiovascular risk factors for CAD in the elderly may be challenging for further investigations.

Study limitations

In this study, the FRS and traditional risk factors for CAD in very elderly people in two departments of internal medicine were examined, but not in very elderly people with CAD in other medical departments. The FRS was calculated after an acute myocardial infarction and preformation of cardiac catheterization to confirm CAD under the assumption that the identified risk factors would have existed 10 years ago. Another limitation was that we were unable to identify very elderly patients with ACS who had not undergone cardiac catheterization for any reason. Moreover, aging itself was considered a risk factor for CAD in previous studies. It is also possible that the risk profiles change over the time among all age groups. The influence of lifestyle and diet in the traditional risk factors were not considered in the very elderly in this study. Therefore, it is difficult to identify the risk profile for CAD in very elderly people. Various causes of the development of CAD have been discussed in the current scientific-medical literature. Most of the very elderly patients had CAD. Therefore, the group of very elderly patients without CAD was small. For this reason, we conducted a two-center study to exclude a statistical error in the limited sample size in the group of very elderly patients without CAD.

Conclusions

We were not able to demonstrate that the FRS has sufficient predictive value in patients over 90 years of age with CAD. In addition, the scoring system with a point for each risk factor for CAD did not have sufficient predictive power for CAD in very elderly people. However, established risk factors such as hypertension, diabetes, hyperlipidemia, obesity, and smoking should be carefully considered in the therapeutic management and prevention of CAD in very elderly people, in addition to treatment for acute and chronic comorbidities.

Author Contributions

Conceived and designed the experiments: YJ. Performed the experiments: YJ. Analyzed the data: YJ. Contributed reagents/materials/analysis tools: YJ. Wrote the paper: YJ.

References

1. Jneid H, Alam M, Virani SS, Bozkurt B (2013) Redefining myocardial infarction: what is new in the ESC/ACCF/AHA/WHF third universal definition of myocardial infarction? Methodist Debakey Cardiovasc J 9: 169–172.

2. Exarchos KP, Exarchos TP, Bourantas CV, Papafaklis MI, Naka KK, et al. (2013) Prediction of coronary atherosclerosis progression using dynamic Bayesian networks. Conf Proc IEEE Eng Med Biol Soc 3889–3892.

3. Schoenhagen P, Tuzcu EM, Apperson-Hansen C, Wang C, Wolski K, et al. (2006) Determinants of arterial wall remodeling during lipid-lowering therapy: serial intravascular ultrasound observations from the Reversal of Atherosclerosis with Aggressive Lipid Lowering Therapy (REVERSAL) trial. Circulation 113: 2826–2834.

4. de Graaf MA, Broersen A, Kitslaar PH, Roos CJ, Dijkstra J, et al. (2013) Automatic quantification and characterization of coronary atherosclerosis with computed tomography coronary angiography: cross-correlation with intravascular ultrasound virtual histology. Int J Cardiovasc Imaging 29: 1177–1190.

5. Priester TC, Litwin SE (2009) Measuring progression of coronary atherosclerosis with computed tomography: searching for clarity among shades of gray. J Cardiovasc Comput Tomogr 3 Suppl 2: S81–90.

6. Martin SS, Abd TT, Jones SR, Michos ED, Blumenthal RS, et al. (2014) American cholesterol treatment guideline: what was done well and what could be done better. J Am Coll Cardio. pii: S0735-1097(14)01579-4.

7. Kavousi M, Leening MJ, Nanchen D, Greenland P, Graham IM, et al. (2014) Comparison of application of the ACC/AHA guidelines, Adult Treatment Panel III guidelines, and European Society of Cardiology guidelines for cardiovascular disease prevention in a European cohort. JAMA 311: 1416–1423.

8. Fihn SD, Gardin JM, Abrams J, Berra K, Blankenship JC, et al. (2012) ACCF/AHA/ACP/AATS/PCNA/SCAI/STS Guideline for the diagnosis and management of patients with stable ischemic heart disease: a report of the American College of Cardiology Foundation/American Heart Association Task Force on Practice Guidelines, and the American College of Physicians, American Association for Thoracic Surgery, Preventive Cardiovascular Nurses Association, Society for Cardiovascular Angiography and Interventions, and Society of Thoracic Surgeons. J AM Coll Cardiol 60: e44–e164.

9. Perk J, De Backer G, Gohlke H, Graham I, Reiner Z, et al. (2012) European guidelines on cardiovascular disease prevention in clinical practice (version 2012). The Fifth Joint Task Force of the European Society of Cardiology and Other Societies on Cardiovascular Disease Prevention in Clinical Practice (constituted by representatives of nine societies and by invited experts). Eur Heart J 33: 1635–1701.

10. Alexander KP, Newby LK, Cannon CP, Armstrong PW, Gibler WB, et al. (2007) Acute coronary care in the elderly, part I: non-ST-segment-elevation acute coronary syndromes: a scientific statement for healthcare professionals from the American Heart Association Council on Clinical Cardiology: in collaboration with the Society of Geriatric Cardiology. Circulation 115: 2549–2569.

11. Lloyd-Jones D, Adams R, Carnethon M, De Simone G, Ferguson TB, et al. (2009) American Heart Association Statistics Committee and Stroke Statistics Subcommittee heart disease and stroke statistics—2009 update. Circulation Jan., 119: 480–486.

12. Third Report of the National Cholesterol Education Program (NCEP) (2002) Expert panel on detection, evaluation, and treatment of high blood cholesterol in adults (Adult Treatment Panel III) final report. Circulation 106: 3143–3421.

13. McPherson R, Frohlich J, Fodor G, Genest J (2006) Canadian Cardiovascular Society position statement: recommendations for the diagnosis and treatment of dyslipidemia and prevention of cardiovascular disease. Can J Cardiol 22: 913–927.

14. Mosca L, Banka CL, Benjamin EJ, Berra K, Bushnell C, et al. (2007) Evidence-based guidelines for cardiovascular disease prevention in women: 2007 update. Circulation 115: 1481–1501.

15. Wood D, De Backer G, Faergeman O, Graham I, Mancia G, et al. (1998) Prevention of coronary heart disease in clinical practice: recommendations of the Second Joint Task Force of European and Other Societies on Coronary Prevention. Atherosclerosis 140: 199–270.

16. Lloyd-Jones DM (2010) Cardiovascular risk prediction, basic concepts, current status, and future directions. Circulation 121: 1768–1777.

17. De Backer G, Ambrosioni E, Borch-Johnsen K, Brotons C, Cifkova R, et al. (2004) European guidelines on cardiovascular disease prevention in clinical practice: Third Joint Task Force of European and Other Societies on Cardiovascular Disease Prevention in Clinical Practice. Atherosclerosis 173: 381–391.

18. Jackson R (2000) Updated New Zealand cardiovascular disease risk-benefit prediction guide. BMJ 320: 709–710.

19. Mahmood SS, Levy D, Vasan RS, Wang TJ (2014) The Framingham Heart Study and the epidemiology of cardiovascular disease: a historical perspective. Lancet 15, 383: 999–1008.

20. Wilson PW, D'Agostino RB, Levy D, Belanger AM, Silbershatz H, et al. (1998) Prediction of coronary heart disease using risk factor categories. Circulation 97: 1837–1847.

21. D'Agostino RB, Grundy SM, Sullivan LM, Wilson P (2001) Validation of the Framingham coronary heart disease prediction scores: results of a multiple ethnic groups investigation. JAMA 286: 180–187.

22. Giampaoli S, Palmieri L, Mattiello A, Panico S (2005) Definition of high risk individuals to optimize strategies for primary prevention of cardiovascular diseases. Nutr Metab Cardiovasc Dis 15: 79–85.

23. NCEP (2001) Executive summary of the third report of the national cholesterol education program (NCEP) expert panel on detection, evaluation, and treatment of high blood cholesterol in adults (Adult Treatment Panel III). JAMA 285: 2486–2497.

24. USPSTF (2008) Aspirin for the prevention of cardiovascular disease: U.S. Preventive Services Task Force recommendation statement. Ann Intern Med 150: 396–404.

25. Conroy RM, Pyorala K, Fitzgerald AP, Sans S, Menotti A, et al. (2003) Estimation of ten-year risk of fatal cardiovascular disease in Europe: the SCORE project. Eur Heart J 24: 987–1003.

26. Assmann G, Cullen P, Schulte H (2002) Simple scoring scheme for calculating the risk of acute coronary events based on the 10-year follow-up of the prospective cardiovascular Munster (PROCAM) study. Circulation 105: 310–315.

27. Rodondi N, Locatelli I, Aujesky D, Bulter J, Vittinghoff E, et al. (2012) Framingham risk score and alternatives for prediction of coronary heart disease in older adults. PLoS One 7: e34287.

28. Psaty BM, Anderson M, Kronmal RA, Tracy RP, Orchard T, et al. (2004) The association between lipid levels and the risks of incident myocardial infarction, stroke, and total mortality: the cardiovascular health study. J Am Geriatr Soc 52: 1639–1647.

29. National Heart, Lung, and Blood Institute (NHLBI) Clinical Practice Guidelines, Cardiovascular Risk Calculator. Available: http://cvdrisk.nhlbi. nih.gov/. Accessed 2014 September 14.

30. National Heart, Lung, and Blood Institute, NHLBI, Estimate of 10-Year for CHD. Available: Nhlbi.nih.gov. Accessed 2014 September 14.

31. Levine GN, Bates ER, Blankenship JC, Bailey SR, Bittl JA, et al. (2011) ACCF/ AHA/SCAI guideline for percutaneous coronary intervention: executive summary: a report of the American College of Cardiology Foundation/ American Heart Association Task Force on Practice Guidelines and the Society for Cardiovascular Angiography and Interventions. Circulation 124: 2574–2609.

32. Expert Dyslipidemia Panel of the International Atherosclerosis Society Panel member (2014) An international atherosclerosis society position paper: global recommendations for the management of dyslipidemia—full report. J Clin Lipidol 8: 29–60.

33. Whitworth JA (2003) World Health Organization, International Society of Hypertension Writing Group. J Hypertens 21: 1983–1992.

34. Rosengran A, Wallentin L, Gitt AK, Behar S, Battler A, et al. (2004) Sex, age, and clinical presentation of acute coronary syndromes. Eur Heart J 5: 663–670.

35. Abbott RD, Curb JD, Rodriquez BL, Masaki KH, Yano K, et al. (2002) Age-related changes in risk factor effects on the incidence of coronary heart disease. Ann Epidemiol 12: 173–181.

36. Rosamond W, Flegal K, Furie K, Go A, Greenlund K, et al. (2008) Heart disease and stroke statistics—2008 update: a report from the American Heart Association Statistics Committee and Stroke Statistics Subcommittee. Circulation 117: e25–146.

37. Greenland P, Knoll MD, Stamler J, Neaton JD, Dyer AR, et al. (2003) Major risk factors as antecedents of fatal and nonfatal coronary heart disease events. JAMA 290: 891–897.

38. Rosengren A, Wallentin L, Simoons M, Gitt AK, Behar S, et al. (2006) Age, clinical presentation, and outcome of acute coronary syndromes in the Euroheart acute coronary syndrome survey. Eur Heart J 27: 789–795.

39. Artigao-Rodenas LM, Carbayo-Herencia JA, Divisón-Garrote JA, Gil-Guillén VF, Massó-Orozco J, et al. (2013) Framingham risk score for prediction of cardiovascular diseases: a population-based study form southern Europe. PLoS One 8: e73529.

40. de Ruijter W, Westendorp RG, Assendelft WJ, den Elzen WP, de Craen AJ, et al. (2009) Use of Framingham risk score and new biomarkers to predict cardiovascular mortality in older people: population based observational cohort study. BMJ 338: a3083.

41. Empana JP, Ducimetière P, Arveiler D, Ferrières J, Evans A, et al. (2003) Are the Framingham and PROCAM coronary heart disease risk functions applicable to different European populations? The PRIME Study. Eur Heart J 24: 1903–1911.

42. Tzoulaki I, Liberopoulos G, Ioannidis JP (2009) Assessment of claims of improved prediction beyond the Framingham risk score. JAMA 302: 2345–2352.

43. Kim DJ, Bergstrom J, Barrett-Connor E, Laughlin GA (2008) Visceral adiposity and subclinical coronary artery disease in elderly adults: Rancho Bernardo Study. Obesity (Silver Spring) 16: 853–858.

44. Gentleman JF, Brown KS, Forbes WF (1978) Smoking and its effect on mortality of the elderly. Am J Med Sci 276: 173–183.

45. Gehnai AA, al-Mulla AW, Chaikhouni A, Ammar AS, Mahrous F, et al. (2001) Myocardial infarction with normal coronary angiography compared with severe coronary artery disease without myocardial infarction: the crucial role of smoking. J Cardiovasc Risk 8: 1–8.

46. Da Costa A, Isaaz K, Faure E, Mourot S, Cerisier A, et al. (2001) Clinical characteristics, aetiological factors and long-term prognosis of myocardial infarction with an absolutely normal coronary angiogram; a 3-year follow-up study of 91 patients. Eur Heart J 22: 1459–1465.

47. Sun YH, Yang YJ, Pei WD, Wu YJ, Gao RL (2006) Patients with low high-density lipoprotein-cholesterol or smoking are more likely to develop myocardial infarction among subjects with a visible lesion or stenosis in coronary artery. Circ J 70: 1602–1605.

3

Screening for Older Emergency Department Inpatients at Risk of Prolonged Hospital Stay: The Brief Geriatric Assessment Tool

Cyrille P. Launay[1], Laure de Decker[2], Anastasiia Kabeshova[1], Cédric Annweiler[1,3], Olivier Beauchet[1,4]*

1 Department of Neuroscience, Division of Geriatric Medicine, UPRES EA 4638, UNAM, Angers University Hospital, Angers, France, 2 Department of Geriatrics, EA 1156–12, Nantes University Hospital, Nantes, France, 3 Robarts Research Institute, Schulich School of Medicine and Dentistry, the University of Western Ontario, London, Ontario, Canada, 4 Biomathics, Paris, France

Abstract

Background: The aims of this study were 1) to confirm that combinations of brief geriatric assessment (BGA) items were significant risk factors for prolonged LHS among geriatric patients hospitalized in acute care medical units after their admission to the emergency department (ED); and 2) to determine whether these combinations of BGA items could be used as a prognostic tool of prolonged LHS.

Methods: Based on a prospective observational cohort design, 1254 inpatients (mean age $\pm$ standard deviation, 84.9 ± 5.9 years; 59.3% female) recruited upon their admission to ED and discharged in acute care medical units of Angers University Hospital, France, were selected in this study. At baseline assessment, a BGA was performed and included the following 6 items: age ≥85years, male gender, polypharmacy (i.e., ≥5 drugs per day), use of home-help services, history of falls in previous 6 months and temporal disorientation (i.e., inability to give the month and/or year). The LHS in acute care medical units was prospectively calculated in number of days using the hospital registry.

Results: Area under receiver operating characteristic (ROC) curves of prolonged LHS of different combinations of BGA items ranged from 0.50 to 0.57. Cox regression models revealed that combinations defining a high risk of prolonged LHS, identified from ROC curves, were significant risk factors for prolonged LHS (hazard ratio >1.16 with $P>0.010$). Kaplan-Meier distributions of discharge showed that inpatients classified in high-risk group of prolonged LHS were discharged later than those in low-risk group ($P<0.003$). Prognostic value for prolonged LHS of all combinations was poor with sensitivity under 77%, a high variation of specificity (from 26.6 to 97.4) and a low likelihood ratio of positive test under 5.6.

Conclusion: Combinations of 6-item BGA tool were significant risk factors for prolonged LHS but their prognostic value was poor in the studied sample of older inpatients.

Editor: Leocadio Rodríguez-Mañas, Hospital Universitario de Getafe, Spain

Funding: The authors report no current funding sources for this study.

Competing Interests: O. Beauchet is affiliated with Biomathics, Paris. There are no patents, products in development or marketed products to declare.

* Email: olbeauchet@chu-angers.fr

Introduction

Older adults are the fastest increasing group of patients admitted to hospital, often through emergency departments (ED) [1,2]. Compared to younger inpatients, multimorbidity and related-disabilities leading to a high disease burden characterize the older inpatients group [3–5]. Because hospital is largely configured for single acute disease rather than multimorbidity and related disability, age-related high burden disease is one of the main challenges faced by hospitals [6]. Thus, assessing and addressing the needs of the growing number of older inpatients with a greater range of acute and chronic diseases causing disability but not mortality is mandatory [6–8].

Adapted care plan of older inpatients are based on multidimensional, interdisciplinary diagnostic process to determine the medical, psychological, and functional capabilities called comprehensive geriatric assessment (CGA) [3]. CGA allows a coordinated and integrated plan for treatment, and thus may prevent complicated medical pathway characterized, for instance, by prolonged length of hospital stay (LHS) [4,3,9]. Early screening of older inpatients at risk of prolonged LHS based on CGA approach is the first step of an adapted care plan of older inpatients because it improves the medical decision-making process, and thus the care pathway [4,10].

Benefits of CGA have been confirmed through a meta-analysis reporting a reduction of admissions and readmissions to hospital [11]. Recently, it has been reported that an early intervention made by geriatricians of a mobile geriatric team (MGT) using a 6-item brief CGA (BGA) reduced LHS in older inpatients [12]. The 6-item BGA has been developed in response to the difficulty of systematic implementation of CGA in daily practice for every older inpatient admitted to ED [4,13,14]. It has been shown that CGA cannot be applied to every older inpatient, and that the best compromise could be the use of two-step approach [15]. The first step is the screening of older inpatients at high risk of adverse outcomes such as prolonged LHS by non-geriatricians using a brief and accurate screening tool applicable during clinical practice, and the second step is a CGA by geriatricians with a diagnostic and therapeutic purpose [15,16].

We recently showed that different combinations of the 6-item BGA tool (i.e., age ≥85 years, gender male, polypharmacy, non-use of home services, history of falls and cognitive decline) were risk factors for prolonged LHS in a cohort of 424 older patients admitted to acute care medical units following ED discharge [16,17]. Among these different combinations, history of falls and cognitive decline were major predictors for prolonged LHS. We also reported that the maximum number of items to predict prolonged LHS was 4. Indeed, the combination of a history of falls, male gender, cognitive impairment and age under 85 years, identified older patients at highest risk of prolonged LHS. These results allowed the identification of 3 levels of risk of prolonged LHS (i.e., high, intermediate and low) according to different combinations of the BGA 6 items. The aims of this study were 1) to confirm that combinations of BGA items were significant risk factors for prolonged LHS among geriatric patients hospitalized in acute care medical units after their admission to the ED; and 2) to determine whether these combinations of BGA items could be used as a prognostic tool of prolonged LHS.

Methods

Recruitment of participants

Between January and December 2012, 2908 older adults aged 75 years and over were admitted to the ED of Angers University Hospital, France. Among them, 1264 (43.5%) were discharged in acute care medical units. None of them declined to be part of the study. Inclusion criteria were: unplanned admissions in ED followed by discharge in acute care medical units, age of 75 years and over, not identified as treatment-limiting decision and willingness to participate. A total of 10 participants have missing data and were excluded form the analysis. In final, 1254 participants (mean age ± standard deviation, 84.9±5.9 years; 59.3% female) were included in the study (Figure 1).

Assessment of participants

The 6-item BGA was performed upon the admission to ED. It was composed of the following items: age coded as a binary variable (i.e.,≥ or <85 years), gender, polypharmacy defined as ≥ 5 drugs per day, use of formal and/or informal home-help services coded as a binary variable (i.e., yes or no), history of falls in previous 6 months coded as a binary variable (i.e., yes or no), and temporal disorientation defined as the inability to give the month and/or year coded as a binary variable (i.e., yes or no). We chose these items because each of them has been separately associated with a prolonged LHS and because we previously reported that their combinations predicted prolonged LHS [16–20]. The place of life (i.e., home versus institution) and the reasons for admission to ED were also recorded because these parameters have both been associated with prolonged LHS [18–20]. Reasons for admission were categorized using two complementary approaches. First, we distinguished acute organ failure versus non-acute organ

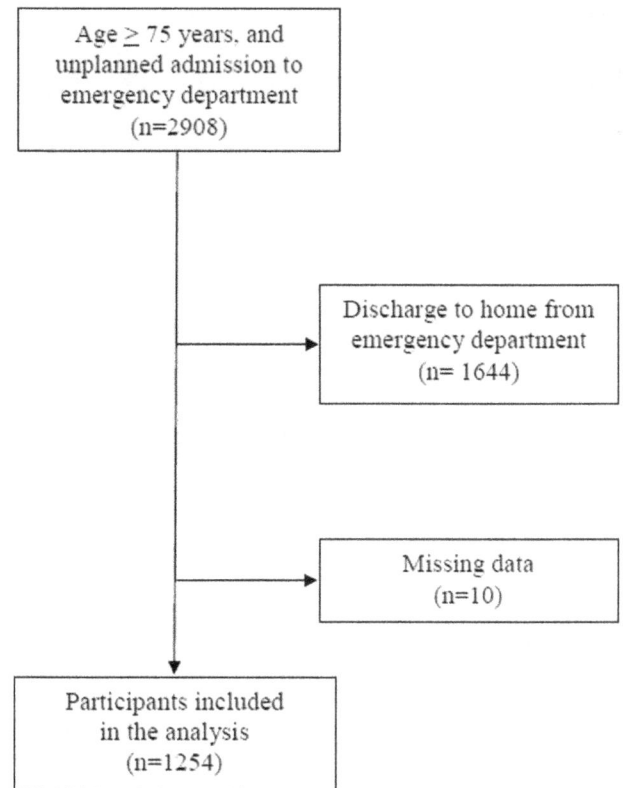

Figure 1. Flow chart showing the selection of participants included in the analysis.

failure. Second, we specified the nature of the acute organ failure in four subgroups based on the prevalence of related diseases in our sample of participants: 19.5% (n = 156) cardio-vascular diseases, 18.4% (n = 147) respiratory diseases, 16.2% (n = 129) digestive diseases, 12.0% (n = 96) neuropsychiatric diseases and 33.9% (n = 271) other acute diseases. In addition, the use of psychoactive drugs including benzodiazepines, antidepressants or neuroleptics was noted.

Definition of endpoints

The risk of prolonged LHS was estimated using two consecutive strategies. First, a priori combinations of BGA items as previously reported to determine 3 levels of risk of prolonged LHS [16,17]. High risk of prolonged LHS was defined by the combination of cognitive decline + history of falls. Intermediate risk was defined by the finding of cognitive decline, or history of falls, or the combination of age ≥85years + male gender + polypharmacy + no use of home services. Low risk of prolonged LHS was defined by the combination of 3 items or less among age ≥85years, male gender male, polypharmacy, and no use of home services. No information was provided to the physicians in charge of the patients. Second, we explored all other possible combinations of BGA items using the receiver operating characteristic (ROC) curve. A new classification into three levels of risk of prolonged LHS was therefore built using areas under ROC separated into three parts (i.e., highest, intermediate and lowest values). The three best combinations for each part were used to define the risk of prolonged LHS. The LHS was prospectively calculated using the administrative registry of the University Hospital and corresponded to the delay in days between the first day of

Table 1. Baseline characteristics of participants (n = 1254).

Characteristics	Value	[95% confidence interval]
Age (years)		
Mean ±SD	84.9±5.9	[84.6–85.3]
≥85 years	671 (53.5)	[50.7–56.3]
Male gender, n (%)	511 (40.7)	[38.0–43.5]
Number of drugs daily taken		
Mean ±SD	6.7±3.2	[6.6–6.9]
≥5, n (%)	929 (74.1)	[71.7–76.5]
Use of psychoactive drugs*, n (%)	646 (51.1)	[48.8–54.3]
History of falls during the past 6 months, n (%)	468 (37.3)	[34.6–40.0]
Temporal disorientation†, n (%)	415 (33.1)	[30.5–35.7]
Non-use of formal and/or informal home services‡	310 (24.7)	[22.3–27.1]
Living at home	875 (69.7)	[67.2–72.3]
Acute organ failure as reason for admission to Emergency Department, n (%)	799 (63.3)	[61.0–66.4]
Cardio-vascular diseases, n (%)	156 (19.5)	[16.8–22.3]
Respiratory diseases, n (%)	147 (18.4)	[15.7–21.1]
Digestive diseases, n (%)	129 (16.2)	[13.6–18.7]
Neuropsychiatric diseases, n (%)	96 (12.0)	[9.8–14.3]
Other diseases, n (%)	271 (33.9)	[30.6–37.2]
Length of hospital stay (days), mean ±SD	8.8±8.4	[8.3–9.2]

SD: standard deviation.
*: Use of benzodiazepines or antidepressants or neuroleptics.
†: Inability to give the month and/or year.
‡: Formal (i.e., health and/or social professional) or informal (i.e., family and/or friends).

admission to ED and the last day of hospitalization in the acute care medical units. Prolonged LHS was defined as being in the highest tertile of LHS (i.e.,>13 days).

Statistical analysis

First, the participants' baseline characteristics were summarized using means and standard deviations or frequencies and percentages, as appropriate. Second, areas under ROC curve of prolonged LHS was calculated for each item and all possible combinations. Third, univariate and multiple Cox regression models were performed to examine the association between prolonged LHS (dependent variable) and the different combinations of BGA items (independent variables) stratified in three risk-levels (low, intermediate, high). For multiple Cox regression models, two types of models were distinguished: those using low-risk level of prolonged LHS as reference and the others. In both cases, there was an adjustment on the place of life and the reasons for admission to ED. Two kind of adjustment were done for reasons of admission using either acute organ failure as independent variable or the nature of acute organ failures (i.e., cardio-vascular diseases, respiratory diseases, digestive diseases, neuropsychiatric diseases and other diseases). Exponential of negative coefficients were calculated for each model. The model produced a survival function that provided the probability of discharge of hospital at a given time for the features supplied for independent variables. Fourth, we studied the elapsed time to discharge from acute care medical units by survival Kaplan-Meier curves and log-rank test. Because only discharge to acute care medical unit was examined, the analysis was censored to 21 days. Fifth, sensitivity, specificity, positive (PPV) and negative (NPV) predictive values, likelihood ratios of positive (LR+) and negative

(LR-) tests of each BGA item and all possible combinations of prolonged LHS were calculated. P-values <0.05 were considered statistically significant. All statistics were performed using SPSS (version 19.0; SPSS, Inc., Chicago, IL) and RStudio.

Standard Protocol Approvals, Registrations, and Participant Consents

The study was conducted in accordance with the ethical standards set forth in the Helsinki Declaration (1983). All participants recruited in this study provided a verbal informed consent because the study did not change the usual clinical practice. The verbal informed consent was obtained from the patients themselves in the presence of their trusted person, usually a family member, who helped them to make decision. The participant consent was recorded in the digital file of patients. The entire study protocol and the consent procedure were approved by the Ethical Committee of Angers, France.

Results

The baseline characteristics of participants are presented in Table 1. More than half of patients were aged 85 years and over. A total of 74.1% took 5 and over different drugs per day. Nearly one third had a history of falls in the past 6 months or had temporal disorientation. One quarter of participants were isolated, and more than two thirds lived at home. A total of 63.3% patients were admitted to ED for an acute organ failure. The main causes of acute organ failure were cardiovascular diseases (19.5%), respiratory diseases (18.4%), digestive diseases (16.2%) and neuropsychiatric diseases (12.0%). The mean LHS was around 9 days. A total of 157 patients (12.5%) died during hospitalization.

Table 2. Area under Receiver operating characteristic curve and prognostic values of brief geriatric assessment items and their combinations* for prolonged length of hospital stay† (n = 1254).

	Area under ROC	Sensitivity(%)	Specify(%)	PPV (%)	NPV (%)	LR+	LR-	Number of individuals classified			
								TP	FP	FN	TN
6 items of the brief geriatric assessment, considered separately											
Age≥85 years	0.50	53.02	46.34	23.55	75.99	0.99	1.01	158	513	140	443
Male gender	0.50	40.94	59.31	23.87	76.31	1.00	1.00	122	389	176	576
Polypharmacy‡	0.51	76.17	26.57	24.43	78.15	1.04	0.90	227	702	71	254
Non-use of home help services§	0.52	27.85	76.26	26.77	77.22	1.17	0.95	83	227	215	729
History of falls¶	0.52	39.93	63.49	25.43	77.23	1.09	0.95	119	349	179	607
Temporal disorientation#	0.55	40.94	69.35	29.40	79.02	1.34	0.58	122	293	176	663
Combinations of the 6 items of the brief geriatric assessment **											
A priori combinations††											
Low risk											
Male + polypharmacy‡ + non-use of home services§	0.54	9.40	91.95	26.67	76.50	1.17	0.99	28	77	270	879
Age≥85 years + polypharmacy‡ + non-use of home services§	0.53	9.06	94.46	33.75	76.92	1.63	0.96	27	53	271	903
Age≥85 years + male + non-use of home services§	0.52	3.69	96.13	22.92	76.20	0.95	1.00	11	37	287	919
Intermediate risk											
History of falls	0.52	39.93	63.49	25.43	77.23	1.09	0.95	119	349	179	607
Temporal disorientation#	0.55	40.94	69.35	29.40	79.02	1.34	0.58	122	293	176	663
Age ≥85years + male + polypharmacy‡ + non-use of home services§	0.54	2.35	97.38	21.88	76.19	0.90	1.00	7	25	291	931
High risk											
History of falls + temporal disorientation#	0.56	18.46	86.30	29.57	77.25	1.35	0.95	55	131	243	825
Newly identified combinations											
Low risk											
Polypharmacy‡ + non-use of home help services§	0.53	17.79	84.21	25.98	76.67	1.13	0.98	53	151	245	805
Polypharmacy‡ + history of falls	0.53	31.88	75.00	28.44	77.93	1.28	0.91	95	239	203	717
Age≥85 years + polypharmacy‡ + history of falls	0.53	17.79	83.89	25.60	76.60	1.10	0.98	53	154	245	802
Intermediate risk											
Age≥85 years + polypharmacy‡ + temporal disorientation#	0.56	15.44	86.72	26.59	76.69	1.16	0.98	46	127	252	829
Male + polypharmacy‡ + temporal disorientation#	0.56	12.08	92.26	32.73	77.10	1.56	0.95	36	74	262	882
Age≥85 years + male + polypharmacy‡ + temporal disorientation#	0.56	5.37	95.26	28.57	76.46	1.28	0.99	16	40	232	915
High risk											
History of falls + temporal disorientation# + Polypharmacy‡	0.57	12.75	91.32	31.40	77.05	1.47	0.96	38	83	260	873

Table 2. Cont.

	Area under ROC	Sensitivity(%)	Specify(%)	PPV (%)	NPV (%)	LR+	LR-	Number of individuals classified			
								TP	FP	FN	TN
History of falls + temporal disorientation# + Polypharmacy‡ + male	0.57	5.03	96.55	31.25	76.53	1.46	0.98	15	33	283	923
Age≥85 years + polypharmacy‡ + non-use of home help services§	0.57	4.03	99.27	63.16	76.84	5.50	0.97	12	7	286	949

ROC: Receiver operating characteristic curve; PPV: Positive predictive value; NPV: Negative predictive value; LR+: Likelihood ration of positive test; LR-: Likelihood ration of negative test; TP: True positive; FP: False positive; TN: True negative; FN: False negative;

*: Only three best models (i.e., highest value of ROC) by level (i.e., Low, intermediate and high risk) are shown;
†: Defined being in the highest tertile of length of hospital saty (i.e.,>13 days);
‡: Defined by a number of drugs taken per day above 4;
§: Living alone without using any formal or informal home services and social help;
#: during the past 6 months;
¶: Inability to give the month and/or year;
***: Only combination involving at least 10 participants were considered;
††: Combinations described in previous published study (Beauchet et al. J Emerg Med. 2013; 45: 739–45).

They were older than those who did not die (mean age ± standard deviation, 86.2±5.4 years versus 84.7±5.9 with P = 0.004) and there were fewer women in this group (49.0% versus 60.4%, P = 0.007). In addition, they had a longer LHS compared to those who did not die (11.3±10.5 days versus 8.4±8.1 days with P< 0.001).

Among BGA items, the best predictor of prolonged LHS was temporal disorientation, this item having the highest value of ROC curve (0.55) (Table 2). The combination 'history of falls' plus 'temporal disorientation', defining the a priori high risk of prolonged LHS identified in our previous publication [16], had the highest value of ROC curve (0.56). Its sensitivity and PPV were low (18.46% and 29.57) but the specificity and NPV were high (86.30% and 77.25). The LR+ and LR- were calculated at 1.35 and 0.95. Compared to this a priori classification, new combinations defining high risk of prolonged LHS had highest values of ROC curve. The sensitivity of all combinations of this level of risk was low under 13.0% but the specificity was high above 90.0%. In addition, the highest LR+ of 5.50 was shown for a combination involving 'age ≥85 years' plus 'polypharmacy' plus 'non-use of home-help services'.

Univariate and Cox regression models adjusted on acute organ failure and place of life showed that patients classified a priori with low risk of prolonged LHS had indeed a significantly shorter LHS (unadjusted Hazard Ratio [HR] = 0.82 with P = 0.001, and adjusted HR = 0.80 with P<0.001), whereas those with high risk of prolonged LHS had a longer LHS (unadjusted HR = 1.27 with P = 0.003, adjusted HR = 1.29 with P = 0.002 and fully adjusted HR = 1.44 with P<0.001) (Table 3). In addition, fully adjusted Cox model (i.e., using the group at low risk of prolonged LHS as reference) shown that patients in intermediate risk group (HR = 1.20 with P = 0.006) had also prolonged LHS. Classification of risk of prolonged LHS based on newly identified combinations underscored that only high risk level predicted a prolonged LHS (unadjusted HR = 1.40 with P<0.001, adjusted HR = 1.43 with P<0.001 and fully adjusted HR = 1.47 with P<0.001). As shown in Table 4, adjustment for the nature of acute organ failures did not alter our results. Indeed, intermediate risk and high risk of prolonged LSH predicted effectively a prolonged LSH with a priori combinations (HR>1.15 and P<0.015), whereas only high risk level predicted prolonged LSH with new combinations (HR> 1.46 and P<0.001).

Generated Kaplan-Meier plot of the probability of discharge from acute care medical units is reported Figures 2 et 3. While using a priori combinations of BGA items (Figure 2), comparison of survival curves showed that inpatients considered at low risk of prolonged LHS were faster discharged from acute care medical units than those in intermediate (P = 0.013) and high-risk groups (P<0.001). Furthermore, patients in intermediate risk of prolonged LHS were also faster discharged from acute care medical units than those in high-risk group (P = 0.026). The new classification showed similar results (Figure 3), except for the comparison of discharge between patients in low-risk group and those in intermediate-risk group which was not significant (P = 0.931). Comparison of survival curves showed that inpatients considered at low risk of prolonged LHS were faster discharged from acute care medical units than those in high-risk group (P< 0.001). Furthermore, patients with intermediate risk of prolonged LHS were also faster discharged from acute care medical units than those in high-risk group (P<0.001).

Table 3. Cox regression models showing the association between the length of hospital stay (dependent variable) and combinations of brief geriatric assessment items (independent variables) separated into three risk-levels (i.e., low risk, intermediate risk, and high risk of prolonged length of hospital stay) (n = 1254).

Combinations of the 6-item brief geriatric assessment, stratified in three levels of risk (low, intermediate, high)	HR [95% CI] (P-Value)		
	Model 1	**Model 2**	**Model 3**
A priori combinations*			
Low-risk level: Three items among age ≥85years, male gender, polypharmacy[†] and non-use of home services[‡]	**0.82** [0.74; 0.92]	**0.80** [0.71; 0.91]	1.00(Ref)
	(0.001)	**(0.001)**	
Intermediate-risk level: History of falls§, or temporal disorientation, or (age ≥85years + male gender + polypharmacy[†] + non-use of home services[‡])	1.06 [0.95; 1.18]	1.06 [0.95; 1.19]	**1.20** [1.05; 1.36]
	(0.325)	(0.323)	**(0.006)**
High-risk level: history of falls§ + temporal disorientation	**1.27** [1.09; 1.49]	**1.29** [1.09; 1.51]	**1.44** [1.20; 1.73]
	(0.003)	**(0.002)**	**(<0.001)**
Newly identified combinations			
Low-risk level: polypharmacy[†] + (non-use of home-help services[‡] or age ≥85years or history of falls§) + (absence of temporal disorientation)	0.93 [0.82; 1.06]	0.90 [0.79; 1.02]	1.00(Ref)
	(0.291)	(0.104)	
Intermediate-risk level: combinations other than low- or high-level combinations	0.91 [0.81; 1.02]	0.93 [0.82; 1.04]	1.05 [0.91; 1.19]
	(0.096)	(0.208)	(0.519)
High-risk level: temporal disorientation + polypharmacy[†] + (history of falls§ or (age ≥85years or non use of home help services[‡]))	**1.40** [1.17; 1.68]	**1.43** [1.19; 1.72]	**1.47** [1.20; 1.81]
	(<0.001)	**(<0.001)**	**(<0.001)**

Model 1: Unadjusted model.
Model 2: Model adjusted on organ failure and place of life.
Model 3: Low risk of prolonged length of hospital stay used as reference, with adjustment on organ failure and place of life.
*: Combinations described previously (Beauchet et al. J Emerg Med. 2013; 45: 739–45).
[†]: Defined by a number of drugs taken per day above 4.
[‡]: Living alone without using any formal or informal home services and social help.
[§]: In past 6 months.
[¶]: Inability to give the month and/or year.
Hazard ratio and p-value significant (i.e., <0.05) indicated in bold.

Discussion

Our results show that combinations of BGA items were significant risk factors for prolonged LHS in geriatric patients admitted to ED and discharged to acute care medical units. However, the prognostic value for prolonged LHS of these combinations of BGA items was poor, whatever the BGA items or their combinations used.

The main findings of our study is the discrepancy between the fact that combinations of BGA items were risk factors for prolonged LHS and their poor prognostic value for this endpoint. Limitations of risk factors as a prognostic tool have been previously reported [21–23]. The conclusions of these publications was that risk factors should exhibit a much stronger association with the studied endpoint (e.g., prolonged LHS in our case) than they ordinarily show in epidemiological studies if it is to provide a basis for prediction in individual patients. Our results are, therefore, in total concordance with this assumption. Indeed, even if HR of certain combinations of BGA items were significant risk factors for prolonged LHS, the magnitude of their values was low below 2, which is consistent with a poor prognostic value for prolonged LHS. This apparent paradoxical result (i.e., a significant risk factor having a poor prognostic value) is in relation with the fact that a risk factor is assessed by comparing the risk of studied outcome at each end of the distribution of the risk factor. While using this statistical approach the effect of being highly exposed to the factor

is compared with the effect of being slightly exposed. Thus, comparison is done on jointly exclusive groups of individuals. The main consequence of this approach is that the group of individuals in the middle of distribution, which represents the majority of individuals, is ignored. Because the aim in screening tool is to identify a group of individuals with a high risk relative to everyone, there is necessary a discrepancy between to be a significant risk factor associated with the studied outcome and to be a poor prognostic risk factor for this outcome.

Combinations of BGA items were significant risk factors for prolonged LHS among studied geriatric inpatients. The strength of this association was greater when specific items were combined underscoring a stronger association while using newly identified combinations compared to *a priori* combinations [16]. This result may be explained by the fact that the BGA items, and specifically the combinations defining the high-risk level, are markers of frailty, which is a status previously identified as a risk factor for prolonged LHS [16,17,5]. Frailty in older adults usually refers to a physiological vulnerability medical that expose to adverse health, functional and social outcomes [24]. Despite the lack of consensus on the definition of frailty, there is a broad agreement that frailty is characterized by an accumulation of deficits related to a combined action of aging and morbidities [25–27]. Under the action of the morbidities and/or ageing that generate disabilities, this dynamic process, occurring from reduced physiological resources, results in

Table 4. Cox regression models showing the association between the length of hospital stay (dependent variable) and combinations of brief geriatric assessment items (independent variables) separated into three risk-levels (i.e., low risk, intermediate risk, and high risk of prolonged length of hospital stay) with separated models for reasons for admission to emergency department (n = 1254).

Combinations of the 6-item brief geriatric Assessment stratified in three levels of risk (low, intermediate, high)	HR [95% CI] (P-Value)*				
	Cardio vascular disease	Respiratory disease	Digestive disease	Neuropsychological disease	Other diseases
A priori combinations†					
Low-risk level: three items among age ≥85years, male gender, polypharmacy‡ and non-use of home-help services§	1.00(Ref)	1.00(Ref)	1.00(Ref)	1.00(Ref)	1.00(Ref)
Intermediate-risk level: history of falls, or temporal disorientation#, or (age ≥85years + male gender + polypharmacy‡ + non-use of home-help services§)	**1.17** [1.04; 1.32]	**1.19** [1.06; 1.35]	**1.18** [1.04; 1.33]	**1.17** [1.04; 1.32]	**1.21** [1.07; 1.37]
	(0.012)	**(0.004)**	**(0.008)**	**(0.010)**	**(0.003)**
High-risk level: history of falls + temporal disorientation#	**1.39** [1.17; 1.65]	**1.44** [1.21; 1.70]	**1.41** [1.19; 1.67]	**1.40** [1.18; 1.65]	**1.46** [1.22; 1.74]
	(<0.001)	**(<0.001)**	**(<0.001)**	**(<0.001)**	**(<0.001)**
Newly identified combinations					
Low-risk level: polypharmacy‡ + (non use of home help services§ or age ≥85years or history of falls) + (absence of temporal disorientation)	1.00(Ref)	1.00(Ref)	1.00(Ref)	1.00(Ref)	1.00(Ref)
Intermediate-risk level: combinations other than low- or high-level combinations	1.05 [0.92; 1.19]	1.03 [0.91; 1.18]	1.04 [0.92; 1.19]	1.05 [0.92; 1.19]	1.04 [0.91; 1.18]
	(0.509)	(0.614)	(0.520)	(0.484)	(0.609)
High-risk level: temporal disorientation# + polypharmacy‡ + (history of falls or (age ≥85years + non-use of home-help services§))	**1.47** [1.19; 1.80]	**1.48** [1.20; 1.81]	**1.48** [1.20; 1.82]	**1.47** [1.20; 1.81]	**1.48** [1.21; 1.82]
	(<0.001)	**(<0.001)**	**(<0.001)**	**(<0.001)**	**(<0.001)**

All models used low-risk level as reference value.
*: adjustment on place of life.
†: Combinations described previously (Beauchet et al. J Emerg Med. 2013; 45: 739–45).
‡: Defined by a number of drugs taken per day above 4.
§: Living alone without using any formal or informal home services and social help.
¶: In past 6 months.
#: Inability to give the month and/or year.
Hazard ratio and p-value significant (i.e., <0.05) indicated in bold.

impaired adaptation to stress such as a hospitalization. As a consequence frail older adults are more prone to prolonged LHS than non-frail older ones [16,25–29].

Our results also show that the risk of prolonged LHS did not increase in a simple cumulative way according to the combination of items. Considered separately, older age, male gender, polypharmacy and the absence of home-help services have been previously associated with prolonged LHS [10,16,28–30]. The highest risk was not reported with the combination of all 6 items. Moreover, high risk of prolonged LHS was found with several combinations rather than one. This results is probably the consequence of a complex interplay of BGA items which are direct or indirect markers of geriatric syndromes, morbidities or functional decline, and where the interaction between medical and change of the environment of an individuals (i.e., hospital and more precisely acute care unit in our study) exposes patients to a major risk of prolonged LHS [16,28,29]. Indeed, the latter parameter underscores the inability of changes of frail individuals due to poor physiological resources. In addition, the heterogeneity of health conditions among geriatric population may also account for the various combinations related to a high risk of prolonged LHS [2,8,16].

Among the BGA items, we confirmed in the studied sample of inpatients that the history of falls and temporal disorientation were strongly related to prolonged LHS, and thus were part of most combinations defining the high risk of prolonged LHS [16–18]. In addition, the risk of prolonged LHS increased when both these items were associated. Falls usually cause and/or result from gait and/or balance disorders, which are themselves identified risk factors for prolonged LHS [31–33]. This specific association has been underscored using Timed Up & Go (TUG), which is a basic assessment of functional mobility and measures the time needed to rise from a chair, walk 3 meters, turn around and return to a seated position [33]. It has been reported that longer TUG was a marker of prolonged LHS in older patients [10,18]. Furthermore, the association between temporal disorientation and prolonged LHS may be explained by the fact that temporal disorientation is a surrogate measure of severe cognitive disorders, either acute (i.e., delirium) and/or chronic (i.e., dementia) [17]. Because these both cognitive disorders have been identified as risk factors for prolonged LHS, they could explain the prolonged LHS reported in our study [10,18]. Our results also highlighted that the risk of prolonged LHS increased when history of falls was combined with temporal disorientation. This is in concordance with previous results showing that individuals combining cognitive decline and

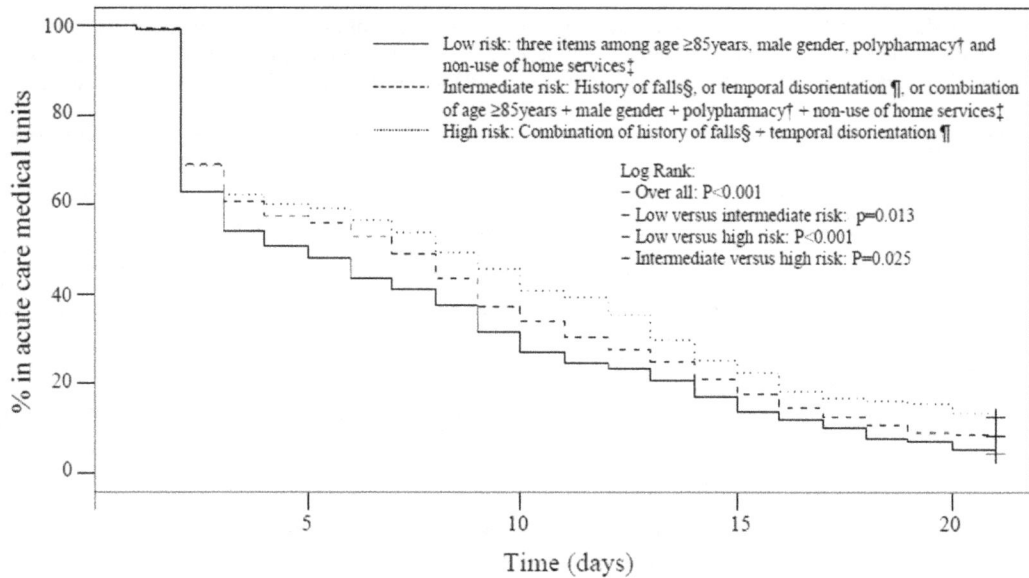

Figure 2. Kaplan-Meier estimates of the probability of discharge from acute care medical units among older inpatients (n = 12,054) using *a priori** combinations of the 6 items of the brief geriatric assessment. *: Combinations described previously (Beauchet et al. J Emerg Med. 2013; 45: 739–45). †: Defined by a number of drugs taken per day above 4. ‡: Living alone without using any formal or informal home services and social help. §: In past 6 months. ¶: Inability to give the month and/or year.

mobility disorders were more at risk of adverse outcomes than those having only one disorder, and that LHS increases with the accumulation of risk factors [18–20]. Finally, this strong association of history of falls and temporal disorientation with prolonged LHS may be explained by the fact that both these disorders are common ways of expression of diseases, whatever their nature. Older adults' health and functional status is heterogeneous because of the various cumulative effects of chronic diseases and physiologic decline, contributing to a vicious cycle of increased

frailty, the frailty being defined as a clinically recognizable state of increased vulnerability [24–27]. The expression of this vulnerability is often a decrease in gait and cognitive performance, the clinical symptoms of this decline being falls and temporal disorientation [24,25].

The poor prognostic value of the 6-item BGA is in concordance with results of previous studies exploring the predictive value of clinical parameters for the occurrence of adverse health events in older adults. Prognostic value of prior tools, such as the

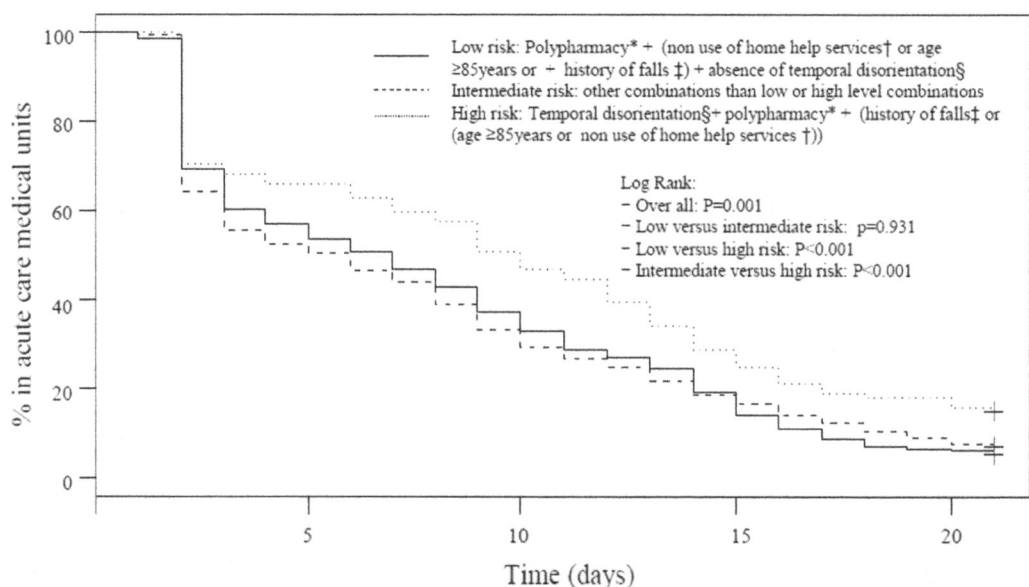

Figure 3. Kaplan-Meier estimates of the probability of discharge from acute care medical units among older inpatients (n = 12,054) using newly identified combinations of the 6 items of the brief geriatric assessment. *: Defined by a number of drugs taken per day above 4. †: Living alone without using any formal or informal home services and social help. ‡: In past 6 months. §: Inability to give the month and/or year.

Identification of Seniors At Risk (ISAR) score and the triage risk stratification tool (TRST), which are the main tools validated in ED users aged 65 years and older, have been examined [34,35]. Like our results, it has been reported that these tools have a poor prognostic value for adverse health outcomes in ED (i.e., death, institutionalisation, readmission) [34,35]. Developing one single tool to predict LHS remains a complex challenge but an objective to reach. A perspective for the prediction of frailty-related adverse outcomes such as prolonged LHS could come from non-linear statistical methods [36–38]. For instance, artificial neural networks (ANNs) are data analysis tools that have been developed to overcome limitations of linear models [36]. Because they apply non-linear statistic to pattern recognition, ANNs are particularly adapted to "chaotic" behavior like frailty-related adverse outcomes. Nowadays, the advance of ANNs combined with improvement of computers technology open new perspectives in diagnostic support aids for helping physicians to take the best decision for their patients [37,38].

Some limitations of this study need to be considered. First, participants were included from a single centre and, thus, they were probably not representative of all older adults admitted to ED. Secondly, although we were able to control for many characteristics likely to modify the LHS, residual potential confounders might still be present. We limited this confounding bias by adjusting our results on organ failure and place of life because these covariables are strong determinants of prolonged LHS [17–18]. Third, there was a potential recall bias about the history of falls, which is well known in the elderly. Falls are usually underreported because of a cognitive decline of fallers who forget to report the falls, and depends on the occurrence of fall-related adverse health outcomes [39].

In conclusion, combinations of 6 BGA items were significant risk factors for prolonged LHS with a risk that did not increase linearly with the accumulation of items, underscoring that some specific combinations of BGA items were greater risk factors than others. Unfortunately, their prognostic value was poor. Further research is required to improve the prognostic value of clinical tools for the identification of adverse events among older adults hospitalized in medical and surgical care units. A perspective may rely on the use of ANNs.

Acknowledgments

The authors would like to thank the patients for their participation in the study.

Author Contributions

Conceived and designed the experiments: CPL OB. Performed the experiments: CPL LDD AK. Analyzed the data: CPL LDD CA AK OB. Contributed reagents/materials/analysis tools: CPL CA AK OB. Wrote the paper: CPL LDD CA AK OB.

References

1. Aminzadeh F, Dalziel WB (2002) Older adults in the emergency department: a systematic review of patterns of use, adverse outcomes, and effectiveness of interventions. Ann Emerg Med 393: 238–247.
2. Xu KT, Nelson BK, Berk S (2009) The changing profile of patients who used emergency department services in the United States: 1996 to 2005. Ann Emerg Med 546: 805–810.
3. Stuck AE, Iliffe S (2011) Comprehensive geriatric assessment for older adults. BMJ 343: 6799.
4. Conroy SP, Ansari K, Williams M, Laithwaite E, Teasdale B, et al (2013) A controlled evaluation of comprehensive geriatric assessment in the emergency department: the 'Emergency Frailty Unit'. Age Ageing 431: 109–114.
5. Drame M, Jovenin N, Novella JL, Lang PO, Somme D, et al. (2008) Predicting early mortality among elderly patients hospitalised in medical wards via emergency department: the SAFES cohort study. J Nutr Health Aging 12: 599–604.
6. Barnett K, Mercer SW, Norbury M, Watt G, Wyke S, et al. (2012) Epidemiology of multimorbidity and implications for health care, research, and medical education: a cross-sectional study. Lancet 380: 37–43
7. Gill TM, Gahbauer EA, Han L, Allore HG (2010) Trajectories of disability in the last year of life. N Engl J Med 362: 1173–1180.
8. Wolff JL, Starfield B, Anderson G (2002) Prevalence, expenditures, and complications of multiple chronic conditions in the elderly. Arch Intern Med 162: 2269–2276.
9. Yoo JW, Seol H, Kim SJ, Yang JM, Ryu WS, et al. (2013) Effects of hospitalist-directed interdisciplinary medicine floor service on hospital outcomes for seniors with acute medical illness. Geriatr Gerontol Int 14: 71–77.
10. Lang PO, Heitz D, Hedelin G, Dramé M, Jovenin N, et al. (2006) Early markers of prolonged hospital stays in older people: a prospective, multicenter study of 908 inpatients in French acute hospitals. J Am Geriatr Soc 547: 1031–1039.
11. Ellis G, Whitehead MA, Robinson D, O'Neill D, Langhorne P (2011) Comprehensive geriatric assessment for older adults admitted to hospital: meta-analysis of randomised controlled trials. BMJ 343: 1034–1036.
12. Launay C, Annweiler C, de Decker L, Kabeshova A, Fantino B at al. (2013) Early hospital discharge of older adults admitted to the emergency department: effect of different types of recommendations made by a mobile geriatric team. J Am Geriatr Soc 616: 1031–1033.
13. Graf CE, Zekry D, Giannelli S, Michel JP, Chevalley T (2010) Efficiency and applicability of comprehensive geriatric assessment in the emergency department: a systematic review. Aging Clin Exp Res 234: 244–254
14. Somme D, Rousseau C (2013) Standardized geriatric assessment or comprehensive gerontological assessment: where do we stand? Rev Med Interne 342: 114–122.
15. McCusker J, Dendukuri N, Tousignant P, Verdon J, Poulin de Courval L, et al. (2003) Rapid two-stage emergency department intervention for seniors: impact on continuity of care. Acad Emerg Med 103: 233–243
16. Beauchet O, Launay CP, Fantino B, Lerolle N, Maunoury F, et al. (2013) Screening for Elderly Patients Admitted to the Emergency Department Requiring Specialized Geriatric Care. J Emerg Med 455: 739–745.
17. Launay C, Haubois G, Hureaux-Huynh R, Gautier J, Annweiler C, et al. (2014) Older adults and emergency department: who is at risk of hospitalization? Geriatr Psychol Neuropsychiatr Vieil 12: 43–49.
18. Lim SC, Doshi V, Castasus B, Lim JK, Mamun K (2006) Factors causing delay in discharge of elderly patients in an acute care hospital. Ann Acad Med Singapore 351: 27–32
19. Byrne DG, Chung SL, Bennett K (2010) Age and outcome in acute emergency medical admissions. Age Ageing 396: 694–698
20. Hastings SN, Whitson E, Purser JL, Sloane RJ, Johnson KS (2009) Emergency department discharge diagnosis and adverse health outcomes in older adults. J Am Geriatr Soc 5710: 1856–1861
21. Wald NJ, Hackshaw AK, Frost CD (1999) When can a risk factor be used as a worthwhile screening test? BMJ 319: 1562–1565.
22. Ware JH (2006) The limitations of risk factors as prognostic tools. N Engl J Med 355: 2615–2617.
23. Pepe MS, Janes H, Longton G, Leisenring W, Newcomb P (2004) Limitations of the odds ratio in gauging the performance of a diagnostic, prognostic, or screening marker. Am J Epidemiol 159: 882–890.
24. Sternberg SA, Wershof Schwartz A, Karunananthan S, Bergman H, Mark Clarfield A (2011) The identification of frailty: a systematic literature review. J Am Geriatr Soc 59: 2129–2138.
25. Berrut G, Andrieu S, Araujo de Carvalho I, Baeyens JP, Bergman H, et al. (2013) Promoting access to innovation for frail old persons. IAGG (International Association of Gerontology and Geriatrics), WHO (World Health Organization) and SFGG (Société Française de Gériatrie et de Gérontologie) Workshop–Athens January 20–21, 2012 Tool (GFST). J Nutr Health Aging 17: 688–693
26. Rockwood K, Bergman H (2012) FRAILTY: A Report from the 3(rd) Joint Workshop of IAGG/WHO/SFGG, Athens, January 2012. Can Geriatr J 15: 31–36.
27. Ravindrarajah R, Lee DM, Pye SR, Gielen E, Boonen S, et al European Male Aging Study Group (2013) The ability of three different models of frailty to predict all-cause mortality: results from the European Male Aging Study (EMAS). Arch Gerontol Geriatr 57: 360–368.
28. Rozzini R, Sleiman I, Maggi S, Noale M, Trabucchi M (2009) Gender differences and health status in old and very old patients. J Am Med Dir Assoc 108: 554–558.
29. Beauchet O, Launay C, de Decker L, Fantino B, Kabeshova A, et al. (2013) Who is at risk of long hospital stay among patients admitted to geriatric acute care unit? Results from a prospective cohort study. J Nutr Health Aging 178: 695–699.
30. de Decker L, Launay C, Annweiler C, Kabeshova A, Beauchet O (2013) Number of drug classes taken per day may be used to assess morbidity burden in older inpatients: a pilot cross-sectional study. J Am Geriatr Soc 617: 1224–1255.

31. Beauchet O, Dubost V, Revel Delhom C, Berrut G, Belmin J (2011) How to manage recurrent falls in clinical practice: guidelines of the French Society of Geriatrics and Gerontology. J Nutr Health Aging 151: 79–84.

32. Rossat A, Fantino B, Nitenberg C, Annweiler C, Poujol L, et al. (2010) Risk factors for falling in community-dwelling older adults: which of them are associated with the recurrence of falls? J Nutr Health Aging 149: 787–791.

33. Podsiadlo D, Richardson S (1991) The timed "Up & Go": a test of basic functional mobility for frail elderly persons. J Am Geriatr Soc 39: 142–148.

34. McCusker J, Bellavance F, Cardin S, Trépanier S, Verdon J, et al. (1999) Detection of older people at increased risk of adverse health outcomes after an emergency visit: the ISAR screening tool. J Am Geriatr Soc 47: 1229–1237.

35. Meldon SW, Mion LC, Palmer RM, Drew BL, Connor JT, et al. (2003) A brief risk-stratification tool to predict repeat emergency department visits and hospitalizations in older patients discharged from the emergency department. Acad Emerg Med 10: 224–232.

36. Akl A, Ghoneim M (2011) Forcasting the Clinical Outcome: Artificial Neural Networks or Multivariate Statistical Models?, Artificial Neural Networks - Methodological Advances and Biomedical Applications, Prof. Kenji Suzuki (Ed.); InTech, ISBN: 978-953-307-243-2.

37. Baxt WG (1995) Application of artificial neural networks to clinical medicine. Lancet 346: 1135–1138.

38. Baxt WG, Skora J (1996) Prospective validation of artificial neural network trained to identify acute myocardial infarction. Lancet 347: 12–15.

39. Cummings SR, Nevitt MC, Kidd S (1988) Forgetting falls. The limited accuracy of recall of falls in the elderly. J Am Geriatr Soc 367: 613–616.

4

Comorbidities among the HIV-Infected Patients Aged 40 Years or Older in Taiwan

Pei-Ying Wu[1], Mao-Yuan Chen[2], Szu-Min Hsieh[2], Hsin-Yun Sun[2], Mao-Song Tsai[3], Kuan-Yeh Lee[4], Wen-Chun Liu[2], Shan-Ping Yang[1], Yu-Zhen Luo[1], Jun-Yu Zhang[1], Wang-Huei Sheng[1,2]*, Chien-Ching Hung[2,5,6]*

1 Center of Infection Control, National Taiwan University Hospital, Taipei, Taiwan, 2 Department of Internal Medicine, National Taiwan University Hospital and National Taiwan University College of Medicine, Taipei, Taiwan, 3 Department of Internal Medicine, Far Eastern Memorial Hospital, New Taipei City, Taiwan, 4 Department of Internal Medicine, National Taiwan University Hospital Hsin-Chu Branch, Hsin-Chu, Taiwan, 5 Department of Medical Research, China Medical University Hospital, Taichung, Taiwan, 6 China Medical University, Taichung, Taiwan

Abstract

Background: With the widespread use of combination antiretroviral therapy (cART), life expectancy of HIV-infected patients has significantly prolonged. An increasing number of HIV-infected patients are aging and concurrent use of medications are not uncommon for management of metabolic complications and cardiovascular diseases related to aging and prolonged exposure to cART.

Methods: We reviewed medical records of all HIV-infected patients aged 40 years or older who had been followed at a university hospital for HIV care in Taiwan between January and December 2013. A standardized case record form was used to collect information on demographics and clinical characteristics, comorbidity, cART, and concurrent medications.

Results: During the study period, 610 patients aged 40 to 49 years (mean, 44.1) and 310 aged 50 years or older (mean, 58.8) sought HIV care at this hospital. Compared with patients aged 40 to 49 years, those aged 50 years or older were significantly more likely to be female (15.9% vs 3.8%); to have received cART (97.7% vs 94.8%) and a lower plasma HIV RNA load (1.6 vs 1.7 $\log_{10}$ copies/ml); and to have diabetes mellitus (18.4% vs 4.6%), hypertension (31.0% vs 10.8%), hyperlipidemia (29.4% vs 11.6%), coronary artery disease (6.8% vs 0.5%), and an estimated glomerular filtration rate <60 ml/min/1.73 m^2 (11.5% vs 2.7%); and were significantly less likely to have syphilis. Other than HIV infection, patients aged 50 years or older were more likely to have been receiving two or more concurrent medications than those aged 40 to 49 years (22.9% vs 6.4%).

Conclusions: Our findings show a significant proportion of the HIV-infected patients aged 50 years or older have multiple comorbidities that may increase the risk for cardiovascular and renal complications. Issues of poly-pharmacy among the HIV-infected patients who are aging should be addressed to ensure adherence and minimize drug-drug interactions.

Editor: Li-Min Huang, National Taiwan University Hospital, Taiwan

Funding: Taiwan Centers for Disease Control (DOH-102-DC-1401). The funders had no role in study design, data collection and analysis, decision to publish, or preparation of the manuscript.

Competing Interests: The authors have declared that no competing interests exist.

* Email: whsheng@ntu.edu.tw (W-HS); hcc0401@ntu.edu.tw (C-CH)

Introduction

The widespread use of combination antiretroviral therapy (cART) has markedly improved the survival of HIV-1-infected patients [1,2]. According to the multinational cohort study, the life expectancy of HIV-infected patients aged 20 years is projected to increase from 36.1 years to 49.4 years [1]. As a result of reduction in AIDS-related mortality, the number of elderly people living with HIV will continue to increase; furthermore, the number of cases of newly diagnosed HIV infection among the elderly people is increasing in many countries [3–5], which will have considerable impact on the future delivery of care in the developed as well as developing countries where cART coverage is increasing.

Prolonged exposure to antiretroviral therapy along with aging may increase risk of developing metabolic complications and cardiovascular diseases among HIV-infected patients. Several studies have provided evidence that comorbidities such as diabetes mellitus [6–11], hypertension [6,8,9,12], coronary artery disease [11], hyperlipidemia [13,14], renal disease [7,11,15], and reduced bone mineral density [16–18] are more common among HIV-infected elderly patients than HIV-uninfected controls. Other than cART, medications for management of metabolic complications and cardiovascular diseases will be needed, which will increase the pill burden and potential for drug-drug interactions in the elderly patients [19,20].

The prevalence of HIV-1 infection continues to increase with improvement of accessibility to HIV testing and care in Taiwan [21,22]. However, the information on comorbidities among the HIV-infected patients has been lacking. The purpose of this study aimed to describe the comorbidity profile and concurrent medications used among the elderly patients with HIV-1 infection who sought care at a referral medical center in Taiwan.

Methods

Study setting and population

After the first case of HIV-1 infection and AIDS was reported in Taiwan in 1984, the number of patients diagnosed as having HIV infection through sexual contacts continued to increase steadily over the next two decades [23]. The outbreak of HIV infection among injecting drug users (IDUs) between 2003 and 2007 had caused a significant change of the landscape of HIV infection in Taiwan, with the proportion of IDUs increasing from less than 2% before 2003 to 27.6% of total cases reported as of 2013. At the end of 2013, a total of 26,457 cases of HIV infection were reported to the Taiwan Centers for Disease Control and 4,171 (15.8%) patients had died. After control of the outbreak of HIV infection among IDUs through harm reduction program, sexual contacts, especially among men who have sex with men (MSM), have re-emerged as the most common route of HIV transmission. As of December 2013, MSM have accounted for 53% of all reported cases of HIV infection and patients aged 50 years or older accounted for 13.6% [21,22].

HIV-infected patients in Taiwan are provided with free medical care at designated hospitals around Taiwan by the government of Taiwan, including cART that was introduced in April 1997, and monitoring of CD4 lymphocyte count and plasma HIV RNA load. As of December 2012, it was estimated that 60% of HIV-infected patients sought HIV-related care and initiated cART after the diagnosis of HIV infection was made.

Study design

This was a cross-sectional study that enrolled HIV-infected patients who were aged 40 years or older and sought HIV care at the HIV clinics of the National Taiwan University Hospital from 1 January, 2013 to 31 December, 2013. Two age groups were identified: patients aged 40–49 years and those aged ≥50 years. We collected information on their baseline demographics, clinical characteristics, and medications including antiretroviral therapy, antihypertensives, lipid-lowering agents, and insulin and oral hypoglycemics. Data on comorbid conditions, including hypertension, diabetes mellitus, chronic viral hepatitis, cardiovascular disease, hyperlipidemia, fracture, malignancy, and osteoporosis and information on smoking status and alcohol use were also collected by interview, which were confirmed by review of medical records. The study was approved by the Research Ethics Committee of the National Taiwan University Hospital (registration number: 200904020R) and participants gave written informed consent.

Clinical measurements

Systolic and diastolic blood pressure was measured after the subjects were seated and rested for at least five minutes. Height was determined without shoes by the same machine. Weight was measured by a digital scale, and patients were fully dressed but without shoes or heavy clothing. Body mass index (BMI) was calculated as weight in kilograms divided by the square of the height in meters. Because diabetes mellitus is considered coronary artery disease-equivalent, we examined the status of diabetes

mellitus control by retrospectively collecting laboratory data of fasting glucose, glycosylated hemoglobin (HbA1C) among those who received a diagnosis of diabetes mellitus from 1 January, 2012 to 31 December, 2013.

Laboratory and radiologic investigations

Total cholesterol, triglyceride, glucose, HbA1C, high-density lipoprotein cholesterol (HDL-C), and low-density lipoprotein-cholesterol (LDL-C) levels were determined after at least an 8-hour fast. The data of most recent plasma HIV RNA load, CD4 lymphocyte count, blood urea nitrogen, serum creatinine, estimated glomerular filtration rate (eGFR) that was calculated with the use of the abbreviated Modification of Diet in Renal Disease (MDRD) equation [24], hemoglobin, and rapid plasma reagin (RPR) (within 6 months of survey) were collected using a standardized case record form. Plasma HIV RNA load was quantified using the Cobas Amplicor HIV-1 Monitor test (Cobas Amplicor version 1.5, Roche Diagnostics Corporation, IN, USA) with a lower detection limit of 20 copies/mL, and CD4 count was determined using FACFlow (BD FACS Calibur, Becton Dickinson, CA, USA). Bone mineral density (BMD) was measured with the use of dual-energy X-ray absorptiometry scan (Lunar Prodigy; GE Healthcare, Belgium) [17].

Definitions

Comorbid conditions were defined by the ICD-9 diagnostic codes or in those who took antihypertensives, hypoglycemics, or lipid-lowering agents. Chronic hepatitis B virus (HBV) infection was defined as presence of HBV surface antigen for 6 months or longer. Hepatitis C virus (HCV) infection was defined as presence of HCV antibody. Osteopenia and osteoporosis were defined on the basis of World Health Organization (WHO) criteria [25]. Patients with a BMD T-score between −1.0 and −2.5 were categorized as having osteopenia, and patients with a BMD T-score less than or equal to −2.5 were categorized as having osteoporosis.

CART was defined as the use of at least 3 agents from at least 2 classes of antiretroviral agents according to the national treatment guidelines for adults with HIV infection. The most commonly prescribed antiretroviral combinations in antiretroviral-naive patients were 2 nucleoside reverse-transcriptase inhibitors (NRTIs) plus 1 non-NRTI (nNRTI), 2 NRTIs plus ritonavir-boosted protease inhibitor (PI), unboosted atazanavir or raltegravir, while triple NRTIs or combination of 3 classes were only infrequently prescribed. Ritonavir was available only in capsule form.

Statistical analysis

Categorical variables were analyzed by using X^2 tests for continuous variables were compared using Student's t test. Baseline and comorbid conditions were compared with two groups. A P-value of <0.05 was considered statistically significant. All P value was two-tailed. Analyses were performed using SAS software (Version 9.3).

Results

During the 12-month study period, 920 patients who were aged 40 years or greater were enrolled, among whom 310 (33.7%) and 610 (66.3%) were aged ≥50 years (elderly group) and 40–49 years (younger group), respectively (Figure 1). Clinical characteristics of the participants, stratified by age, are shown in Table 1. Of the 815 patients with available data, 304 (37.3%) were classified as overweight with a BMI >24 according to the criteria of the National Bureau of Health Promotion, Ministry of Health and

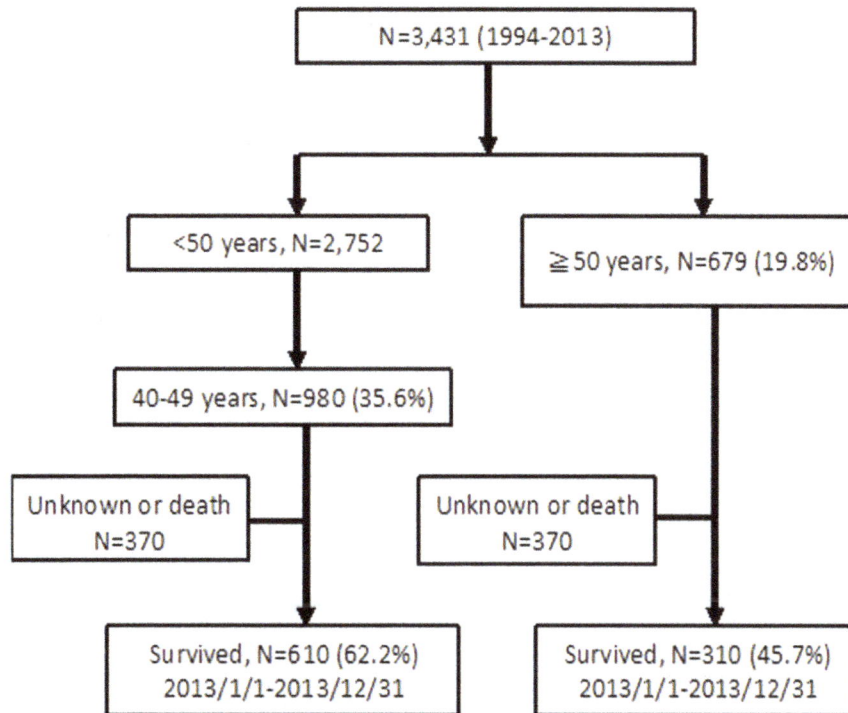

Figure 1. Study flow.

Welfare, Taiwan; 31.0% (231/745) had fasting glucose levels ≥100 mg/dl, 51.5% (456/885) triglyceride levels ≥150 mg/dl, 20.0% (112/561) HbA1C levels ≥6.0%, and 5.7% (49/854) eGFR levels <60 mL/min/1.73 m².

The two groups of patients differed significantly in many characteristics examined (Table 1). Compared with patients in the younger group, HIV-infected patients in the elderly group were more likely to be female (15.9% vs 3.8%) and have a higher fasting glucose level (106 vs 97 mg/dl), HbA1C level (5.9 vs 5.6%) and systolic blood pressure (130 vs 126 mmHg), and have a lower eGFR (88.5 vs 98.9 ml/min/1.73 m2), plasma HIV RNA load (1.6 vs 1.7 $\log_{10}$ copies/ml) and BMI (22.9 vs 23.4 Kg/m²) (Table 1). Compared with the younger group, there was a statistically significantly higher prevalence of comorbidities in the elderly patients (59.0 vs 36.4%) (Table 2), such as hypertension (31.0 vs 10.8%), hyperlipidemia (29.4 vs 11.6%), diabetes mellitus (18.4 vs 4.6%), and coronary artery disease (6.8 vs 0.5%); furthermore, HIV-infected patients in the elderly group were more likely to have 2 or more comorbidities (30.6 vs. 8.7%).

Of the 920 patients, 76 (8.3%) were taking oral hypoglycemic agents or receiving insulin replacement for control of diabetes mellitus, 102 (11.1%) lipid-lowering agents, 142 (15.4%) antihypertensives, and 159 (17.3%) hypnotics drugs (Table 2). More than 95% of the patients (95.8%) were receiving cART during the study period. The antiretroviral agents to which the patients had been exposed and the cumulative exposure duration for each antiretroviral agent are shown in Table 3. Patients in the elderly group had significantly longer exposure durations to PIs, nNRTIs, and NRTIs than those in the younger group (Table 3). The antiretroviral agents and exposure durations for patients with at least 1 metabolic, cardiovascular, renal or hepatic comorbidity and those without any comorbidity are shown in Table 4.

Compared with those in the younger group, HIV-infected patients in the elderly group were more likely to take medications for management of comorbidities: oral hypoglycemic agents or insulin replacement (16.5% vs 4.1%), lipid-lowering agents (19.4% vs 6.9%), and antihypertensives (26.5% vs 9.8%) (Table 2). Other than therapy for HIV infection, patients in the elderly group were more likely to have receiving 2 or more concurrent medications than those in the younger group (22.9% vs 6.4%). Patients in the younger group had a higher prevalence of syphilis (RPR titer ≥4) than those in the elderly group (26.3% vs. 11.4%).

The comparisons of clinical characteristics of 85 patients (9.2%) with diabetes mellitus and 835 patients (90.8%) without diabetes mellitus are shown in Table S1. Compared with those patients without diabetes mellitus, the patients with diabetes mellitus were more likely to be aged 50 years or greater (67.1 vs 30.3%) and to have a higher BMI (24.2 vs 23.2 Kg/m²), higher systolic blood pressure (134 vs 127 mmHg), higher triglyceride level (260 vs 195 mg/dl), lower eGFR (82.7 vs 96.7 mL/min), and lower plasma HIV RNA load (1.5 vs 1.7 $\log_{10}$ copies/ml).

Because diabetes mellitus is related to long-term metabolic, cardiovascular and renal complications, we examined the status of control by assessing the fasting glucose and HbA1C data of the patients with diabetes mellitus. All of the available results of blood sampling in fasting state (n = 270) of 85 patients with diabetes mellitus over the 12-month follow-up were stratified into 4 groups (Figure S1): group 1, HbA1C>6.5% and fasting glucose> 110 mg/dl (53.3%; 144/270); group 2, HbA1C>6.5% and fasting glucose<110 mg/dl (6.7%; 18/270); group 3, HbA1C<6.5% and fasting glucose>110 mg/dl (21.9%; 59/270) and group 4, HbA1C<6.5% and fasting glucose<110 mg/dl (18.1%; 49/270).

Discussion

In this cross-sectional study, we found that HIV-1-infected Taiwanese patients who were aged 50 years or older had significantly more comorbidities than those who were aged 40–

Table 1. Comparisons of demographic and clinical characteristics of the two study populations according to age.

Variable	≥50 years, N=310	40–49 years, N=610	P
Male, n (%)	262 (84.5)	587 (96.2)	<.0001
Age, mean (SD), years	58.8 (7.8)	44.1 (2.9)	<.0001
Risk behavior, n (%)			<.0001
MSM	152 (49.0)	521 (85.4)	
Heterosexual	139 (44.8)	64 (10.5)	
IDU	12 (3.9)	22 (3.6)	
Other	7 (2.3)	3 (2.3)	
Smoking status, n (%) (N=290, 550)			
Never	149 (51.4)	269 (48.9)	0.50
Past	64 (22.1)	80 (14.6)	<.01
Current	77 (26.6)	201 (36.6)	<.01
Body mass index, mean (SD), Kg/m^2	22.9 (3.3)	23.4 (3.4)	0.02
(N=287, 552)			
Systolic blood pressure, mean (SD), mm Hg (N=286, 540)	130 (18.7)	126 (15.5)	<0.001
Diastolic blood pressure, mean (SD), mm Hg,	78 (11.9)	80 (11.4)	0.01
(N=286, 540)			
Plasma HIV RNA load, mean (SD), log$_{10}$ copies/ml (N=306, 603)	1.6 (0.7)	1.7 (1.0)	0.006
CD4, mean (SD), cells/µl, (N=308, 602)	525 (273)	552 (278)	0.2
TG, mean (SD), mg/dl (N=300, 585)	199 (148.2)	203 (177.8)	0.73
TG≥150 mg/dl, n (%)	162 (54.0)	294 (50.3)	0.29
T-cholesterol, mean(SD), mg/dl (N=300, 579)	180 (39.7)	178 (37.0)	0.34
T-cholesterol≥220 mg/dl, n (%)	54 (18.0)	75 (13.0)	0.05
HDL, mean (SD), mg/dl (N=26, 87)	44 (15.2)	40 (10.1)	0.24
HDL<40 mg/dl, n (%)	12 (46.2)	46 (52.9)	0.55
LDL, mean (SD), mg/dl (N=38, 74)	105 (40.7)	104 (31.9)	0.85
Fasting glucose, mean (SD), mg/dl (N=261, 484)	106 (32.8)	97 (25.3)	<.001
Fasting glucose≥100 mg/dl, n (%)	116 (44.4)	115 (23.8)	<.0001
Fasting glucose≥110 mg/dl, n (%)	59 (22.6)	51 (10.5)	<.0001
HbA1C, mean (SD) (N=215, 346)	5.9 (1.0)	5.6 (0.9)	<.0001
HbA1C≥6.5%, n (%)	32 (14.9)	18 (5.2)	<.0001
BUN, mean (SD) (N=214, 395)	18.1 (13.2)	14.5 (6.7)	<.001
Serum creatinine, mean (SD) (N=297, 553)	1.1 (1.2)	0.9 (0.8)	0.12
eGFR, mean (SD), ml/min/1.73 m^2 (N=297, 557)	88.5 (27.4)	98.9 (24.9)	<.0001
eGFR <60 ml/min/1.73 m^2, n (%)	34 (11.5)	15 (2.7)	<.0001
On cART, n (%)	303 (97.7)	578 (94.8)	0.03
Current exposure to PI	185 (59.7)	325 (53.3)	0.06
Current exposure to TDF	92 (29.7)	246 (40.3)	0.002

Note: The numbers in the parenthesis presented after each variable indicate the number of patients with data for the elderly and younger groups of patients, respectively.
Abbreviations: BUN, blood urea nitrogen; cART, combination antiretroviral therapy; eGFR, estimated glomerular filtration rate; HbA1C, glycosylated hemoglobin, HDL, high-density lipoprotein cholesterol; IDU, injecting drug use; LDL, low-density lipoprotein cholesterol; MSM, men who have sex with men; PI, protease inhibitor; SD, standard deviation; TDF, tenofovir disoproxil fumarate; TG, triglyceride.

49 years. Polypharmacy was not uncommon in that more than 20% of the elderly patients were taking 2 or more concurrent medications in addition to cART for HIV infection.

The prevalence of the elderly group with 2 or more comorbidities is higher than younger group in our study (30.6 vs. 8.6%), which is similar to what have been observed in HIV-infected elderly patients with access to cART in many Western countries [6–9,13]. The types of comorbid diseases in our study are also similar to those reported among the HIV-infected elderly patients in Western countries, such as hypertension [7,9,12,13] and hyperlipidemia [13]. Previous studies comparing the prevalence of comorbidities between HIV-infected and HIV-uninfected individuals showed discrepant results, however. The prospective cross-sectional study by Onen et al showed that HIV-infected patients in the US had a higher prevalence of hypertension and hypertriglyceridemia than HIV-uninfected individuals [18], while the VACS study by Oursler et al showed that HIV-uninfected

Table 2. Comorbid conditions of the two study populations.

Variable	≥50 years, N = 310 (%)	40–49 years, N = 610 (%)	P
At least one comorbidity, n (%)	183 (59.0)	222 (36.4)	<.0001
Diabetes mellitus	57 (18.4)	28 (4.6)	<.0001
Hypertension	96 (31.0)	66 (10.8)	<.0001
Anti-HCV-positivity	18 (5.8)	46 (7.6)	0.33
Chronic HBV infection	21 (6.8)	63 (10.3)	0.08
Hyperlidemia	91 (29.4)	71 (11.6)	<.0001
Cancer	12 (3.9)	13 (2.1)	0.12
CAD	21 (6.8)	3 (0.5)	<.0001
Fracture	3 (1.0)	1 (0.2)	0.08
Osteoporosis (N = 99, 99)	7 (7.1)	2 (2.0)	0.09
Active drinking (N = 288, 551)	13 (4.5)	18 (3.3)	0.36
RPR ≥ 4, n (%)	31 (11.4)	148 (26.3)	<.0001
Concurrent medications, n (%)			
Lipid-lowering agent	60 (19.4)	42 (6.9)	<.0001
Hypoglycemic agent	51 (16.5)	25 (4.1)	<.0001
Anti-hypertensives	82 (26.5)	60 (9.8)	<.0001
Hypnotics	59 (19.0)	100 (16.4)	0.31

Note: The numbers in the parenthesis presented after each variable indicate the number of patients with data for the elderly and younger groups of patients, respectively.
Abbreviations: CAD, coronary artery disease; HBV, hepatitis B virus; HCV, hepatitis C virus; RPR, rapid plasma regain.

individuals in the US had a higher prevalence of hypertension and diabetes mellitus than HIV-infected patients [12].

With the increasing prevalence of comorbidities, it is not surprising that, other than antiretroviral therapy, use of concomitant medications for management of comorbid diseases were common in our patients. It is therefore important to note some of the negative consequences as a result of polypharmacy. The patients taking multiple drugs for many chronic medical conditions are at potentially increased risk of drug-drug interactions and adverse drug events [20,26]. Consistent with findings reported in the literature (range, 82–96%) [20,26,27], 52.3% of our patients aged ≥ 50 years and 29.2% of the patients aged 40–49 years in this study were receiving 1 or more concurrent medications.

Table 3. The cumulative exposure durations of antiretroviral agents of the two study populations.

Drug class and duration	≥50 years, N = 310	40–49 years, N = 610	P
PI, mean (SD), months	64.40 (46.6)	56.1 (40.8)	0.02
Lopinavir/ritonavir	50.26 (37.9)	46.10 (37.1)	0.41
Atazanavir	45.94 (29.7)	43.96 (29.9)	0.51
Darunavir	24.43 (24.5)	17.21 (15.8)	0.22
Indinavir	23.56 (25.9)	21.21 (19.6)	0.59
Saquinavir	19.10 (19.5)	17.48 (13.7)	0.74
NRTI, mean (SD), months	103.0 (57.7)	78.04 (55.1)	<.0001
Zidovudine	68.88 (53.8)	58.70 (48.8)	0.03
d4T/ddl/ddC	36.79 (41.1)	33.87 (37.7)	0.52
Abacavir/lamivudine	59.08 (37.1)	50.54 (32.6)	0.006
Tenofovir	21.29 (9.8)	18.60 (9.4)	0.02
nNRTI, mean (SD), months	71.35 (56.8)	54.88 (52.0)	0.0003
Efavirenz	75.73 (55.7)	56.17 (51.9)	0.0002
Nevirapine	45.79 (54.5)	35.36 (45.8)	0.17
Integrase inhibitor, mean (SD), months	27.65 (23.2)	17.93 (11.8)	0.07

Abbreviations: d4T, stavudine; ddl, didanosine; ddC, deoxycytidine; NRTI, nucleoside reverse-transcriptase inhibitors; nNRTI, non-nucleoside reverse-transcriptase inhibitors; PI, protease inhibitor.

Table 4. The cumulative exposure durations of antiretroviral agents of the two study populations.

Drug class and duration	Presence of any comorbidity (+), N = 405	Without any comorbidity(-), N = 515	P
PI, mean(SD) months	64.67 (45.9)	54.52 (40.2)	0.004
Lopinavir/ritonavir	50.63 (34.7)	45.51(38.9)	0.29
Atazanavir	46.78 (30.3)	42.78 (29.2)	0.16
Darunavir	22.24 (20.0)	16.27 (17.2)	0.17
Indinavir	25.46 (27.9)	18.76 (14.8)	0.11
Saquinavir	19.46 (19.4)	16.19 (11.0)	0.45
NRTI, mean (SD), months	99.78 (59.1)	75.99 (53.4)	<.0001
Zidovudine	69.73 (52.4)	55.93 (48.5)	0.003
d4T/ddI/ddC	35.75 (40.6)	34.43 (37.6)	0.77
Abacavir/lamivudine	57.75 (36.5)	50.29 (32.7)	0.01
Tenofovir	20.07 (9.6)	18.83 (9.5)	0.23
nNRTI, mean (SD), months	71.27 (64.8)	51.90 (52.6)	<.0001
Efavirenz	73.36 (54.6)	54.0 (51.9)	0.0001
Nevirapine	45.33 (51.7)	34.50 (47.1)	0.15
Integrase inhibitor, mean (SD), months	24.97 (18.7)	16.93 (14.3)	0.06

Note: The comorbidities include hypertension, diabetes mellitus, hyperlipidemia, coronary artery disease, chronic kidney disease (eGFR<60 ml/min/1.73 m^2), malignancy, osteoporosis, and chronic viral hepatitis.
Abbreviations: d4T, stavudine; ddI, didanosine; ddC, deoxycytidine; NRTI, nucleoside reverse-transcriptase inhibitors; nNRTI, non-nucleoside reverse-transcriptase inhibitors; PI, protease inhibitor.

The prevalence and incidence of diabetes mellitus are increasing worldwide, especially in the elder patients regardless of the status of HIV infection [10,28–30]. Presence of diabetes mellitus is associated with a higher mortality rate among HIV-uninfected patients [31–34] because of increased risk of cardiovascular diseases, nephropathy, retinopathy, and neuropathy [35,36]. Whether the incidence of diabetes mellitus is higher in HIV-infected patients than HIV-uninfected individuals remains controversial. In the French study, Capeau et al found a markedly higher incidence of diabetes mellitus in HIV-infected than HIV-uninfected population (14.1 vs. 4-6/1000 person-years) [37]. In the Denmark study, Rasmussen et al found HIV-infected individuals did not have an increased risk of developing diabetes mellitus compared to HIV-uninfected population (3.70 vs. 3.87/1000 person-years) [38]. The discrepancy of incidence of DM in the published studies may be due to differences in demographic factors such as age, gender and race, exposure duration to cART and regimens of cART used [39,40].

Using Taiwan National Health Insurance data, Jiang et al have found that the prevalence of DM among women and men aged 40 to 59 years increased from 4.63% to 5.47% and from 4.97% to 7.56%, respectively, between 2000 and 2009 [33]; the prevalence of DM among women and men aged 60 to 79 years increased from 17.17 to 21.97% and from 13.60 to 13.97%, respectively, between 2000 and 2009. In this study that was conducted in 2013, we found that the prevalence of DM in HIV-infected males (N = 749) and females (N = 41) aged 40–59 years was 7.48% and 7.32%, respectively; for the patients who were aged 60 years or older (N = 130), the prevalence of DM in males (N = 100) and females (N = 30) was 21.0% and 16.67%, respectively. However, given the small sample size of the patients in our study, the interpretation of the data should be cautious.

In our study, we found that diabetes mellitus was associated with older age and higher BMI, which are consistent with other studies [10,28,29]. The finding that more than 50% of the blood sampling

among HIV-infected patients with diabetes mellitus showed HbA1C >6.5% and fasting glucose levels >110 mg/dl suggests that better strategies with multidisciplinary approach are urgently needed to improve the quality of care in terms of diabetic control to prevent the occurrence or delay the progression of metabolic, cardiovascular, and renal complications in the patients enrolled in this study.

Renal function in terms of eGFR usually decreases with age. The prevalence of eGFR<60 mL/min/1.73 m^2 in our elderly patients was 11.5%, which is higher than those in other studies among the HIV-infected population from Brazil (3.9%) [8] and Taiwan (7.03%) [41], but is lower than the studies from the UK (15.5%) [15] and Japan (15.4%) [42]. The difference between ours and other studies may be explained by the study populations. In our study population, the mean age was 49 years, which is greater than the other study from Taiwan (36.9 years). In the US study, Onen et al. found approximately 50% of the overall elderly study population had renal impairment with chronic kidney disease in 11% and 7% of HIV-infected persons and HIV-uninfected patients, respectively [18].

While most of patients in this study were receiving cART with good control of HIV infection, the finding of a high prevalence of syphilis is of particular concerns, especially in the patients aged 40 to 49 years [43,44]. Acquisition of syphilis indicates unprotected sex, which may increase the risk of HIV transmission to sexual partners or superinfection with HIV resistant to the regimens the patients were receiving; furthermore, several studies have demonstrated that syphilis is associated with acquisition of other sexually transmitted hepatotrophic virus infections such as hepatitis B, C and D virus [45–48].

There are several limitations of our study. First, it is a cross-sectional survey of patients who sought HIV care at a university hospital. The information examined is mainly from laboratory data that were accumulated during the clinical care. Many other comorbidities were not systematically examined, such as osteoporosis and malignancy. Second, the exposure duration to cART was not taken into consideration in comparisons made between the two age groups. Third, we did not have an HIV-uninfected population for comparison in terms of the frequency of comorbidity. Therefore, it is not known whether the frequency of any comorbidity examined in this study is higher in HIV-infected patients than in HIV-uninfected patients in Taiwan, although several studies have suggested that cART and HIV infection may accelerate aging and increase risk of metabolic, cardiovascular and renal complications [10,14,15,39,40,42].

In conclusion, our findings show that a significant proportion of the HIV-infected elderly patients In Taiwan have multiple comorbidities that may increase risk for cardiovascular and renal complications. Issues of poly-pharmacy among the elderly with HIV infection should be addressed to ensure adherence and minimize drug-drug interactions. Comprehensive approach to the management of metabolic, cardiovascular and renal comorbidities cannot be overemphasized in the long-term successful management of HIV-infected elderly population.

Supporting Information

Figure S1 The scattered plot of glycosylated hemoglobin (HbA1C) and fasting glucose data collected from the 85 patients with diabetes mellitus during the 12-month study period. PI, protease inhibitor-containing regimens.

Table S1 Comparisons of demographic and clinical characteristics of the patients with and those without diabetes mellitus.

Acknowledgments

Footnote: Preliminary analyses of these data were presented as abstract no. PE15/13 at the 14th *European AIDS Conference*, Brussels, Belgium, 16–19 October, 2013.

Author Contributions

Conceived and designed the experiments: WHS CCH PYW. Performed the experiments: PYW MYC SMH HYS MST KYL WCL SPY YZL JYZ. Analyzed the data: PYW MYC SMH HYS MST KYL. Contributed reagents/materials/analysis tools: WCL SPY YZL JYZ. Contributed to the writing of the manuscript: CCH PYW WHS.

References

1. Antiretroviral Therapy Cohort C (2008) Life expectancy of individuals on combination antiretroviral therapy in high-income countries: a collaborative analysis of 14 cohort studies. Lancet 372: 293–299.
2. Sterne JA, Hernan MA, Ledergerber B, Tilling K, Weber R, et al. (2005) Long-term effectiveness of potent antiretroviral therapy in preventing AIDS and death: a prospective cohort study. Lancet 366: 378–384.
3. Lazarus JV, Nielsen KK (2010) HIV and people over 50 years old in Europe. HIV Med 11: 479–481.
4. Linley L, Prejean J, An Q, Chen M, Hall HI (2012) Racial/ethnic disparities in HIV diagnoses among persons aged 50 years and older in 37 US States, 2005–2008. Am J Public Health 102: 1527–1534.
5. Wallrauch C, Barnighausen T, Newell ML (2010) HIV prevalence and incidence in people 50 years and older in rural South Africa. S Afr Med J 100: 812–814.
6. Hasse B, Ledergerber B, Furrer H, Battegay M, Hirschel B, et al. (2011) Morbidity and aging in HIV-infected persons: the Swiss HIV cohort study. Clin Infect Dis 53: 1130–1139.
7. Vance DE, Mugavero M, Willig J, Raper JL, Saag MS (2011) Aging with HIV: a cross-sectional study of comorbidity prevalence and clinical characteristics across decades of life. J Assoc Nurses AIDS Care 22: 17–25.
8. Torres TS, Cardoso SW, Velasque Lde S, Marins LM, de Oliveira MS, et al. (2013) Aging with HIV: an overview of an urban cohort in Rio de Janeiro (Brazil) across decades of life. Braz J Infect Dis 17: 324–331.
9. Chu C, Umanski G, Blank A, Meissner P, Grossberg R, et al. (2011) Comorbidity-related treatment outcomes among HIV-infected adults in the Bronx, NY. J Urban Health 88: 507–516.
10. Lo YC, Chen MY, Sheng WH, Hsieh SM, Sun HY, et al. (2009) Risk factors for incident diabetes mellitus among HIV-infected patients receiving combination antiretroviral therapy in Taiwan: a case-control study. HIV Med 10: 302–309.
11. Guaraldi G, Orlando G, Zona S, Menozzi M, Carli F, et al. (2011) Premature age-related comorbidities among HIV-infected persons compared with the general population. Clin Infect Dis 53: 1120–1126.
12. Oursler KK, Goulet JL, Crystal S, Justice AC, Crothers K, et al. (2011) Association of age and comorbidity with physical function in HIV-infected and uninfected patients: results from the Veterans Aging Cohort Study. AIDS Patient Care STDS 25: 13–20.
13. Manrique L, Aziz M, Adeyemi OM. (2010) Successful immunologic and virologic outcomes in elderly HIV-infected patients. J Acquir Immune Defic Syndr 54: 332–333.
14. Wu PY, Hung CC, Liu WC, Hsieh CY, Sun HY, et al. (2012) Metabolic syndrome among HIV-infected Taiwanese patients in the era of highly active antiretroviral therapy: prevalence and associated factors. J Antimicrob Chemother 67: 1001–1009.
15. Ibrahim F, Hamzah L, Jones R, Nitsch D, Sabin C, et al. (2012) Comparison of CKD-EPI and MDRD to estimate baseline renal function in HIV-positive patients. Nephrol Dial Transplant 27: 2291–2297.
16. Bonjoch A, Figueras M, Estany C, Perez-Alvarez N, Rosales J, et al. (2010) High prevalence of and progression to low bone mineral density in HIV-infected patients: a longitudinal cohort study. AIDS 24: 2827–2833.

17. Tsai MS, Hung CC, Liu WC, Chen KL, Chen MY, et al. (2014) Reduced bone mineral density among HIV-infected patients in Taiwan: prevalence and associated factors. J Microbiol Immunol Infect 47: 109–115.
18. Onen NF, Overton ET, Seyfried W, Stumm ER, Snell M, et al. (2010) Aging and HIV infection: a comparison between older HIV-infected persons and the general population. HIV Clin Trials 11: 100–109.
19. Marzolini C, Back D, Weber R, Furrer H, Cavassini M, et al. (2011) Ageing with HIV: medication use and risk for potential drug-drug interactions. J Antimicrob Chemother 66: 2107–2111.
20. Tseng A, Szadkowski L, Walmsley S, Salit I, Raboud J (2013) Association of age with polypharmacy and risk of drug interactions with antiretroviral medications in HIV-positive patients. Ann Pharmacother 47: 1429–1439.
21. Centers for Disease Control ROC, (2013) Taiwan. Statistics of HIV/AIDS. In 2013;http://www.cdc.gov.tw/english/submenu.aspx?treeid=00ed75d6c887bb27&nowtreeid=f6f562fd95fd8df9.
22. Huang YF, Chen CH, Chang FY (2013) The emerging HIV epidemic among men who have sex with men in Taiwan. J Formos Med Assoc 112: 369–371.
23. Yang CH, Huang YF, Hsiao CF, Yeh YL, Liou HR, et al. (2008) Trends of mortality and causes of death among HIV-infected patients in Taiwan, 1984-2005. HIV Med 9: 535–543.
24. Levey AS, Coresh J, Greene T, Stevens LA, Zhang YL, et al. (2006) Using standardized serum creatinine values in the modification of diet in renal disease study equation for estimating glomerular filtration rate. Ann Intern Med 145: 247–254.
25. Kanis JA (1994) Assessment of fracture risk and its application to screening for postmenopausal osteoporosis: synopsis of a WHO report. WHO Study Group. Osteoporos Int 4: 368–381.
26. Nachega JB, Hsu AJ, Uthman OA, Spinewine A, Pham PA (2012) Antiretroviral therapy adherence and drug-drug interactions in the aging HIV population. AIDS 26 Suppl 1:S39–53.
27. Gleason LJ, Luque AE, Shah K (2013) Polypharmacy in the HIV-infected older adult population. Clin Interv Aging 8: 749–763.
28. De Wit S, Sabin CA, Weber R, Worm SW, Reiss P, et al. (2008) Incidence and risk factors for new-onset diabetes in HIV-infected patients: the Data Collection on Adverse Events of Anti-HIV Drugs (D:A:D) study. Diabetes Care 31: 1224–1229.
29. Ledergerber B, Furrer H, Rickenbach M, Lehmann R, Elzi L, et al. (2007) Factors associated with the incidence of type 2 diabetes mellitus in HIV-infected participants in the Swiss HIV Cohort Study. Clin Infect Dis 45: 111–119.
30. Butt AA, McGinnis K, Rodriguez-Barradas MC, Crystal S, Simberkoff M, et al. (2009) HIV infection and the risk of diabetes mellitus. AIDS 23: 1227–1234.
31. Gregg EW, Gu Q, Cheng YJ, Narayan KM, Cowie CC (2007) Mortality trends in men and women with diabetes, 1971 to 2000. Ann Intern Med 147: 149–155.
32. Preis SR, Hwang SJ, Coady S, Pencina MJ, D'Agostino RB, et al.(2009) Trends in all-cause and cardiovascular disease mortality among women and men with and without diabetes mellitus in the Framingham Heart Study, 1950 to 2005. Circulation 119: 1728–1735.
33. Jiang YD, Chang CH, Tai TY, Chen JF, Chuang LM (2012) Incidence and prevalence rates of diabetes mellitus in Taiwan: analysis of the 2000–2009 Nationwide Health Insurance database. J Formos Med Assoc 111: 599–604.

34. Li HY, Jiang YD, Chang CH, Chung CH, Lin BJ, et al. (2012) Mortality trends in patients with diabetes in Taiwan: a nationwide survey in 2000–2009. J Formos Med Assoc 111: 645–650.

35. Stratton IM, Adler AI, Neil HA, Matthews DR, Manley SE, et al. (2000) Association of glycaemia with macrovascular and microvascular complications of type 2 diabetes (UKPDS 35): prospective observational study. BMJ 321: 405–412.

36. Alberti KG, Zimmet PZ (1998) Definition, diagnosis and classification of diabetes mellitus and its complications. Part 1: diagnosis and classification of diabetes mellitus provisional report of a WHO consultation. Diabet Med 15: 539–553.

37. Capeau J, Bouteloup V, Katlama C, Bastard JP, Guiyedi V, et al. (2012) Ten-year diabetes incidence in 1046 HIV-infected patients started on a combination antiretroviral treatment. AIDS 26: 303–314.

38. Rasmussen LD, Mathiesen ER, Kronborg G, Pedersen C, Gerstoft J, et al. (2012) Risk of diabetes mellitus in persons with and without HIV: a Danish nationwide population-based cohort study. PLoS One 7:e44575.

39. Brown TT, Cole SR, Li X, Kingsley LA, Palella FJ, et al. (2005) Antiretroviral therapy and the prevalence and incidence of diabetes mellitus in the multicenter AIDS cohort study. Arch Intern Med 165: 1179–1184.

40. Tien PC, Schneider MF, Cole SR, Levine AM, Cohen M, et al. (2007) Antiretroviral therapy exposure and incidence of diabetes mellitus in the Women's Interagency HIV Study. AIDS 21: 1739–1745.

41. Hsieh MH, Lu PL, Kuo MC, Lin WR, Lin CY, et al. (2013) Prevalence of and associated factors with chronic kidney disease in human immunodeficiency virus-infected patients in Taiwan. J Microbiol Immunol Infect.

42. Yanagisawa N, Ando M, Ajisawa A, Imamura A, Suganuma A, et al. (2011) Clinical characteristics of kidney disease in Japanese HIV-infected patients. Nephron Clin Pract 118:c285–291.

43. Chang YH, Liu WC, Chang SY, Wu BR, Wu PY, et al. (2013) Associated factors with syphilis among human immunodeficiency virus-infected men who have sex with men in Taiwan in the era of combination antiretroviral therapy. J Microbiol Immunol Infect.

44. de Coul EO, Warning T, Koedijk F, Dutch STIc (2014) Sexual behaviour and sexually transmitted infections in sexually transmitted infection clinic attendees in the Netherlands, 2007–2011. Int J STD AIDS 25: 40–51.

45. Sun HY, Chang SY, Yang ZY, Lu CL, Wu H, et al. (2012) Recent hepatitis C virus infections in HIV-infected patients in Taiwan: incidence and risk factors. J Clin Microbiol 50: 781–787.

46. van de Laar T, Pybus O, Bruisten S, Brown D, Nelson M, et al. (2009) Evidence of a large, international network of HCV transmission in HIV-positive men who have sex with men. Gastroenterology 136: 1609–1617.

47. Hung CC, Wu SM, Lin PH, Sheng WH, Yang ZY, et al. (2014) Increasing incidence of recent hepatitis D virus infection in HIV-infected patients in an area hyperendemic for hepatitis B virus infection. Clin Infect Dis 58: 1625–1633.

48. Sun HY, Cheng CY, Lee NY, Yang CJ, Liang SH, et al. (2014) Seroprevalence of hepatitis B virus among adults at high risk for HIV transmission two decades after implementation of nationwide hepatitis B virus vaccination program in Taiwan. PLoS One 9:e90194.

5

A Wearable Proprioceptive Stabilizer (Equistasi®) for Rehabilitation of Postural Instability in Parkinson's Disease: A Phase II Randomized Double-Blind, Double-Dummy, Controlled Study

Daniele Volpe[1]*, Maria Giulia Giantin[1], Alfonso Fasano[2]

1 Department of Physical Medicine & Rehabilitation, S. Raffaele Arcangelo Fatebenefratelli Hospital, Venice, Italy, 2 Morton and Gloria Shulman Movement Disorders Clinic and the Edmond J. Safra Program in Parkinson's Disease, Toronto Western Hospital and Division of Neurology, University of Toronto, Toronto, Ontario, Canada

Abstract

Background: Muscle spindles endings are extremely sensitive to externally applied vibrations, and under such circumstances they convey proprioceptive inflows to the central nervous system that modulate the spinal reflexes excitability or the muscle responses elicited by postural perturbations. The aim of this pilot study is to test the feasibility and effectiveness of a balance training program in association with a wearable proprioceptive stabilizer (Equistasi) that emits focal mechanical vibrations in patients with PD.

Methods: Forty patients with PD were randomly divided in two groups wearing an active or inactive device. All the patients received a 2-month intensive program of balance training. Assessments were performed at baseline, after the rehabilitation period (T1), and two more months after (T2). Posturographic measures were used as primary endpoint; secondary measures of outcome included the number of falls and several clinical scales for balance and quality of life.

Results: Both groups improved at the end of the rehabilitation period and we did not find significant between-group differences in any of the principal posturographic measures with the exception of higher sway area and limit of stability on the instrumental functional reach test during visual deprivation at T1 in the Equistasi group. As for the secondary outcome, we found an overall better outcome in patients enrolled in the Equistasi group: 1) significant improvement at T1 on Berg Balance Scale (+45.0%, p = .026), Activities-specific Balance Confidence (+83.7, p = .004), Falls Efficacy Scale (−33.3%, p = .026) and PDQ-39 (−48.8%, p = .004); 2) sustained improvement at T2 in terms of UPDRS-III, Berg Balance Scales, Time Up and Go and PDQ-39; 3) significant and sustained reduction of the falls rate.

Conclusions: This pilot trial shows that a physiotherapy program for training balance in association with focal mechanical vibration exerted by a wearable proprioceptive stabilizer might be superior than rehabilitation alone in improving patients' balance.

Trial Registration: EudraCT 2013-003020-36 and ClinicalTrials.gov (number not assigned)

Editor: Terence J. Quinn, University of Glasgow, United Kingdom

Funding: The authors have no support or funding to report.

Competing Interests: The authors have declared that no competing interests exist.

* Email: dott.dvolpe@libero.it

Introduction

Parkinson's disease (PD) is a progressive neurological condition associated with reduced physical activity and poor mobility. Postural instability severely affects the conditions of these patients because it is associated with an increased risk of falls, immobility, hospitalization and the need for long-term care [1,2], overall reducing the health-related quality of life [3].

The pathophysiology of postural instability in PD is not fully understood as it probably depends from a complex interaction between compensatory strategies and the impairment caused by the disease at different levels of the nervous system [4,5]. Several posturographic studies investigating the centre of pressure (COP),

in both static and dynamic conditions, have showed that PD patients sway significantly more than healthy subjects because they tend to exceed their limits of stability to a much greater extent [6]. On the other hand, early [7] and recent [8] studies have demonstrated that PD patients have a reduced limit of stability particularly during dynamic conditions, thus supporting the hypothesis that an important role is played by an impairment in appropriately scaling the postural reactions in response to perturbations [9].

In a gravity environment, with a firm base of support, healthy subjects mainly rely on somatosensory information in order to maintain an upright posture [10]. Accordingly, artificially impairing proprioception worsens postural stability and particularly reduces the COP displacements in response to external perturbations during visual deprivation [11]. Muscle spindles endings are extremely sensitive to externally applied vibrations, and under such circumstances they convey proprioceptive inflows to the central nervous system that modulate the spinal reflexes excitability [12,13,14] as well as posture [15,16,17] or the muscle responses elicited by postural perturbations [9,18,19]. Similar protocols have been applied in PD patients during either static [20] or dynamic [21] conditions, obtaining responses similar to healthy subjects, in keeping with a normal integration of the proprioceptive inflow. Notwithstanding, it is known that the postural control of PD patients mainly relies on visual cues, possibly compensating for a proprioceptive impairment [22]. In keeping with a role for proprioceptive impairment in PD, Valkovic et al. [23,24] documented a defective scaling and habituation of postural reactions during either neck or legs vibration, the extent of these abnormalities being correlated with disease progression.

Although there is growing evidence showing that physical activity and exercise programs can improve strength [25], balance [26,27], mobility [28] and quality of life [3,29] in patients with PD, most studies have shown limited long-term benefits despite short-term gains [30,31,32]. Therefore, there is a cogent need to find effective and innovative methods for training balance in people with this debilitating and progressive disease [33,34].

Alternate vibratory stimulation on trunk muscles has been used for therapeutic purposes in PD, providing an improvement of trunk sway [35] or gait [21]. In particular, Nanhoe-Mahabier et al. [35] have recently investigated the effect of balance training combined with artificial vibrotactile biofeedback on the trunk sway of PD patients and have found that feedback group had a significantly greater reduction in roll and pitch sway angular velocity, thus resulting in a beneficial effects on trunk stability; authors concluded that further studies should examine if these effects increase further after more intensive training and how long these persist after training has stopped [35]. Therefore, we can argue that combining a perturbation-based training in association with a wearable postural stabilizer (WPS) providing prolonged muscle mechanical vibrations could improve postural stability in PD.

The present phase II double-blind, double-dummy randomized controlled trial (RCT) tests the feasibility, safety and effectiveness of a standard balance training program combined with the use of a WPS (Equistasi, Milan, Italy). Equistasi is a registered (class 1, ministerial code n. 342577 on 05/08/2010) medical device consisting in a rectangular plate measuring $10 \times 20 \times 0.5$ mm and with a weight of 0.17 gr (Figure 1). The device is exclusively composed by nanotechnology fibers that transform the body temperature into mechanical vibratory energy (<0.8N, 9000 Hz) able to generate a variation of muscle length of max 0.02 mm [36], by far within the safety limit (0.12 mm) found to be harmful for human muscles [37].

The present RCT will enable us to examine whether enhancing balance training using a WPS in a rehabilitation setting leads to a clinically meaningful effect in PD patients with balance impairment and is safe, i.e. it does not worsen postural stability.

Methods

Design

We conducted a double-blind, double-dummy, parallel group RCT with a focus on clinical measures of balance as primary outcome. The study protocol and supporting CONSORT checklist are available as supporting information (see Protocol S1 and Checklist S1). After screening and enrolment, forty patients

were monitored for 2 months in order to record the falls rate. Afterward, participants were randomized to receive a 2-month intensive (see below) program of balance training while wearing a WPS (Equistasi) or the identical training program while wearing a placebo device identical to the active one (Figure 2). Patients were recruited from the Neurorehabilitation Unit of "S. Raffaele Arcangelo" Hospital in Venice, Italy. The trial was approved by the hospital ethics committee (C.E.O.C. Brescia Italy, ref 35/2013) and was registered online at EudraCT (n. 2013-003020-36) and at ClinicalTrials.gov (number not assigned and delayed in being posted online due to the FDA restrictions for devices unapproved in U.S.). Written informed consent was obtained from the participants or from their spouses if they scored less than 25/30 on the Mini Mental State Examination (MMSE) [38].

Participants

Participants were eligible for inclusion if they consented to participation, had PD diagnosed according to the current criteria [39], Hoehn and Yahr [40] stage ≥ 2 on levodopa, and history of at least one fall in the past. Exclusion criteria were: medication-induced dyskinesias (to avoid confounding effects on force platform assessments), presence of co-morbidities preventing mobility or safe exercise (including clinically evident neuropathy and major medical conditions such as malignancies), history of deep brain stimulation (DBS) surgery or other conditions affecting stability (e.g. poor visual acuity or vestibular dysfunction), Hoehn and Yahr stage ≥ 4 on levodopa, and inability to travel to the physiotherapy venues.

Randomization and blindness

A blocked stratified randomization procedure conducted by a third party and based on the Hoehn & Yahr score was used to allocate participants to one of the two treatment groups (i.e.

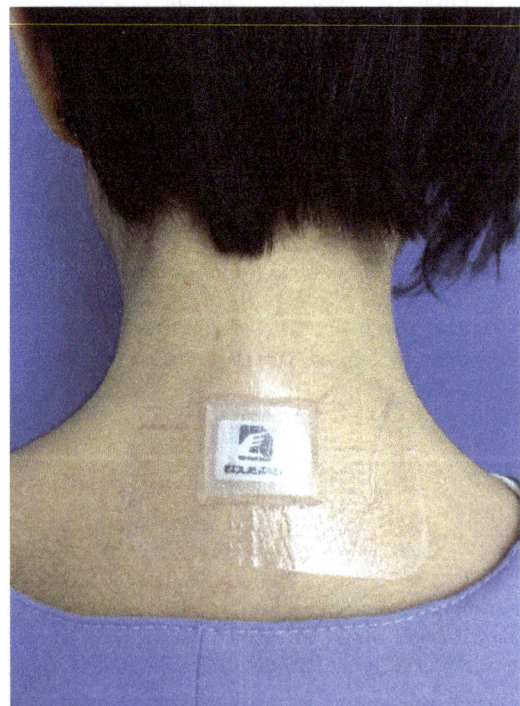

Figure 1. The wearable postural stabilizer (Equistasi) employed in the present study.

physiotherapy with or without an active WPS). The two trained assessors and patients were blinded to the group allocation during the whole duration of the study. The study coordinator responsible for WPS placing (M.G.G.) was not blinded to group allocation, but she was not involved in rehabilitation procedures or outcome assessment. The therapists providing the interventions were blinded and not involved in other aspects of the trial (i.e., aims, hypotheses or predictions of the study were not disclosed). Both active and placebo WPSs were identical and did not cause any recognizable sensory sensation, thus guarantying patients' blindness. To test the quality of blinding procedures, the trained assessors were asked to guess the group allocation at the end of the trial and they only guessed 40% of the group assignments.

Intervention

Participants of the two groups received the same 60-minute physiotherapy daily session 5 days a week for 2 months at the S. Raffaele Hospital of Venice, Italy. Table S1 details the type of daily physiotherapy provided by the hospital physiotherapists. The physiotherapy protocol included 40 minutes' individual sessions designed to improve balance with a perturbation-based balance training program, where patients were asked to voluntary reach their limit of stability in protected conditions and taught how to correctly activate the postural responses to external perturbations. Exercises were preceded by warming up and stretching exercises and followed by cooling down, each epoch lasting 10 minutes. At the beginning of each session, participants were required to sign a form in order to attest their attendance.

While receiving the same physiotherapy, participants were allocated to two groups:

– **"Equistasi"**: each patient wore 3 Equistasi devices (Figure 1), applied over the 7th cervical vertebra and on each soleus muscle tendons. These sites were chosen on the basis of previous studies showing changes of the centre of pressure (COP) induced by either leg or paraspinal muscle vibration [16,20,41].
– **"Placebo"**: each patient wore 3 inactive devices, applied on the same body sites chosen for the active group.

During the first three weeks of rehabilitation, both groups wore the devices six days a week, 60 (1st week), 120 (2nd week) and 180 (3rd week) minutes a day; during the fourth week onward, they wore the devices for 5 days a week, four hours a day. Devices application was held in the morning, prior to the physiotherapy program; devices were removed on the same day after the necessary time was elapsed, meaning that patients waited in the hospital area after the training session. Medications were unchanged during the whole trial period.

Outcome Measures

We assessed outcomes at three time points. Baseline (T0) measures were taken within 1 week prior to enrolling. The second assessment (T1) occurred within 1 week after the two-month therapy period. The last assessment (T2) was undertaken two months after T1. T1 and T2 were chosen in order to evaluate the attainment and retention of skills learned during physiotherapy classes [42].

Instrumental assessment.   As primary measures of outcome for balance, static posturography (stabilometry) was assessed in keeping with current guidelines [43]. The COP sway in the antero-posterior (AP) and medio-lateral (ML) directions was recorded on a force platform (Milletrix model 2.0– Rome, Italy) with an acquisition frequency of 50 Hz. Acquisition was performed during upright stance with the patient barefoot with the feet splayed out at 30 degrees, while keeping the arms alongside the body and staring at a fixed point marked on the wall at a distance of one meter at the height of the glabella of each individual. Data acquisition was performed for 51.2 seconds under each condition [with eyes open (EO) or closed (EC)]. The following parameters were taken into account: mean COP velocity (m/s) and sway area (mm^2) and path (mm).

The same equipment was used to evaluate an instrumental version of the functional reach test (FRT) [44], by asking the subject to bend forward while maintaining feet planted in a standing position during both EO and EC conditions. The sway area (mm^2) and the displacement along the AP axis were taken into account; displacements along the ML axis were also recorded but not taken into account for the analysis, given the notion that PD patients display instability principally along the AP one [45] and considering that patients were asked to bend forward along the AP axis.

Clinical assessment.   Motor impairment was assessed with the parts II (activities of daily living) and III (motor examination) of the Unified PD Rating Scale [46], the Timed Up and Go (TUG) [47], and the Berg Balance Scale (BBS) [48]. Falls Efficacy Scale (FES) [49] and the Activities-specific Balance Confidence (ABC) [50] were administered to measure the fear of falling. Falls were recorded by means of fall diaries of the previous two months. We also quantified health-related quality of life in all participants using the PDQ-39 [51]. Other data collected at baseline included age, gender, body mass index (BMI), disease duration, anti-PD medications expressed as levodopa-equivalent daily dose [52], cognitive status assessed with the MMSE. All adverse events such as injuries, distress and hospital admissions were verified by phone interview and recorded during the trial period.

Statistical Analysis

This clinical trial used a sample of convenience, with the assumption that 40 participants would be ample to explore safety and feasibility. Given the small sample and the lack of normal distribution of most of the variables on Shapiro-Wilk test, non-parametric statistics were used. Absolute values and magnitude of change were compared in both groups at the three time points by means of Mann-Whitney U test. Treatment effect across time points in each group were explored by means of the Friedman analysis of variance by ranks, and in case of statistical significance post-hoc comparisons were carried out with the Wilcoxon signed-rank test. Categorical variables were compared by means of chi-square test. All values were expressed as median (25th and 75th percentiles), with the exception of figures, where mean and standard deviation were chosen to improve clarity of data presentation. IBM SPSS Statistics ver. 20.0 was used for all statistical analyses. All tests were two-sided with a level of significance set at P<0.05.

Results

Twenty subjects were enrolled in each study arm and they did not differ in any of the demographic and baseline clinical and instrumental data (Tables 1–2 and Figures 3–4). For the sample as a whole, 95.6% of intervention sessions were delivered without differences across study arms (2160 and 2220 minutes on average for Equistasi and placebo group, respectively); sessions were not delivered due to personal reasons or due to illnesses not related to PD. No major adverse event or death was observed during the study period.

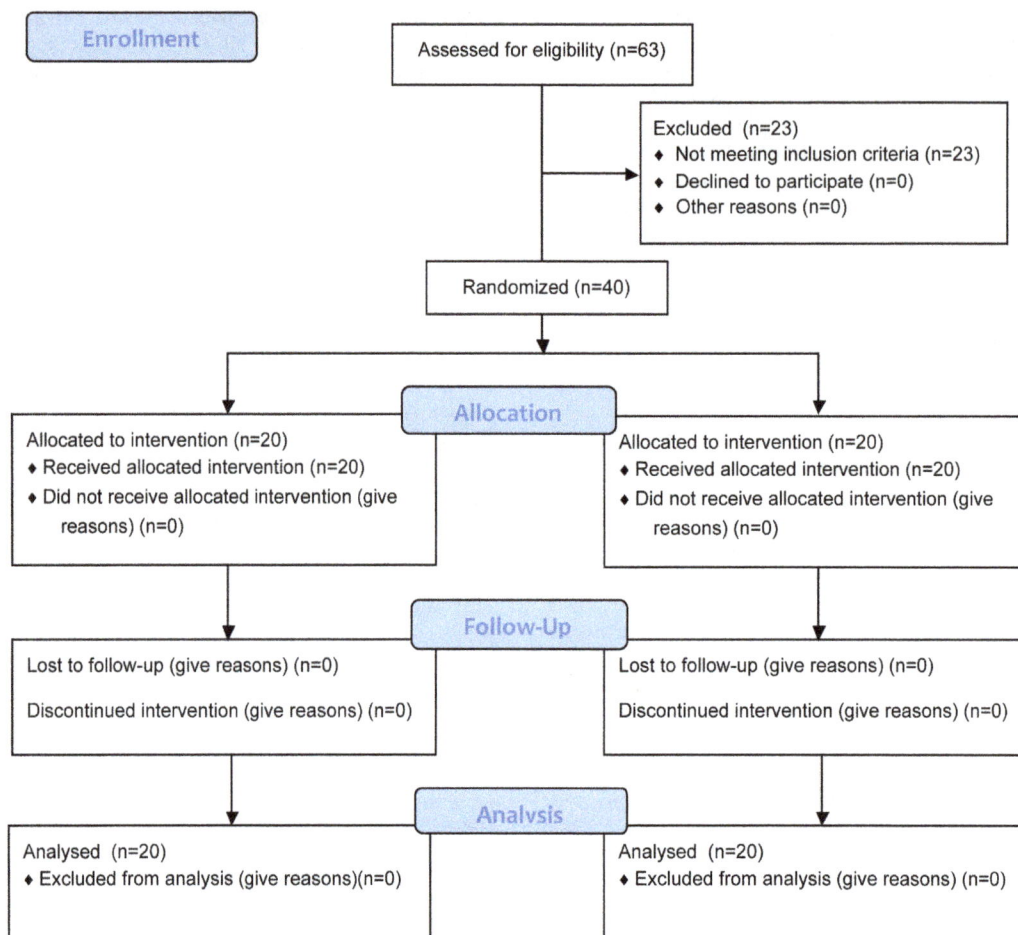

Figure 2. The CONSORT flow diagram for this study.

Therapy outcomes in the Equistasi group

The combined intervention of balance training plus Equistasi did not modify the parameters of static posturography with the exception of the sway area during EO condition (p = 0.005); on post-hoc T2 these values were significantly lower than T0 (p = 0.008; Table 2). By contrast, a profound effect was found for both the sway area (p = 0.049) and the displacement along the AP axis (p = 0.039) at the instrumental FRT during the EC

Table 1. Baseline demographic and clinical variables of the two groups enrolled in the study.

	Active group	Placebo group	P
	(n = 20)	(n = 20)	value*
Gender	7M/13F	9M/11F	.747
Age	66.5 (64.0; 78.0)	69.5 (65.0; 73.8)	.947
BMI	24.6 (22.9; 27.0)	27.7 (24.4; 29.0)	.060
H&Y	3.0 (3.0; 3.0)	3.0 (2.0; 3.0)	.429
Disease duration	6.0 (4.0; 10.8)	6.5 (4.0; 9.0)	.862
≥1 fall during the observation period at T0	16	12	.300
MMSE	26.1 (24.0; 27.7)	26.4 (25.3; 27.2)	.000
Total LEDD	667.1 (500; 780)	700.0 (356.3; 900.0)	.551
L-dopa LEDD	487.5 (315.0; 690.0)	450.0 (293.8; 600.0)	.892
DA LEDD	120.0 (0.0; 275.0)	175.0 (0.0; 300.0)	.721

Abbreviations: * Mann-Witney U test was used for the comparisons except gender, which was compared with chi-square; H&Y: Hoehn & Yahr stage; LEDD: levodopa equivalent daily dose; MMSE: mini-mental state examination.

Table 2. Static stabilometry values of the two groups enrolled in the study at each time point.

		Equistasi			Control			T1-T0		T2-T0		T2-T1	
		T0	T1	T2	T0	T1	T2	Equistasi	Control	Equistasi	Control	Equistasi	Control
Sway area (mm²)	EO	**130.6 (97.6; 400.2)**	192.0 (95.2; 486.4)	**298.9 (175.2; 473.6)***	181.3 (84.6; 351.8)	165.7 (73.6; 743.4)	149.1 (62.9; 331.6)	25.2 (−141.2; 99.6)	−15.7 (−126.5; 377.1)	**155.0 (88.2; 244.0)**	**−74.3 (−139.7; 115.8)****	105.2 (−21.3; 299.4)	−38.9 (−345.2; 50.8)
	EC	337.5 (90.3 803.8)	257.9 (116.3; 892.5)	275.9 (142.5; 565.7)	163.2 (73.3; 664.1)	246.9 (60.7; 595.9)	217.1 (105.7; 384.0)	6.0 (−314.4; 189.2)	15.8 (−157.5; 212.9)	41.6 (−289.4; 191.5)	31.6 (−96.2; 240.8)	73.8 (−587.0; 172.9)	−8.8 (−207.2; 160.8)
Sway path (mm)	EO	418.2 (278.9; 498.0)	353.5 (274.2; 623.6)	409.3 (309.0; 567.6)	347.1 (295.0; 543.1)	351.9 (275.2; 516.7)	314.2 (224.5; 606.8)	−22.4 (−113.6; 160.7)	2.2 (−111.2; 79.5)	51.3 (−92.0; 136.7)	−35.7 (−153.5; 103.6)	31.0 (−66.9; 82.4)	5.8 (−68.6; 78.8)
	EC	571.8 (321.6; 717.2)	530.3 (357.0; 850.2)	461.1 (304.3; 774.7)	440.0 (308.4; 704.6)	453.0 (294.7; 744.9)	414.0 (290.2; 883.6)	−13.7 (−146.6; 80.5)	−8.2 (−110.9; 138.0)	30.1 (−195.3; 91.2)	49.5 (−119.1; 121.4)	35.1 (−110.3; 59.4)	22.8 (−46.8; 93.2)
Mean COP Velocity (m/s)	EO	8.2 (5.4; 9.7)	6.9 (5.4; 12.2)	8.0 (6.0; 11.1)	6.8 (5.8; 10.6)	6.9 (5.4; 10.1)	6.1 (4.4; 11.9)	−0.4 (−2.2; 3.1)	0.0 (−2.2; 1.5)	1.0 (−1.8; 2.7)	−0.7 (−3.0; 2.1)	0.6 (−1.3; 1.6)	0.1 (−1.3; 1.6)
	EC	11.2 (6.3; 14.0)	10.3 (7.0; 16.6)	9.0 (5.9; 15.1)	8.6 (6.0; 13.7)	8.8 (5.7; 14.5)	8.1 (5.7; 17.2)	−0.2 (−2.9; 1.6)	−0.2 (−2.2; 2.7)	0.6 (−3.8; 1.8)	1.0 (−1.7; 2.4)	0.7 (−2.2; 1.2)	0.9 (−0.9; 1.8)

Abbreviations: *: significantly different than T0 (p = .008); **: significantly different than Equistasi (p = .011); COP: centre of pressure; EC: eyes closed; EO: eyes open.

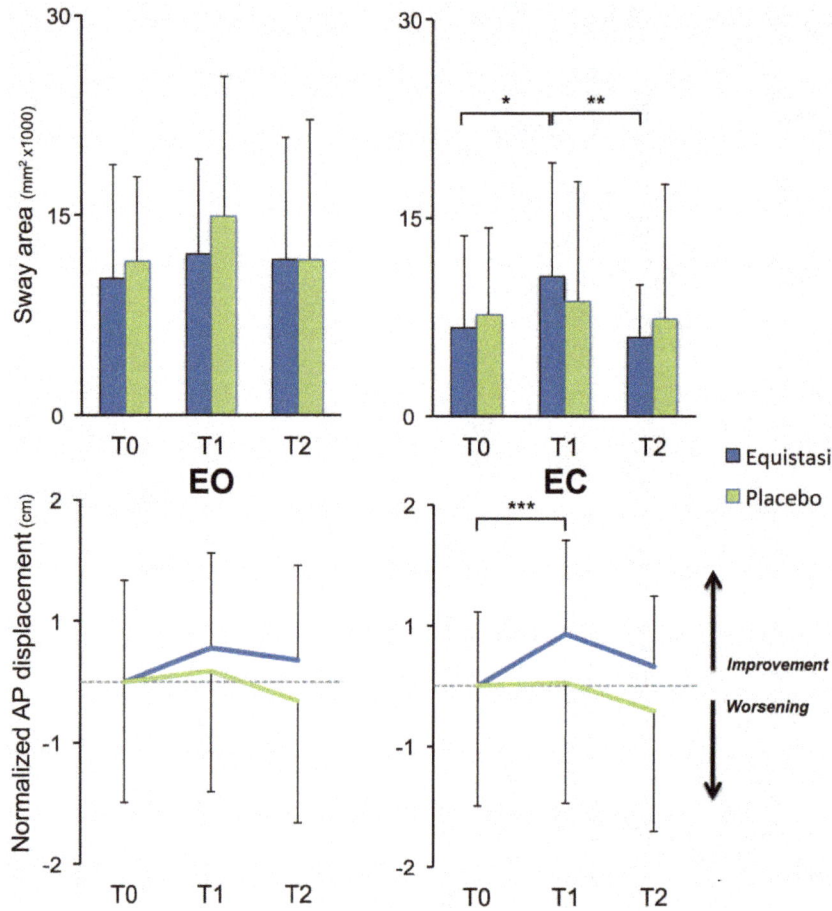

Figure 3. The sway area and the displacement along the AP axis (expressed as value normalized to the baseline) at the instrumental FRT during EO (left panels) and EC (right panels) conditions. Data are presented as mean ± standard deviation. Abbreviations: AP: antero-posterior; EC: eyes closed; EO: eyes open; *: p = .006; **: p = .02; ***: p = .01 (Wilcoxon signed-rank test).

condition; on post-hoc, these were significantly higher at T1 than T0 (Figure 3).

As for the other clinical measures, a significant effect was found for UPDRS-II (p<0.001), UPDRS-III (p<0.001), BBS (p<0.001), TUG (p<0.001), ABC (p<0.001), FES (p<0.001), and PDQ-39

(p<0.001). Table 3 details the post-hoc results: overall, a significant improvement was observed at T1 for all the aforementioned scales; at T2 the improvement was retained for the UPDRS-III, BBS, TUG and PDQ-39 whereas UPDRS-II, ABC and FES were comparable than T0 and significantly worse than

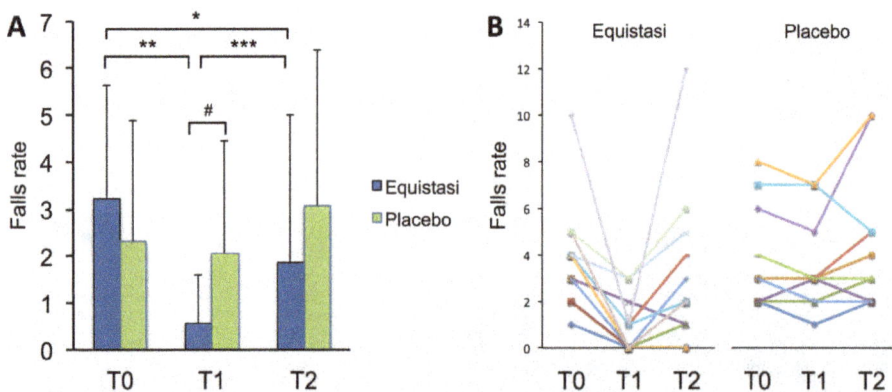

Figure 4. The Falls rate over the 2-month observation period. Data are presented as mean ± standard deviation (A) and individual trends excluding patients with no baseline history of falls (B). Abbreviations: *: p = .03; **: p = .0001; ***: p = .003 (Wilcoxon signed-rank test); #: p = .03 (Mann-Whitney U test).

T1. Finally, a significant effect was found for the falls rate (p< 0.001); on post-hoc analysis a significant improvement was found when comparing T1 and T2 with T0 (Figure 4A).

Therapy outcomes in the Control group

The combined intervention of balance training plus placebo devices did not modify the parameters of static posturography nor of the instrumental FRT (Table 2 and Figure 3).

As for the other clinical measures, a significant effect was found for UPDRS-II (p<0.001), UPDRS-III (p<0.001), BBS (p<0.001), TUG (p<0.001), ABC (p = 0.006), FES (p = 0.004), and PDQ-39 (p<0.001). Table 3 details the post-hoc results: overall, a significant improvement was observed at T1 for all the aforementioned scales; at T2 the improvement was retained for the UPDRS-II and BBS, whereas FES, UPDRS-III and ABC were comparable to T0, being the last two also significantly worse than T1; TUG and PDQ-39 at T2 were significantly worse than T1 and T0 (Table 3).

No significant effect was found for the falls rate.

Comparisons between Equistasi and Control groups

At T1, Equistasi group significantly presented less falls (Figure 4A). The same effect was detected when considering only fallers at T0 (p<.0001): in the Equistasi group median falls rate dropped from 4 (3; 4) at T0 to 0 (0; 1) at T1 and worsened again at T2 [4 (1; 3.75)]; by contrast, in the Control group median falls rate did not change, being 3 (2; 5.5), 3 (2; 4.5) and 3 (2; 5) at T0, T1 and T2, respectively (Figure 4B).

When comparing the between-group magnitude of change, Equistasi patients showed a significant improvement of at T1 in terms of BBS (+45.0%, p = .026), ABC (+83.7, p = .004), FES (−33.3%, p = .026) and PDQ-39 (−48.8%, p = .004) (Table 3). No other significant differences were found.

Discussion

The present RCT has shown that enhancing balance training using a WPS in a rehabilitation setting is safe and might lead to some clinically meaningful effect in PD patients with balance impairment. Although both groups with an active and placebo WPS improved at the end of the rehabilitation period and we did not find significant between-group differences in the principal posturographic measures with the exception of higher sway area and limit of stability on the instrumental functional reach test during visual deprivation at T1, we found an overall improvement in many secondary endpoints only in patients enrolled in the Equistasi group. Specifically, we found a significant improvement at T1 on BBS, ABC, FES and PDQ-39, a sustained improvement at T2 of UPDRS-III, BBS, TUG and PDQ-39, and a significant and sustained reduction of the falls rate. By contrast, patients enrolled in the control group did not experience any falls rate reduction and at T2 only retained the improvement of UPDRS-II and BBS, whereas TUG and PDQ-39 were also significantly worse than baseline.

The rehabilitative programs were delivered successfully with high adherence in both groups and, in keeping with the current knowledge [27], balance training significantly improved the key clinical variables in both groups.

Posturography measurements were the principal endpoint of this RCT, given the higher sensitivity and reliability of instrumental results in trials with small sample size. The lack of between-groups differences at the baseline confirms the goodness of randomization already seen on clinical scales. Noteworthy, at the end of rehabilitation statistically significant differences arose in

the Equistasi group only. The significant reduction at T2 of the sway area in static-EO condition is difficult to comment in absence of a group of healthy controls and, more importantly, in light of the lack of conclusive data linking static posturography with balance performance and falls in PD patients [53]. In fact, studies have shown either increased, normal or reduced spontaneous body sway [54,55], indicating that reliability of postural sway during static conditions could be influenced by many factors such as the progression of the disease, pharmacological and non-pharmacological interventions, bradykinesia [56] or postural deformities [57]. Notwithstanding, the significant reduction of the sway area is in keeping with the reduction of the falls rate, since greater postural sway has shown to be a predictor of falls in PD patients [58].

PD patients have a reduced limit of stability particularly during dynamic conditions, thus pointing to dynamic posturography as a better instrument to capture improvement of balance [7,8]. Accordingly, our RCT did show a significant increase of the limits of stability in the AP plane at T1 and only in the Equistasi group. Interestingly, the effect was only noticeable in the EC condition, a setting relying on the integrity of the vestibular and proprioceptive system, in keeping with the notion that bilateral Achilles tendon vibration applied in healthy subjects results in a profound effect on trunk, hips and knees displacement in the absence of vision [41]. The limit of stability mainly depends on the size of anticipatory postural adjustments, which have been found to be increased by Achilles tendon vibration in rectus femoris, biceps femoris and erector spinae muscles prior to a fast arm movement [59].

Spindles respond to vibrations as if the muscle is stretched, thus producing a tonic contraction on the stimulated muscle [60,61]. Muscle vibration does not only impact on local spinal cord circuits but it also provides a substantial proprioceptive inflow to different parts of the central nervous system, thus influencing the accuracy of calibrations of action selection and execution of voluntary movement [62]. Accordingly, vibration of axial muscles has been proved to produce systematic changes in standing posture [16] and body orientation (the so-called "vibratory myesthetic illusions") [63].

From the aforementioned studies, eliciting proprioceptive inflow by means of vibration has a biological plausibility in patients with PD, although the mechanism for its beneficial effect is largely speculative. Our findings are in keeping with previous researches using vibratory stimulation on trunk muscles for therapeutic purposes in PD, providing an improvement of trunk sway [35] or gait [21]. These studies have proved that patterned muscle vibrations are able to improve weight transfer along AP or ML axes, whose impairment is a core feature of axial control of PD patients [64]. In order to deliver vibration trains to the muscles, available studies have adopted battery-operated custom-made systems (generally consisting in vibrating units fixed on the distal tendons by elastic bands and connected to a wearable control unit) [21,35]; by contrast, the WPS used in our protocol can be worn for days given the small dimension and the lack of power supply. Therefore, our experimental set up shows for the first time the effects of prolonged chronic externally applied vibrations. On the other hand, PD patients with postural instability respond hyperactively to proprioceptive sensory manipulation when a mechanical vibration is applied to the soleus muscles [24], thus raising the possibility that the prolonged use of vibration could have impaired balance. In addition, vibration has been shown to change spatial body orientation very fast [41], thus resulting in a postural response known as a "vibration-induced falling" [15], especially when vibration is used to experimentally impair

Table 3. Clinical variables of the two groups enrolled in the study and their comparisons at each time point.

	Equistasi						Control						T1 - T0			T2 - T0			T2 - T1		
	T0	T1	T2	T1 vs. T0	T2 vs. T0	T2 vs. T1	T0	T1	T2	T1 vs. T0	T2 vs. T0	T2 vs. T1	Equistasi	Control	p	Equistasi	Control	p	Equistasi	Control	p
UPDRS-II*	20.5 (15.5; 25.3)	15.5 (12.0; 19.8)	17.5 (15.0; 22.8)	**.001**	.058	**.001**	18.5 (15.3; 22.8)	14.5 (10.0; 18.0)	18.0 (12.0; 20.0)	**.001**	**.004**	**.001**	-3.0 (-7.0; -1.3)	-4.0 (-6.8; -4.0)	.050	-2.0 (-4.0; 1.0)	-2.0 (-3.0; -1.0)	.659	2.5 (1.3; 4.8)	3.0 (1.0; 4.0)	.730
UPDRS-III*	42.0 (36.3; 48.3)	36.0 (24.0; 39.8)	37.0 (28.0; 43.8)	**.001**	**.015**	**.001**	39.5 (31.3; 51.0)	33.5 (23.5; 40.5)	38.0 (32.0; 43.0)	**.001**	.071	**.001**	-7.0 (-11.8; -3.3)	-8.0 (-11.0; -4.3)	1.0	-2.0 (-7.3; 0.0)	-3.0 (-5.0; 1.0)	.756	6.0 (2.0; 8.0)	4.0 (1.0; 9.0)	.621
BBS^	43.5 (35.3; 45.0)	52.0 (48.0; 54.0)	47.0 (39.0; 49.0)	**.001**	**.002**	**.001**	45.5 (40.0; 48.0)	51.0 (47.5; 53.8)	49.0 (45.0; 51.0)	**.001**	**.001**	**.001**	**10.0 (6.0; 13.0)**	**5.5 (4.0; 7.8)**	**.026**	4.0 (1.0; 6.0)	3.0 (1.0; 4.0)	.745	-5.0 (-9.0; -1.0)	-2.0 (-4.0; -2.0)	.052
TUG*	14.6 (12.2; 19.1)	12.4 (10.7; 15.0)	12.7 (12.2; 15.6)	**.001**	**.004**	**.005**	12.8 (10.5; 14.7)	11.9 (10.2; 13.3)	12.5 (10.9; 13.9)	**.001**	**.022**	**.021**	-1.4 (-6.3; -0.2)	-0.8 (-1.4; -0.4)	.752	-0.8 (-4.8; -0.2)	-0.6 (-1.0; 0.1)	.516	0.7 (0.1; 1.6)	0.4 (0.1; 1.0)	.330
ABC^	51.6 (42.6; 61.5)	66.3 (57.2; 82.2)	51.3 (41.3; 73.1)	**.001**	.398	**.001**	56.2 (52.5; 64.7)	59.1 (53.8; 67.5)	51.3 (41.9; 62.5)	**.012**	.444	**.002**	**15.3 (5.9; 22.7)**	**2.5 (-0.5; 7.3)**	**.004**	1.4 (-8.1; 13.6)	-1.9 (-11.3; 8.1)	.516	-12.8 (-18.4; -8.1)	-3.3 (14.4; -0.9)	.194
FES*	12.5 (9.5; 17.5)	6.5 (3.3; 11.8)	12.0 (6.0; 14.0)	**.001**	.063	**.006**	10.0 (6.3; 15.0)	7.0 (5.0; 12.0)	10.0 (4.0; 14.0)	**.001**	.358	.405	**-6.0 (-8.8; -2.5)**	**-2.0 (-3.0; -1.0)**	**.026**	-2.0 (-6.0; 1.0)	0.0 (-5.0; 2.0)	.745	3.0 (1.0; 7.0)	2.0 (-2.0; 3.0)	.194
PDQ-39*	66.0 (48.8; 73.3)	39.0 (32.5; 60.5)	53.0 (40.0; 68.0)	**.001**	**.039**	**.007**	63.0 (36.3; 85.0)	58.0 (35.0; 82.5)	59.0 (40.0; 84.0)	**.001**	**0.039**	**.001**	**-13.5 (-30.5; -9.3)**	**-7.0 (-9.8; -3.5)**	**.004**	-6.0 (-20.0; 0.0)	-3.0 (-6.0; 0.0)	.737	11.0 (6.0; 20.0)	3.0 (1.0; 7.0)	.052

Bold-typed values represent significant improvement; abbreviations: *: score reduction means improvement; ^: score increase means improvement; ABC: Activities-specific Balance Confidence; BBS: Berg balance scale; FES: Falls Efficacy Scale; TUG: timed up and go, UPDRS: unified PD rating scale.

proprioception. In contrast with such assumptions, we found a significant reduction of the falls rate, thus confirming that the positive effects found on the instrumental FRT are clinically meaningful and that the high-frequency and small-amplitude vibration induced by the WPS used in our protocol does not exert detrimental effects on proprioception. PD patients display an impairment of scaling and habituation of postural reactions triggered by lower leg proprioception, whereas they do not seem to present deficits in proprioceptive afferent or central integrative functions [24]. Notwithstanding, PD-related abnormalities in proprioception might manifest as alteration of kinesthesia, defined as the conscious awareness of body and limb position, motion and orientation in space (for a review see [65]). In addition, PD patients have an impaired sense of the timing [66] and discrimination [67] of proprioceptive inputs, which can also lead to deficient compensation of mechanical perturbations. The enhancement of the proprioceptive inflow, as that induced by the present vibration protocol with Equistasi, might overcome the subtle impairment in kinesthesia, as previously argued [20]. Another potential mechanism of action could be related to the influence on muscular tone, since tendon vibration has been successfully applied in healthy subjects to change muscular tone during voluntary contraction [68] or to improve muscle velocity and strength after training [69].

The improvement of falls rate was retained 2 months after rehabilitation, thus supporting a strong and synergic effect between Equistasi and balance training. Falling is a major determinant of quality and quantity of life in PD patients, but it is often resistant to classic antiparkinsonian treatment and different approaches are currently tried, ranging from medications enhancing the central cholinergic pathways to DBS targeting brainstem nuclei (for a review see [5]). Since rehabilitation still remains the main treatment for balance problems, but it is often ineffective in the long-term, the sustained benefit on the falls rate detected by our experimental protocol deserves attention and needs to be replicated by future studies.

This pilot study has a number of limitations. First, even if testing occurred at peak dose of the morning medications, we cannot rule out the bias introduced by fluctuations in levodopa plasmatic concentration; however, this limitation plays a marginal role in the study results because: 1) it applies to both groups, 2) it is well known that levodopa does not hugely impact on posturography, 2) we excluded patients with dyskinesias, and 4) instrumental changes were paralleled by changes in other clinical measures relying on historical data. Second, though the sample size allowed the detection of significant changes, it is small and our results have to be replicated by larger trial, possibly enrolling patients with an higher number of falls at baseline. Third, even if the physiotherapy program for balance training was conducted in according with published guidelines, the execution of exercises were influenced by

therapists expertise and patients' motivation, meaning that our protocol does not necessarily reflect the clinical practice in other parts of the world. Finally, WPS were only tested on the neck and soleus muscles and not in other muscles involved in posture control; in fact, it had been demonstrated that vibration applied to the ankle or trunk muscles alone produces different effects on posture or gait [70]; in addition, it is known that these effects are modulated by the frequency of stimulation (typically 100–200 Hz) and to the best of our knowledge no study has employed the very high frequency delivered by Equistasi. Future protocols should compare the effects of vibrations applied on different muscles as well as different frequencies of vibration.

In conclusion, this pilot RCT shows that a physiotherapy program based on perturbation-based training in association with focal mechanical vibration exerted by a wearable postural stabilizer appears to be safe and tolerated; in addition, although it fails to prove superiority in most of primary endpoints, it resulted effective in improving clinical variables assessing self-confidence of balance, disability and falls rate, overall positively impacting on the health related quality of life. This preliminary investigation provides encouraging data on the feasibility and safety of our protocol, thus supporting the development of a large scale RCT. Future studies are certainly needed and will expand our knowledge on the mechanisms of action of WPS, on the exposure time needed to achieve a meaningful improvement and on its long-term duration.

Acknowledgments

The members staff of Equistasi are gratefully acknowledged for having provided the active and placebo devices. We also thank the patients who so graciously participated in this trial.

Author Contributions

Conceived and designed the experiments: DV AF. Performed the experiments: MGG. Analyzed the data: AF. Contributed reagents/materials/analysis tools: DV MGG. Wrote the paper: DV AF. Conceived the study: DV.

References

1. Lamont RM, Morris ME, Woollacott MH, Brauer SG (2012) Community walking in people with Parkinson's disease. Parkinsons Dis 2012: 856237.
2. Tan D, Danoudis M, McGinley J, Morris ME (2012) Relationships between motor aspects of gait impairments and activity limitations in people with Parkinson's disease: a systematic review. Parkinsonism Relat Disord 18: 117–124.
3. Soh SE, Morris ME, McGinley JL (2011) Determinants of health-related quality of life in Parkinson's disease: a systematic review. Parkinsonism Relat Disord 17: 1–9.
4. Benatru I, Vaugoyeau M, Azulay JP (2008) Postural disorders in Parkinson's disease. Neurophysiol Clin 38: 459–465.
5. Fasano A, Plotnik M, Bove F, Berardelli A (2012) The neurobiology of falls. Neurol Sci 33: 1215–1223.
6. Menant JC, Latt MD, Menz HB, Fung VS, Lord SR (2011) Postural sway approaches center of mass stability limits in Parkinson's disease. Mov Disord 26: 637–643.
7. Schieppati M, Hugon M, Grasso M, Nardone A, Galante M (1994) The limits of equilibrium in young and elderly normal subjects and in parkinsonians. Electroencephalogr Clin Neurophysiol 93: 286–298.
8. Nonnekes J, de Kam D, Geurts A, Weerdesteyn V, Bloem BR (2013) Unraveling the mechanisms underlying postural instability in Parkinson's disease using dynamic posturography. Expert Rev Neurother 13: 1303–1308.
9. Beckley DJ, Bloem BR, Remler MP (1993) Impaired scaling of long latency postural reflexes in patients with Parkinson's disease. Electroencephalogr Clin Neurophysiol 89: 22–28.
10. Peterka RJ (2002) Sensorimotor integration in human postural control. J Neurophysiol 88: 1097–1118.

11. Mohapatra S, Krishnan V, Aruin AS (2012) Postural control in response to an external perturbation: effect of altered proprioceptive information. Exp Brain Res 217: 197–208.

12. Schieppati M, Crenna P (1984) From activity to rest: gating of excitatory autogenetic afferences from the relaxing muscle in man. Exp Brain Res 56: 448–457.

13. Desmedt JE, Godaux E (1978) Mechanism of the vibration paradox: excitatory and inhibitory effects of tendon vibration on single soleus muscle motor units in man. J Physiol 285: 197–207.

14. Burke D, Hagbarth KE, Lofstedt L, Wallin BG (1976) The responses of human muscle spindle endings to vibration during isometric contraction. J Physiol 261: 695–711.

15. Eklund G (1972) General features of vibration-induced effects on balance. Ups J Med Sci 77: 112–124.

16. Courtine G, De Nunzio AM, Schmid M, Beretta MV, Schieppati M (2007) Stance- and locomotion-dependent processing of vibration-induced proprioceptive inflow from multiple muscles in humans. J Neurophysiol 97: 772–779.

17. Smiley-Oyen AL, Cheng HY, Latt LD, Redfern MS (2002) Adaptation of vibration-induced postural sway in individuals with Parkinson's disease. Gait Posture 16: 188–197.

18. Nardone A, Schieppati M (2005) Reflex contribution of spindle group Ia and II afferent input to leg muscle spasticity as revealed by tendon vibration in hemiparesis. Clin Neurophysiol 116: 1370–1381.

19. Bove M, Nardone A, Schieppati M (2003) Effects of leg muscle tendon vibration on group Ia and group II reflex responses to stance perturbation in humans. J Physiol 550: 617–630.

20. De Nunzio AM, Nardone A, Picco D, Nilsson J, Schieppati M (2008) Alternate trains of postural muscle vibration promote cyclic body displacement in standing parkinsonian patients. Mov Disord 23: 2186–2193.

21. De Nunzio AM, Grasso M, Nardone A, Godi M, Schieppati M (2010) Alternate rhythmic vibratory stimulation of trunk muscles affects walking cadence and velocity in Parkinson's disease. Clin Neurophysiol 121: 240–247.

22. Demirci M, Grill S, McShane L, Hallett M (1997) A mismatch between kinesthetic and visual perception in Parkinson's disease. Ann Neurol 41: 781–788.

23. Valkovic P, Krafczyk S, Saling M, Benetin J, Botzel K (2006) Postural reactions to neck vibration in Parkinson's disease. Mov Disord 21: 59–65.

24. Valkovic P, Krafczyk S, Botzel K (2006) Postural reactions to soleus muscle vibration in Parkinson's disease: scaling deteriorates as disease progresses. Neurosci Lett 401: 92–96.

25. Li F, Harmer P, Fitzgerald K, Eckstrom E, Stock R, et al. (2012) Tai chi and postural stability in patients with Parkinson's disease. N Engl J Med 366: 511–519.

26. Hirsch MA, Toole T, Maitland CG, Rider RA (2003) The effects of balance training and high-intensity resistance training on persons with idiopathic Parkinson's disease. Arch Phys Med Rehabil 84: 1109–1117.

27. Allen NE, Sherrington C, Paul SS, Canning CG (2011) Balance and falls in Parkinson's disease: a meta-analysis of the effect of exercise and motor training. Mov Disord 26: 1605–1615.

28. Ashburn A, Fazakarley L, Ballinger C, Pickering R, McLellan LD, et al. (2007) A randomised controlled trial of a home based exercise programme to reduce the risk of falling among people with Parkinson's disease. J Neurol Neurosurg Psychiatry 78: 678–684.

29. Goodwin VA, Richards SH, Henley W, Ewings P, Taylor AH, et al. (2011) An exercise intervention to prevent falls in people with Parkinson's disease: a pragmatic randomised controlled trial. J Neurol Neurosurg Psychiatry 82: 1232–1238.

30. Morris ME, Iansek R, Kirkwood B (2009) A randomized controlled trial of movement strategies compared with exercise for people with Parkinson's disease. Mov Disord 24: 64–71.

31. Munneke M, Nijkrake MJ, Keus SH, Kwakkel G, Berendse HW, et al. (2010) Efficacy of community-based physiotherapy networks for patients with Parkinson's disease: a cluster-randomised trial. Lancet Neurol 9: 46–54.

32. Rochester L, Rafferty D, Dotchin C, Msuya O, Minde V, et al. (2010) The effect of cueing therapy on single and dual-task gait in a drug naive population of people with Parkinson's disease in northern Tanzania. Mov Disord 25: 906–911.

33. Morris ME (2006) Locomotor training in people with Parkinson disease. Phys Ther 86: 1426–1435.

34. Morris ME, Martin CL, Schenkman ML (2010) Striding out with Parkinson disease: evidence-based physical therapy for gait disorders. Phys Ther 90: 280–288.

35. Nanhoe-Mahabier W, Allum JH, Pasman EP, Overeem S, Bloem BR (2012) The effects of vibrotactile biofeedback training on trunk sway in Parkinson's disease patients. Parkinsonism Relat Disord 18: 1017–1021.

36. Equistasi website. Available: http://www.equistasi.com/en/. Accessed 2013 Dec 13.

37. Necking LE, Lundstrom R, Dahlin LB, Lundborg G, Thornell LE, et al. (1996) Tissue displacement is a causative factor in vibration-induced muscle injury. J Hand Surg Br 21: 753–757.

38. Folstein MF, Folstein SE, McHugh PR (1975) "Mini-mental state". A practical method for grading the cognitive state of patients for the clinician. J Psychiatr Res 12: 189–198.

39. Berardelli A, Wenning GK, Antonini A, Berg D, Bloem BR, et al. (2013) EFNS/MDS-ES/ENS [corrected] recommendations for the diagnosis of Parkinson's disease. Eur J Neurol 20: 16–34.

40. Hoehn MM, Yahr MD (1967) Parkinsonism: onset, progression and mortality. Neurology 17: 427–442.

41. Thompson M, Medley A (2007) Forward and lateral sitting functional reach in younger, middle-aged, and older adults. J Geriatr Phys Ther 30: 43–48.

42. Nieuwboer A, Rochester L, Muncks L, Swinnen SP (2009) Motor learning in Parkinson's disease: limitations and potential for rehabilitation. Parkinsonism Relat Disord 15 Suppl 3: S53–58.

43. Scoppa F, Capra R, Gallamini M, Shiffer R (2013) Clinical stabilometry standardization: basic definitions-acquisition interval–sampling frequency. Gait Posture 37: 290–292.

44. Duncan PW, Weiner DK, Chandler J, Studenski S (1990) Functional reach: a new clinical measure of balance. J Gerontol 45: M192–197.

45. Abdo WF, Borm GF, Munneke M, Verbeek MM, Esselink RA, et al. (2006) Ten steps to identify atypical parkinsonism. J Neurol Neurosurg Psychiatry 77: 1367–1369.

46. Fahn S, Elton R, Members of the UPDRS Development Committee (1987) Recent developments in Parkinson's disease. Fahn S, Marsden C, Calne D, Goldstein M, editors. Folorham Park, NJ: Macmillan Health Care Information. 153–163, 293–304 p.

47. Podsiadlo D, Richardson S (1991) The timed "Up & Go": a test of basic functional mobility for frail elderly persons. J Am Geriatr Soc 39: 142–148.

48. Berg K, Wood-Dauphinee S, Williams JI (1995) The Balance Scale: reliability assessment with elderly residents and patients with an acute stroke. Scand J Rehabil Med 27: 27–36.

49. Tinetti ME, Richman D, Powell L (1990) Falls efficacy as a measure of fear of falling. J Gerontol 45: P239–243.

50. Powell LE, Myers AM (1995) The Activities-specific Balance Confidence (ABC) Scale. J Gerontol A Biol Sci Med Sci 50A: M28–34.

51. Peto V, Jenkinson C, Fitzpatrick R, Greenhall R (1995) The development and validation of a short measure of functioning and well being for individuals with Parkinson's disease. Qual Life Res 4: 241–248.

52. Tomlinson CL, Stowe R, Patel S, Rick C, Gray R, et al. (2010) Systematic review of levodopa dose equivalency reporting in Parkinson's disease. Mov Disord 25: 2649–2653.

53. Nardone A, Schieppati M (2006) Balance in Parkinson's disease under static and dynamic conditions. Mov Disord 21: 1515–1520.

54. Schieppati M, Nardone A (1991) Free and supported stance in Parkinson's disease. The effect of posture and 'postural set' on leg muscle responses to perturbation, and its relation to the severity of the disease. Brain 114 (Pt 3): 1227–1244.

55. Horak FB, Nutt JG, Nashner LM (1992) Postural inflexibility in parkinsonian subjects. J Neurol Sci 111: 46–58.

56. Paul SS, Canning CG, Sherrington C, Fung VS (2012) Reproducibility of measures of leg muscle power, leg muscle strength, postural sway and mobility in people with Parkinson's disease. Gait Posture 36: 639–642.

57. Latt MD, Lord SR, Morris JG, Fung VS (2009) Clinical and physiological assessments for elucidating falls risk in Parkinson's disease. Mov Disord 24: 1280–1289.

58. Kerr GK, Worringham CJ, Cole MH, Lacherez PF, Wood JM, et al. (2010) Predictors of future falls in Parkinson disease. Neurology 75: 116–124.

59. Slijper H, Latash ML (2004) The effects of muscle vibration on anticipatory postural adjustments. Brain Res 1015: 57–72.

60. Roll JP, Vedel JP (1982) Kinaesthetic role of muscle afferents in man, studied by tendon vibration and microneurography. Exp Brain Res 47: 177–190.

61. Marsden CD, Meadows JC, Hodgson HJ (1969) Observations on the reflex response to muscle vibration in man and its voluntary control. Brain 92: 829–846.

62. Kording KP, Wolpert DM (2006) Bayesian decision theory in sensorimotor control. Trends Cogn Sci 10: 319–326.

63. Lackner JR, Levine MS (1979) Changes in apparent body orientation and sensory localization induced by vibration of postural muscles: vibratory myesthetic illusions. Aviat Space Environ Med 50: 346–354.

64. Rocchi L, Chiari L, Mancini M, Carlson-Kuhta P, Gross A, et al. (2006) Step initiation in Parkinson's disease: influence of initial stance conditions. Neurosci Lett 406: 128–132.

65. Conte A, Khan N, Defazio G, Rothwell JC, Berardelli A (2013) Pathophysiology of somatosensory abnormalities in Parkinson disease. Nat Rev Neurol 9: 687–697.

66. Fiorio M, Stanzani C, Rothwell JC, Bhatia KP, Moretto G, et al. (2007) Defective temporal discrimination of passive movements in Parkinson's disease. Neurosci Lett 417: 312–315.

67. Jacobs JV, Horak FB (2006) Abnormal proprioceptive-motor integration contributes to hypometric postural responses of subjects with Parkinson's disease. Neuroscience 141: 999–1009.

68. Cordo P, Gurfinkel VS, Bevan L, Kerr GK (1995) Proprioceptive consequences of tendon vibration during movement. J Neurophysiol 74: 1675–1688.

69. Bosco C, Colli R, Introini E, Cardinale M, Tsarpela O, et al. (1999) Adaptive responses of human skeletal muscle to vibration exposure. Clin Physiol 19: 183–187.

70. Ivanenko YP, Grasso R, Lacquaniti F (2000) Influence of leg muscle vibration on human walking. J Neurophysiol 84: 1737–1747.

6

Age Effects on Mediolateral Balance Control

L. Eduardo Cofré Lizama[1], Mirjam Pijnappels[1], Gert H. Faber[1], Peter N. Reeves[2], Sabine M. Verschueren[3], Jaap H. van Dieën[1]*

1 MOVE Research Institute Amsterdam, Faculty of Human Movement Sciences, VU University Amsterdam, Amsterdam, The Netherlands, 2 College of Osteopathic Medicine, Michigan State University, East Lansing, Michigan, United States of America, 3 Department of Rehabilitation Sciences, Faculty of Kinesiology and Rehabilitation Sciences, Katholieke Universiteit Leuven, Leuven, Belgium

Abstract

Background: Age-related balance impairments, particularly in mediolateral direction (ML) may cause falls. Sufficiently sensitive and reliable ML balance tests are, however, lacking. This study is aimed to determine (1) the effect of age on and (2) the reliability of ML balance performance using Center of Mass (CoM) tracking.

Methods: Balance performance of 19 young (26±3 years) and 19 older (72±5 years) adults on ML-CoM tracking tasks was compared. Subjects tracked predictable and unpredictable target displacements at increasing frequencies with their CoM by shifting their weight sideward. Phase-shift (response delay) and gain (amplitude difference) between the CoM and target in the frequency domain were used to quantify performance. Thirteen older and all young adults were reassessed to determine reliability of balance performance measures. In addition, all older adults performed a series of clinical balance tests and conventional posturography was done in a sub-sample.

Results: Phase-shift and gain dropped below pre-determined thresholds (−90 degrees and 0.5) at lower frequencies in the older adults and were even lower below these frequencies than in young adults. Performance measures showed good to excellent reliability in both groups. All clinical scores were close to the maximum and no age effect was found using posturography. ML balance performance measures exhibited small but systematic between-session differences indicative of learning.

Conclusions: The ability to accurately perform ML-CoM tracking deteriorates with age. ML-CoM tracking tasks form a reliable tool to assess ML balance in young and older adults and are more sensitive to age-related impairment than posturography and clinical tests.

Editor: Kevin Paterson, University of Leicester, United Kingdom

Funding: This research was funded by the European Commission through MOVE-AGE, an Erasmus Mundus Joint Doctorate program (2011-0015). Experimental set-up was supported by MOTEK Medical BV, Amsterdam, The Netherlands. Mirjam Pijnappels was financially supported by a TOP-NIG grant (#91209021) from the Dutch Organization for Scientific Research (NWO). The European Union as well as The Dutch Organization for Scientific Research (NWO) had no role in study design, data collection and analysis, decision to publish, or preparation of the manuscript.

Competing Interests: With regards to the role of MOTEK Medical BV, this company only provided the software for data collection.

* Email: j.van.dieen@vu.nl

Introduction

It is widely accepted that, in our aging society, falls and fall-related injuries are a major problem with high personal and economic impact [1]. Balance impairments form one of the main risk factors for falls, not only in patient populations but also in community-dwelling older adults [2]. Most of the individuals older than 60 years exhibit some degree of balance impairment, which gradually affects mobility and increases dependency [3]. Therefore, early and adequate assessment of balance impairments is of paramount importance to identify those individuals in need of preventive care [4] and to monitor effects of preventive interventions [5].

Mediolateral (ML) balance impairments have in particular been associated with an increased risk of falling in the older population [6–8]. For instance, in prospective and retrospective studies,

postural sway parameters in the ML direction have been shown to be higher (i.e. larger area and excursion of the centre of pressure) in fallers than in non-fallers [7]. Nevertheless, as balance control declines gradually with aging, current clinical tools are not sensitive enough to detect early stage impairments in community-dwelling older adults, as these tests exhibit ceiling effects [5]. For instance, Berg and POMA scales have shown ceiling effects even in older adults who exhibit moderate to severe limitations of function (i.e. inability to climb stairs without assistance) [9]. Also conventional posturography, does not consistently discriminate between young and older adults [10]. It appears that ability of balance performance measurements to predict fall risk can be improved over that of conventional posturography by adding a more dynamic component, which involves center of mass (CoM) movements or weight shifting [11]. In line with this, slow lateral stepping responses have been associated with fall risk in older adults [6] and based on videos of real-life falls, inadequate weight shifting accounted for 41% of the falls [12]. Although the latter study focused on older adults living in long-term care facilities, previous studies in community-dwelling older adults also suggest that a considerable proportion of falls can be attributed to incorrect weight-shifting or daily-life tasks that challenge ML balance [13,14].

Sufficient sensitivity to detect age-related impairments in ML balance control, even in relatively fit and healthy community-dwelling older, can be reached by utilizing tests with incremental difficulty, which can probe the limits of the responsiveness of the balance control system in relation to the demands of the task. The responsiveness can be expressed as control bandwidth, i.e. the range of frequencies over which one can operate within some tolerated error level. For example, a low frequency sinusoidal target signal can be tracked closely, but as the frequency of the signal increases, limits in control bandwidth result in growing tracking errors. Bandwidth of ML balance control can be reduced by slower central and peripheral processing of sensory information [15] and reduced ability to execute motor commands due to muscle weakness (reduced strength and power) [16].

Recent work by our group showed that a mediolateral balance assessment task (coined MELBA), using the center of pressure (CoP) for tracking a visual target allows determining limits in control bandwidth even in healthy young adults [17]. In the current study, we used a modified version of MELBA, in which the subject tracks a target with his or her body CoM, instead of CoP. We believe that using CoM instead of CoP is more meaningful and intuitive, since the CoM is the controlled variable in balancing and weight shifting [18].

The aim of this study was to determine the effect of age on balance responsiveness (control bandwidth) using MELBA. We hypothesized that older adults would have a narrower control bandwidth than young adults. To compare sensitivity of MELBA with conventional methods, we also used posturography. In addition, we investigated test-retest reliability of the modified MELBA. Based on results obtained with CoP tracking [17], we hypothesized that test-retest reliability would be similar or better than CoP-tracking.

Methods

Participants

Nineteen healthy older and 19 healthy younger subjects were recruited for this study. To further characterize the older participants, the mini mental state examination MMSE, the Quickscreen (QS) [19], short physical performance battery (SPPB) [20], Berg balance scale (BBS) [21], miniBEST (MB) [22], performance-oriented mobility assessment balance section (POMA-B) [23] and timed up-and-go (TUG) [24] were used. Performance during the timed up-and-go with dual task (DTUG) was extracted from the MB. This research was approved by the Ethical Committee of the Faculty of Human Movement Sciences, VU University, Amsterdam (2011-48M), in accordance with the ethical standards of the declaration of Helsinki. All participants were informed of the experimental procedures and signed informed consent was obtained prior to the experiment.

Task and Procedure

Each participant performed a series of ML-CoM tracking tasks, while standing barefoot and with the arms crossed in a quiet and low-intensity lit room (for set-up details, see Figure 1). Body CoM was calculated with a 9-markers frontal plane model (forehead,

shoulder, anterior-superior iliac spines, knees and ankles) using an Optotrak Certus motion capture system (Northern Digital Instruments, Canada). Gender specific CoM calculations were performed using scaling of anthropometric data and inertial parameters described by de Leva [25]. D-flow 3.10.0 software (Motek Medical, The Netherlands) was used to produce target signals as well as to record (60 samples/s) and display target and CoM data on a screen 2.5 m in front of the participant. ML-CoM tracking consisted of tracking a predictable and unpredictable target signal using the ML displacement of the CoM projected on the screen. The target signal and CoM were represented by white and red spheres of 11 and 9 cm diameter, respectively. CoP data were collected using a Kistler-9281B force plate (Kistler Instruments AG, Winterthur, Switzerland) sampled at 60 samples/s.

The *predictable* target signal was constructed using 2 blocks of 20 seconds, 1 block of 10 seconds and 17 blocks of 5 seconds, each composed by one sine wave, which increased in frequency from 0.1 to 2.0 Hz in steps of 0.1 Hz. This information was enhanced using a metronome synchronized with the maximum displacement of the target in order to increase sensory input abundance. The total ML-CoM tracking time for this target signal was 135 seconds.

The *unpredictable* target signal was constructed using 15 blocks composed by the sum of 6 consecutive sine waves separated by 0.1 Hz. A pseudorandom phase-shift between sine waves between –1 to 1 period was introduced in order to avoid predictability. After each block the lowest frequency, which started at 0.1 Hz, was increased by 0.1 Hz until it reached 1.5 Hz. Duration was 40 s for block 1, 20 s for block 2, 10 s for block 3, 8 s for blocks 4 and 5, 6 s for blocks 6 and 7, and 4 seconds for blocks 8 to 15. Duration of the blocks was chosen to obtain a minimum of 2 cycles per frequency contained in the block. The total ML-CoM tracking time for this target signal was 132 seconds. Examples of the two target signals are depicted in Figure 1.

Each participant performed 6 ML-CoM tracking trials: 3 with the predictable and 3 with the unpredictable target. Before performing the test, one practice trial was allowed for each of the conditions. To determine test-retest reliability, all younger and 13 of the older adults repeated the test in a second session 7 days later at the same time of the day. Trials were performed with at least 1 minute of rest in between. Since stance width alters lower limb neuromechanical responses when displacing CoM and CoP in the ML direction [26], stance width was standardized by setting the heel distance to 11% of body height. A fixed 14° stance angle was used across all participants (Figure 1). These stance measures have been shown to be within the values of normal stance [27]. Target maximum side-to-side displacement for both target signals was normalized for each subject at 50% of stance width; allowing ML-CoM displacements to be within the base of support. On average, older participants stood on the force plate with 19.0x±1.0 cm distance between heels, which determined a maximum target displacement of 9.5x±0.5 cm whereas younger participants stood on the force plate with 18.9x±1.1 cm distance between heels, which determined a maximum target displacement of 9.4±0.5 cm. Between groups displacement differences were not significant. Additionally, a subsample of 10 older adults and all younger participants performed 3 standing still trials of 50 seconds with the eyes open and 3 with eyes closed for comparison with ML-CoM non-tracking postural sway measures and conventional posturographic measures (i.e. CoP sway area). No data was discarded and the use of subsamples for the re-test session and posturography measures was imposed by the time constraints of the participants who were unable to attend two sessions.

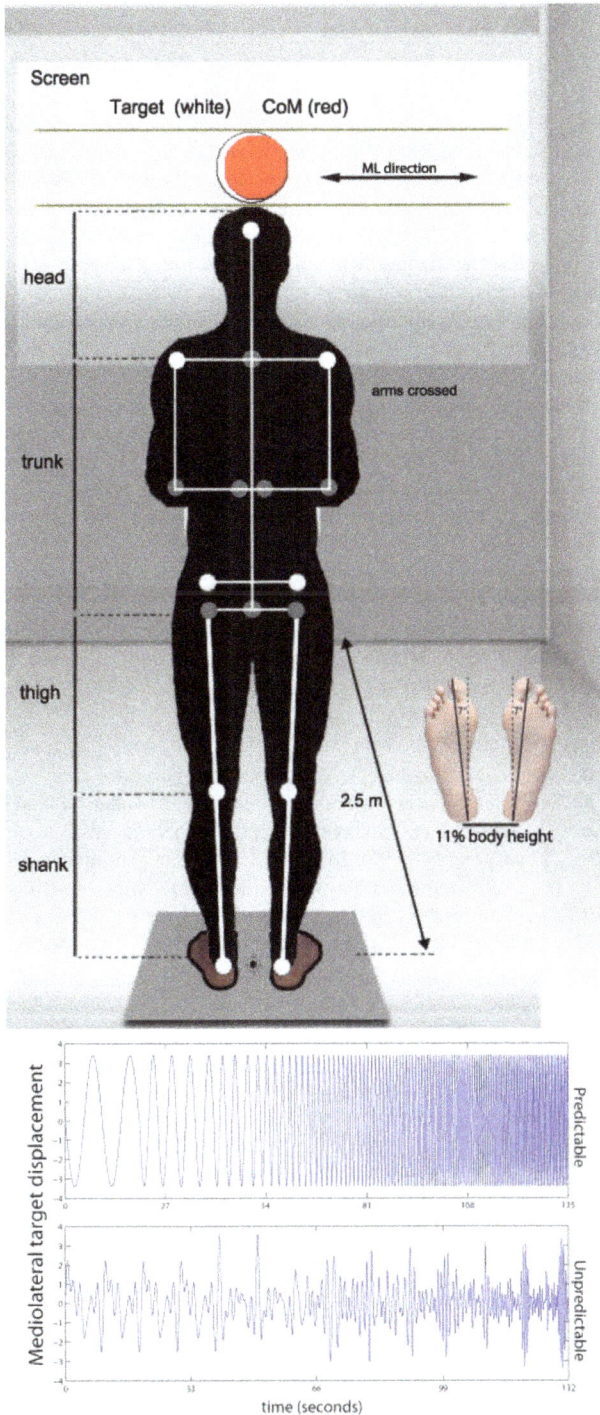

Figure 1. Illustration of the set-up and the model for Center of Mass (CoM) calculation utilized in this experiment, showing a silhouette of a subject standing in the middle of a forceplate with marker placement superimposed (in white actual makers and in grey estimated joint centers) and the display of the CoM feedback (red sphere). The white sphere in the centre represents target which moved in the mediolateral (ML) direction following the patterns depicted in the bottom panel: predictable (top) and unpredictable (bottom). An insertion of foot soles is presented showing foot positioning during the experiments (stance width and angle).

Data analysis

All data analysis was performed using custom-made software in Matlab R2011a (Mathworks, Natick MA, USA). Balance performance over the frequency ranges in the target signal was described by the gain of the linear constant coefficient transfer function between CoM and target signal. This analysis was performed using the Welch algorithm over windows of 0.25 times the length of the target (per block) with 90% overlap between windows [17]. For the unpredictable target, phase-shift, gain and coherence were calculated as the average of the values at each frequency over blocks with overlapping frequency content. The phase-shift (PS) reflects the delay (in degrees) between target and CoM whereas gain (G) reflects the ratio between the target and CoM amplitudes; both in the frequency domain. Perfect performance implies $PS = 0$ and $G = 1$ over all frequencies comprising the target signal. In addition, the coherence (Coh) was determined, as a measure of the correspondence between the target and CoM in the frequency domain, which in this study was used to corroborate the assumption of input (target)/output (CoM) linearity and therewith the validity of estimates of PS and G. Perfect linearity produces $Coh = 1$ over all frequencies comprising the target signal.

To characterize balance performance, 4 descriptors were calculated. First, the values at which PS dropped below 90 degrees and G dropped below 0.5 were determined as the cutoff frequencies (coined f_{PS} and f_G, respectively). Second, PS_{mean} and G_{mean} were computed as the average of the G and PS values within the bandwidth determined by f_{PS} and f_G, respectively.

For the posturographic measures (eyes open and eyes closed), CoP sway area and mean velocity, maximal velocity, total excursion and standard deviation of the CoP in the anterioposterior (AP) and ML directions were calculated. Additionally the sum of energies across the .05–2.0 Hz power spectrum of the ML-CoM postural sway was analyzed. This range was chosen since it contains the frequencies present in both targets used in the tracking tasks. Although conventional posturography uses CoP to asses balance, it has been shown that during unperturbed upright standing there is a direct relation between CoP and CoM [18].

Statistical Analysis

Repeated measures ANOVAs were performed on the dependent variables f_{PS}, PS_{mean}, f_G, and G_{mean} with age as a between-subject factor (younger versus older), and target (predictable and unpredictable target) as a within-subject factor. For this analysis the averaged values over three trials performed in session 1 were used. The strength of the age-effect was quantified by calculating the effect size (eta squared).

To analyze test-retest reliability, the data of all subjects participating in both sessions were used. First, to assess systematic differences, a repeated measures ANOVA with age as a between-subject factor (younger versus older), target (predictable and unpredictable target), trial number (1 to 3) and session (1 or 2) as within-subject factors. In view of multiple testing, α was set at .0125 (.05/4). To determine reliability of performance descriptors, intraclass correlations (ICC 2, 1) of the measured variables were calculated for the whole group. To better determine reliability of the measures when applied in a specific age range, ICC was also performed for each age group separately. Measures were considered to exhibit excellent reliability when ICC>.74, good = .60–.74 and fair = .40–.59 [28].

A univariate ANOVA with age as a random factor was performed to determine the effect of age on ML-CoM non-tracking postural sway (conventional posturography). Separate univariate ANOVAs with age as a random factor were used to determine the effect of age on CoP sway measures with eyes open and closed. To better compare age effect on MELBA and conventional posturography, α was also set at 0.0125 and the effect size of age was quantified using eta-squared. Statistical analyses were performed using IBM SPSS (Statistics 21).

Results

Subjects

Demographics for all subjects and results of clinical balance tests for the older adults are presented in Table 1. No differences in height and weight were found between groups. Participants did not report any musculoskeletal or neurological condition or use of medication that could affect balance. The older adults scored close to the maximum in all clinical tests and scores were above the cut-off scores for the highest (best balance performance) category defined for each test.

ML-CoM tracking

For all balance performance measures (f_{PS}, PS_{mean}, f_G and G_{mean}), significant main effects of age were found (p<.001), indicating a narrower control bandwidth in the older compared to the younger adults (Figure 2; Table 2). In addition, a significant main effect of target was found, with all measures exhibiting lower values when tracking the unpredictable target (Figure 2; Table 2). No interactions between age and target were found. Although lower than for the target main effect, the effect size of age for all measures was medium ($\eta^2 \le 0.13$) to large ($\eta^2 \le 0.38$).

A moderate to high linearity between ML-CoM and the displacement of both targets was found as expressed by mean coherences (0.1 to 2.0 Hz range) >0.4 and >0.6 for unpredictable and predictable ML-CoM tracking, respectively. This supports characterization of balance control using gain and phase-shift. Overall, subjects performed better when tracking the predictable target, reflected by gain values closer to 1 and phase shifts closer to

0, compared to tracking the unpredictable target, especially for input frequencies below 0.8 Hz. For the unpredictable target, near-optimal values for gain and phase were not observed, underlining the challenging nature of this task.

When testing over repeated sessions, significant main effects of session were found for all balance performance measures (all p≤ 0.01), with a slightly better performance during the second session (Figure 2). Furthermore, we found interactions of session and target for f_G and G_{mean} ($p \le 0.01$), indicating more improved performance over sessions, when tracking the predictable target. A significant main effect of trial was found only for f_{PS} ($p < 0.01$) with a consistent improvement over trials in the younger adults mainly, as indicated by an age-by-trial interaction ($p = 0.01$). A significant interaction of trial and age was also found for PS_{mean} ($p = 0.01$), here with the older adults exhibiting more improved performance over trials. Finally, a significant target-by-trial interaction was found for f_{PS} ($p = 0.01$), with more improved performance over trials when tracking the unpredictable target. In spite of these systematic between-session effects, ICCs showed that for all subjects pooled, reliability of all balance performance descriptors was excellent, with ICC values ranging from 0.77 for G_{mean} when tracking the predictable target to 0.91 for f_{PS} when tracking the unpredictable target (Table 3). As expected, stratified analysis by age group showed lower ICC values, but reliability still ranged from fair to excellent.

Posturography

No age effect on ML-CoM non-tracking postural sway, as expressed by the energy across the 0.05–2.0 Hz range in quiet standing, was found (younger: $0.27 \pm .09$ m^2/Hz and older: $0.27 \pm .22$ m^2/Hz, $p = 0.91$). In addition, no significant differences were found conventional posturography (CoP sway measures) measures. The largest effect sizes were found for the maximum sway velocity in the ML direction for both, eyes-open and eyes-

Table 1. Top part of the table shows demographics for all participants.

			Older adults		Young	
			mean	sd	mean	sd
Demo-graphics	Age	(years)	72.0	4.6	26.0	3.3
	Height	(m)	1.7	.1	1.7	.1
	Weight	(kg)	76.6	15.2	67.0	12.0
Clinical measures in Older Adults						
			mean	sd	95% confidence interval	
time	TUG	(seconds)	6.16	1.05	5.65	6.67
	DTUG	(seconds)	7.29	1.75	6.45	8.13
			median			
scores	QS	(min 0)	2		0	4
	BBS	(max 56)	56		53	56
	SPPB	(max 12)	12		10	12
	MiniBEST	(max 28)	26		23	28
	POMA-B	(max 16)	16			

Bottom part of the table shows the descriptive statistics (mean, ± sd, median, lowest and highest scores) for the clinical measures of balance in the older participants: Quickscreen (QS), short physical performance battery (SPPB), Berg balance scale (BBS), miniBEST test (MB) and performance-oriented mobility assessment balance section (POMA-B). For the timed up-and-go (TUG) and dual-task timed up-and-go (DTUG), the mean ± sd and 95% confidence interval are presented.

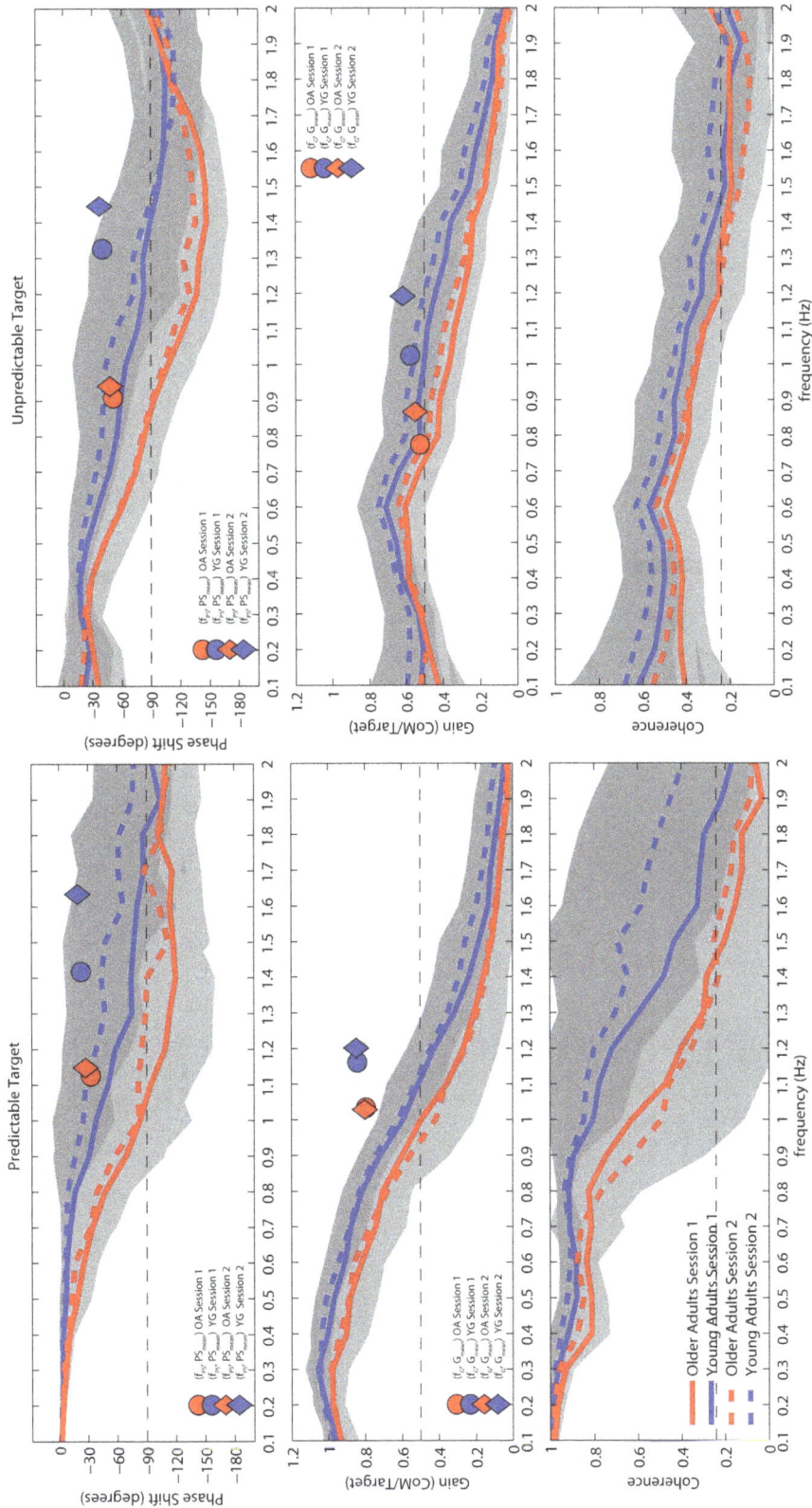

Figure 2. Averaged curves (± sd) for phase shift (top panel), gain (mid panel) and coherence (bottom panel) measures using both, predictable target (left) and unpredictable (right) targets, during first (continuous line) and second (dashed line) sessions and for the younger (in black) and the older adults (in dark grey). Grey shading indicates the ± sd for all subjects and for all trials. Markers inserted in the plots indicate means for performance descriptors for the first session (circular markers) and second session (diamond markers) for the younger (in black) and the older adults (in dark grey).

Table 2. Descriptive statistics for MELBA performance descriptors (f_{PS}, PS_{mean}, f_G and G_{mean}) for the predictable and unpredictable targets.

| | | PREDICTABLE | | | | UNPREDICTABLE | | | | RMANOVA (effects of age and target in 1st session) | | | | | |
| | | Session 1 | | Session 2 | | Session 1 | | Session 2 | | p | | | η^2 | | |
		mean	sd	mean	sd	mean	sd	mean	sd	age	tar	tar*age	age	tar	tar*age
f_{PS} (Hz)	Young	1.42	.34	1.64	.32	1.33	.39	1.45	.34	**<.01**	**<.01**	.11	.26	.35	.08
	Older	1.13	.31	1.15	.33	.91	.17	.94	.20						
PS_{mean} (°)	Young	−23.04	7.08	−19.33	6.77	−40.18	10.07	−37.18	9.21	**<.01**	**<.01**	.72	.36	.87	<.01
	Older	−33.00	5.58	−27.58	5.38	−51.03	6.98	−47.89	9.53						
f_G (Hz)	Young	1.16	.10	1.20	.13	1.02	.25	1.19	.27	**<.01**	**<.01**	.14	.34	.45	.07
	Older	1.03	.15	1.03	.16	.77	.15	.87	.14						
G_{mean}	Young	.84	.05	.85	.04	.58	.08	.62	.08	**.01**	**<.01**	.83	.20	.92	<.01
	Older	.79	.06	.80	.04	.52	.06	.55	.07						

Right part of the table summarizes the p-values and effect sizes (η^2) of the repeated measures ANOVAs for the between-subjects comparison ('age': older vs young adults) the main effect of target ('tar': unpredictable and predictable) and age-by-target interaction. Statistically significant p-values are presented in bold.

Table 3. Intraclass correlations (absolute agreement) for the performance descriptors (f_{PS}, PS_{mean}, f_G and G_{mean}) for both visual tracking tasks (predictable and unpredictable) for all subjects and stratified by age group.

| | Intraclass correlations | | | | | | | |
| | Predictable | | | | Unpredictable | | | |
	f_{PS}	PS_{mean}	f_G	G_{mean}	f_{PS}	PS_{mean}	f_G	G_{mean}
All (32)	**.86**	**.83**	**.86**	**.77**	**.91**	**.88**	**.84**	**.87**
Young (19)	.74	**.83**	.74	.62	**.85**	**.89**	.78	**.85**
Elderly (13)	**.95**	.57	**.87**	.64	**.85**	.68	.74	**.85**

Descriptors exhibiting excellent reliability are shown in bold.

closed conditions (with p = 0.03, NS after Bonferroni correction), with, however, lower velocities for the older adults.

Discussion

We studied the effects of age on ML balance control using a ML balance assessment task (MELBA), which consists of tracking predictable and unpredictable visual targets with the body's CoM. These tasks were used to assess the responsiveness of the balance control system, expressed in terms of control bandwidth. We found a significant effect of age for all descriptors of control bandwidth even though our older participants scored near maximum values on all clinical balance tests. The gradual increase in phase shift and decrease in gain with increasing frequency observed in both groups and for both targets (Figure 2) shows that MELBA tasks are challenging enough to avoid ceiling effects. In contrast, no age effect on ML-CoM postural sway and CoP postural sway during quiet standing were found. The reliability of descriptors of ML balance control bandwidth was also studied. Although small but significant learning effects between sessions, were present, reliability of the descriptors was fair to excellent with ICCs ranging from 0.57 to 0.95.

Although widely used, the evidence for the association of posturographic measures and fall risk in the elderly is inconclusive [29] and age-related changes in postural sway are controversial [10]. In the present study we found overall no age effect and only a trend towards a lower CoP-sway velocity in the ML direction in the older adults. While lower velocity would conventionally be interpreted as reflecting better balance performance, this may be attributed to a reduced exploratory behavior in the older adults, affecting functional variability hence stability [30]. Conversely, it may also reflect the reduced control bandwidth in our older participants revealed by MELBA.

Clinical measures of balance and mobility for older adults were used in the present study, to characterize the subject sample. The near-maximum scores obtained corroborate the ceiling effects reported in community-dwelling older adults [9] and underline that our sample was relatively healthy and fit. For all subjects tested, scores fell within the maximum ranges of the tests. On average, subjects were predicted to have a low risk of falling (QS = 0–1 points [19], BBS = 43–56 points [21]; MB = 19–28 points [31] and TUG and even DTUG<13.5 s [24]), no balance impairments (POMA-B = 14–16 points) [23] and no risk of developing a future disability (SPPB = 10–12 points) [20]. The clinical tests used in this study, are thus not sensitive to subtle impairments of balance that the ML-CoM tracking tasks revealed.

Different factors may account for the lower control bandwidth observed in the older adults. The gluteus medius muscles are strongly involved in ML weight-shifting tasks [32]. When target frequency increases, faster changes in hip torques are required, which could be limited by the rate of force development of the hip abductors [33] possibly due to a selective atrophy of type-II (fast-twitch) fibers [34] and due to a reduced number of fast motor units [35]. Furthermore, tendons become more compliant with age, which can further delay force transmission and thus slow down ML balance responses [36]. It is also plausible that an increased co-activation of antagonist muscles acting in the frontal plane during the tracking tasks may hamper CoM displacement in the ML direction [37], as increased co-activation coinciding with greater stiffness and damping during ML perturbations was found in older adults [38].

In addition to changes at the effector level, impairments of the visual, vestibular, proprioceptive and somatosensory systems may affect balance control. Even though ML-CoM tracking tasks are based on, visual inputs that direct voluntary movements resulting in ML-CoM displacements, accurate online information of CoM position and velocity is needed for execution of accurate motor outputs. Deterioration of the somatosensory system due to aging may provide less accurate proprioceptive information into the balance control system [39]. Proprioceptive impairments due to aging at the hip joint have been reported [40] and may contribute to reducing ML balance control in the older adults. In addition to proprioceptive information, cutaneous plantar receptors and the vestibular organ are involved in providing sensory information into the balance control system even in the presence of explicit visual feedback on CoM movement [41]. Increased perception thresholds of cutaneous plantar receptors with aging have been reported [42] and have been associated with fall risk [19]. Also a reduced function of the vestibular system has been observed with aging [42]. The relevance of this impairment was questioned, because it was not associated with balance impairment as assessed with the POMA [42], but this may be explained by this scale not being sufficiently sensitive, as shown by the results of our study. Effects of decreased vestibular function may be more pronounced when balance is assessed with MELBA, since faster and higher amplitude body movements are made, which would rely more on vestibular information than small-amplitude and slow movements [43].

Multisensory integration is the process by which information arising from different sensory modalities is simultaneously collected [44]. Parallel weighting of sensory inputs occurs in order to control balance according to the demands imposed for a given task. For instance, impairment or absence of a sensory modality causes an up-weighting of other more reliable sources [45]. It has been proposed that the ability to re-weight sensory information as well as to perform parallel cognitive tasks is affected by aging [46,47]. Inability to properly weight sensory information and altered sensorimotor integration [48] might therefore partially explain the lower balance performance in our older adults. This is in line with previous studies that reported increased processing delays during visuomotor tasks with stepping responses [49]. Similarly, slow reactions during stepping responses have been observed in fallers who exhibited longer gluteus medius onset times [6].

Comparisons between predictable and unpredictable ML-CoM tracking tasks showed a smaller phase shift and higher gain when tracking the predictable target. This may indicate more involvement of cognitive components and more reliance upon feedback mechanisms when performing the unpredictable task [17]. Dual-tasks, used to determine the relationship between cognition and balance and balance-recovery, have shown a decreased balance performance in older adults [47]. This cognition-balance interference could be expected to cause a lower performance in the older adults, especially when tracking the unpredictable target. However, we did not find an interaction of age and task suggesting that other neuro-musculoskeletal factors, as those mentioned above, are more likely to affect ML balance performance than the decline of cognitive resources in the healthy older adults.

Although significant between-sessions differences were found, the ICC values for ML-CoM tracking performance descriptors show these to be reliable measures. All cut-off frequency descriptors (f_{PS} and f_G) had excellent reliability also in the older adults. This indicates that the bandwidth at which performance is above the thresholds (PS>−90° and G>0.5) highly correlates over sessions. The somewhat lower ICC and higher mean values for PS_{mean} and G_{mean} indicate that, within this bandwidth, performance is more variable, especially for PS and for the predictable target. Compared to the previous version of MELBA, in which CoP instead of CoM feedback was used, reliability was better in the present study, especially for the unpredictable target [17]. This may be due to the fact that ML-CoP tracking is less constrained and could allow different motor strategies, which may vary across trials and between-sessions.

The occurrence of learning effects (except for f_{PS}) between, but not within sessions, has previously been interpreted as dissociation between the ongoing learning process and the adaptation after exposure to a novel task [50]. The results partly support the premise that visuomotor processing delay can be improved by training [51]. Although no interaction effects of session-by-age were found, differences in the average ML-CoM tracking performance between the first and second sessions were larger in the younger subjects for all descriptors except PS_{mean}, for which improvements were larger in the older adults in both tracking tasks. Overall this indicates that also older adults are able to improve ML balance through training. However, correlations with daily-life ML balance performance using accelerometers should be assessed to explore the relevance of such training effects.

MELBA tasks aim to assess weight-shifting ability, which has been found to be deteriorated and associated to falls in older adults [12]. Performance on the predictable ML-CoM tracking may indicate maximal capacities within the requirements of the task, whereas performance on the unpredictable ML-CoM tracking can give insights into the sensorimotor integration in a more reactive manner [17]. The later may be more associated to stressing situations as those observed when internal or external perturbations are applied. Although the tracking tasks imposed do not simulate daily-life dynamic balance demands, MELBA challenges

mediolateral balance control to one's maximal capacities, thereby yielding highly sensitive outcomes. Further longitudinal research needs, however, to assess the predictive value of ML balance performance on MELBA for fall risk. Finally, the utilization of less expensive and more user-friendly motion capture systems should be explored to simplify MELBA's setup to make it more clinically available.

Conclusions

In conclusion, the ability to accurately track predictable and unpredictable targets deteriorates with age. This indicates a deterioration of ML balance in apparently healthy older adults. MELBA appears to be a sensitive and reliable tool to assess ML balance performance in younger and community-dwelling older adults.

Acknowledgments

The authors of this paper would like to thank to Josine van Dorsselaer MSc and Georgia Andreopoulou PT MSc for their help with data collection and clinical assessments.

Author Contributions

Conceived and designed the experiments: LECL MP GF PR SV JVD. Performed the experiments: LECL. Analyzed the data: LECL MP GF JVD. Contributed to the writing of the manuscript: LECL MP GF PR SV JVD.

References

1. World Health Organization (2007) Global report on falls prevention in older age.
2. Maki BE, Sibley KM, Jaglal SB, Bayley M, Brooks D, et al. (2011) Reducing fall risk by improving balance control: development, evaluation and knowledge-translation of new approaches. Journal of safety research 42: 473–485.
3. Close JCT, Lord SR (2011) Clinical Review Fall assessment in older people. British Medical Journal 343.
4. Dionyssiotis Y (2012) Analyzing the problem of falls among older people. International journal of general medicine 5: 805–813.
5. Pardasaney PK, Latham NK, Jette AM, Wagenaar RC, Ni P, et al. (2012) Sensitivity to change and responsiveness of four balance measures for community-dwelling older adults. Physical Therapy 92: 388–397.
6. Brauer SG, Burns YR, Galley P (2000) A Prospective Study of Laboratory and Clinical Measures of Postural Stability to Predict Community-Dwelling Fallers. The Journals of Gerontology Series A: Biological Sciences and Medical Sciences 55: M469–M476.
7. Maki BE, Holliday PJ, Topper AK (1994) A prospective-study of postural balance and risk of falling in an ambulatory and independent elderly population. Journals of Gerontology 49: M72–M84.
8. Hilliard MJ, Martinez KM, Janssen I, Edwards B, Mille M-L, et al. (2008) Lateral Balance Factors Predict Future Falls in Community-Living Older Adults. Archives of Physical Medicine and Rehabilitation 89: 1708–1713.
9. Pardasaney PK, Latham NK, Jette AM, Wagenaar RC, Ni PS, et al. (2012) Sensitivity to Change and Responsiveness of Four Balance Measures for Community-Dwelling Older Adults. Physical Therapy 92: 388–397.
10. van Wegen EEH, van Emmerik REA, Riccio GE (2002) Postural orientation: Age-related changes in variability and time-to-boundary. Human Movement Science 21: 61–84.
11. Tucker MG, Kavanagh JJ, Morrison S, Barrett RS (2009) Voluntary sway and rapid orthogonal transitions of voluntary sway in young adults, and low and high fall-risk older adults. Clinical Biomechanics 24: 597–605.
12. Robinovitch SN, Feldman F, Yang YJ, Schonnop R, Leung PM, et al. (2013) Video capture of the circumstances of falls in elderly people residing in long-term care: an observational study. Lancet 381: 47–54.
13. Topper AK, Maki BE, Holliday PJ (1993) Are activity-based assessments of balance and gait in the elderly predictive of risk of falling and or type of fall. Journal of the American Geriatrics Society 41: 479–487.
14. Nevitt MC, Cummings SR, Black D, Genant HK, Arnaud C, et al. (1993) Type of fall and risk of hip and wrist fractures - the study of osteoporotic fractures. Journal of the American Geriatrics Society 41: 1226–1234.
15. Teasdale N, Simoneau M (2001) Attentional demands for postural control: the effects of aging and sensory reintegration. Gait & Posture 14: 203–210.

16. Orr R (2010) Contribution of muscle weakness to postural instability in the elderly A systematic review. European Journal of Physical and Rehabilitation Medicine 46: 183–220.
17. Cofré Lizama LE, Pijnappels M, Reeves NP, Verschueren SMP, van Dieën JH (2013) Frequency domain mediolateral balance assessment using a center of pressure tracking task. Journal of biomechanics 46: 2831–2836.
18. Winter DA, Patla AE, Frank JS (1990) Assesment of balance control in humans. Medical Progress through Technology 16: 31–51.
19. Tiedemann A, Lord SR, Sherrington C (2010) The Development and Validation of a Brief Performance-Based Fall Risk Assessment Tool for Use in Primary Care. Journals of Gerontology Series a-Biological Sciences and Medical Sciences 65: 893–900.
20. Guralnik JM, Simonsick EM, Ferrucci L, Glynn RJ, Berkman LF, et al. (1994) A short physical performance battery assessing lower extremity function: association with self-reported disability and prediction of mortality and nursing home admission. J Gerontol A: Biol Sci Med Sci 49: 85–94.
21. Thorbahn LDB, Newton RA (1996) Use of the Berg balance test to predict falls in elderly persons. Physical Therapy 76: 576–583.
22. Franchignoni F, Horak F, Godi M, Nardone A, Giordano A (2010) Using psychometric techniques to improve the balance evaluation systems test: the mini-bestest. Journal of Rehabilitation Medicine 42: 323–331.
23. Harada N, Chiu V, Damronrodriguez J, Fowler E, Siu A, et al. (1995) Screening for balance and mobility impairment in elderly individuals living in residential care facilities. Physical Therapy 75: 462–469.
24. Barry E, Galvin R, Keogh C, Horgan F, Fahey T (2014) Is the Timed Up and Go test a useful predictor of risk of falls in community dwelling older adults: a systematic review and meta- analysis. BMC geriatrics 14: 14–14.
25. de Leva P (1996) Adjustments to Zatsiorsky-Seluyanov's segment inertia parameters. Journal of biomechanics 29: 1223–1230.
26. Bingham JT, Choi JT, Ting LH (2011) Stability in a frontal plane model of balance requires coupled changes to postural configuration and neural feedback control. Journal of Neurophysiology 106: 437–448.
27. McIlroy WE, Maki BE (1997) Preferred placement of the feet during quiet stance: Development of a standardized foot placement for balance testing. Clinical Biomechanics 12: 66–70.
28. Cicchetti DV, Sparrow SA (1981) Developing criteria for establishing interrater reliability of specific items - Applications to assessment of adaptive-behavior. American Journal of Mental Deficiency 86: 127–137.
29. Piirtola M, Era P (2006) Force platform measurements as predictors of falls among older people - A review. Gerontology 52: 1–16.

30. van Emmerik REA, van Wegen EEH (2002) On the functional aspects of variability in postural control. Exercise and Sport Sciences Reviews 30: 177–183.

31. Mak MKY, Auyeung MM (2013) The mini-BESTest can predict parkinsonian recurrent fallers: a 6-month prospective study. Journal of Rehabilitation Medicine 45: 565–571.

32. Egerton T, Brauer SG, Cresswell AG (2010) Dynamic postural stability is not impaired by moderate-intensity physical activity in healthy or balance-impaired older people. Human Movement Science 29: 1011–1022.

33. Chang SHJ, Mercer VS, Giuliani CA, Sloane PD (2005) Relationship between hip abductor rate of force development and mediolateral stability in older adults. Archives of Physical Medicine and Rehabilitation 86: 1843–1850.

34. Nilwik R, Snijders T, Leenders M, Groen BBL, van Kranenburg J, et al. (2013) The decline in skeletal muscle mass with aging is mainly attributed to a reduction in type II muscle fiber size. Experimental Gerontology 48: 492–498.

35. Lexell J (1995) Human aging, muscle mass, and fiber-type composition. Journals of Gerontology Series a-Biological Sciences and Medical Sciences 50: 11–16.

36. Narici MV, Maffulli N, Maganaris CN (2008) Ageing of human muscles and tendons. Disability and Rehabilitation 30: 1548–1554.

37. Hortobagyi T, DeVita P (2006) Mechanisms responsible for the age-associated increase in coactivation of antagonist muscles. Exercise and Sport Sciences Reviews 34: 29–35.

38. Cenciarini M, Loughlin PJ, Sparto PJ, Redfern MS (2010) Stiffness and Damping in Postural Control Increase With Age. Ieee Transactions on Biomedical Engineering 57: 267–275.

39. Shaffer SW, Harrison AL (2007) Aging of the somatosensory system: A translational perspective. Physical Therapy 87: 193–207.

40. Wingert JR, Welder C, Foo P (2014) Age-Related Hip Proprioception Declines: Effects on Postural Sway and Dynamic Balance. Archives of Physical Medicine and Rehabilitation 95: 253–261.

41. Cofré Lizama LE, Pijnappels M, Reeves NP, Verschueren SMP, van Dieën JH Can visual feedback efface the effects of sensory manipulations on mediolateral balance performance? *Submitted*.

42. Baloh RW, Ying SH, Jacobson KM (2003) A longitudinal study of gait and balance dysfunction in normal older people. Archives of Neurology 60: 835–839.

43. Goodworth AD, Peterka RJ (2009) Contribution of sensorimotor integration to spinal stabilization in humans. J Neurophysiol 102: 496–512.

44. Freiherr J, Lundstrom JN, Habel U, Reetz K (2013) Multisensory integration mechanisms during aging. Frontiers in Human Neuroscience 7.

45. Peterka RJ (2002) Sensorimotor integration in human postural control. Journal of Neurophysiology 88: 1097–1118.

46. Hay L, Bard C, Fleury M, Teasdale N (1996) Availability of visual and proprioceptive afferent messages and postural control in elderly adults. Experimental Brain Research 108: 129–139.

47. Maki BE, McIlroy WE (2007) Cognitive demands and cortical control of human balance-recovery reactions. Journal of Neural Transmission 114: 1279–1296.

48. Horak FB (2006) Postural orientation and equilibrium: what do we need to know about neural control of balance to prevent falls? Age and Ageing 35: 7–11.

49. Sparto PJ, Jennings JR, Furman JM, Redfern MS (2014) Lateral step initiation behavior in older adults. Gait & Posture 39: 799–803.

50. King BR, Fogel SM, Albouy G, Doyon J (2013) Neural correlates of the age-related changes in motor sequence learning and motor adaptation in older adults. Frontiers in Human Neuroscience 7.

51. Young WR, Hollands MA (2012) Evidence for age-related decline in visuomotor function and reactive stepping adjustments. Gait & Posture 36: 477–481.

7

Patient Age and the Prognosis of Idiopathic Membranous Nephropathy

Makoto Yamaguchi[1], Masahiko Ando[2], Ryohei Yamamoto[3], Shinichi Akiyama[1], Sawako Kato[1], Takayuki Katsuno[1], Tomoki Kosugi[1], Waichi Sato[1], Naotake Tsuboi[1], Yoshinari Yasuda[1], Masashi Mizuno[1], Yasuhiko Ito[1], Seiichi Matsuo[1], Shoichi Maruyama[1]*

1 Department of Nephrology, Nagoya University Graduate School of Medicine, Nagoya, Japan, 2 Center for Advanced Medicine and Clinical Research, Nagoya University Hospital, Nagoya, Japan, 3 Department of Geriatric Medicine and Nephrology, Osaka University Graduate School of Medicine, Suita, Japan

Abstract

Background: Idiopathic membranous nephropathy (IMN) is increasingly seen in older patients. However, differences in disease presentation and outcomes between older and younger IMN patients remain controversial. We compared patient characteristics between younger and older IMN patients.

Methods: We recruited 171 Japanese patients with IMN, including 90 (52.6%) patients <65 years old, 40 (23.4%) patients 65–70 years, and 41 (24.0%) patients ≥71 years. Clinical characteristics and outcomes were compared between younger and older IMN patients.

Results: During a median observation period of 37 months, 103 (60.2%) patients achieved complete proteinuria remission, which was not significantly associated with patient age ($P = 0.831$). However, 13 (7.6%) patients were hospitalized because of infection. Multivariate Cox proportional hazards models identified older age [adjusted hazard ratio (HR) = 3.11, 95% confidence interval (CI): 1.45–7.49, per 10 years; $P = 0.003$], prednisolone use (adjusted HR = 11.8, 95% CI: 1.59–242.5; $P = 0.014$), and cyclosporine used in combination with prednisolone (adjusted HR = 10.3, 95% CI: 1.59–204.4; $P = 0.012$) as significant predictors of infection. A <25% decrease in proteinuria at 1 month after immunosuppressive therapy initiation also predicted infection (adjusted HR = 6.72, 95% CI: 1.51–37.8; $P = 0.012$).

Conclusions: Younger and older IMN patients had similar renal outcomes. However, older patients were more likely to develop infection when using immunosuppressants. Patients with a poor response in the first month following the initiation of immunosuppressive therapy should be carefully monitored for infection and may require a faster prednisolone taper.

Editor: Giuseppe Remuzzi, Mario Negri Institute for Pharmacological Research and Azienda Ospedaliera Ospedali Riuniti di Bergamo, Italy

Funding: This study was supported by a Grant-in-Aid for Progressive Renal Diseases Research, Research on Rare and Intractable Disease, from the Ministry of Health, Labor, and Welfare of Japan. The funders had no role in study design, data collection and analysis, decision to publish, or preparation of the manuscript.

Competing Interests: The authors have declared that no competing interests exist.

* Email: marus@med.nagoya-u.ac.jp

Introduction

In Japan, the elderly population (i.e., those aged 65 and over) comprised 24.1% of the total population as of October 2012, a figure that is expected to increase to 39.9% by 2060 [1]. With increases in life expectancy, greater numbers of elderly patients with chronic kidney diseases are surviving longer. Membranous nephropathy (MN) is the most important cause of nephrotic syndrome in elderly patients [2,3]. The incidence of MN is higher in the elderly than in younger adults. Although little information is available regarding the natural course of MN in elderly patients, Zent et al. [4] reported similar clinical presentations between older and younger patients. However, clinical information such as the prevalence of leg edema or pleural effusion was not included. Thus, the clinical severity associated with nephrotic syndrome could not be adequately evaluated.

Most randomized trials of immunosuppressive therapy for MN included few, if any, patients older than 65 [5–9], and only a few retrospective studies and case series specifically reported immunosuppressive therapy outcomes [4,10,11]. Consequently, the optimal immunosuppressive regimen for elderly idiopathic membranous nephropathy (IMN) patients remains controversial.

Based on our clinical experience, our impression is that compared to younger IMN patients, older patients have more severe symptoms associated with nephrotic syndrome and are more susceptible to infection. It can therefore be difficult to weigh the risks and benefits of initiating immunosuppressive therapy, especially among elderly patients.

To understand the clinical characteristics of elderly IMN patients and identify patients at high risk for infection, we conducted a retrospective multicenter observational cohort study that was organized as part of the Nagoya Nephrotic Syndrome

Cohort Study (N-NSCS), a study based in 10 major nephrology centers in Nagoya, Japan.

Subjects and Methods

Study Population and Data Sources

Participants in the present study were included in our previous multicenter retrospective cohort study, N-NSCS, which identified cigarette smoking as a risk factor for kidney dysfunction for IMN [12]. The study design of N-NSCS was described in detail elsewhere [12]. Briefly, this study included patients older than 18 years who were diagnosed with MN based on kidney biopsy results at Nagoya University, Chubu Rosai Hospital, Japanese Red Cross Nagoya Daiichi Hospital, Tsushima City Hospital, Kasugai Municipal Hospital, Nagoya Kyoritsu Hospital, Anjo Kosei Hospital, Ichinomiya Municipal Hospital, Handa City Hospital, or Tosei General Hospital between January 2003 and December 2012. Out of 272 identified MN patients, we excluded those with conditions generally considered to cause secondary MN [10]. Furthermore, we excluded seven patients (3.9%) because of loss to follow-up (n = 6) and missing data (n = 1). Ultimately, 171 (62.9%) IMN patients were enrolled and followed up until September 2013.

Our study was conducted by using linkable anonymous data set. No informed consent was obtained. The study protocol and consent procedure were approved by the ethics committees of Nagoya University, Chubu Rosai Hospital, Japanese Red Cross Nagoya Daiichi Hospital, Tsushima City Hospital, Kasugai Municipal Hospital, Nagoya Kyoritsu Hospital, Anjo Kosei Hospital, Ichinomiya Municipal Hospital, Handa City Hospital, and Tosei General Hospital.

Data Collection

Baseline characteristics were collected retrospectively from patients' medical records. Clinical characteristics at the time of kidney biopsy were considered to represent baseline if the patient had not received immunosuppressive therapy or received immunosuppressive therapy only after a kidney biopsy. For patients who received immunosuppressive therapy before biopsy, the clinical characteristics at the time of initiating immunosuppressive therapy were used as baseline. Baseline characteristics included age, gender, body mass index, systolic and diastolic blood pressure, serum total cholesterol, serum creatinine, glomerular filtration rate [GFR; estimated using the equation recently developed by the Japanese Society of Nephrology: eGFR (mL/min/ 1.73 m^2) = 194×Scr$^{-1.094}$×Age$^{-0.287}$×0.739 (if female) (13)], serum albumin, 24-hour urinary protein excretion or urinary protein/creatinine ratio, smoking status, antihypertensive drug use, and initial use of corticosteroids and/or other immunosuppressive agents.

Antihypertensive drugs used in this cohort included angiotensin-converting enzyme (ACE) inhibitors or angiotensin II receptor blockers (ARB), calcium channel blockers, β-blockers, and thiazides. Information regarding therapeutic interventions was also collected, including the use of ACE inhibitors/ARBs and corticosteroids or other immunosuppressive agents that were prescribed during the observation period.

Nephrotic syndrome was defined as a urinary protein excretion ≥3.5 g/day (or a urinary protein/creatinine ratio ≥3.5) and a serum albumin level <3.0 mg/dL.

Complete remission (CR) from proteinuria was defined as a urinary protein excretion <0.3 g/day, a urinary protein/creatinine ratio <0.3, and/or a negative/trace result for urinary protein on a dipstick test. Partial remission (PR) from proteinuria was

defined as a urinary protein excretion <3.5 g/day and a urinary protein/creatinine ratio <3.5. Relapse was defined as a urinary protein excretion ≥1.0 g/day, a urinary protein/creatinine ratio ≥1.0, or a urinary protein dipstick result ≥2+ on at least two occasions after CR had been achieved.

The rate of eGFR decline per year (mL/min per 1.73 m^2/year) was determined by plotting eGFR against the observation time.

The anonymous data set is available in the **Table S7 in File S2**.

Outcomes

Our primary outcome was the first CR. Secondary outcomes were hospitalization due to infection and a 30% decline in the eGFR before end-stage renal disease (ESRD). Patients who died before achieving either outcome were censored at the time of death. The eGFR was measured as required for each patient at 1–3 month intervals. Patients were followed up until September 2013 and censored at the time of their death before ESRD or as of their last serum creatinine measurement before September 2013.

Statistical Analyses

We stratified patients into three age categories: <65, 65–70, and ≥71 years old. Clinical characteristics were compared between these three groups using a Wilcoxon rank-sum test or Fisher's exact test. To determine predictors independently associated with each outcome, potential covariates were assessed using a log-rank test and/or univariate and multivariate Cox proportional hazards (CPH) models. For continuous variables, a Wilcoxon rank-sum test was used to assess the significance of intergroup differences. Results for categorical variables were expressed as percentages and compared by using Fisher's exact test. The cumulative probabilities of achieving a first CR and hospitalization due to infection were determined using the Kaplan-Meier method and log-rank tests. Predictors of these outcomes were identified using univariate and multivariate CPH models. The proportional hazards assumption for covariates was tested using scaled Schoenfeld residuals. A −2 log likelihood value for fitting a model with all explanatory variables was determined for individual CPH models that included 25%, 50%, or 75% decreases in proteinuria in the first month after initial immunosuppressive therapy, and was used to compare the performance of these three models. A likelihood ratio test was used to determine whether the fit of a model that included a 25% decrease rate was the best model for the present study. The trend in the outcome with respect to the decreases in proteinuria in the first month after initial immunosuppressive therapy was examined statistically by scoring ≥50% decrease as 0 and 25–50% decrease, 0–25% decrease, and exacerbation as 1, 2, and 3, respectively; the resulting scores were then included in the regression model. Least squares mean±95% confidence intervals for urinary protein and eGFR during follow-up period were compared between three age categories using linear mixed-effect models.

The level of statistical significance was set at $P<0.05$. All statistical analyses were performed using JMP version 10.0.0 (SAS Institute, Cary, NC, USA; www.jmp.com), SAS version 9.4 (SAS Institute, Cary, NC; www.sas.com), and STATA version 13.0 (STATA Corp, www.stata.com).

Results

Clinical Characteristics

A total of 171 patients were diagnosed with IMN after appropriate clinical and laboratory screening for secondary causes.

Table 1. Baseline characteristics of 171 IMN patients.

	<65 years	65–70 years	≥71 years	P-value
Number	90	40	41	
Baseline characteristics				
Age (years)	57 (50–62)	68 (66–69)	75 (74–78)	
Male [n (%)]	63 (70.0)	28 (70.0)	27 (65.9)	0.882
Body mass index (kg/m²)	23.2 (21.2–25.8)	23.2 (22.0–25.7)	22.6 (21.1–24.6)	0.440
Systolic blood pressure (mmHg)	129 (120–140)	135 (125–158)	138 (122–147)	0.028
Diastolic blood pressure (mmHg)	77 (70–86)	80 (70–86)	76 (70–84)	0.502
Serum creatinine (mg/dL)	0.77 (0.68–0.90)	0.80 (0.68–0.99)	0.95 (0.7–1.2)	0.011
eGFR (mL/min/1.73 m²)	81 (70–97)	73 (58–86)	59 (46–81)	<0.001
Serum albumin (g/dL)	2.8 (2.1–3.5)	2.5 (2.0–3.1)	2.3 (1.9–2.8)	0.014
Urinary protein (g/day)	4.2 (2.6–7.0)	3.6 (2.6–7.6)	5.1 (3.3–7.7)	0.275
Urinary protein >3.5 (g/day) [n (%)]	29 (32.2)	17 (42.5)	11 (26.8)	0.310
Total cholesterol (mg/dL)	279 (229–382)	284 (239–400)	297 (249–367)	0.859
Leg edema [n (%)]	64 (71.1)	29 (72.5)	38 (92.7)	0.020
Pleural effusion [n (%)]	12 (13.3)	8 (20.0)	13 (31.7)	0.048
Treatment				
ACE inhibitor or ARB therapy [n (%)]	80 (88.9)	39 (97.5)	47 (90.2)	0.268
Immunosuppressive therapy				0.893
No immunosuppressants	36 (40.0)	17 (42.5)	17 (41.5)	
Prednisolone [n (%)]	17 (18.9)	10 (25.0)	8 (19.5)	
Prednisolone+Cyclosporine [n (%)]	37 (41.1)	13 (32.5)	16 (39.0)	
Observational period (months)	44 (20–86)	31 (15–63)	25 (11–54)	0.021

NOTE: Median (interquartile range), Conversion factors for units: SCr in mg/dL to μmol/L, ×88.4; eGFR (mL/min/1.73 m2) = 194×Scr$^{-1.094}$×Age$^{-0.287}$×0.739 (if female), total cholesterol in mg/dL to mmol/L, ×0.02586.
Abbreviations: IMN, idiopathic membranous nephropathy; eGFR, estimated glomerular filtration rate; ACE inhibitor/ARB, angiotensin-converting enzyme inhibitor/angiotensin receptor blocker.

Baseline characteristics stratified by the three age categories are shown in Table 1.

The cohort included 90 (52.6%) patients <65 years old, 40 (23.4%) aged 65–70 years, and 41 (24.0%) ≥71 years old. Compared with younger patients, older patients had lower serum albumin levels (P = 0.014), lower eGFRs (P<0.001), higher serum creatinine levels (P = 0.011), higher systolic blood pressure (P = 0.028), and a higher prevalence of leg edema and pleural effusion (P = 0.020 and P = 0.048, respectively). This suggested a greater severity of symptoms associated with nephrotic syndrome in older patients than in younger patients. The prevalence of pleural effusion was determined by chest radiography results at the time of kidney biopsy. No trends were found for initial immunosuppressive therapy among the different age categories. The observation periods were shorter in the elderly group (P = 0.021).

Treatment During the Observation Period

During follow-up, 156 (91.2%) patients used ACE inhibitors or ARBs. Patients were divided into three groups according to the type of treatment they received during the observation period: (1) a prednisolone group comprising 35 patients (20.5%) who received prednisolone alone; (2) a cyclosporine group comprising 66 patients (38.6%) who received prednisolone and cyclosporine; and (3) a supportive therapy group comprising 70 patients (40.9%) who did not receive prednisolone or other immunosuppressive drugs. One patient in the cyclosporine group (0.6%) developed a

50% serum creatinine increase over baseline and was prescribed mizoribine.

The median initial prednisolone dose was 30 mg (interquartile range: 20–40 mg/day) and was tapered according to treatment response. Most patients in the cyclosporine group were started on cyclosporine at 1–2 mg/kg and prednisolone at 0.4–0.6 mg/kg. Cyclosporine dosing was modified by monitoring whole-blood trough levels, while prednisolone was tapered according to treatment response. The time from kidney biopsy to immunosuppressive therapy initiation was 0.7 months (interquartile range: 0.3–3.3 months).

Outcomes

Primary outcome: first complete remission. Outcome data are shown in Table 2. The median observation period for the entire cohort was 37 months (interquartile range: 15–72 months). CR from proteinuria was achieved by 103 (60.2%) patients. The mean time to CR was 14 months (interquartile range: 6–25 months).

The cumulative probabilities of achieving a CR within 1, 5, and 10 years were, respectively, 0.37, 0.74, and 0.81 for patients <65 years old; 0.45, 0.79, and 0.79 for those 65–70 years old; and 0.32, 0.86, and 0.86 for those ≥71 years old. There were no significant differences in CR from proteinuria according to patient age (P = 0.831; **Figure 1**).

Furthermore, the changes in average proteinuria over time did not differ among the various age groups (P = 0.458; **Figure S1**).

Table 2. Outcomes of 171 IMN patients.

	<65 years	65–70 years	≥71 years	P-value
Number	90	40	41	
30% reduction in eGFR [n (%)]	17 (18.9)	9 (22.5)	11 (26.8)	0.591
Decline in eGFR (mL/min per 1.73 m² per year)	2.37 (0.25–7.43)	3.06 (−2.17–8.33)	4.10 (−0.58–8.31)	0.956
ESRD [n (%)]	1 (1.1)	0 (0.0)	1 (2.4)	1.000
Death [n (%)]	1 (1.1)	3 (7.5)	7 (17.1)	0.003
Death due to infection [n (%)]	0 (0.0)	1 (2.5)	6 (14.6)	<0.001
Hospitalization due to infection [n (%)]	2 (2.2)	3 (7.5)	8 (19.5)	0.003
Hospitalization due to cardiovascular disease [n (%)]	1 (1.1)	0 (0.0)	2 (4.9)	0.197
Venous thrombotic events [n (%)]	0 (0.0)	0 (0.0)	0 (0.0)	1.000
Malignancy [n (%)]	2 (2.2)	2 (5.0)	1 (2.4)	0.671
Steroid psychosis [n (%)]	1 (1.1)	1 (2.5)	1 (2.4)	0.756
Use of antidiabetic agents [n (%)]	8 (8.9)	3 (7.5)	2 (4.9)	0.724
Aseptic osteonecrosis with surgical treatment [n (%)]	0 (0.0)	0 (0.0)	0 (0.0)	1.000
Remission				
Complete remission [n (%)]	56 (62.2)	26 (65.0)	21 (51.2)	0.383
Partial remission [n (%)]	81 (90.0)	36 (90.0)	33 (80.5)	0.270
Relapse [n (%)]	17 (24.3)	2 (6.7)	7 (21.9)	0.120

NOTE: Median (interquartile range), Conversion factors for units: SCr in mg/dL to µmol/L, ×88.4; eGFR (mL/min/1.73 m2) = 194×Scr$^{-1.094}$×Age$^{-0.287}$×0.739 (if female), total cholesterol in mg/dL to mmol/L, ×0.02586.
Abbreviations: IMN, idiopathic membranous nephropathy; eGFR, estimated glomerular filtration rate; ESRD, end-stage renal disease.

Among patients who achieved a first remission, 26 (25.2%) relapsed at least once.

Secondary outcomes: hospitalization due to infection and a 30% decline in eGFR level. During follow-up, 37 (21.6%) patients developed a 30% decline in eGFR before ESRD. In all 37 patients, eGFR levels did not improve by the last follow-up visit.

Although there were no significant differences according to patient age in 30% eGFR declines and eGFR decline rates, the average eGFR over time in patients <65 years old was significantly higher than that in ≥71 years old (P = 0.046; **Figure S2**).

Infection caused 13 (7.6%) individual patient hospitalizations and 7 (4.1%) deaths. The older age categories were significantly associated with hospitalization and death due to infection (P = 0.003). The cumulative probabilities of hospitalization due to infection within 1, 5, and 10 years were, respectively, 0.02, 0.02, and 0.02 for those <65 years old; 0.05, 0.08, and 0.08 for those 65–70 years old; and 0.16, 0.28, and 0.28 for those ≥71 years old. There were significant differences in hospitalization due to infection according to patient age (P = 0.002; **Figure 2**).

Causes of infection were tuberculosis pleuritis (n = 1), bacterial pneumonia (n = 7), *Pneumocystis jiroveci* pneumonia (n = 1), vertebral osteomyelitis (n = 1), methicillin-resistant *Staphylococcus aureus* bacteremia (n = 1), fungemia (n = 1), and pyelonephritis (n = 1).

After excluding seven patients who died because of infection, the remaining causes of death were acute subdural hematoma (n = 1), traffic accident (n = 1), sudden death (n = 1), and intestinal bleeding (n = 1). Malignancy occurred in five (2.9%) patients, whose diagnoses included esophageal cancer (n = 1), stomach cancer (n = 1), colon cancer (n = 1), prostate cancer (n = 1), and malignant lymphoma (n = 1). Only three (1.8%) patients were hospitalized for cardiovascular disease, and no patient had a venous thromboembolic event.

Treatment and clinical characteristics: comparison of patients in different treatment groups

Clinical characteristics of the three groups including (1) the prednisolone monotherapy group, (2) the combined cyclosporine group, and (3) the supportive therapy group are shown in **Tables S1 and S2 in File S1**. The serum albumin level in the supportive therapy group was significantly higher than that in the immuno-

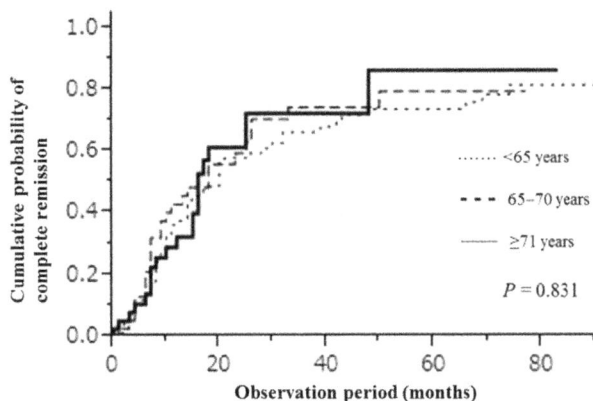

Number at risk					
<65 years	90	34	17	13	6
65–70 years	40	12	5	2	0
≥71 years	41	8	3	2	1

Figure 1. Cumulative probability of complete remission in 171 IMN patients stratified by age.

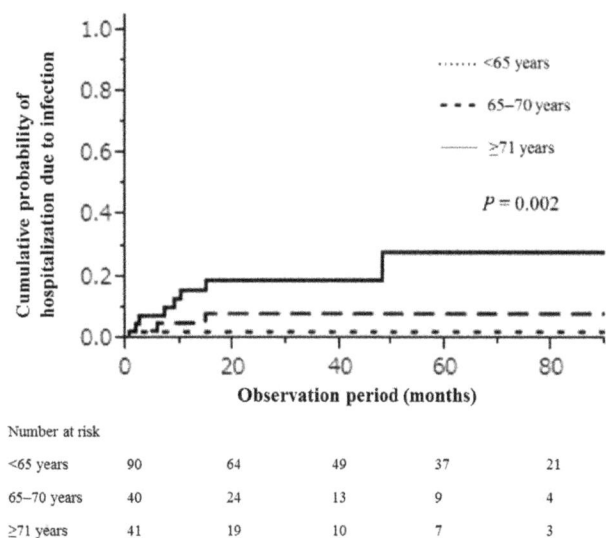

Figure 2. Cumulative probability of hospitalization due to infection in 171 IMN patients stratified by age.

Number at risk

<65 years	90	64	49	37	21
65–70 years	40	24	13	9	4
≥71 years	41	19	10	7	3

suppressive therapy groups (prednisolone monotherapy and combined cyclosporine groups) ($P<0.001$), and the urinary protein level in the supportive therapy group was significantly lower than that in the immunosuppressive therapy group ($P<0.001$). With respect to outcomes, the proportion of patients achieving a 30% eGFR decrease was not significantly different among the three groups ($P = 0.591$), whereas the proportion of patients achieving CR and the rate of hospitalization due to infection were significantly higher in the immunosuppressive therapy groups than the supportive group ($P = 0.031$ and $P = 0.032$, respectively).

Predictors of First Complete Remission

Univariate CPH models showed that a lower serum creatinine level, initial use of prednisolone monotherapy, and initial use of cyclosporine in combination with prednisolone were significantly associated with a first CR from proteinuria (**Table 3**). After adjusting for clinically relevant factors, the initial use of prednisolone monotherapy [adjusted hazard ratio (HR) = 1.78, 95% confidence interval (CI): 1.01–3.10; $P = 0.045$) and cyclosporine in combination with prednisolone (adjusted HR = 1.95. 95% CI: 1.16–3.26; $P = 0.011$) remained as significant predictors of a first CR from proteinuria.

Predictors of Infection

A total of 13 (7.6%) patients had at least one infection that required hospitalization. Of these, 12 (92.3%) received immuno-suppressive therapy before developing an infection. The median time from immunosuppressive therapy initiation to first hospitalization due to infection was 3 months (interquartile range: 1–5 months). When examining all hospitalizations due to infections, univariate analyses identified several statistically significant predictors of increased infection risk: older age, higher serum creatinine levels, and immunosuppressive therapy use, namely prednisolone monotherapy and cyclosporine combination therapy (**Table 4**).

After adjusting for clinically relevant factors, older age (adjusted HR = 3.11, 95% CI: 1.45–7.49; $P = 0.003$), prednisolone use (adjusted HR = 11.8, 95% CI: 1.59–242.5; $P = 0.014$), and cyclosporine used in combination with prednisolone (adjusted

HR = 10.3, 95% CI: 1.59–204.4; $P = 0.012$) were identified as significant predictors for the development of infection. This suggests that among older IMN patients, immunosuppressive therapy was a more important predictor of infection risk.

Because immunosuppressive therapy use may have been affected by patient age, biasing our estimate of the predictive power of age, we assessed potential associations between patient age and immunosuppressive therapy during the observation period, i.e., the cumulative dose of prednisolone and cyclosporine used during the observation period.

Compared with younger patients, the cumulative dose of prednisolone was lower in elderly patients at 3, 6, and 12 months ($P<0.001$, $P<0.001$, and $P = 0.002$, respectively; **Table S3 in File S1**). No significant trend between patient age and cyclosporine use emerged at 1, 3, 6, and 12 months ($P = 0.163$, $P = 0.740$, $P = 0.447$, and $P = 0.387$, respectively).

The median times to reach doses of 20, 15, 10, and 7.5 mg/day were shorter in elderly patients than in younger patients ($P = 0.015$, $P = 0.006$, $P<0.001$, and $P<0.001$, respectively; **Table S4 in File S1**). The cumulative doses of prednisolone to reach 20, 15, 10, and 7.5 mg/day were also lower in elderly patients than in younger patients ($P = 0.006$, $P = 0.005$, $P<0.001$, and $P<0.001$, respectively).

These results strongly suggest that the higher incidence of infections in elderly patients was not attributable to the prednisolone dose or to the type of immunosuppressive therapy.

Predictors of Infections in Patients who Received Immunosuppressive Therapy

In patients who received immunosuppressive therapy (n = 101), we evaluated predictors of infection using clinical data obtained within 1 month from initial immunosuppressive therapy including age, sex, serum creatinine, serum albumin, urinary protein at the time of initiating immunosuppressive therapy, use of immunosuppressive therapy within 1 month after treatment, initial daily dose of prednisolone, and a <25% decrease in proteinuria in the first month after immunosuppressive therapy initiation (**Table 5**).

Univariate CPH models showed that age, serum creatinine, and a <25% decrease in proteinuria in the first month after immunosuppressive therapy initiation were significant risk factors for developing infection. A multivariate CPH model adjusted for age, sex, creatinine, proteinuria at the time of initiating immunosuppressive therapy, use of immunosuppressive therapy within 1 month after starting therapy, and initial daily dose of prednisolone, was then applied. In the multivariate analysis, older age (adjusted HR = 2.80, 95% CI: 1.20–7.83; $P = 0.016$) and a < 25% decrease in proteinuria in the first month after immunosuppressive therapy initiation (adjusted HR = 7.27, 95% CI: 1.74–37.7; $P = 0.007$) were identified as significant risk factors. The −2 log likelihood values with all explanatory variables were 39.32, 39.93, and 39.96, respectively, for Cox models that included a 25% decrease, 50% decrease, and 75% decrease in proteinuria in the first month after immunosuppressive therapy initiation. Because the degrees of freedom were the same for these three models, these results indicate that the Cox model that included a 25% decrease in proteinuria was the best fit to the observed infection events.

We further stratified the decreasing rate of proteinuria in the first month after the initial multivariate analysis, and found that patients with a poor response to initial therapy had a nearly linear high risk for infection ($P = 0.006$, **Table 6**).

Because the decrease in proteinuria in the first month after initial immunosuppressive therapy may have affected subsequent treatment, resulting in bias, we evaluated the associations between

Table 3. Predictors of first CR.

	Univariate model		Multivariate model	
	HR (95% CI)	P-value	HR (95% CI)	P-value
Age (per 10 years)	0.99 (0.83–1.19)	0.886	0.98 (0.79–1.23)	0.759
Male (versus female)	0.69 (0.46–1.04)	0.075	0.77 (0.47–1.27)	0.302
Systolic blood pressure (per 10 mmHg)	1.00 (0.91–1.09)	0.959	1.06 (0.96–1.17)	0.276
Serum albumin (per 1.0 g/dL)	0.86 (0.67–1.11)	0.249	1.04 (0.74–1.45)	0.818
Serum creatinine (per 1.0 mg/dL)	0.47 (0.21–0.96)	0.037	0.25 (0.03–1.68)	0.163
Urinary protein excretion (per 1.0 g/day)	1.01 (0.95–1.06)	0.730	1.16 (0.29–4.18)	0.823
ACE inhibitor or ARB therapy	0.66 (0.44–1.02)	0.061	0.56 (0.26–1.31)	0.170
Immunosuppressive treatment during follow-up period				
No immunosuppressive agents	Reference		Reference	
Prednisolone	1.76 (1.00–2.96)	0.048	1.78 (1.01–3.10)	0.045
Prednisolone+cyclosporine	2.18 (1.41–3.36)	<0.001	1.95 (1.16–3.26)	0.011

NOTE: HR, hazard ratio; CI, confidence interval.
Data are the HR, 95% CI, and P-value from Cox proportional hazard regression analyses.
Adjusted for baseline characteristics (age, sex, systolic pressure, serum albumin level, serum creatinine level, urinary protein, use of immunosuppressive therapy).
Abbreviations: CR, complete remission; IMN, idiopathic membranous nephropathy.

proteinuria decreases (<25% vs. ≥25%) and immunosuppressive therapy during the observation period, namely, the cumulative dose of prednisolone and immunosuppressive agent use during the observation period (**Table S5 in File S1**). There were no significant differences between patients achieving <25% and ≥ 25% decreases in proteinuria with respect to the initial prednisolone dose, cyclosporine use in the first month, and the cumulative dose of prednisolone at 3, 6, and 12 months ($P = 0.164$, $P = 0.553$, and $P = 0.678$, respectively). No significant trend was between age and cyclosporine use was observed at 3, 6, and 12 months ($P = 0.526$, $P = 0.139$, and $P = 0.675$, respectively).

The median times to reach 20, 15, 10, and 7.5 mg/day doses did not between the two groups ($P = 0.143$, $P = 0.349$, $P = 0.431$, and $P = 0.650$, respectively; **Table S6 in File S1**). The cumulative doses of prednisolone to reach 20, 15, 10, and

7.5 mg/day were not different between these two groups ($P = 0.138$, $P = 0.277$, $P = 0.958$, and $P = 0.871$, respectively).

These results suggest that patients with a <25% decrease in proteinuria at 1 month did not subsequently receive a higher dose of prednisolone.

Discussion

In the current study, we investigated the clinical characteristics and outcomes of older IMN patients as compared with younger IMN patients. Furthermore, this is the first study to have examined predictors of infection in a large cohort of IMN patients.

Consistent with a previous study [2], we found that the remission rate, a 30% decline in eGFR, and the rate of decline in renal function after the onset of MN were similar in older and

Table 4. Predictors of hospitalization due to infection (n = 171).

	Univariate model		Multivariate model	
	HR (95% CI)	P-value	HR (95% CI)	P-value
Age (per 10 years)	3.07 (1.56–6.58)	<0.001	3.11 (1.45–7.49)	0.003
Male (versus female)	1.49 (0.45–6.63)	0.533	1.34 (0.37–6.29)	0.666
Serum albumin (per 1.0 g/dL)	0.73 (0.33–1.50)	0.394	1.24 (0.47–3.21)	0.662
Serum creatinine (per 1.0 mg/dL)	5.27 (1.81–12.5)	0.004	2.62 (0.83–7.70)	0.098
Urinary protein excretion (per 1.0 g/day)	0.96 (0.79–1.12)	0.613	0.92 (0.71–1.13)	0.468
Immunosuppressive treatment during follow-up period				
No immunosuppressive agents	Reference		Reference	
Prednisolone	9.54 (1.54–182.6)	0.014	11.8 (1.59–242.5)	0.014
Prednisolone+cyclosporine	7.26 (1.29–135.8)	0.022	10.3 (1.59–204.4)	0.012

NOTE: HR, hazard ratio; CI, confidence interval.
Data are the HR, 95% CI, and P-value from Cox proportional hazard regression analyses.
Adjusted for baseline characteristics (age, sex, systolic pressure, serum albumin level, serum creatinine level, urinary protein, use of immunosuppressive therapy).
Abbreviations: IMN, idiopathic membranous nephropathy.

Table 5. Predictors of hospitalization due to infection in patients treated with immunosuppressive therapy.

	Univariate model		Multivariate model	
	HR (95% CI)	P-value	HR (95% CI)	P-value
Age (per 10 years)	2.71 (1.42–5.55)	0.002	2.80 (1.20–7.83)	0.016
Male (versus female)	1.16 (0.34–5.21)	0.827	1.65 (0.39–8.46)	0.500
Serum albumin (per 1.0 g/dL)	1.12 (0.46–2.55)	0.792	2.15 (0.64–7.99)	0.217
Serum creatinine (per 1.0 mg/dL)	4.15 (1.42–9.53)	0.013	1.15 (0.31–3.88)	0.830
Urinary protein excretion (per 1.0 g/day)	0.92 (0.73–1.09)	0.374	0.94 (0.70–1.19)	0.633
Immunosuppressive treatment within 1 month after kidney biopsy				
Prednisolone	Reference		Reference	
Prednisolone+cyclosporine	1.45 (0.46–4.89)	0.524	3.22 (0.74–16.9)	0.119
Initial dose of PSL/mg/day	0.97 (0.92–1.01)	0.162	1.00 (0.94–1.07)	0.943
25% decrease of proteinuria within 1 month after initial immunosuppressive therapy	5.78 (1.67–26.4)	0.005	7.27 (1.74–37.7)	0.007

NOTE: HR, hazard ratio; CI, confidence interval.
Data are the HR, 95% CI, and P-value from Cox proportional hazard regression analyses.
This analysis is based on data from 100 patients because the decrease rate of proteinuria was missing for one patient.
Adjusted for baseline characteristics (age, sex, systolic/diastolic pressure, serum albumin level, serum creatinine level, urinary protein, use of immunosuppressive therapy, initial dose of PSL (mg)/day, 25% decrease of proteinuria within 1 month after initial immunosuppressive therapy).
Abbreviations: IMN, idiopathic membranous nephropathy.

younger IMN patients. However, our elderly patients may have died before developing a 30% decline in eGFR because the relationship between age and renal dysfunction may have been underestimated.

Our study included older patients than previously published cohort studies. Nevertheless, both remission and renal survival rates in the present study were higher than those reported by Ponticelli et al. and Jha et al. [5,6]. This indicates that Japanese patients achieve a benign course compared to patients in other countries.

Unlike previous studies [4,10], we observed that compared to younger patients, older patients presented with more severe clinical findings such as lower serum albumin levels, leg edema, and pleural effusion. In elderly patients, edema is often attributed to heart failure or venous insufficiency of the lower limbs. Edema occurs more readily in elderly patients because of reduced

elasticity of the skin and interstitial tissues. Thus, edema may coincide with higher serum albumin levels in the elderly [14].

With regard to immunosuppressive therapy, the recently published Kidney Disease Improving Global Outcomes (KDIGO) guidelines for IMN recommended a restrictive treatment strategy for IMN patients [15]. According to these guidelines, initial therapy should be started only if proteinuria is persistently >4 g/day after 6 months of conservative therapy and does not show a tendency to decline, if the serum creatinine concentration increases by >30%, or if severe, disabling, or life-threatening symptoms related to nephrotic syndrome are present. However, the KDIGO recommendations were based on studies that included only a small number of elderly patients. Therefore, the optimal immunosuppressive regimen for elderly IMN patients remains unclear.

Two retrospective studies involving 115 patients older than 60–65 years found little evidence for the benefits of glucocorticoid

Table 6. Predictors of hospitalization due to infection.

	Univariate model		Multivariate model	
	HR (95% CI)	P-value	HR (95% CI)	P-value
Decrease of proteinuria within 1 month (%)				
≥50% decrease	Reference		Reference	
25–50% decrease	0.60 (0.03–3.17)	0.609	2.27 (0.10–25.3)	0.535
0–25% decrease	7.98 (1.56–57.6)	0.014	6.52 (0.99–54.3)	0.051
Exacerbation	6.05 (1.18–43.6)	0.031	14.4 (1.87–145.6)	0.011
Test for trend		0.011		0.006

NOTE: HR, hazard ratio; CI, confidence interval.
Data are the HR, 95% CI, and P-value from Cox proportional hazard regression analyses. This analysis is based on data from 100 patients because the decrease rate of proteinuria was missing for one patient. Adjusted for baseline characteristics (age, sex, systolic/diastolic pressure, serum albumin level, serum creatinine level, urinary protein, use of immunosuppressive therapy, initial dose of PSL (mg)/day, 25% decrease of proteinuria within 1 month after initial immunosuppressive therapy).

monotherapy along with a higher incidence of adverse effects such as infection, peptic ulcer, and gastrointestinal disturbances [4,16]. Furthermore, many patients with mild-to-moderate disease achieve a spontaneous remission [17]. These studies therefore suggest that in older patients, immunosuppressive therapy should be considered only for those who are at high risk for progression and only after maximum conservative therapy has failed [11,18,19]. However, these studies provide no information regarding clinical presentation, including the prevalence of pleural effusion or the corticosteroid dose used during the follow-up period, which are important points for consideration in the elderly.

In the present study, the time from kidney biopsy to immunosuppressive therapy initiation was shorter than that recommended in the KDIGO guidelines [15]. However, our results show that elderly patients had more clinically severe symptoms than younger patients. Thus, Japanese doctors may consider that in patients with clinically severe symptoms, immunosuppressive therapy should be started as soon as possible, exhibiting different practice patterns than those observed in other countries.

As in previous studies, our elderly patients were significantly predisposed to infection. The infection incidence in our cohort did not greatly differ from those observed previously [20,21]. We found that the higher incidence of infection among elderly patients was unlikely to be due to more intensive immunosuppressive therapy because the cumulative corticosteroid dose in this age group was lower than that in younger patients. Elderly IMN patients were found to be at a higher risk for infection than younger patients.

Interestingly, we found that a <25% decrease in proteinuria at 1 month after starting immunosuppressive therapy was a significant predictor of infection. Furthermore, the higher incidence of infection associated with a <25% decrease in proteinuria in the first month after initial immunosuppressive therapy was not attributable to the prednisolone dose or the type of immunosuppressive therapy. These results suggest that poor responders after the first month of immunosuppressive therapy are vulnerable to the development of infection.

Therefore, it might be well advised to taper prednisolone more quickly among patients with a poor response to 1 month of initial immunosuppressive therapy.

However, it has also been postulated that severe nephrotic syndrome is associated with an immunologic deficit that predisposes to the development of infection. Susceptibility to bacterial infections in patients with a nephrotic syndrome has been attributed to decreased levels of IgG and the alternative complement factor B [11]. Compared with younger patients, older IMN patients had more severe symptoms of nephrotic syndrome, which may contribute to subsequent infections after the initiation of immunosuppressive therapy. Admittedly, this is a complicated subject, and it is unlikely that this retrospective analysis can address all the issues necessary to reach a conclusion whether the treatment should be intensified or not.

Our study had several limitations. First, our patients may not be representative of IMN patients in other countries. Therefore, we advise caution when interpreting and generalizing our results. Second, due to the retrospective nature of this study, the criteria used to select patients' therapeutic regimens are unknown. Selected regimens may vary across different centers, eras, or physicians. These potential biases should be included in the analyses. In actuality, we could carry out only patient-level analysis adjusted for clinically relevant factors but could not carry out a facility-level analysis to reduce confounding by indication concerning therapy selection. This is because the present study

included as many as 10 nephrology centers, some of which treated a patient number too small to evaluate using Cox proportional hazard models. Furthermore, it was difficult to add era as a covariate in our models. Third, our practice patterns are different from those recommended by the KDIGO guidelines. Namely, we often use cyclosporine in combination with corticosteroids for the first-line treatment of IMN patients. The 2012 KDIGO clinical practice guidelines for IMN recommend a cytotoxic agent (cyclophosphamide) for patients at high risk of progression [15]. However, no patients in our study were treated with cyclophosphamide. Therefore, our results should be interpreted carefully. Fourth, because the time from IMN diagnosis to immunosuppressive therapy initiation was relatively short, we did not evaluate whether nephrotic syndrome itself would predispose to infection by observing patients without immunosuppressive therapy.

Allowing for these methodological issues, our study has several advantages. It is one of the largest multicenter adult Japanese MN cohorts ever reported. Additionally, to the best of our knowledge, this is the first study to evaluate predictors of infection in IMN patients.

In conclusion, our retrospective cohort study of IMN patients showed that elderly patients were similar to younger patients in terms of renal outcomes. However, the use of immunosuppressive therapy and poor response to initial immunosuppressive therapy were significant predictors of infection among elderly IMN patients. Therefore, care should be taken when selecting a treatment strategy for these patients.

Supporting Information

Figure S1 The course of proteinuria during the follow-up period (comparison of the three age categories).

Figure S2 The course of eGFR during the follow-up period (comparison of the three age categories).

File S1 Table S1 in File S1, Baseline characteristics of 171 IMN patients: comparison of patients in different treatment groups. **Table S2,** Outcomes of 171 IMN patients: comparison of patients in different treatment groups. **Table S3,** Immunosuppressive treatment during the observation period (comparison of the three age categories). **Table S4,** Duration and cumulative dose of prednisolone (comparison of the three age categories). **Table S5,** Immunosuppressive treatment during the observation period (comparison of the decrease in proteinuria (<25% vs. ≥ 25%) in the first month after starting immunosuppressive therapy). **Table S6,** Duration and cumulative dose of prednisolone (comparison of the decrease in proteinuria (<25% vs. ≥25%) in the first month after starting immunosuppressive therapy).

File S2 Table S7, The anonymous data set of 171 patients with IMN.

Acknowledgments

We are grateful for the time and efforts of the nephrologists who supported the present study: Dr. Shizunori Ichida, Dr. Hideaki Shimizu, Dr. Junichiro Yamamoto, Dr. Tomohiko Naruse, Dr. Hirofumi Tamai, Dr. Kei Kurata, Dr. Hirotake Kasuga, Dr. Arimasa Shirasaki, and Dr. Makoto Mizutani.

Author Contributions

Conceived and designed the experiments: MY MA SK S. Maruyama. Performed the experiments: MY MA RY SA SK T. Katsuno T. Kosugi WS NT YY MM YI S. Matsuo S. Maruyama. Analyzed the data: MY MA RY. Contributed reagents/materials/analysis tools: MY MA RY SK S. Maruyama. Contributed to the writing of the manuscript: MY MA S. Maruyama.

References

1. White Book of Aging from the Government of Japan. Available: http://www8.cao.go.jp/kourei/whitepaper/w-2013/gaiyou/pdf/1s1s.pdf.
2. Cameron JS (1996) Nephrotic syndrome in the elderly. Semin Nephrol 16: 319–329.
3. Yokoyama H, Sugiyama H, Sato H, Taguchi T, Nagata M, et al. (2012) Renal disease in the elderly and the very elderly Japanese: analysis of the Japan Renal Biopsy Registry (J-RBR). Clin Exp Nephrol 16: 903–920.
4. Zent R, Nagai R, Cattran DC (1997) Idiopathic membranous nephropathy in the elderly: a comparative study. Am J Kidney Dis 29: 200–206.
5. Ponticelli C, Zucchelli P, Passerini P, Cesana B, Locatelli F, et al. (1995) A 10-year follow-up of a randomized study with methylprednisolone and chlorambucil in membranous nephropathy. Kidney Int 48: 1600.
6. Jha V, Ganguli A, Saha TK, Kohli HS, Sud K, et al. (2007) A randomized, controlled trial of steroids and cyclophosphamide in adults with nephrotic syndrome caused by idiopathic membranous nephropathy. J Am Soc Nephrol 18: 1899.
7. Ponticelli C, Altieri P, Scolari F, Passerini P, Roccatello D, et al. (1998) A randomized study comparing methylprednisolone plus chlorambucil versus methylprednisolone plus cyclophosphamide in idiopathic membranous nephropathy. J Am Soc Nephrol 9: 444.
8. Cattran DC, Appel GB, Hebert LA, Hunsicker LG, Pohl MA, et al. (2001) North America Nephrotic Syndrome Study Group Cyclosporine in patients with steroid-resistant membranous nephropathy: a randomized trial. Kidney Int 59: 1484.
9. Cattran DC, Greenwood C, Ritchie S, Bernstein K, Churchill DN, et al. (1995) A controlled trial of cyclosporine in patients with progressive membranous nephropathy. Canadian Glomerulonephritis Study Group. Kidney Int 47: 1130.
10. Hofstra JM, Wetzels JF (2012) Management of patients with membranous nephropathy. Nephrol Dial Transplant 27: 6–9.
11. Rollino C, Roccatello D, Vallero A, Basolo B, Piccoli G (1995) Membranous glomerulonephritis in the elderly. Is therapy still worthwhile? Geriatr Nephrol Urol 5: 97–104.
12. Makoto Y, Masahiko A, Ryohei Y, et al. (2014) Smoking is a risk factor for the progression of idiopathic membranous nephropathy. PLoS One, in press.
13. Matsuo S, Imai E, Horio M, Yasuda Y, Tomita K, et al. (2009) Collaborators developing the Japanese equation for estimated GFR. Revised equations for estimated GFR from serum creatinine in Japan. Am J Kidney Dis 53: 982–992.
14. Deegens JK, Wetzels JF (2007) Membranous nephropathy in the older adult: epidemiology, diagnosis and management. Drugs Aging 24: 717–732.
15. KDIGO Working Group: (2012) KDIGO clinical practice guideline for glomerulonephritis. Kidney Int Suppl 2 186–197.
16. Passerini P, Como G, Viganò E, Melis P, Pozzi C, et al. (1993) Idiopathic membranous nephropathy in the elderly. Nephrol Dial Transplant 8: 1321.
17. Philibert D, Cattran D (2008) Remission of proteinuria in primary glomerulonephritis: we know the goal but do we know the price? Nat Clin Pract Nephrol 4: 550.
18. Glassock RJ (1998) Glomerular disease in the elderly population. Geriatr Nephrol Urol 8: 149–154.
19. Bernard DB (1988) Extrarenal complications of the nephrotic syndrome. Kidney Int 33: 1184–1202.
20. Eriguchi M, Oka H, Mizobuchi T, Kamimura T, Sugawara K, et al. (2009) Long-term outcomes of idiopathic membranous nephropathy in Japanese patients treated with low-dose cyclophosphamide and prednisolone. Nephrol Dial Transplant 24: 3082–3088. doi: 10.1093/ndt/gfp251. Epub 2009 May 22.
21. Yoshimoto K, Yokoyama H, Wada T, Furuichi K, Sakai N, et al. (2004) Pathologic findings of initial biopsies reflect the outcomes of membranous nephropathy. Kidney Int 65: 148–153.

8

Comorbidities and Disease Severity as Risk Factors for Carbapenem-Resistant *Klebsiella pneumoniae* Colonization: Report of an Experience in an Internal Medicine Unit

Antonio Nouvenne[1,2]*, **Andrea Ticinesi**[1,2], **Fulvio Lauretani**[3], **Marcello Maggio**[2], **Giuseppe Lippi**[4], **Loredana Guida**[1], **Ilaria Morelli**[1], **Erminia Ridolo**[1,2], **Loris Borghi**[1,2], **Tiziana Meschi**[1,2]

1 Internal Medicine and Critical Subacute Care Unit, Parma University Hospital, Parma, Italy, 2 Department of Clinical and Experimental Medicine, University of Parma, Parma, Italy, 3 Geriatrics Unit, Parma University Hospital, Parma, Italy, 4 Laboratory of Clinical Chemistry and Hematology, Parma University Hospital, Parma, Italy

Abstract

Background: Carbapenem-resistant *Klebsiella pneumoniae* (CRKP) is an emerging multidrug-resistant nosocomial pathogen, spreading to hospitalized elderly patients. Risk factors in this setting are unclear. Our aims were to explore the contribution of multi-morbidity and disease severity in the onset of CRKP colonization/infection, and to describe changes in epidemiology after the institution of quarantine-ward managed by staff-cohorting.

Methods and Findings: With a case-control design, we evaluated 133 CRKP-positive patients (75 M, 58 F; mean age 79±10 years) and a control group of 400 CRKP-negative subjects (179 M, 221 F; mean age 79±12 years) admitted to Internal Medicine and Critical Subacute Care Unit of Parma University Hospital, Italy, during a 10-month period. Information about comorbidity type and severity, expressed through Cumulative Illness Rating Scale-CIRS, was collected in each patient. During an overall 5-month period, CRKP-positive patients were managed in an isolation ward with staff cohorting. A contact-bed isolation approach was established in the other 5 months. The effects of these strategies were evaluated with a cross-sectional study design. CRKP-positive subjects had higher CIRS comorbidity index (12.0±3.6 vs 9.1±3.5, p<0.0001) and CIRS severity index (3.2±0.4 vs 2.9±0.5, p<0.0001), along with higher cardiovascular, respiratory, renal and neurological disease burden than control group. CIRS severity index was associated with a higher risk for CRKP-colonization (OR 13.3, 95%CI6.88–25.93), independent of comorbidities. Isolation ward activation was associated with decreased monthly incidence of CRKP-positivity (from 16.9% to 1.2% of all admissions) and infection (from 36.6% to 22.5% of all positive cases; p=0.04 derived by Wilcoxon signed-rank test). Mortality rate did not differ between cases and controls (21.8% vs 15.2%, p=0.08). The main limitations of this study are observational design and lack of data about prior antibiotic exposure.

Conclusions: Comorbidities and disease severity are relevant risk factors for CRKP-colonization/infection in elderly frail patients. Sanitary measures may have contributed to limit epidemic spread and rate of infection also in internal medicine setting.

Editor: Hiroshi Nishiura, The University of Tokyo, Japan

Funding: The authors have no support or funding to report.

Competing Interests: The authors have declared that no competing interests exist.

* Email: antonio.nouvenne@alice.it

Introduction

In the era of antibiotic resistance and multi-drug resistant bacteria, the emergence and spread of carbapenem-resistant *Klebsiella pneumoniae* (CRKP), also known as carbapenemase-producing *Klebsiella pneumoniae*, has rapidly become a major health concern for hospitalized patients in industrialized countries [1]. Carbapenemases are β-lactamases that can hydrolyze carbapenems. Their outbreak in clinical isolates of Gram negative bacteria has been appreciated since the late 1990 s, with an increasing number of carbapenem-affine types identified ever since [2–3]. *Klebsiella pneumoniae* is the most frequent bacterial species associated with production of high-affinity carbapenemases. Their

genes typically reside on transferable plasmids and are conventionally known as KPC. The first in vivo isolation of a CRKP strain dates back to 2000 in an intensive care unit of North Carolina [4]. During the following years, CRKP has been responsible of a large number of nosocomial outbreaks in many hospitals of Northeastern United States, causing a large number of deaths due to septic shock [5]. CRKP had reached all developed countries worldwide by the end of the 2000 s. In Europe, CRKP has an heterogeneous distribution, with some countries such as Poland and Greece, where CRKP infection is currently considered as endemic, and others such as Sweden and Portugal, where only few sporadic cases have been identified [6]. The first Italian CRKP isolation was recorded in Florence in 2009 in a patient with complicated intra-abdominal infection [7]. Since then, CRKP has rapidly spread throughout the country. This explains why Italy, that was classified only a few years ago as a nation with sporadic isolations, has been recently upgraded to an endemic country [6,8]. Moreover, recent national data showed that CRKP is more frequently isolated from patients outside intensive care units (ICU), often admitted to geriatric or internal medicine wards [9–11].

CRKP is generally transmitted by contact and primarily colonizes lower intestinal tract and inguinal or perineal skin, so that active microbiological screening is regarded as an effective measure to prevent the onset of infection [12]. The main risk factors for colonization or infection identified in literature are critical illness and chronic diseases such as respiratory failure, prior antibiotic therapy and prior hospitalization [13–15]. When the infection occurs, it is generally associated with a bloodstream bacteremia followed by quick development of septic shock. Blood culture isolation of CRKP is an independent predictor of death, and the overall mortality ranges from 41% to 80% despite the establishment of appropriate antibiotic therapy [16–18]. Therapeutic options are indeed very limited, and include aminoglycosides, tigecycline, colistin, fosfomycin or even carbapenems themselves, when the minimal inhibitory concentrations (MICs) are ≤4 mg/L [19–21].

Few studies have investigated the characteristics of CRKP outbreaks in populations of elderly frail hospitalized patients with multi-morbidity. However, the quick spread of this pathogen in general internal medicine and geriatric wards around the globe may suggest that chronic diseases could play a major role as risk factors.

Aims

We carried out a case-control study to explore the contribution of multi-morbidity and disease severity, measured through literature-validated indexes, in the onset of CRKP colonization/infection in a population of hospitalized, elderly and frail patients. With a cross-sectional study design, we have then described the changes in CRKP epidemic trend and rate of infection occurred after the institution of special sanitary measures, namely quarantine ward with staff cohorting management.

Setting and Methods

The University Hospital of Parma, Italy, is a 1218-bed tertiary referral facility with approximately 51300 admissions per year. From August 2011 to May 2012, it has been the scenario of a pandemic outbreak of CRKP colonization and infection. This phenomenon especially involved older patients admitted to general internal medicine units. In order to limit the diffusion of CRKP, Healthcare Hospital Direction arranged an immediate transfer of all patients with a CRKP positivity to Internal Medicine and Critical Subacute Care Unit. This unit, a 94-bed large internal medicine area, split in smaller wards and organized by intensity of care, is mainly dedicated to the care of elderly frail patients.

All CRKP-positive patients were managed by contact isolation precautions. They received antibiotic therapy only in the presence of clinical or laboratory signs of infection. Colonized patients with no signs of infection were not treated.

Following the recommendations issued by Italian Health Ministry and Emilia-Romagna Region Health Authority [22], all high-risk patients admitted to our unit and all patients with clinical signs of infection underwent an active microbiological surveillance program consisting of a weekly rectal swab for CRKP detection. A patient was considered at high risk of CRKP infection if he/she

had been transferred from another hospital or from a community nursing home, hospitalized in the previous 60 days, transferred from an intensive care unit, in contact (i.e., in the same room) with a CRKP-positive patient or completely bedridden for at least 3 days. In case of clinical signs of infection, other microbiological tests, such as blood or urine culture, were prescribed whenever appropriate and according to the clinical characteristics of each patient. Surveillance was continued until the patient was discharged or had 3 consecutive rectal swabs negative for CRKP detection.

Moreover, given the high number of CRKP-positive patients, from October 2011 (two months after the beginning of the outbreak) to February 2012, under the indication of Healthcare Hospital Direction, a 14-bed isolation ward with a staff-cohorting management was activated. This ward was reserved only to CRKP-positive patients with dedicated health care professionals that could not come to contact with other CRKP-negative patients. A simple model validated in the literature and already used to control multi-drug resistant infection outbreaks was used [23–24]. This 14-bed isolation ward was closed at the end of February 2012, since its maintenance was considered no longer cost-effective by Healthcare Hospital Direction, due to the rapid and consistent decrease of new cases of CRKP positivity. Colonized or infected patients admitted thereafter were only managed by contact isolation precautions until the end of the observation period. Active microbiological surveillance was continued throughout the study period, regardless of the management by staff cohorting or contact isolation.

To assess whether comorbidity number and severity is a risk factor for CRKP colonization/infection, we carried out a case-control study (Figure 1). We reviewed all clinical records of patients admitted to our unit from August 2011 to May 2012 (1897 subjects) to check CRKP status. CRKP positivity was defined as the presence of at least one biological sample positive for CRKP. All patients admitted to our unit who failed to meet the requirements for epidemiological surveillance program or who had microbiological analysis (i.e., all rectal swabs) negative for CRKP were considered as CRKP-negative. For the study purposes, all consecutive CRKP-positive patients (133 subjects) who were identified during the study period were considered as cases. We also randomly selected 400 clinical records of CRKP-negative patients and considered them as controls.

Moreover, subjects in whom CRKP was isolated only in rectal swabs performed for epidemiological surveillance reasons and with other biological samples resulted negative for CRKP, were considered as CRKP-colonized. Subjects who had clinical signs of infection and at least one biological sample, other than rectal swab, positive for CRKP were considered as CRKP-infected, irrespective of their rectal swab status.

In both cases and controls, a well-trained physician recorded age, primary diagnosis, type and severity of comorbidities according to the Cumulative Illness Rating Scale (CIRS) score [25], overall hospital length of stay, biological sample of CRKP isolation and genotypic characteristics when available, possible clinical signs of CRKP infection and final outcome (discharge or death).

To describe changes in epidemiologic trend after the institution of the staff cohorting quarantine ward, we also carried out a cross-sectional study (Figure 1). We considered only CRKP-positive patients, classified as colonized or infected according to the above criteria. Incidence of CRKP-positivity was calculated as the number of newly diagnosed cases per month related to the overall number of admissions in the same month. Outbreak control was defined as a persistent decline or stability in the trend of monthly

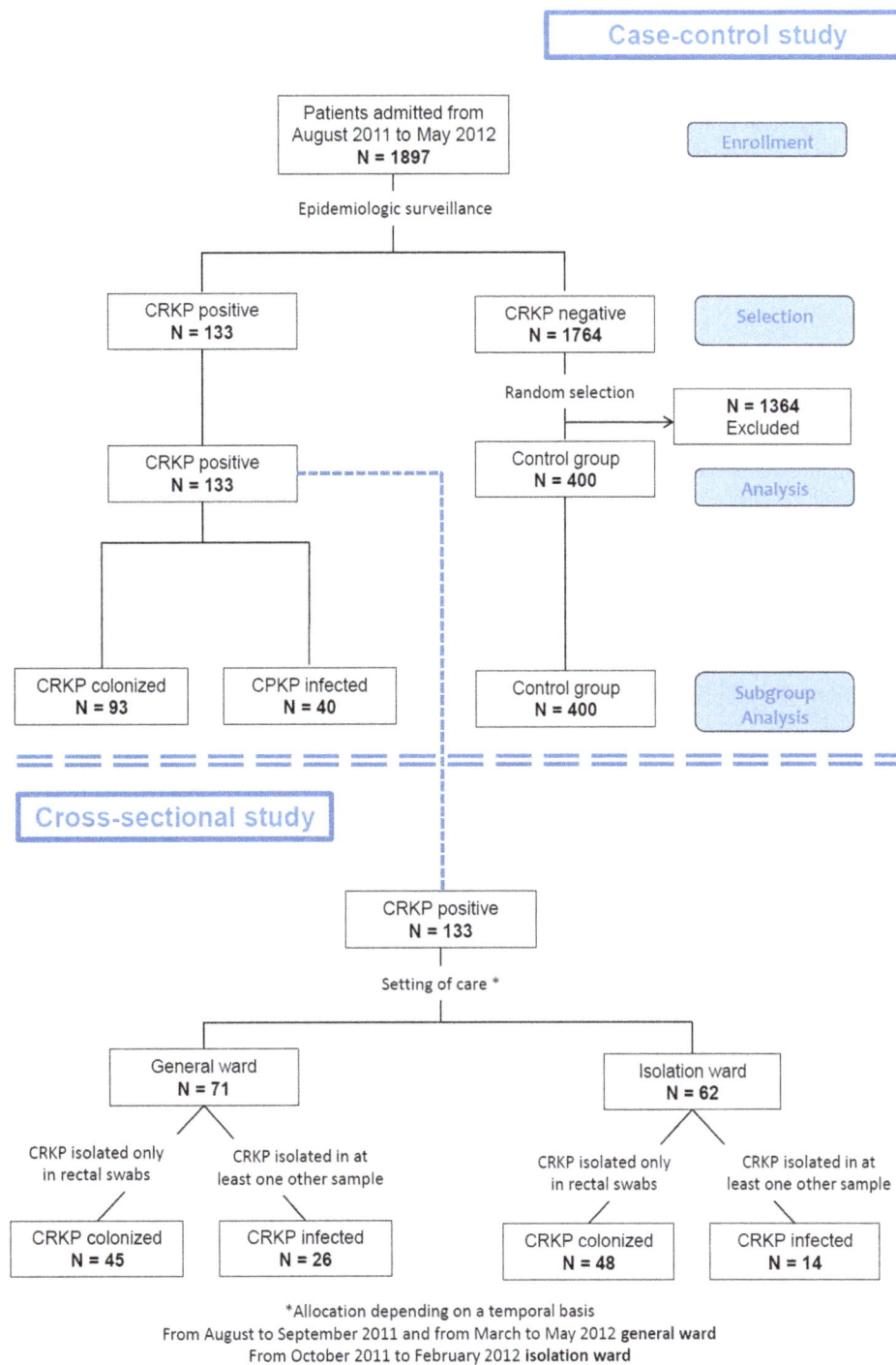

Figure 1. Summary of the study design.

incidence. The rate of infection was calculated as the percentage of CRKP-infected patients related to the overall number of CRKP-positive patients. Data about CRKP genotype was also recorded for each patient whenever available.

The protocol was authorized by the Ethics Committee of Healthcare Hospital Direction of Parma University Hospital, that is also supported by a Scientific Research Board and a specific Research Plan approved by Geriatric-Rehabilitation Department. All patients signed a specific informed consent form at time of admission, stating that the patient authorizes personal and clinical data treatment and analysis in aggregate way for scientific-statistic research purposes according to Italian legislation. All the clinical investigations were performed according to the principles expressed in the Declaration of Helsinki.

For descriptive purposes, baseline characteristics of cases and controls were compared using a χ^2 test (Mantel-Haenszel method) and ANOVA model for categorical and continuous variables, respectively.

Bivariate tests were used: χ^2 for dichotomic variables was used to test the significance of categorical covariates. Parametric (ANOVA) and non-parametric test, the Wilcoxon signed-rank test, were used to assess the significance of continuous covariates. Logistic regression analysis was used to examine the relationship between CIRS category in the case group compared to control group.

All analyses were performed using SAS (version 8.2, SAS Institute, Inc., Cary, NC) with a statistical significance level set at $p < 0.05$.

Results

The total number of CRKP-positive patients observed from August 2011 to May 2012 (42 weeks) was 133 (75 M, 58 F; mean age 79 ± 12 years). The control group (400 patients) included 179 males and 221 females, with a mean age of 79 ± 10 years. In the same period, the overall number of patients admitted to our unit was 1897, so that the overall incidence of CRKP positivity was 7%.

As also shown in Figure 1, 93 patients out of 133 cases (70%), were classified as simply CRKP-colonized, while 40 patients (30%) were CRKP-infected. The biological samples, other than rectal swabs, in which CRKP was first isolated in infected subjects were blood or vascular catheters in 21 cases (52.5%), urine in 13 cases (32.5%), phlegm in 3 cases (7.5%) and surgical wound swabs in other 3 cases (7.5%).

CRKP-positive patients had a large number of comorbidities with a high degree of clinical complexity, as attested by high values of CIRS comorbidity and CIRS severity indexes (Table 1). Both indexes were significantly higher in CRKP-positive patients than in controls (comorbidity index 12.0 ± 3.6 vs 9.1 ± 3.5; $p < 0.0001$; severity index 3.2 ± 0.4 vs 2.9 ± 0.5; $p < 0.0001$) (Table 1). The comparison of the mean values of each CIRS score item between cases and controls is shown in Table 2. CRKP-positive patients had a significantly higher burden of cardiovascular, respiratory, renal, neurological and musculoskeletal disorders than CRKP-negative patients. Cardiovascular and respiratory diseases were indeed the most frequent among the case group, with a prevalence of 64% and 54%, respectively. The role of cardiovascular, respiratory, neurological and renal diseases as risk factors for CRKP colonization was confirmed by logistic regression analysis, and appeared to be independent of age, sex, head and neck, upper and lower gastrointestinal, hepatic, urological, endocrine and psycho-behavioral diseases (Table 3). Moreover, a high CIRS severity index was found to be the leading risk factor for CRKP positivity (odds ratio 13.3; 95% CI 6.88–25.93; $p < 0.0001$).

A subgroup analysis performed on infected vs colonized patients showed that neither the CIRS comorbidity score (11.5 ± 3.1 vs 12.2 ± 3.8, $p = 0.36$), nor the CIRS severity index (3.1 ± 0.3 vs 3.2 ± 0.4, $p = 0.55$) were statistically different between these two groups.

Mean hospital length of stay was significantly longer in CRKP-positive patients than in the control group (35 ± 24 vs 18 ± 12 days, $p < 0.001$), as also shown in Table 1.

Twenty-nine CRKP-positive patients out of 133 died during hospitalization (21.8%). However, the mortality rate was not significantly different compared to that observed in the control group (61/400 subjects, 15%; $p = 0.08$). When only CRKP-infected patients were considered, the hospital mortality rate was 47.5%, while it was much lower in CRKP-colonized patients (10 patients out of 93; 10.7%).

A total number of 71 CRKP-positive patients was managed in the general medical ward with simple contact bed isolation precautions (from August to September 2011 and from March to May 2012). Sixty-two CRKP-positive patients were managed with staff cohorting approach in the isolation ward (from October 2011 to February 2012), as shown in Figure 1. The highest monthly incidence was observed in the first two months of the epidemic outbreak (23 and 18 new cases per month, with a 16.9% and a 13.2% monthly incidence, respectively). After the activation of the staff cohorting isolation ward, a net decrease in incidence of new cases was observed, with an average of 8 cases per month (range 3–13). A statistical analysis performed with Wilcoxon signed-rank test demonstrated that the decrease between the first (August–September 2011) and the second period (October 2011–February 2012) was statistically significant ($p = 0.04$). After closure of the quarantine ward at the end of February 2012, an increased incidence of new CRKP cases was recorded, although not statistically significant (second period October 2011–February 2012 vs third period March–May 2012, $p = 0.08$). The overall monthly incidence trend is shown in Figure 2. The mean monthly incidence during the period of quarantine ward management was 4.0%, whereas it was 10.3% in the period of general ward management. This difference was statistically significant ($p = 0.03$), as also shown in Figure 3.

The rate of CRKP-infected patients was similar in the subgroup managed by contact isolation approach in general ward (26 subjects out of 71, 36.6%) and in the subgroup managed by staff cohorting approach in isolation ward (14 subjects out of 62, 22.5%, $p = 0.07$ with Mantel-Haenszel chi-square). Mortality was also not statistically different in the two groups (16.1% in quarantine ward vs 26.7% in general ward, $p = 0.14$ with Mantel-Haenszel chi-square).

Information about the CRKP genotype was available in 102 out of 133 patients. In 76 patients (74%) the strain was positive for blaKPC or other type A carbapenemases, in 12 patients (12%) the strain was positive for type B carbapenemases, namely New Delhi metallo-beta-lactamase (NDM-1), whereas in the remaining 14 patients (14%) the isolated CRKP strain was genotypically classified as not carbapenemase producer. The infection and mortality rates were higher in patients positive for NDM-1-producing strains (50% and 42%, respectively) than in patients positive for type A carbapenemase-producing strains (25% and 17%, respectively) and in patients positive for non-carbapenemase-producing strains (29% and 7%, respectively). The groups exhibited also similar CIRS comorbidity score and severity index.

Discussion

CRKP has rapidly emerged as a notable cause of nosocomial infections in Italy, with a high potential for developing large pandemic outbreaks [9,11,18,26–28]. In this study, we have demonstrated that chronic comorbidities, namely cardiovascular, respiratory, renal and neurological impairments, along with disease severity, play a relevant role as risk factors for CRKP colonization/infection in elderly hospitalized subjects. To our knowledge, this is the first study in a population of frail elderly with a large number of comorbidities admitted to an internal medicine setting. The present investigation is also one of the few that considered this health issue from a genuine clinical perspective, more focused on disease-related risk factors for CRKP colonization/infection rather than on microbiological or molecular issues. The main limitations are the retrospective design, the lack of data about prior antibiotic exposure and functional status of patients before admission. Moreover, comorbidities were assessed through CIRS, which is not completely objective even when performed by a trained physician, although well-validated in medical literature.

Table 1. Characteristics of the study population.

	CASES n = 133	CONTROLS n = 400	p*
Age (years) (mean ± SD)	79±12	79±10	0.50
Men (n, %)	75 (56.4)	221 (55.3)	0.94
CIRS comorbidity Score**	**12.0±3.6**	**9.1±3.5**	**<0.0001**
CIRS severity Index***	**3.2±0.4**	**2.9±0.5**	**<0.0001**
Number of comorbidities****	**3.8±1.2**	**3.3±1.5**	**<0.0001**
Hospital length of stay (days)	**35±24**	**18±12**	**<0.0001**

* Age- and sex-adjusted (where possible).
** CIRS comorbidity Score was calculated as the sum of each of the first 13 items of organ or system disease, excluding only psycho-behavioral disease item. For each item, a score ranging from 0 to 4 can be given. 0 means absence of disease, while 4 means a potential life-threatening disease.
*** CIRS severity Index represents the number of times that a patient ranks 3 or 4 points in each of the 14 items of CIRS (psycho-behavioral disease included).
**** Number of comorbidities was calculated as the number of acute or chronic illnesses that were recorded during the hospital stay for each patient.
CIRS = Cumulative Index Rating Scale.

Some risk factors for CRKP colonization and infection have already been investigated in the literature. For example, the importance of prior antibiotic exposure, especially to carbapenems, has been earlier emphasized [13–15].

Few studies have assessed the role of specific comorbidities as risk factors for developing a CRKP colonization or infection. There is actually only one study, performed in an ICU setting, that has associated a specific chronic disease, namely chronic obstructive pulmonary disease (COPD), with the risk of CRKP positivity [14]. Our data seem to confirm this finding, since CRKP-positive patients do have a higher degree of respiratory impairment than control subjects, although we also showed that cardiovascular, neurological and kidney disease may represent other substantial risk factors. Therefore, in our experience, a high number of comorbidities is an outstanding element influencing the risk of becoming CRKP-positive (Tables 2–3).

As also shown in an ICU context [13–16], disease severity is another relevant risk factor, irrespective of the number of comorbidities. According to our data, patients with a high CIRS severity index actually have an impressive 13-fold risk of becoming CRKP-positive, regardless of single organs or systems involved in disease. Thus, we can argue that CRKP, both in ICUs and in internal medicine wards, mainly affects frail complex patients with severe prognosis. In this subset of patients, in whom the clinical course is often difficult to manage, CRKP provides a new, sometimes fatal, element of clinical complexity. However, it is also noteworthy that a higher risk for infection is a finding common to resistant organisms in these patients. CRKP has actually epidemiologic features similar to the ones of other emerging nosocomial pathogens.

Therefore, it should be no longer only considered a typical ICU concern, but also a pathogen that internal medicine health care professionals and physicians need to deal with.

Table 2. Differences between singular CIRS categories in the cases compared to controls.

CIRS CATEGORY*	CASES n = 133	CONTROLS n = 400	p**
Heart disease	**2.12±1.52**	**1.13±1.42**	**<0.0001**
Hypertension	**1.34±1.12**	**0.73±0.91**	**<0.0001**
Vascular, hematological disease	0.84±1.55	0.67±1.31	0.20
Respiratory disease	**1.97±1.78**	**1.05±1.54**	**<0.0001**
Eye, ear, nose, and throat disease	0.12±0.68	0.10±0.43	0.73
Upper gastrointestinal disease	0.30±1.02	0.37±0.99	0.53
Lower gastrointestinal disease	0.47±1.23	0.50±1.22	0.76
Liver disease	0.12±0.67	0.15±0.62	0.62
Kidney disease	**1.03±1.55**	**0.61±1.23**	**0.001**
Other genitourinary disease	0.14±0.71	0.21±0.74	0.28
Musculoskeletal, skin disease	**0.27±1.00**	**0.58±1.23**	**0.009**
Neurological disease	**1.30±1.72**	**0.96±1.51**	**0.03**
Endocrine, metabolic disease	0.72±1.20	0.77±1.44	0.70
Psychiatric or cognitive disease	1.30±1.81	1.29±1.53	0.73

* All the single CIRS items are listed in this Table. For each item, a score ranging from 0 to 4 can be given. 0 means absence of disease, while 4 means a potential life-threatening disease.
** Age- and sex-adjusted.
CIRS = Cumulative Index Rating Scale.

Table 3. Odds of association between CIRS category in the case group (n = 133) compared to control group (n = 400).

	ODDS RATIO	95% CI	p*
CIRS severity Index	**13.3**	**6.88–25.93**	**<0.0001**
Hypertension	1.96	1.43–2.70	<0.0001
Heart disease	1.68	1.36–2.09	<0.0001
Respiratory disease	1.46	1.25–1.70	<0.0001
Vascular, hematological disease	1.39	1.16–1.66	0.0004
Kidney disease	1.37	1.14–1.64	<0.0001
Neurological disease	1.33	1.12–1.57	0.001

* Also adjusted for age; sex; eye, ear, nose and throat disease; upper and lower gastrointestinal disease; liver disease; other genitourinary diseases; endocrine and metabolic disease; psychiatric and cognitive diseases.
CIRS = Cumulative Index Rating Scale.

However, despite the high comorbidity burden of our patients, the recorded mortality rate was surprisingly not as high as that reported in literature [16–18]. As a matter of fact, the number of deaths was not significantly different in all CRKP-positive patients than those recorded in the control group of CRKP-free patients. However, when the CRKP infection occurs, the mortality rises due to the high risk of fatal septic shock. The mortality rate that we have recorded in CRKP-infected subjects is actually very similar to that previously reported in our country by Tumbarello and colleagues in a multicenter study [18]. We can hypothesize that simple rectal colonization by CRKP does not significantly modify the clinical course of frail elderly patients with multiple comorbidities. However, when the infection occurs, it significantly threatens survival of these patients, similarly to what has been shown in ICU patients. Further research is needed to better understand factors that induce the transformation of colonization into infection, both in intensive care and internal or geriatric medicine settings.

In our experience, we have also observed the effects of an isolation ward activation with a staff cohorting management, as an attempt to limit the contacts of CRKP-negative patients with colonized or infected patients. However, the cross-sectional design of the study does not allow to establish whether or not the variations in incidence of CRKP positivity are causally related to different management strategies. Moreover, patients were managed by staff cohorting or by contact bed precautions on a temporal basis and not on a random assignment. However, the remarkable decrease of monthly incidence observed after the institution of these measures, combined with the new increase detected after the isolation ward was closed (Figure 2), indirectly suggests that this approach may be related to a decrease in the incidence of new cases. Our data also indicate that this strategy may help reducing the rate of CRKP-positive patients that develop a clinical infection by CRKP. Further research is needed to confirm these hypotheses. Staff cohorting management is a simple sanitary measure, which was proven effective in other nosocomial pandemics [24–25]. Some recent studies in Greece demonstrated that the implementation of basic hand hygiene and contact precautions by health care professionals, isolation of CRKP-positive patients in dedicated rooms and staff cohorting are effective, either alone or in combination, to limit the spread of CRKP, although in surgical and intensive care settings [29–30]. There are also reports in which even more strict hygienic measures have been applied, such as daily chlorhexidine baths for positive patients, environmental surveillance for CRKP detection on surfaces at high risk for contamination and meticulous daily environmental cleaning [31–32]. These measures are obviously

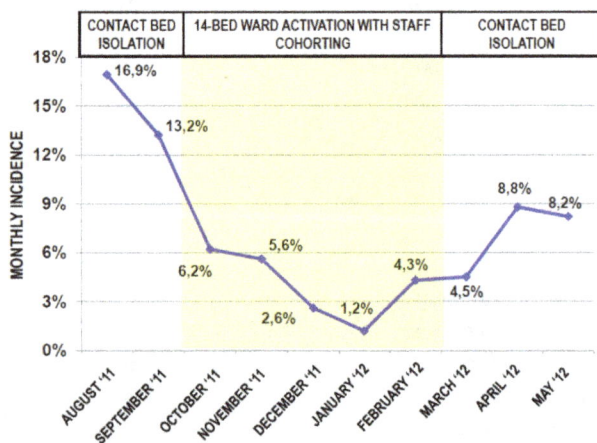

Figure 2. Trend in monthly incidence of CRKP positive cases in the period studied. (CRKP = Carbapenemase-resistant *Klebsiella pneumoniae*).

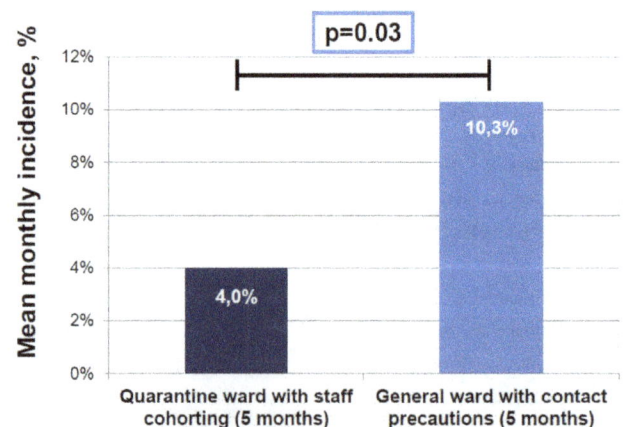

Figure 3. Comparison of mean monthly incidence of new cases of CRKP positivity between quarantine ward management period and general ward management period. Statistical analysis performed with analysis of variance. (CRKP = Carbapenemase-resistant *Klebsiella pneumoniae*).

more difficult to be established in a non-ICU setting. Nevertheless, it is plausible that the higher number of hygienical precautions are established, the more effective is the prevention protocol for limiting multi-drug resistant outbreaks, even in geriatric frail patients.

However, possible biases should also be taken into account for the interpretation of our results. For example, considering that the lowest incidence in our experience was reported during winter months, we cannot exclude that CRKP colonization/infection outbreaks exhibit a seasonal periodicity. Our data are in agreement with those from a large multicenter epidemiologic study that some years ago evaluated non-multidrug-resistant *Klebsiella pneumoniae* strains [33]. Interestingly, opposite data emerged from a subsequent study conducted in a temperate climate area of the United States [34].

Conclusions

CRKP outbreaks are becoming a relevant health issue, not only in an intensive care setting, but also in internal medicine and geriatric wards. Special sanitary measures, such as epidemiologic surveillance with weekly rectal swabs, bed isolation and quarantine ward activation with staff cohorting management may play a role in controlling the epidemic spread.

Our experience clearly suggests that a high number of comorbidities, and particularly cardiovascular, respiratory, renal and neurological disease, and high disease severity represent relevant risk factors for colonization and infection in elderly frail patients. Therefore these data open new scenarios for the most suitable strategies for issuing effective preventive measures in those patients at higher risk, not only admitted in ICU setting but also in general internal medicine wards. The clinicians' awareness and knowledge of this problem will therefore be crucial in the future for management of these severe hospital pandemics. Future research is needed to assess the relationships between the domains of frailty and chronic illness and the risk for CRKP colonization or infection.

Acknowledgments

We are grateful to Prof. Matteo Goldoni for his smart advice in the phase of manuscript preparation and revision.

Author Contributions

Conceived and designed the experiments: AN AT LB TM. Performed the experiments: LG IM ER. Analyzed the data: AN AT FL MM. Wrote the paper: AN AT GL TM.

References

1. Chen LF, Anderson DJ, Paterson DL (2012) Overview of the epidemiology and the threat of *Klebsiella pneumoniae* carbapenemases (KPC) resistance. Infect Drug Resist 5: 133–141.
2. Nordmann P, Poirel L (2002) Emerging carbapenemases in Gram-negative aerobes. Clin Microbiol Infect 8: 321–331.
3. Cornaglia G, Giamarellou H, Rossolini GM (2011) Metallo-β-lactamases: a last frontier for β-lactams? Lancet Infect Dis 11: 381–393.
4. Yigit H, Queenan AM, Anderson GJ, Domenech-Sanchez A, Biddle JW, et al. (2001) Novel carbapenem-hydrolyzing β-lactamase, KPC-1, from a carbapenem-resistant strain of *Klebsiella pneumoniae*. Antimicrob Agents Chemother 45: 1151–1161.
5. Lomaestro BM, Tobin EH, Shang W, Gootz T (2006) The spread of *Klebsiella pneumoniae* carbapenemase-producing *K. pneumoniae* to upstate New York. Clin Infect Dis 43: e26–e28.
6. Munoz-Price LS, Poirel L, Bonomo RA, Schwaber MJ, Daikos GL, et al. (2013) Clinical epidemiology of the global expansion of *Klebsiella pneumoniae* carbapenemases. Lancet Infect Dis 13: 785–796.
7. Giani T, D'Andrea MM, Pecile P, Borgianni L, Nicoletti P, et al. (2009) Emergence in Italy of *Klebsiella pneumoniae* sequence type 258 producing KPC-3 carbapenemase. J Clin Microbiol 47: 3793–3794.
8. Nordmann P, Cuzon G, Naas T (2009) The real threat of *Klebsiella pneumoniae* carbapenemase-producing bacteria. Lancet Infect Dis 9: 228–236.
9. Gaibani P, Ambretti S, Berlingeri A, Gelsomino F, Bielli A, et al. (2011) Rapid increase of carbapenemase-producing Klebsiella pneumoniae strains in a large Italian hospital: surveillance period 1 March-30 September 2010. Euro Surveill 12: pii 19800.
10. Giani T, Pini B, Arena F, Conte V, Bracco S, et al. (2013) Epidemic diffusion of KPC carbapenemase-producing *Klebsiella pneumoniae* in Italy: results of the first countrywide survey, 15 May to 30 June 2011. Euro Surveill 18: pii 20489.
11. Gagliotti C, Ciccarese V, Sarti M, Giordani S, Barozzi A, et al. (2013) Active surveillance for asymptomatic carriers of carbapenemase-producing *Klebsiella pneumoniae* in a hospital setting. J Hosp Infect 83: 330–332.
12. Nordmann P, Gniadkowski M, Giske CG, Poirel L, Woodford N, et al. (2012) Identification and screening of carbapenemase-producing *Enterobacteriaceae*. Clin Microbiol Infect 18: 432–438.
13. Gasink LB, Edelstein PH, Lautenbach E, Synnestvedt M, Fishman NO (2009) Risk factors and clinical impact of *Klebsiella pneumoniae* carbapenemase-producing *K. pneumoniae*. Infect Control Hosp Epidemiol 30: 1180–1185.
14. Papadimitriou-Olivgeris M, Marangos M, Fligou F, Christofidou M, Bartzavali C, et al. (2012) Risk factors for KPC-producing *Klebsiella pneumoniae* enteric colonization upon ICU admission. J Antimicrob Chemother 67: 2976–2981.
15. Armand-Lefèvre L, Angebault C, Barbier F, Hamelet E, Defrance G, et al. (2013) Emergence of imipenem-resistant Gram-negative bacilli in intestinal flora of intensive care patients. Antimicrob Agents Chemother 57: 1488–1495.
16. Mouloudi E, Protonotariou E, Zagorianou A, Iosifidis E, Karapanagiotou A, et al. (2010) Bloodstream infections caused by metallo-β-lactamase/*Klebsiella pneumoniae* carbapenemase-producing *K. pneumoniae* among intensive care unit patients in Greece: risk factors for infection and impact of type of resistance on outcomes. Infect Control Hosp Epidemiol 31: 1250–1256.

17. Zarkotou O, Pournaras S, Tselioti P, Dragoumanos V, Pitiriga V, et al. (2011) Predictors of mortality in patients with bloodstream infections caused by KPC-producing *Klebsiella pneumoniae* and impact of appropriate antimicrobial treatment. Clin Microbiol Infect 17: 1798–1803.
18. Tumbarello M, Viale P, Viscoli C, Trecarichi EM, Tumietto F, et al. (2012) Predictors of mortality in bloodstream infections caused by *Klebsiella pneumoniae* carbapenemase-producing *K. pneumoniae*: importance of combination therapy. Clin Infect Dis 55: 943–950.
19. Livermore DM, Warner M, Mushtaq S, Doumith M, Zhang J, et al. (2011) What remains against carbapenem-resistant Enterobacteriaceae? Evaluation of chloramphenicol, ciprofloxacin, colistin, fosfomycin, minocycline, nitrofurantoin, temocillin and tigecycline. Int J Antimicrob Agents 37: 415–419.
20. Hirsch EB, Guo B, Chang KT, Cao H, Ledesma KR, et al. (2013) Assessment of antimicrobial combinations for *Klebsiella pneumoniae* carbapenemase-producing *K. pneumoniae*. J Infect Dis 207: 786–793.
21. Daikos GL, Markogiannakis A (2011) Carbapenemase-producing *Klebsiella pneumoniae*: (when) might we still consider treating with carbapenems? Clin Microbiol Infect 17: 1135–1141.
22. Gagliotti C, Cappelli V, Carretto E, Pan A, Sarti M, et al. Indicazioni pratiche e protocolli operativi per la diagnosi, la sorveglianza e il controllo degli enterobatteri produttori di carbapenemasi nelle strutture sanitarie e socio-sanitarie. Regione Emilia-Romagna, Agenzia Sanitaria e Sociale Regionale. Bologna, January 2013. http://assr.regione.emilia-romagna.it/it/servizi/pubblicazioni/rapporti-documenti. Accessed on December 2nd, 2013. Italian language.
23. Jochimsen EM, Fish L, Manning K, Young S, Singer DA, et al. (1999) Control of vancomycin-resistant enterococci at a community hospital: efficacy of patient and staff cohorting. Infect Control Hosp Epidemiol 20: 106–109.
24. Chitnis AS, Caruthers PS, Rao AK, Lamb J, Lurvey R, et al. (2012) Outbreak of carbapenem-resistant Enterobacteriaceae at a long-term acute care hospital: sustained reductions in transmission through active surveillance and targeted interventions. Infect Control Hosp Epidemiol 33: 984–992.
25. Miller MD, Paradis CF, Houck PR, Mazumdar S, Stack JA, et al. (1992) Rating chronic medical illness burden in geropsychiatric practice and research: application of the Cumulative Illness Rating Scale. Psychiatry Res 41: 237–248.
26. Agodi A, Voulgari E, Barchitta M, Politi L, Koumaki V, et al. (2011) Containment of an outbreak of KPC-3-producing *Klebsiella pneumoniae* in Italy. J Clin Microbiol 49: 3986–3989.
27. Giuffrè M, Bonura C, Geraci DM, Saporito L, Catalano R, et al. (2013) Successful control of an outbreak of colonization by *Klebsiella pneumoniae* carbapenemase-producing *K. pneumoniae* sequence type 258 in a neonatal intensive care unit, Italy. J Hosp Infect 85: 233–236.
28. Aschbacher R, Giani T, Corda D, Conte V, Arena F, et al. (2013) Carbapenemase-producing Enterobacteriaceae during 2011-12 in the Bolzano area (Northern Italy): incresing diversity in a low-endemicity setting. Diagn Microbiol Infect Dis 77: 354–356.
29. Spysa V, Psichogiou M, Bouzala GA, Hadjihannas L, Hatzakis A, et al. (2012) Transmission dynamics of carbapenemase-producing Klebsiella pneumoniae

and anticipated impact of infection control strategies in a surgical unit. PLoS One 7: e41068.

30. Poulou A, Voulgari E, Vrioni G, Xidopoulos G, Pliagkos A, et al. (2012) Imported *Klebsiella pneumoniae* carbapenemase-producing *K. Pneumoniae* clones in a Greek hospital: impact of infection control measures for restraining their dissemination. J Clin Microbiol 50: 2618–2623.

31. Munoz-Price LS, Hayden MK, Lolans K, Won S, Calvert K, et al. (2010) Successful control of an outbreak of *Klebsiella pneumoniae* carbapenemase-producing *K. pneumoniae* at a long-term acute care hospital. Infect Control Hosp Epidemiol 31: 341–347.

32. Munoz-Price LS, De La Cuesta C, Adams S, Wyckoff M, Cleary T, et al. (2010) Successful eradication of a monoclonal strain of *Klebsiella pneumoniae* carbapenemase-producing *K. pneumoniae* outbreak in a surgical intensive care unit in Miami, Florida. Infect Control Hosp Epidemiol 31: 1074–1077.

33. Anderson DJ, Richet H, Chen LF, Spelman DW, Hung YJ, et al. (2008) Seasonal variation in *Klebsiella pneumoniae* bloodstream infection on 4 continents. J Infect Dis 197: 752–756.

34. Al-Hasan MN, Lahr BD, Eckel-Passow JE, Baddour LM (2010) Epidemiology and outcome of *Klebsiella* species bloodstream infection: a population-based study. Mayo Clin Proc 85: 139–144.

9

Postural Instability Detection: Aging and the Complexity of Spatial-Temporal Distributional Patterns for Virtually Contacting the Stability Boundary in Human Stance

Melissa C. Kilby[1]*, Semyon M. Slobounov[1,2], Karl M. Newell[1,2]

1 Department of Kinesiology, The Pennsylvania State University, University Park, Pennsylvania, United States of America, 2 Center for Sport Concussion Research and Services, The Pennsylvania State University, University Park, Pennsylvania, United States of America

Abstract

Falls among the older population can severely restrict their functional mobility and even cause death. Therefore, it is crucial to understand the mechanisms and conditions that cause falls, for which it is important to develop a predictive model of falls. One critical quantity for postural instability detection and prediction is the instantaneous stability of quiet upright stance based on motion data. However, well-established measures in the field of motor control that quantify overall postural stability using center-of-pressure (COP) or center-of-mass (COM) fluctuations are inadequate predictors of instantaneous stability. For this reason, 2D COP/COM virtual-time-to-contact (VTC) is investigated to detect the postural stability deficits of healthy older people compared to young adults. VTC predicts the temporal safety margin to the functional stability boundary (= limits of the region of feasible COP or COM displacement) and, therefore, provides an index of the risk of losing postural stability. The spatial directions with increased instability were also determined using quantities of VTC that have not previously been considered. Further, Lempel-Ziv-Complexity (LZC), a measure suitable for on-line monitoring of stability/instability, was applied to explore the temporal structure or complexity of VTC and the predictability of future postural instability based on previous behavior. These features were examined as a function of age, vision and different load weighting on the legs. The primary findings showed that for old adults the stability boundary was contracted and VTC reduced. Furthermore, the complexity decreased with aging and the direction with highest postural instability also changed in aging compared to the young adults. The findings reveal the sensitivity of the time dependent properties of 2D VTC to the detection of postural instability in aging, availability of visual information and postural stance and potential applicability as a predictive model of postural instability during upright stance.

Editor: Ramesh Balasubramaniam, University of California, Merced, United States of America

Funding: These authors have no support or funding to report.

Competing Interests: The authors have declared that no competing interests exist.

* Email: mck18@psu.edu

Introduction

Falls, in particular among the elderly, are a serious threat to their functional mobility in activities of daily living [1–2]. It is crucial to understand what mechanisms and processes cause falls in the elderly. To do so, there is a pressing need for fall prediction and detection algorithms [3–5] and more generally for methods that identify groups of people at a higher risk of falling due to disease or aging [1,6–8]. Previous research has considered numerous factors such as diabetes mellitus, history of falls, fear of falling, visual impairment, depression or postural control deficits (increased postural sway) as fall predictors in the elderly [9–12]. Postural sway, that is, the amount of whole body postural motion (center-of-pressure (COP) or center-of-mass (COM) fluctuations) in quiet standing is a well-established measure in the field of motor control [13–15]. It has been shown that healthy aging progressively increases postural motion when standing still over time periods of 20-30 s up to several min [2,16]. However, the commonly reported overall postural motion appears to be an inadequate predictor of instantaneous stability in quiet upright stance, because even if an overall greater amount of postural motion happens to coincide with reduced overall stability, this measure may not provide an estimate of the level of instantaneous stability [17–20]. Yet, quantification of the instantaneous postural stability is pivotal in developing applicable on-line falls prediction algorithms.

Mechanical inverted pendulum models of upright stance [18,20] and virtual time-to-contact (VTC) approaches [21–24] appear to be more relevant in the regard of dynamic prediction. VTC quantifies the temporal proximity to the stability boundary, which is commonly defined geometrically as the outside edge of the feet that coincides with the limits of the base of support [18,20]. Thus, VTC is highly relevant to postural stability from a mechanical point of view. The general emphasis in this view is the temporal safety margin to the stability boundary based on the current spatial position, velocity and acceleration of the COM or COP [22–23,25] rather than the spatial and/or temporal departure from a presumed fixed point in the center of the postural stability region [15]. A direct implication is that a close position of the COM to the stability boundary together with a high velocity away from the nearest boundary can indeed reflect a relatively stable state. Among older people VTC has been shown to be a viable predictor of the instant of taking a step after a perturbation [25] and Slobounov et al. [22] also showed that 2D VTC was reduced with aging due to increased postural motion that takes place within a reduced stability boundary region [26].

The novelty of our study here was to implement the 2D VTC approach of Slobounov et al. [22] as a predictive model of postural instability in the elderly using dynamic quantities of VTC that have not been previously considered. More specifically, we aimed to quantify not only the temporal proximity to the stability boundary, but also to address the related fundamental question as to the direction of postural motion in which instability is increased [5,27–28]. The directional information is critical in characterizing weaknesses or limitations of the postural control system and has the potential to being a direct indicator of an increased risk of falls into specific directions [3,5]. To extract the directional information, we analyzed the spatial location on the 2D boundary of the stability region at which the virtual second order trajectory of COP or COM intersected the boundary. The stability boundary was divided into different segments in order to perform a distributional analysis of the probability of virtual contacts and the associated magnitude of VTC across the boundary segments. These polar distributions hold theoretical and clinical implications because actual and simulated falls have been reported with the indication of the direction of falling [3–5].

To our knowledge previous studies of quiet upright stance have solely analyzed postural responses more generally in anterior-posterior (AP) and medial-lateral (ML) directions, showing that AP usually exceeds ML motion [15,29–30]. However, a more direct examination of postural instability in specific directions, for example, in the forward, backward or forward sideways directions has mostly been carried out in perturbation or leaning studies [23,27–28]. Our study examined this new feature of VTC in young and old adults through removing visual information feedback [6] and enhancing postural motion near the lateral stability boundary by increasing the loading of one leg [31–33]. Furthermore, a dynamic sway condition allowed us to test the effect of this in contrast to the typical quiet stance condition. Of particular interest was whether the dynamic condition would channel the minimum VTC to a lower level than occurs in quiet stance through being dynamical closer (in a temporal limit sense) to the stability boundary.

The analysis of the time-dependent structure of VTC was included into the here introduced predictive model of postural instability as it has long been recognized that the temporal structure of postural adjustments quantifies a critical, non-mechanical property of postural stability [19,34–35]. A reduced temporal structure, commonly termed complexity, is traditionally interpreted as a functional decline of the regulation of the postural control system – a feature that would enhance the likelihood of losing postural stability. Previous research has shown that the age related increase of postural motion in quiet stance occurs concomitantly with a reduction in the time- and frequency-dependent structure of the postural motion [35–37]. These patterns of change in the motor control of posture with aging have been shown to relate to the *loss of complexity* of the output of the motor system [36,38] in that there is an age-related inverse relation between the dispersion and structure/complexity of postural motion [34–35,37], that is hypothesized to be dependent on the task and the emergent attractor dynamics [36].

Here we investigate whether aging reduces the complexity of the spatial-temporal distributional patterns for virtually contacting the postural stability boundary. To study the complexity of VTC we applied the Lempel-Ziv-Complexity (LZC) algorithm [39]. As opposed to the generally applied non-linear time series analysis tools in the field of postural control [19,34–35,37] we applied LZC as this algorithm is applicable for on-line monitoring [40], requires a shorter minimum data length and finally the computational cost is lower. The basic idea of this algorithm is to detect repetitive patterns in a given sequence and dates back to finding algorithms to compress any given data set and, therefore, saving storage space. It is interpreted that if there are such recurrent patterns, there is redundant information and the shortest description of the critical information contained in the sequence must be shorter than the sequence length and thus can be compressed. A lower information content/complexity or higher consistency/structure links to increased predictability. Recognizing the degree of predictability of a system is an ambitious goal in many research fields [41], in that: 1) quantifying the predictability may correct the assumption of an at first sight random looking human process [6,42] and 2: improving the ability to predict in our case human postural performance through algorithms may help to reveal in advance extended periods of postural instability based on previous performance.

The primary purpose of this study was to validate and extend 2D VTC as an approach to construct an applicable predictive model of postural instability during upright stance in the elderly. Therefore, aside from investigating the effects of aging, we also tested the effects of the availability of visual information (vision and no vision) and different loadings of the legs on the spatial-temporal distribution and complexity properties of VTC during two footed upright side by side stance. We hypothesized that VTC depends on age, and that this dependency would be influenced by the visual feedback condition and weight distributions between the legs. We predicted that: 1) the removal of visual information and aging would decrease the area of the stability region and the magnitude of VTC; 2) with aging, the withdrawal of vision and the manipulation of the weight loading on each foot would produce less stable spatial-temporal distributional patterns for virtually contacting the stability boundary; and 3) that the complexity of VTC dynamics will be reduced by aging, the withdrawal of visual information and the unequal load weighting on the legs.

Methods

Participants

Two age groups were recruited for this study, one group of twelve young adults (22.2 ± 2.6 years, 5 males and 7 females) and one group of twelve old adults (69.7 ± 2.3 years, 6 males and 6 females). All participants were self-reported non-fallers. In addition, based on self-report all participants were free from any neurological or neuromotor disorders and musculoskeletal injuries that could affect balance. The experimental protocol was approved by the Institutional Review Board of the Pennsylvania State University. After giving written informed consent, participants started with the experimental procedures.

Apparatus

Whole body motion capture was realized using Qualisys Track Manager Software (Qualisys AB, Gothenburg, Sweden) and six ProReflex cameras that tracked the 3D coordinates of 22 passive reflective skin markers. Ground reaction force and moment signals were collected using two adjacent AMTI (American Mechanical Technology, Inc., Watertown, MA) strain gauge force platforms. The kinematic and kinetic data were synchronized and sampled at 100 Hz.

Experimental procedures

There were two manipulations: vision and leg weight loading. Each loading condition was performed with and without vision (eyes open and eyes closed). The 4 different load weightings of the legs were: approximately equal weight on both feet (EqWe), more weight on the left leg (LWe) or on the right leg (RWe), and dynamically shifting the weight between legs during the trial (Dyn). Except for the dynamic trials, the task goal was to stand as still as possible for the entire duration of the trial. For the dynamic condition a 0.15 Hz metronome was implemented as an acoustic cue for shifting load on the feet. When shifting the weight to one leg, participants were asked to load one leg as much so that the posture was most comfortable. The trunk, however, should not be bent sideways.

Prior to data collection markers were attached to the skin at the following landmarks: Distal Phalanges, 5th metatarsal, heel, lateral malleolus, lateral femoral epicondyle, greater trochanter, iliac crest, acromion process, lateral humeral epicondyle, dorsal wrist (between radial and ulnar styloid), and the lateral aspect of the head (anterior to ear canal). Participants were then asked to adopt a comfortable double leg standing posture on both force platforms (one foot on each of the two platforms) with the feet approximately hip width apart. A trace of this foot position was taken, so that the foot placement was the same for each trial.

Initially, the functional stability boundaries with eyes open and eyes closed were recorded. Participants were asked to maximally lean forward, backward and to either side without raising heels [22]. Subsequently the experimental trial blocks (3 trials of 30 s each condition) were conducted.

Data processing

Data were processed in Matlab (MathWorks, Natick, MA). Postural center of pressure (COP) excursions were derived from the digitally low-pass filtered (10 Hz cutoff) ground reaction force and moment time series and whole body center of mass (COM) excursions were derived from the low-pass filtered (6 Hz cutoff) marker coordinates. The COM position was calculated as the weighted sum of segmental center of mass positions. We modeled the human body as 13 rigid segments (head, the upper arms and forearms/hands, thorax/abdomen, pelvis, and thighs, shanks and feet) using constant Dempster's body segment parameters to be consistent with previous work [15].

Data analysis

The magnitude of the COP stability boundary was assessed through the area of the stability boundary model (Figure 1) and the amount of COP motion through the 2D path length. The analysis of the COM motion was limited to the motion in anterior-posterior (AP) and medial-lateral (ML) directions. Input data for VTC calculation in custom written Matlab code were the 2D position of the COP or COM along with the instantaneous velocity and acceleration vectors, respectively. In addition, the matching experimental boundary trial (for example boundary trial with removed vision for all no vision trials) was loaded simultaneously.

From this boundary trial a multi-segment polygon consisting of 40 line segments (Figure 1) was derived to model the coordinates of the functional stability boundary. The extrema of the functional stability boundary ellipse were based on the maximum motion of the COP or COM to the front, back and either side during the experimental boundary trials. Each segment of the boundary spans a sector of 9°. The supplementary video animation (Video S1) can be accessed for visualization of how the functional stability boundary was modelled.

Subsequently, the virtual time (τ) the COP or COM would need to contact with the stability boundary if it were to continue from the current position ($\vec{r} = [r_x, r_y]T$) with instantaneous initial velocity ($\vec{v} = [v_x, v_y]T$) and instantaneous constant acceleration ($\vec{a} = [a_x, a_y]T$) was extracted. Thus, we used a second order approximation to the virtual trajectory as it has been proposed to more appropriately represent the postural dynamics [17,22].

The VTC (τ) at each time instant (30 s at 100 Hz) was computed as follows [Haibach et al. 2007]. Let (x_c, y_c) denote the point on the stability boundary where the virtual trajectory intersects it for the first time. If the end points of the corresponding boundary line segment are (x_1, y_1) and (x_2, y_2) the slope (s) of the line connecting the two points is

$$s = (y_2 - y_1)/(x_2 - x_1) \tag{1}$$

Assuming constant slope in the differential segment between (x_1, y_1) and (x_2, y_2), the slope can also be computed as

$$s = (y_c - y_1)/(x_c - x_1) \tag{2}$$

Assuming a point mass model for the COM and constant acceleration, the point of virtual contact can be written as,

$$x_c(\tau) = r_x + v_x \cdot \tau + a_x \cdot \frac{\tau^2}{2} \tag{3}$$

$$y_c(\tau) = r_y + v_y \cdot \tau + a_y \cdot \frac{\tau^2}{2} \tag{4}$$

Substituting x_c and y_c from equations 3–4 in 2, and equating it to 1, gives a quadratic equation in τ. VTC (τ) is the lowest positive solution of this quadratic equation. In the case where both velocity and acceleration were zero, VTC would be infinity.

The mean and minimum values of VTC were computed. Furthermore, the VTC time series was decomposed into as many time series as boundary segments, yielding a separate VTC time series for each of the 40 boundary segments. This representation related the VTC properties to the spatial location for virtually contacting the stability boundary. On this basis, we studied the distributional patterns across boundary segments for the mean VTC magnitude and the probability of virtual contacts.

The sequence of the virtually contacted boundary segments (Boundary) over time was further processed with non-parametric tools. We computed the algorithmic information theory-based Lempel Ziv complexity (LZC) of these sequences [39]. This complexity measure characterizes the time evolutionary development of spatial-temporal patterns in nonlinear systems. To our knowledge this measure has previously not been used for analysis of postural sway data. However, it has been extensively used for analyzing other physiological measures, such as EEG data [40]. LZC is based on the number of distinct subsequences contained in the given sequence when scanning the finite sequence from left to right. The reader can refer to Zhang et al. [40] for a detailed description of the implemented LZC code. According to Kaspar and Schuster [43] the LZC was normalized to the upper theoretical limit that is based on the sample length and number

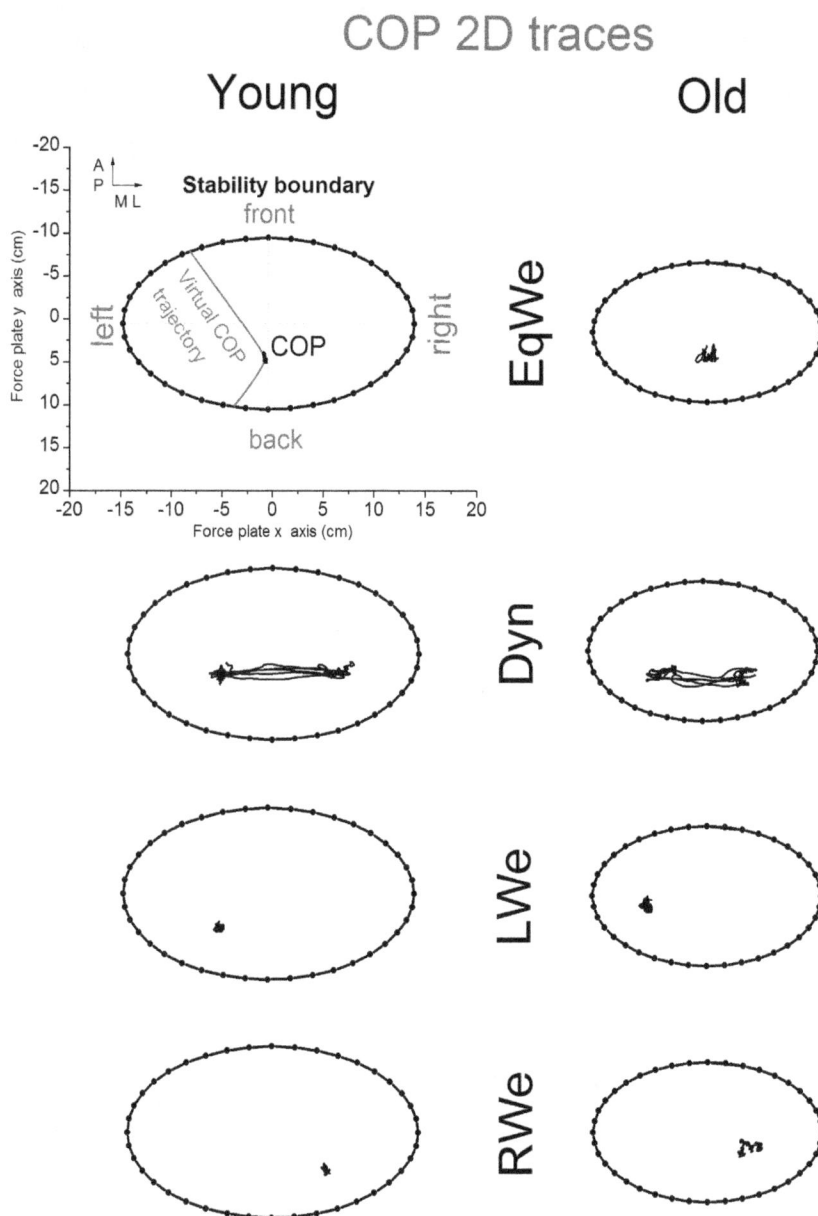

Figure 1. In the upper left panel the 2D COP path of one single representative trial with normal vision, the respective polygon representation of the 2D functional stability boundary and two virtual COP trajectories at arbitrary time instants are illustrated in original aspect ratio, resolved in the force platform coordinate system. Each boundary segment represented one specific direction in relation to the COP (e.g. front or back segments). Additional representative 2D traces of the COP with the functional stability boundary as a function of age and loading (with normal vision) are also illustrated.

of symbols contained in the sequence. Higher LZC values are indicative of greater complexity and the normalized LZC in biological signals is usually less than 1 [40].

Statistics

The statistical analysis was performed using an Age (2 levels) by Vision (2 levels) by Loading (4 levels) ANOVA with repeated measures on the last two factors. The significance level was set at $p<0.05$. Post hoc pairwise multiple comparisons were made with the Bonferroni correction procedure. We used R software for the statistical analysis.

Results

COP displacement and COP stability boundary

Figure 2 shows the mean COP path length as a function of age, vision and leg loading condition. There were main effects of vision ($F_{1,22} = 20.98$, $p<0.01$), loading ($F_{1.09,24.15} = 234.72$, $p<0.01$), and a significant age × loading interaction ($F_{1.09,24.15} = 3.80$, $p<0.05$).

Post hoc analysis showed that COP path length significantly increased under no vision. The age × loading interaction showed that COP path length only significantly increased for the old compared to the young group during the EqWe and LWe conditions. Further the age × loading interaction revealed that for both age groups COP path length was highest under Dyn

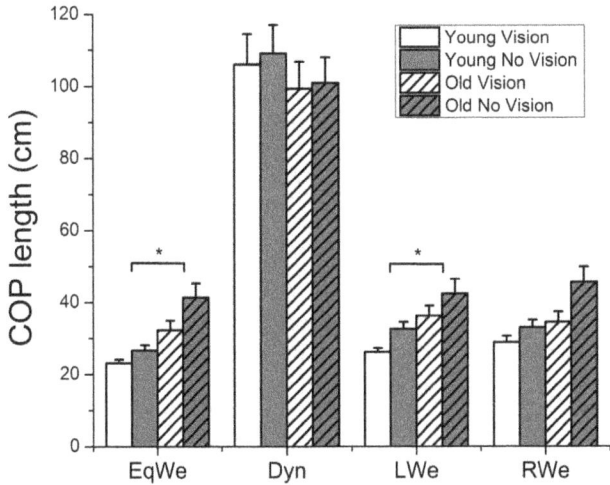

Figure 2. Group mean ± SE (N = 12) 2D COP path length as a function of age, vision and loading. The asterisks * illustrate the significant age × loading interaction with regard to age.

compared to all other conditions. For the young adults the COP path length was also higher under either RWe or LWe in contrast to EqWe.

The functional COP stability boundary was significantly reduced with aging ($F_{1,22} = 33.63$, p<0.01) and when vision was removed ($F_{1,22} = 36.10$, p<0.01). Figure 1 shows representative 2D COP displacement traces for each of the 4 leg loading conditions with the respective stability boundary.

Standard statistical properties of VTC (using COP)

The upper two panels of Figure 3 show the mean VTC mean and min values using the 2D COP data. The main effects of age (VTC min $F_{1,22} = 11.97$, p<0.01; VTC mean $F_{1,22} = 23.92$, p< 0.01), vision (VTC min $F_{1,22} = 22.60$, p<0.01; VTC mean $F_{1,22} = 60.92$, p<0.01), loading (VTC min $F_{3,66} = 99.54$, p<0.01; VTC mean $F_{3,66} = 82.82$, p<0.01), and the age × vision (VTC min $F_{1,22} = 8.53$, p<0.01) and age × loading (VTC min $F_{3,66} = 3.40$, p<0.05) interactions were significant.

VTC mean values generally decreased with the withdrawal of vision, whereas VTC min decreased with the withdrawal of vision only for the old adults. The VTC mean values were significantly reduced for the old compared to the young group. In addition, the VTC min age × loading interaction revealed that the VTC min values were only significantly reduced for the old compared to the

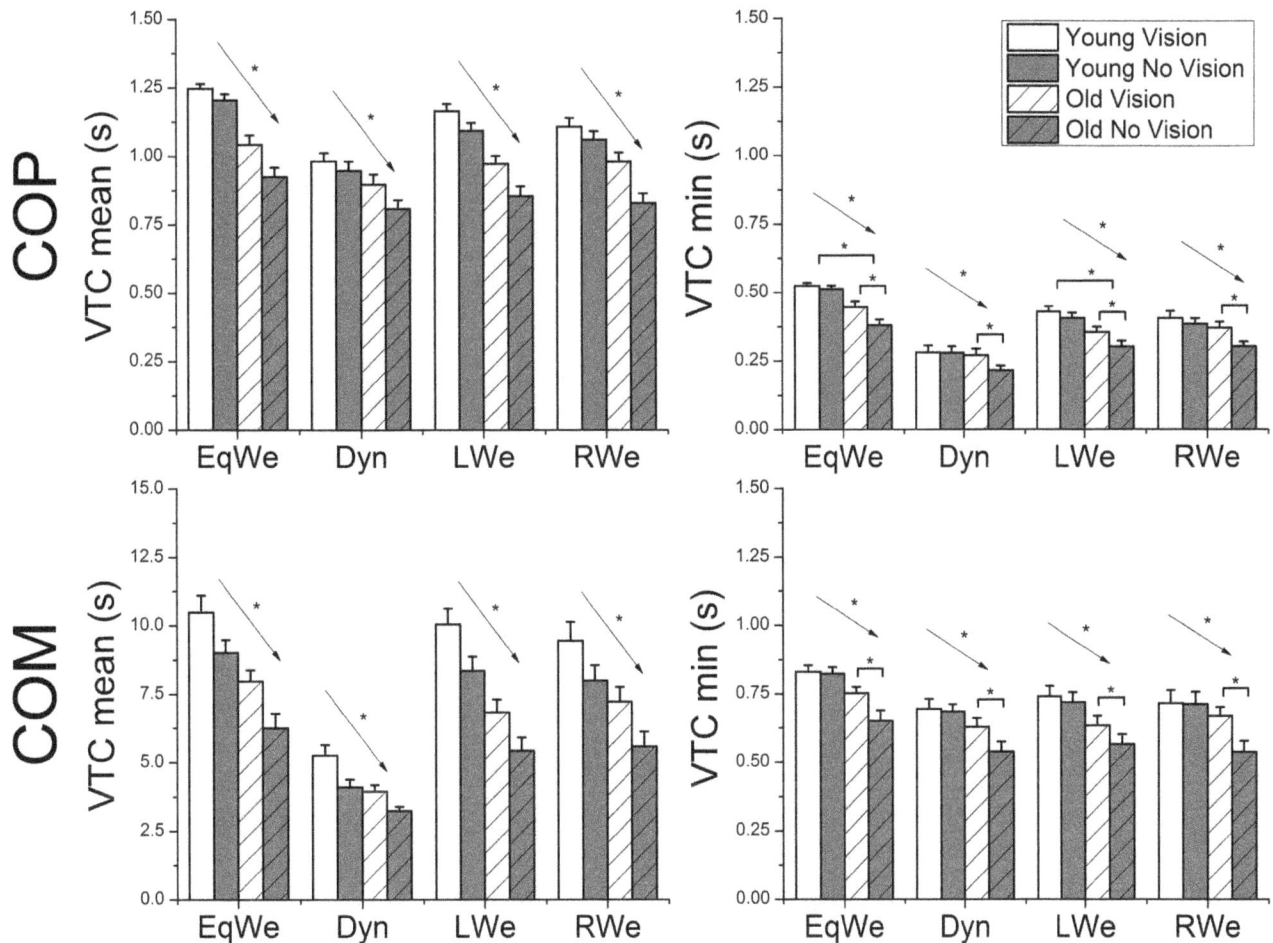

Figure 3. Group mean ± SE (N = 12) VTC mean and minimum values for both COP and COM as a function of age, vision and loading. The asterisks * illustrate the significant age × vision interaction with regard to vision and the age × loading interaction with regard to age. The arrow with asterisk indicates significant main effects of age and vision.

young adults during EqWe and LWe. Further, post hoc analysis of the main effect of loading for both VTC mean and min values showed that either LWe or RWe reduced the VTC values compared to EqWe. Dyn had the lowest VTC values compared to the remaining conditions.

Standard statistical properties of VTC (using COM)

The lower two panels of Figure 3 show the mean VTC mean and min values using the 2D COM data. The main effects of age (VTC min $F_{1,22} = 8.68$, p<0.01; VTC mean $F_{1,22} = 16.12$ p< 0.01), vision (VTC min $F_{1,22} = 12.78$, p<0.01; VTC mean $F_{1,22} = 65.33$ p<0.01), loading (VTC min $F_{3,66} = 21.23$, p<0.01; VTC mean $F_{2.08,45.94} = 121.65$ p<0.01), and the age × vision (VTC min $F_{1,22} = 8.26$, p<0.01) and age × loading (VTC mean $F_{2.08,45.94} = 121.65$ p<0.01) interactions were significant. VTC mean values were significantly decreased with the withdrawal of vision, whereas VTC min values decreased with the withdrawal of vision only for the old adults. Further, the VTC mean and min

values were significantly reduced for the old compared to the young group.

The VTC mean age × loading interaction revealed that for the old both LWe and RWe induced lower VTC values compared to EqWe. Dyn showed the lowest VTC compared to the remaining loading conditions. For the young group EqWe had significantly higher VTC than RWe. Dyn also showed the lowest VTC compared to all remaining conditions. Finally, post hoc analysis for the VTC min main effect of loading showed that EqWe was significantly higher than Dyn or RWe or LWe.

Spatial-temporal distributional patterns of VTC

Figures 4, 5, 6, and 7 show the mean VTC mean values and the mean probability of virtual contacts for each of the 40 boundary segments. The polar distributions are displayed separately for both COP and COM data with vision available and under the removal of vision.

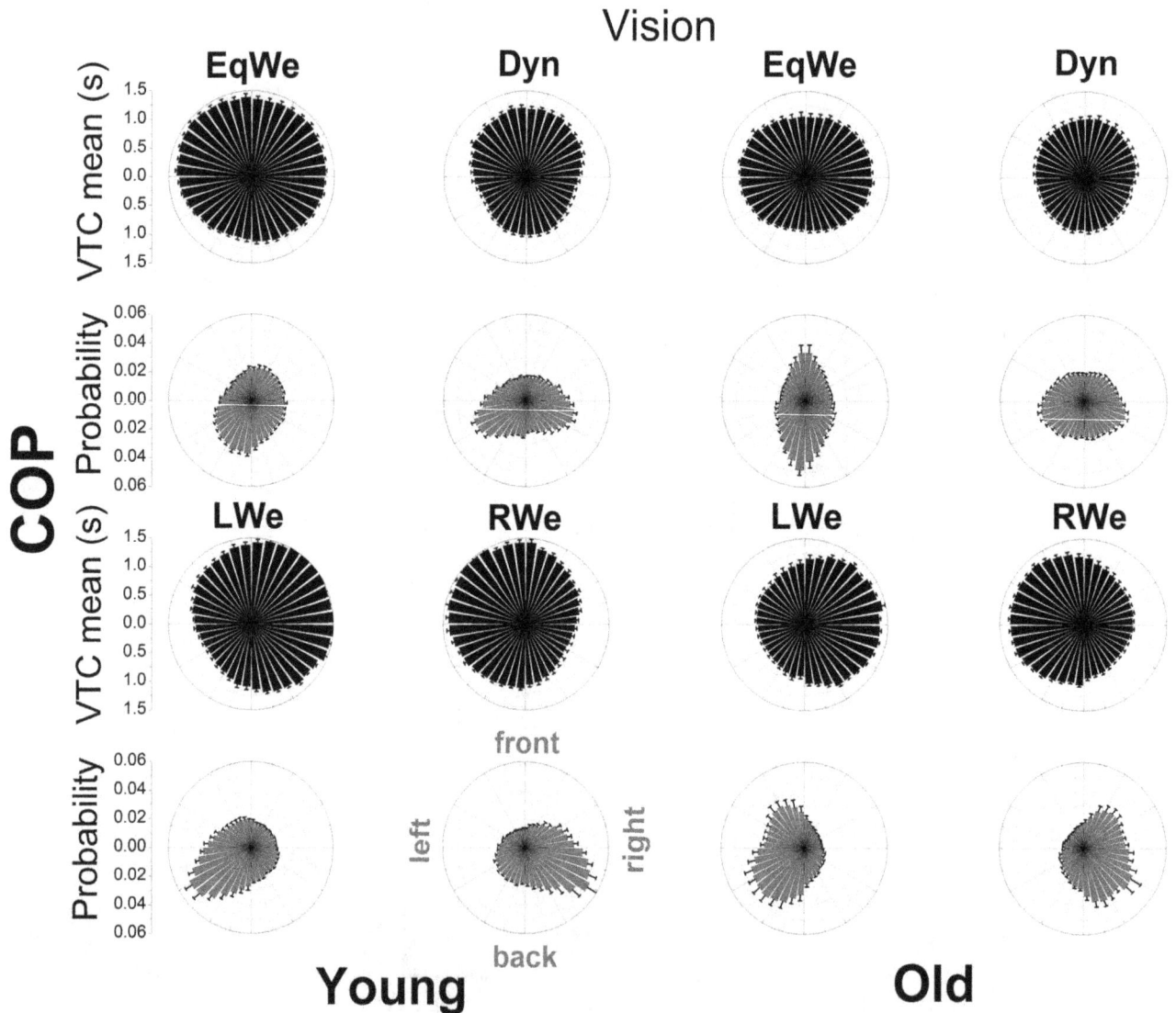

Figure 4. Polar distributions of VTC mean magnitude and probability of a virtual contact across the 40 boundary segments as a function of age and loading (with normal vision) using COP data. Each bar represents the group mean value ± SE (N = 12) for the respective boundary segment.

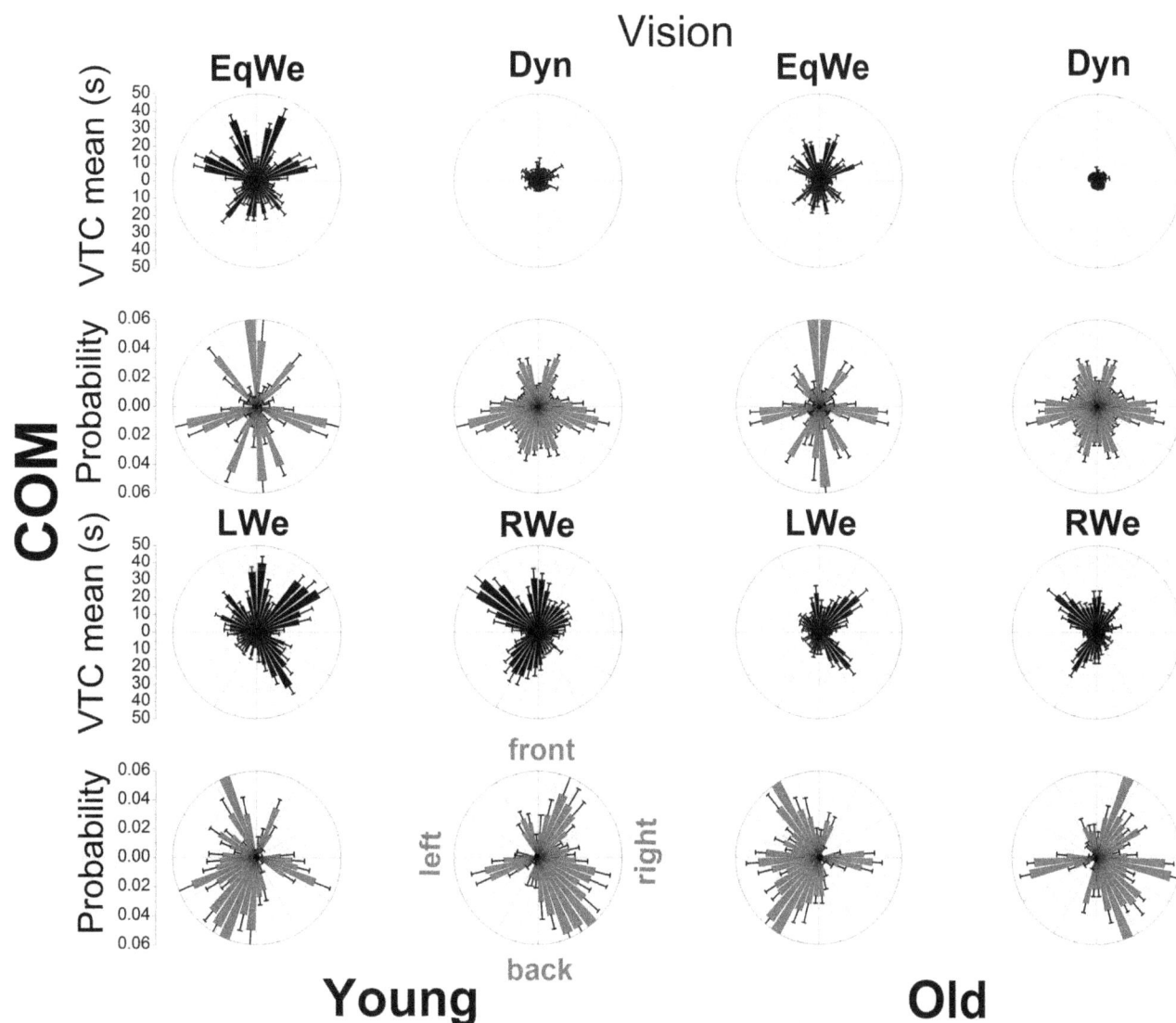

Figure 5. Polar distributions of VTC mean magnitude and probability of a virtual contact across the 40 boundary segments as a function of age and loading (with normal vision) using COM data. Each bar represents the group mean value ± SE (N = 12) for the respective boundary segment.

For both COP and COM data there is a clear qualitative change in the shape of the distributions across loading conditions and age groups. When visual information was removed the overall shape of the distributions does not appear to change. In addition, the relatively smooth COP distributions contrast with the COM distributions that show discrete segmented distributions within prevalent spatial regions. The individual distributions of the COM appear to be even sharper.

We examined the general relationship of the mean magnitude of VTC and the probability of a virtual contact for each age group and experimental condition through a quadratic function. For the COP data the significant inverse relationships of VTC and probability were well fitted by a quadratic function (R^2 values ranging from 0.82 to 0.94), showing that for low VTC mean values the probability of a virtual contact was highest and that this probability was reduced as the mean magnitude of VTC increases. The R^2 values for the COM ranged from 0.14 to 0.51.

Complexity (LZC) of Boundary (using COP)

Table 1 shows the results of the Boundary complexity analysis. Furthermore, typical boundary segment sequences are provided in the supplementary video material (Video S1). Age ($F_{1,22} = 6.51$, $p<0.05$), vision ($F_{1,22} = 12.10$, $p<0.01$) and loading ($F_{2.08,45.67} = 19.90$, $p<0.01$) significantly affected LZC. The interactions of age × vision ($F_{1,22} = 4.75$, $p<0.05$) and age × loading ($F_{2.08,45.67} = 6.02$, $p<0.01$) were also found to be significant. Pairwise comparisons of age × vision showed that only for the old group were the complexity values reduced when vision was removed compared to available vision. The age × loading interaction revealed that the old showed decreased complexity compared to the young adult group during EqWe and LWe. Further, for both age groups both LWe and RWe conditions were less complex than EqWe. In addition, in the young group complexity was significantly lower during Dyn compared to EqWe and LWe.

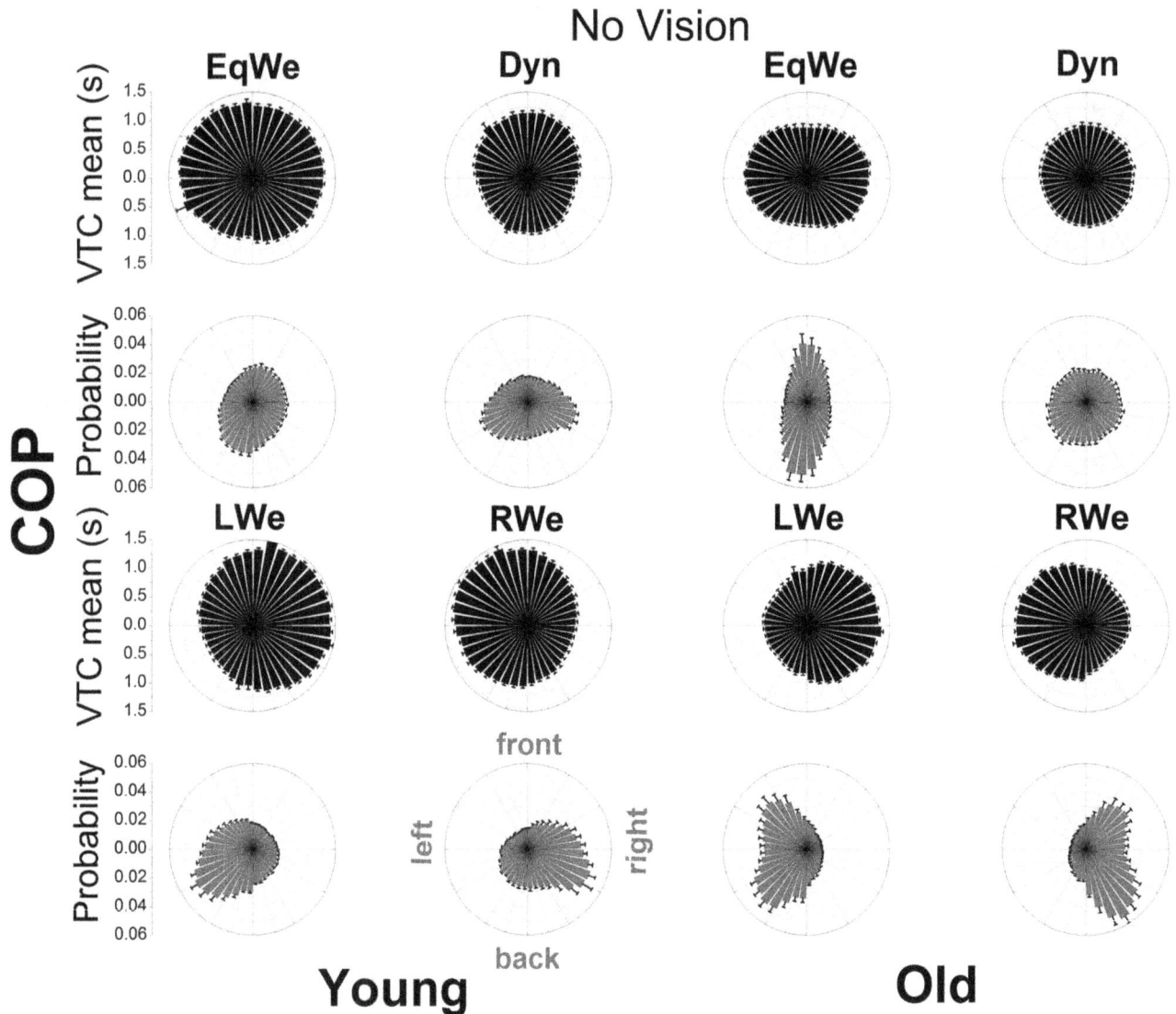

Figure 6. Polar distributions of VTC mean magnitude and probability of a virtual contact across the 40 boundary segments as a function of age and loading (visual information removed) using COP data. Each bar represents the group mean value ± SE (N = 12) for the respective boundary segment.

Complexity (LZC) of Boundary (using COM)

Vision ($F_{1,22} = 38.50$, p<0.01) and loading ($F_{3,66} = 752.00$, p< 0.01) significantly affected LZC complexity (Tab. 1). The Boundary complexity was higher when removing vision than when vision was available. Post hoc analysis of the main effect of loading showed that all multiple comparisons, except LWe vs. RWe were significant. Complexity was lowest for EqWe and highest for Dyn.

Surrogate data analysis for Boundary complexity

An additional Boundary complexity analysis was performed with a lower resolution of boundary segments (20 instead of 40 segments) to test for artifacts due to a specific number of boundary segments. The mixed ANOVA showed that the reported findings regarding the Boundary complexity remained unchanged.

In addition, the sequences were randomly shuffled in order to check whether the obtained complexity values resulted from a random process or are due to nonlinearity. The t-tests (COP Boundary: $|t_{23}| = 27.12$; COM Boundary: $|t_{23}| = 42.15$) showed

that the shuffled sequences produced throughout significantly higher complexity values, p<0.01.

Discussion

This study investigated virtual-time-to-contact (VTC) and Lempel-Ziv-Complexity (LZV) in the study of human stance to quantify the risk of potentially losing postural stability (taking a step or falling). We examined the influence of aging, visual information and leg loading on the regulation of upright two-leg stance. In particular, we investigated whether the spatial-temporal distributional patterns for virtually contacting the stability boundary lost complexity [36,38] with aging and whether these distributions were influenced by the availability of vision and load weighting of the legs. The boundary distributional patterns of VTC provide theoretical insight into the control of posture and hold relevance to the risk of losing postural stability in aging [3,24].

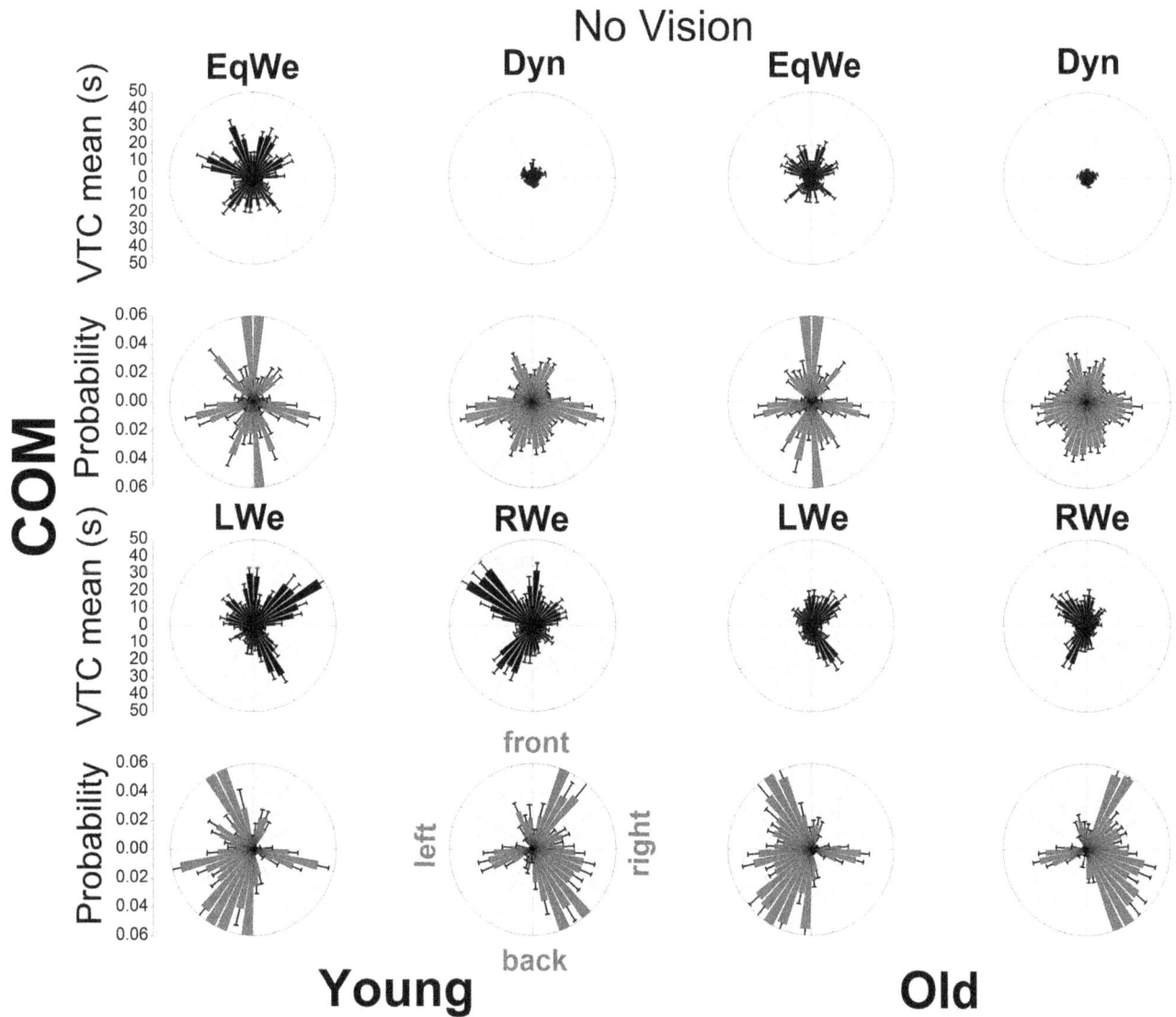

Figure 7. Polar distributions of VTC mean magnitude and probability of a virtual contact across the 40 boundary segments as a function of age and loading (visual information removed) using COM data. Each bar represents the group mean value ± SE (N = 12) for the respective boundary segment.

Magnitude of postural motion and stability boundary

The COP path length was analyzed as a traditional measure of postural control and indicator of stability. As anticipated the COP path length increased with aging [16], when visual information was removed [37], when posture was more challenged by unequal loading on the legs [32], and during the dynamic in contrast to the quiet standing trials. These results confirm that the overall magnitude of COP displacement reveals how the postural control system handles increasingly difficult constraints to standing still. However, no conclusions in terms of the instantaneous stability can be drawn [17–20].

Our results also confirm that the area of the functional stability boundary ellipse decreased in the old compared to young adults [8]. Determining a functional boundary as shown here has the advantage that one can scale the coordinates of the stability boundary to influencing factors such as the availability of vision or aging. It can also help to define the ratio of the region of postural motion and the region of stability, thus emphasizing an interpretation of the amount of postural motion with respect to the individual maximum stability tolerance [17].

Virtual time-to-contact (VTC) and distributional patterns of VTC with the functional stability boundary

The VTC approach in this study offers one feasible solution to relate postural motion to the individual maximum stability tolerance from a mechanical point of view. This study focused on the temporal safety margin when virtually interpolating the COP or COM to the functional stability boundary. The VTC mean values in particular confirmed previous findings [8,21,23,44], that is, the VTC mean decreased with aging, when visual information was removed and when challenging posture through leg loading - just the reverse trend of the COP path length. The reduced VTC values indicate that the postural control system has a lower temporal safety margin or less potential time for adequately balancing the unstable human body.

Table 1. Group mean ± SE (N = 12) Lempel Ziv complexity values (LZC) for the Boundary segment sequence for both COP and COM as a function of age, vision and loading.

	Young adults				Old adults			
	EqWe	Dyn	LWe	RWe	EqWe	Dyn	LWe	RWe
Boundary Complexity – Vision								
COP	.78571	.74253	.76697	.75663	.75533	.73772	.73471	.74287
	±.0016	±.0063	±.0043	±.0066	±.011	±.007	±.0086	±.0111
COM	.49753	.60669	.50177	.50170	.50127	.61702	.51608	.51058
	±.0067	±.0048	±.0060	±.0090	±.0060	±.0036	±.0045	±.0056
Boundary Complexity – No Vision								
COP	.78216	.74092	.75886	.75441	.73703	.72816	.71952	.71864
	±.0026	±.0055	±.0045	±.0049	±.0145	±.0076	±.0138	±.0136
COM	.50108	.61981	.51366	.51247	.50635	.61789	.51623	.51557
	±.0084	±.0044	±.0075	±.0065	±.0062	±.0027	±.0054	±.0061

A unique approach of the VTC analysis here was the decomposition of VTC into the different spatial regions of the stability boundary in order to quantify and gain deeper insight into the probabilistic properties of losing postural stability. In the old adults during regular two-legged stance (EqWe) the probability distribution of virtual contacts (COP) showed a clear symmetrical bimodal distribution with the peaks at the front and back boundary segments. In particular the probability for the back segments with reduced VTC magnitude was highest for the old adults. The geometry of the feet may drive the channeling of COP motion in AP direction. However, in the young adults these patterns were not replicated, in fact the probability distribution appears to be more uniform. VTC and probability are inversely related; considered together; distributions of the VTC magnitude and the probability of a virtual contact also intuitively link the postural motion to the risk of falls or losing postural stability [1]. The strong inverse relationship between VTC magnitude and probability raises the question as to whether there might be a simple mechanistic relationship between these two quantities. Further research is needed to investigate this relationship.

In the EqWe stance the highest risk of losing postural stability (taking a step or falling) was in the backwards direction. This direction of motion has also been shown to be even more critical or unstable in Parkinson's disease [27] and studies on real-world falls in the elderly have shown that in particular forward and especially backward falls were reported more frequently than sideward falls [3–4,45]. Van Wegen et al. [23] also found the largest effects of aging on VTC during a backward lean condition. The generally increased risk of falling motion in AP direction in the old adults may also indicate an associated postural control strategy that requires less demanding cortical resources [46]. In addition, it should be noted that the lateral postural stability has also been shown to be a valid predictor of future risk of falling in aging adults [47].

In the probability distribution (COP) for loading on either the right (RWe) or left (LWe) leg [31] there was one main peak at the corresponding lateral boundary segments (e.g. left boundary segments for LWe). These patterns possibly emerged, because the postural control system constantly needs to correct for not losing stability to the side the body is inclined to. Interestingly, the corrections towards the other directions are more uniform. In addition, for the elderly the virtual contacts are more broadly distributed along the boundary segments that the body is inclined to which might reflect the need to produce more counterbalanced mechanical stress at the lower extremities or simply an increased imbalance.

We conclude that approaching the complexity of postural dynamics through virtual interpolations to the stability boundary reveals the risk of losing postural stability as a function of the direction of postural motion and that the risk of losing postural stability in any particular direction depends on age [28] and the task constraints to posture. When examining these distributions for the COM many features of the COP distributions seem to be similar, although the distributions for the COM are segmented into discrete regions of the stability boundary. The prevalent regions and dead spaces across the stability boundary segments for COM are attributed to be a reflection of the body's inertia in contrast to the massless COP. It appears that COP is exerting continuous control on discontinuous spatial/temporal dynamics of COM – a postulation that warrants further investigation. The higher COM VTC mean values in contrast to the COP VTC also reflect the damping of the controlled variable, the COM [15].

Complexity and increased consistency with advanced age

We used the Lempel Ziv compression algorithm [39] to approximate the Kolmogorov complexity of a symbolic sequence representing postural dynamics. We applied this measure to the postural data to quantify not only the information content, but also the consistency in performance. Our proposed analysis of system complexity adds to other sensitive nonlinear tools for postural analysis [19,48–49], however, the computational speed is much faster and it is suitable for on-line implementation for example in medical assistive devices [40,50].

For the COP the LZC of the Boundary sequence decreased when vision was removed only in the old adults and was also lower in the old compared to the young during EqWe and LWe. It appears that with aging and when visual information is removed the spatial-temporal solutions of the postural control system in exploring the workspace are reduced, supporting the *loss of complexity* with aging hypothesis [36,38]. Exploring the workspace may keep adaptability high, therefore, the more frequent recurrent patterns in the elderly could be one of the reasons why the ability to adaptively compensate perturbations deteriorates with aging

[51]. However, the increased predictability with aging may enhance the possibility to assist postural control with artificial systems [50].

In addition, the complexity generally decreased under the unequal weight loading conditions in contrast to EqWe and was lowest in the Dyn condition. This shows that when task difficulty is higher or when more voluntary directed motion (Dyn) is involved complexity decreases. The Boundary complexity values using the COM were in general lower than those on COP. Also, there was no effect of aging with COM. However, the main effects of vision and loading were similar, except that Boundary complexity was higher when vision was removed and lowest for EqWe and highest for Dyn. This finding is the reverse of the VTC COP complexity, which has been attributed to be a reflection of damping mechanisms in human upright stance [15].

Finally, it should be noted that our previous work in isometric force control has shown a bidirectional change of movement complexity in aging adults [36] as a function of task and the attractor dynamics of force output, opening the conjecture that the general issue may be loss of adaptability in aging rather than necessarily a loss of complexity. The findings here in the quiet stance EqWe condition showed the aging loss of complexity effect. There was not, however, an increment of complexity in VTC at the boundary in the dynamic postural task (Dyn) as would be expected from the parallels to the intrinsic dynamics of the isometric force conditions [36]. This may be because the dynamics of the time series of the amplitude of COP or COM motion was not analyzed as was in effect the case in the isometric force studies.

Concluding remarks on VTC boundary control framework for falls assessment

This study revealed that VTC as a time function based on COP/COM dynamics provides a basis to assess future instability in terms of temporal-spatial risk of losing postural stability and the direction of potentially losing postural stability. The computational cost of the implemented algorithms is low and thus suitable for on-line applications [40]. We found that aging, vision and the postural task are critical in determining the characteristics of the risk of losing postural stability. In particular, we showed that the instantaneous postural stability is compromised in aging adults and that the complexity of the postural dynamics, as estimated by LZC of VTC is decreased in aging. Broader impacts of our research include the possibility of implementing the here introduced method of analyzing VTC in the clinical setting [3,45] for assessing instantaneous postural instability in relation to the functional stability boundary.

Author Contributions

Conceived and designed the experiments: MCK SMS KMN. Performed the experiments: MCK. Analyzed the data: MCK. Wrote the paper: MCK SMS KMN.

References

1. Cumming RG, Klineberg RJ (1994) Fall frequency and characteristics and the risk of hip fractures. J Am Geriatr Soc 42: 774–8.
2. Maki BE, Holliday PJ, Topper AK (1994) A prospective study of postural balance and risk of falling in an ambulatory and independent elderly population. J Gerontol 49:M72–84.
3. Bagalà F, Becker C, Cappello A, Chiari L, Aminian K, et al. (2012) Evaluation of accelerometer-based fall detection algorithms on real-world falls. PLoS One 7: e37062.
4. Klenk J, Becker C, Lieken F, Nicolai S, Maetzler W, et al. (2011) Comparison of acceleration signals of simulated and real-world backward falls. Med Eng Phys 33: 368–73.
5. Tolkiehn M, Atallah L, Lo B, Yang GZ (2011) Direction sensitive fall detection using a triaxial accelerometer and a barometric pressure sensor. Conf Proc IEEE Eng Med Biol Soc 2011: 369–72.
6. Collins JJ, De Luca CJ (1995) The effects of visual input on open-loop and closed-loop postural control mechanisms. Exp Brain Res 103: 151–63.
7. Duarte M, Zatsiorsky VM (2000) Long-range correlations in human standing. Physics Lett A 283: 124–128.
8. Slobounov SM, Moss SA, Slobounova ES, Newell KM (1998) Aging and time to instability in posture. J Gerontol A Biol Sci Med Sci 53:B71–8.
9. Maurer MS, Burcham J, Cheng H (2005) Diabetes mellitus is associated with an increased risk of falls in elderly residents of a long-term care facility. J Gerontol A Biol Sci Med Sci 60: 1157–62.
10. Tromp AM, Pluijm SM, Smit JH, Deeg DJ, Bouter LM, et al. (2001) Fall-risk screening test: a prospective study on predictors for falls in community-dwelling elderly. J Clin Epidemiol 54: 837–44.
11. Stalenhoef PA, Diederiks JP, Knottnerus JA, Kester AD, Crebolder HF (2002) A risk model for the prediction of recurrent falls in community-dwelling elderly: a prospective cohort study. J Clin Epidemiol 55: 1088–1094.
12. Close JC, Lord SL, Menz HB, Sherrington C (2005) What is the role of falls? Best Pract Res Clin Rheumatol 19: 913–935.
13. Massion J (1994) Postural control system. Curr Opin Neurobiol 4: 877–87.
14. Rothwell JC (1993) Control of human voluntary movement. New York: Springer.
15. Winter DA (2009) Biomechanics and Motor Control of Human Movement. New Jersey: John Wiley & Sons.
16. Sheldon JH (1963) The effect of age on the control of sway. Gerontol Clin 5: 129–38.
17. Haibach PS, Slobounov SM, Slobounova ES, Newell KM (2007) Virtual time-to-contact of postural stability boundaries as a function of support surface compliance. Exp Brain Res 177: 471–82.
18. Hof AL, Gazendam MG, Sinke WE (2005) The condition for dynamic stability. J Biomech 38: 1–8.
19. Newell KM, van Emmerik REA, Lee D, Sprague RL (1993) On postural stability and variability. 4: 225–230.
20. Patton JL, Pai Y, Lee WA (1999) Evaluation of a model that determines the stability limits of dynamic balance. Gait Posture 9: 38–49.
21. Haddad JM, Van Emmerik RE, Wheat JS, Hamill J (2008) Developmental changes in the dynamical structure of postural sway during a precision fitting task. Exp Brain Res 190: 431–41.
22. Slobounov SM, Slobounova ES, Newell KM (1997) Virtual Time-to-Collision and Human Postural Control. J Mot Behav 29: 263–281.
23. van Wegen EE, van Emmerik RE, Riccio GE (2002) Postural orientation: age-related changes in variability and time-to-boundary. Hum Mov Sci 21: 61–84.
24. Riccio GE (1993) Information in movement variability about the qualitative dynamics of posture and orientation. In: Newell KM, Corcos DM, editors. Variability and motor control. Champaign: Human Kinetics. pp. 317–358.
25. Hasson CJ, Caldwell GE, Van Emmerik RE (2009) Scaling of plantarflexor muscle activity and postural time-to-contact in response to upper-body perturbations in young and older adults. Exp Brain Res 196: 413–27.
26. King MB, Judge JO, Wolfson L (1994) Functional base of support decreases with age. J Gerontol 49:M258–63.
27. Horak FB, Dimitrova D, Nutt JG (2005) Direction-specific postural instability in subjects with Parkinson's disease. Exp Neurol 193: 504–21.
28. Allum JH, Carpenter MG, Honegger F, Adkin AL, Bloem BR (2002) Age-dependent variations in the directional sensitivity of balance corrections and compensatory arm movements in man. J Physiol 542: 643–63.
29. Park JW, Jung M, Kweon M (2014) The Mediolateral CoP Parameters can Differentiate the Fallers among the Community-dwelling Elderly Population. J Phys Ther Sci 26: 381–4.
30. Lin D, Seol H, Nussbaum MA, Madigan ML (2008) Reliability of COP-based postural sway measures and age-related differences. Gait Posture 28: 337–42.
31. Blaszczyk JW, Prince F, Raiche M, Hébert R (2000) Effect of ageing and vision on limb load asymmetry during quiet stance. J Biomech 33: 1243–8.
32. Kazennikov OV, Kireeva TB, Shlykov VY (2013) Characteristics of the maintenance of the vertical posture during standing with an asymmetrical load on the legs. Human Physiol 39: 392–399.
33. Prado JM, Dinato MC, Duarte M (2011) Age-related difference on weight transfer during unconstrained standing. Gait Posture 33: 93–7.
34. Costa M, Goldberger AL, Peng CK (2005) Multiscale entropy analysis of biological signals. Phys Rev E Stat Nonlin Soft Matter Phys 71: 021906.

35. Newell KM, Vaillancourt DE, Sosnoff JJ (2006) Aging, complexity and motor performance: Healthy and disease states. In: Birren JE, Schaie KW, editors. Handbook of the psychology of aging. Amsterdam: Elsevier. pp. 182–183.

36. Vaillancourt DE, Newell KM (2002) Changing complexity in human behavior and physiology through aging and disease. Neurobiol Aging 23: 1–11.

37. Newell KM (1998) Degrees of freedom and the development of postural center of pressure profiles. In: Newell KM, Molenaar PCM, editors. Applications of nonlinear dynamics to development process modeling. New Jersey: Lawrence Erlbaum Associates. pp. 63–84.

38. Lipsitz LA, Goldberger AL (1992) Loss of 'complexity' and aging. Potential applications of fractals and chaos theory to senescence. JAMA 267: 1806–9.

39. Lempel A, Ziv J (1976) On the complexity of finite sequences. IEEE Trans. Inform. Theory 22: 75–81.

40. Zhang XS, Roy RJ, Jensen EW (2001) EEG complexity as a measure of depth of anesthesia for patients. IEEE Trans Biomed Eng 48: 1424–1433.

41. Song C, Qu Z, Blumm N, Barabási AL (2010) Limits of predictability in human mobility. Science 327: 1018–1021.

42. Newell KM, Slobounov SM, Slobounova ES, Molenaar PC (1997) Stochastic processes in postural center-of-pressure profiles. Exp Brain Res 113: 158–64.

43. Kaspar F, Schuster HG (1987) Easily calculable measure for the complexity of spatiotemporal patterns. Phys Rev A 36: 842–848.

44. Forth KE, Metter EJ, Paloski WH (2007) Age associated differences in postural equilibrium control: a comparison between EQscore and minimum time to contact (TTC(min)). Gait Posture 25: 56–62.

45. Manckoundia P, Mourey F, Pérennou D, Pfitzenmeyer P (2008) Backward disequilibrium in elderly subjects. Clin Interv Aging 3: 667–72.

46. Slobounov S, Hallett M, Cao C, Newell K (2008) Modulation of cortical activity as a result of voluntary postural sway direction: an EEG study. Neurosci Lett 442: 309–13.

47. Maki BE, Holliday PJ, Topper AK (1994) A prospective study of postural balance and risk of falling in an ambulatory and independent elderly population. J Gerontol 49:M72–84.

48. King AC, Wang Z, Newell KM (2012) Asymmetry of recurrent dynamics as a function of postural stance. Exp Brain Res 220: 239–50.

49. Roerdink M, De Haart M, Daffertshofer A, Donker SF, Geurts AC, et al. (2006) Dynamical structure of center-of-pressure trajectories in patients recovering from stroke. Exp Brain Res 174: 256–69.

50. Dubowsky S, Genot F, Godding S, Kozono H, Skwersky A, et al. (2000) PAMM - a robotic aid to the elderly for mobility assistance and monitoring: a "helping-hand" for the elderly. Proc ICRA IEEE 1: 570–576.

51. Gu MJ, Schultz AB, Shepard NT, Alexander NB (1996) Postural control in young and elderly adults when stance is perturbed: dynamics. J Biomech 29: 319–29.

10

Patterns, Predictors, and Outcomes of Falls Trajectories in Older Adults: The MOBILIZE Boston Study with 5 Years of Follow-Up

Achille E. Tchalla[1,2,3,4], **Alyssa B. Dufour**[1,2,3], **Thomas G. Travison**[1,2,3], **Daniel Habtemariam**[3], **Ikechukwu Iloputaife**[3], **Brad Manor**[1,2,3], **Lewis A. Lipsitz**[1,2,3]*

1 Harvard Medical School, Boston, Massachusetts, United States of America, 2 Division of Gerontology, Beth Israel Deaconess Medical Center, Boston, Massachusetts, United States of America, 3 Institute for Aging Research, Hebrew SeniorLife, Boston, Massachusetts, United States of America, 4 Department of Geriatric Medicine, University Hospital Center of Limoges, University of Limoges; EA 6310 HAVAE (Disability, Activity, Aging, Autonomy and Environment), Limoges, France

Abstract

Background: Falls may occur as unpredictable events or in patterns indicative of potentially modifiable risks and predictive of adverse outcomes. Knowing the patterns, risks, and outcomes of falls trajectories may help clinicians plan appropriate preventive measures. We hypothesized that clinically distinct trajectories of falls progression, baseline predictors and their coincident clinical outcomes could be identified.

Methods: We studied 765 community-dwelling participants in the MOBILIZE Boston Study, who were aged 70 and older and followed prospectively for falls over 5 years. Baseline demographic and clinical data were collected by questionnaire and a comprehensive clinic examination. Falls, injuries, and hospitalizations were recorded prospectively on daily calendars. Group-Based Trajectory Modeling (GBTM) was used to identify trajectories.

Results: We identified 4 distinct trajectories: No Falls (30.1%), Cluster Falls (46.1%), Increasing Falls (5.8%) and Chronic Recurring Falls (18.0%). Predictors of Cluster Falls were faster gait speed (OR 1.69 (95CI, 1.50–2.56)) and fall in the past year (OR 3.52 (95CI, 2.16–6.34)). Predictors of Increasing Falls were Diabetes Mellitus (OR 4.3 (95CI, 1.4–13.3)) and Cognitive Impairment (OR 2.82 (95CI, 1.34–5.82)). Predictors of Chronic Recurring Falls were multi-morbidity (OR 2.24 (95CI, 1.60–3.16)) and fall in the past year (OR 3.82 (95CI, 2.34–6.23)). Symptoms of depression were predictive of all falls trajectories. In the Chronic Recurring Falls trajectory group the incidence rate of Hospital visits was 121 (95% CI 63–169) per 1,000 person-years; Injurious falls 172 (95% CI 111–237) per 1,000 person-years and Fractures 41 (95% CI 9–78) per 1,000 person-years.

Conclusions: Falls may occur in clusters over discrete intervals in time, or as chronically increasing or recurring events that have a relatively greater risk of adverse outcomes. Patients with multiple falls, multimorbidity, and depressive symptoms should be targeted for preventive measures.

Editor: Antony Bayer, Cardiff University, United Kingdom

Funding: Grant P01 AG04390 and R37 AG25037 from the US National-Institute on Aging. The funders had no role in study design, data collection and analysis, decision to publish, or preparation of the manuscript.

Competing Interests: The authors have declared that no competing interests exist.

* Email: lipsitz@hsl.harvard.edu

Introduction

Falls are common among older persons [1,2] and rank among the 10 leading causes of death in the United States, resulting in more than $19 billion in health care costs annually [3]. Falls account for approximately 10% of visits to an emergency department and 6% of hospitalizations among Medicare beneficiaries [4].

Although scientific evidence supports associations between a number of risk factors and falls [5], efforts to translate these findings into effective fall prevention strategies have been limited [6]. A Cochrane review showed that multifactorial interventions significantly reduce the rate of falls in varying degrees [7,8] but it may be difficult to identify the appropriate group to target for interventions. It is possible that some people may experience falls as random, unpredictable events, while others may have patterns of falls that are indicative of potentially modifiable risks factors and are predictive of adverse outcomes. Knowing the patterns, risks, and outcomes of falls trajectories may help clinicians plan appropriate preventive measures. To our knowledge there are no longitudinal studies that have observed long-term trajectories of falls and determined their predictors and outcomes.

We hypothesized that: 1- there are distinct clinical patterns of falls trajectories ranging from no falls, random falls, clusters of falls, progressively increasing numbers of falls, and chronic recurring falls; 2- baseline "predictive factors", such as chronic illnesses associated with these patterns could be identified; and 3- clinically important health outcomes would be worse in those with chronically elevated fall rates. Therefore, we examined a unique longitudinal database from the MOBILIZE Boston Study (which stands for The Maintenance Of Balance, Independent Living, Intellect, and Zest in Elderly (MBS)), which rigorously collected falls calendar data from a cohort of community-dwelling elderly people over a 5 year period. We used this database to identify subgroups of people with distinct falls trajectories, identify baseline characteristics associated with these trajectories, and determine their coincident clinical outcomes.

Materials and Methods

Ethics Statement

The MOBILIZE Boston Study Trajectory (MBSTraj), Protocol Number: 13-029 was reviewed and approved by the Hebrew SeniorLife Institutional Review Board (IRB) at the Hebrew Rehabilitation Center (HRC) in Boston. Written informed consent was obtained from each participant at each phase of MOBILIZE Boston Study. The study was conducted according to the principles of Helsinki Declaration.

Study participants

Study participants were women and men aged 70 years and older living in the community in Boston and nearby suburbs. Recruitment and enrollment took place from September 2005 to January 2008 within a defined geographic area bounded by a 5-mile radius around the Institute for Aging Research at HRC in Boston. The sampling area was chosen to capture a diverse urban and suburban population, to increase likelihood of recognition of the study center, and to minimize transportation burden. Details of the study methods were published previously [9,10]. Initial eligibility was based on age 70 years or older, ability to walk 20 feet without personal assistance, ability to communicate in English, and the expectation of staying in the area for 2 years. Following the initial recruitment visit, study staff contacted prospective enrollees by telephone to confirm eligibility and schedule the baseline home and clinic visits. During the home visit, written informed consent was obtained and participants were screened and excluded for moderate or severe cognitive impairment using the Mini-Mental State Examination (MMSE score, <18) [11,12].

Falls and Clinical Outcomes Assessments

During the Follow-up, a fall was defined as unintentionally coming to rest on the ground or other lower level not as a result of a major intrinsic event (e.g., myocardial infarction, stroke, or seizure) or an overwhelming external hazard (e.g., hit by a vehicle) [13]. Participants were instructed to complete and return monthly

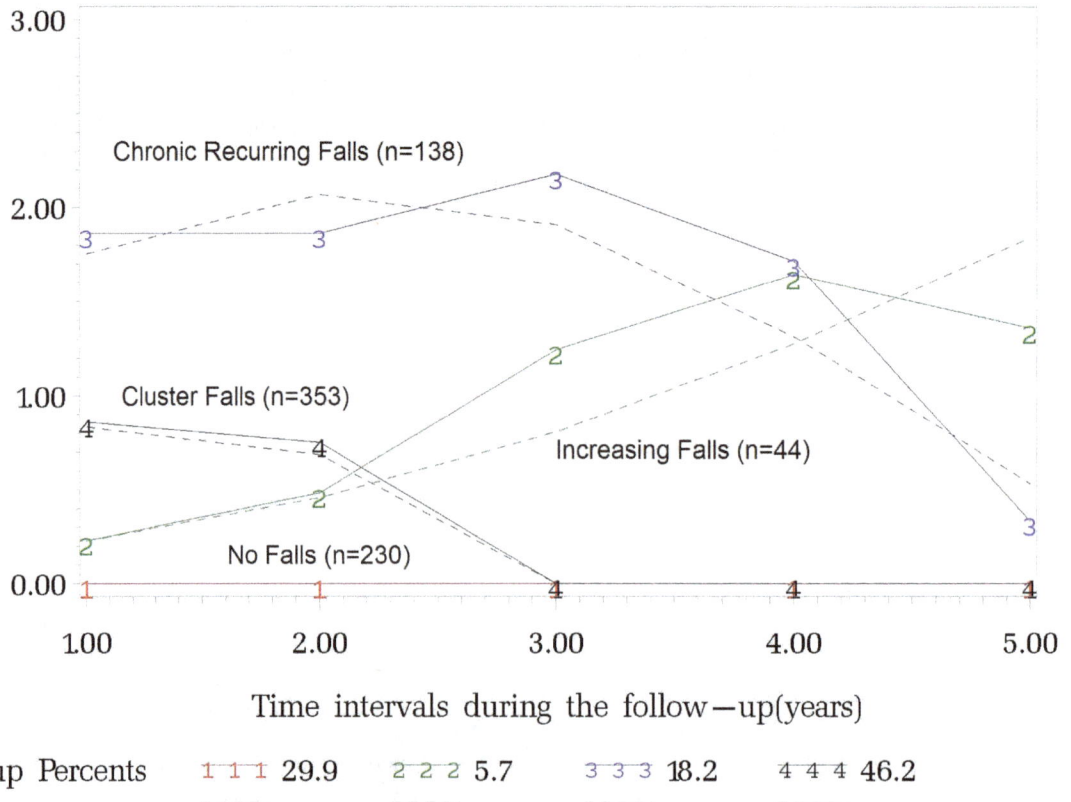

Figure 1. Patterns of Falls Trajectories over 5 years in Older Adults (The MOBILIZE Boston Study). —Solid lines are estimated trajectories. ---- Dashed lines are observed trajectories for each group.

Table 1. Summary of Baseline Characteristics (The MOBILIZE Boston Study).

Demographic Characteristics and Risk Factors	Total sample n = 765[a]	
	No.	%
Age, mean (SD), y	78.1	(5.4)
Women,	488	63.8
Race,		
White	609	79.6
Nonwhite	156	20.4
Years of Education, mean (SD), y	14.8	(6.1)
Body mass index, kg/m², [b]		
<25	233	30.4
25–29.9	297	38.8
≥30	206	26.9
Fell in past year,	289	37.8
Comorbidities ≥2,	491	64.2
Hypertension,	607	79.3
Previous stroke,	72	9.4
Diabetes mellitus,	172	22.5
Hyperlipidemia,	469	61.3
Congestive heart failure,	38	5.0
Mini-Mental State Examination score <24, [c]	154	20.1
CES-D Revised score, mean (SD), points	11.0	(11.2)
Physical activity score, [d]		
0–66	245	32.0
66.01–124	262	34.3
124.01–559	258	33.7
Impaired balance, score <4 out 7, [e]	318	41.6
Slow gait speed, <0.78 m/s, [f]	189	24.7
Slow chair stands, >16.37 s, [g]	95	12.4

[a]Forty four of the 809 older adults were missing data and therefore excluded from the analysis.
[b]Body mass index is calculated as weight in kilograms divided by height in meters squared.
[c]Mini-Mental State Examination (MMSE) cut off point for cognitive impairment [11,12].
[d]Physical activity tertiles measured using the Physical Activity Scale for the Elderly [15].
[e]Balance score was based on 4 progressively difficult stands: feet side by side, semi-tandem, tandem, and 1-leg stand [17].
[f]Slow gait speed (m/s) is the lowest 25% based on time of lowest of 2 usual-paced 4-meter walks [17].
[g]Highest quartile (slowest performance) of time to complete 5 repeated chair stands [17].

falls calendar postcards designed to be posted on a refrigerator. On the postcards, participants were to record an *F* for each fall on the day it occurred and an *N* on days when No Falls occurred. This approach has been well-validated for use in epidemiological cohort studies [14]. The calendar postcards also included questions about whether the participant experienced a hospitalization during the preceding month. Research staff monitored the return of the calendars and on any given month, approximately one-third of participants were called for missing or incomplete calendars. All subjects who reported falls were also called to determine the circumstances of the fall and clinical outcomes whether any injuries (e.g. fractures) and hospital visits were incurred.

Covariates

Covariates included sociodemographic characteristics, physiologic risk factors, health status, and amount of physical activity. Sociodemographic characteristics assessed in the home interview included age, sex, race (self-identified), and years of education.

Cognitive status was assessed using the MMSE, scored 0–30 [12]. We used the validated Physical Activity Scale for the Elderly (PASE) to measure physical activity in the previous week [15]. Participants were asked about physician-diagnosed major medical conditions. Details of the study methods were published previously [9,10]. During the clinic visit, several measures were calculated. Diabetes was defined using an algorithm based on self-reported diabetes, use of antidiabetic medications, and laboratory measures from the baseline clinic visit including random glucose (200 mg/dL) and hemoglobin A_{1c} (7%). Depression was assessed using the Eaton method based on a modification of the 20-item Centers for Epidemiologic Studies Depression scale [16]. Body mass index (calculated as weight in kilograms divided by height in meters squared) was calculated from measured height and weight. Standing balance was scored using 4 timed tests (side-by-side, semi-tandem, tandem, and 1-leg stands) [17]. For the timed chair stands test, participants were asked to fold their arms across their chest and stand up and down from a chair 5 times as quickly as

Table 2. Bayesian Information Criterion (BIC) Values and Predicted Group Proportions for Group-Based Trajectory Models.

Model	No. of Groups	BIC	Predicted Group Proportions				
			Group 1	Group 2	Group 3	Group 4	Group 5
1	3	−2385.99	0.272	0.495	0.233		
2	4	−2350.01	0.302	0.465	0.058	0.175	
3	5	−2350.87	0.318	0.452	0.044	0.074	0.112

possible [17]. Gait speed was based on the shortest time of 2 trials of a usual-paced 4-meter walk [17].

Data Analysis

To identify clinically distinct trajectories of falls, we use Group-Based Trajectory Modeling (GBTM) [18]. This method allowed us to simultaneously estimate probabilities for multiple trajectories rather than a single mean for the population, as is the case for traditional regression or growth-curve models. We used SAS software, and the PROC TRAJ macro (http://www.andrew.cmu.edu/user/bjones) [19,20], a closed-source module developed specifically for use with SAS software, which fits a semiparametric mixture model to longitudinal data with the use of the maximum-likelihood method. It is possible that some people may experience falls as random, unpredictable events, while others may have patterns of falls that are indicative of potentially modifiable risks factors and are predictive of adverse outcomes. Knowing the patterns, risks, and outcomes of falls trajectories may help clinicians plan appropriate preventive measures. The metric for defining the trajectory was years into the study. The number of falls that each participant reported each month was summated for each year over the 5 years study period and quantified as a "Falls Per Year of Aging" Score (FPYA Score). For each one year time interval, No Falls equaled FPYA 0, one fall equaled FPYA 1, two falls equaled FPYA 2 (recurrent falls), and three or more falls equaled FPYA 3 (high number of recurrent falls). FPYA scores were examined as a function of different time periods from 1 to 5 years long, independent of the chronological time at which these periods started (e.g., a 3 year period could start at year 1 and include years 1–3, year 2 and include years 2–4, or year 3 and include years 3–5 of the study). PROC TRAJ was used with the follow-up time metric from 1 to 5 years long independent of their age. So interval time was 1-year and Falls Per Year Aging (FPYA) was scored with 1-year follow-up time metric. FPYA (Falls per year aging) as the y-axis in Figure 1 represents the average of fall rate per year as a function of different intervals in time (shown on the x-axis). These scores were modeled as a censored normal distribution. We used the Bayesian Information Criterion (BIC) to test from three to six trajectories and to determine whether each trajectory was best fit by intercept only (i.e., constant) or by linear, quadratic, or cubic terms [21]. The final model was selected based on a combination of the Bayesian information criterion (BIC; where the value closest to 0 indicates the best-fitting model) and by estimated trajectory group proportions that were sufficiently large (e.g., 0.05) [22]. These analyses were repeated after adjustment for age, sex, race or ethnic group, years of education, chronic conditions such as hypertension, stroke, diabetes mellitus, hyperlipidemia, cognitive status and previous falls at baseline using the Proc Traj software "risk" command. The proportions of older adults classified according to each trajectory, the mean probability of assignment, and the proportions with poor fit were based on the original data, and 95% confidence intervals were estimated with the use of 1000 bootstrap samples [18]. Missing data on the trajectory modeling and on time-varying variables were handled with a maximum likelihood approach [18] together with the missing-at-random assumption, which assumes that for each individual, the likely values for missing data on the trajectory and time-varying variables can be estimated from other available observed data. This approach uses available information on each case for constructing the trajectories rather than deleting individuals with missing observations.

After determining the most appropriate GBTM, group status for each individual was obtained to identify relevant predictors of each falls trajectory group. An individual was assigned to the

Table 3. Summary of Baseline Characteristics by Falls Trajectory Profiles Derived From Group-Based Trajectory Modeling (The MOBILIZE Boston Study, No. = 765[a]).

Characteristics and Risk Factors	Trajectory Group[b]								P Value[c]
	No Falls n=230, 30.1%		Cluster Falls n=353, 46.1%		Increasing Falls n=44, 5.8%		Chronic Recurring Falls n=138, 18.0%		
	No.	%	No.	%	No.	%	No.	%	
Age, mean (SD), y	78.1	(5.4)	77.9	(5.4)	76.5	(4.7)	78.8	(5.6)	0.71
Women,	142	61.6	232	65.7	29	66.7	85	61.5	0.73
Race,									
White	155	67.2	282	79.9	35	79.5	137	99.1	<0.001
Nonwhite	75	32.8	71	20.1	9	20.5	1	0.9	
Years of Education	14.3	(8.3)	15.0	(5.2)	14.3	(2.4)	15.8	(2.3)	0.27
Body mass index, kg/m²,[d]									
<25	71	31.0	108	30.6	3	7.7	51	37.3	<0.05
25–29.9	97	42.1	116	40.8	22	50.0	62	45.2	
≥30	62	26.9	101	28.6	19	42.3	24	17.5	
Fell in past year,	28	11.9	153	43.3	6	13.7	102	73.9	<0.001
Comorbidities ≥2,	121	52.6	231	65.5	32	73.7	107	77.5	<0.01
Hypertension,	183	79.6	276	78.2	37	83.3	111	80.4	0.08
Stroke,	23	10.0	31	8.8	0	0.0	18	12.8	0.24
Diabetes mellitus,	54	23.3	75	21.3	30	68.4	13	9.4	<0.001
Hyperlipidemia,	136	59.2	223	63.3	37	83.3	73	52.9	<0.01
Congestive heart failure,	10	4.4	20	5.7	0	0.0	8	5.5	0.6
Mini-Mental State Examination score <24,[e]	36	15.7	44	12.5	7	16.7	67	4.9	<0.05
CES-D Revised score, mean (SD), points[f]	6.2	(6.8)	11.6	(11.6)	16.3	(14.8)	14.7	(11.7)	<0.001
Physical activity score,[f]									
0–66	67	29.1	122	34.6	24	53.9	32	23.1	<0.01
66.01–124	70	30.4	129	36.5	15	34.6	48	35.0	
124.01–559	93	40.5	102	28.9	5	11.5	58	41.9	
Impaired balance, score <4 out 7,[g]	86	37.6	158	44.7	8	19.1	66	47.6	<0.05
Slow gait speed, <0.78 m/s,[h]	73	31.7	72	20.5	7	15.9	37	27.1	<0.01
Slow chair stands, >16.37 s,[i]	23	10.1	55	15.6	4	9.5	13	9.4	0.11

[a]Forty four of the 809 older adults were missing data and therefore excluded from the analysis;
[b]Estimated from Group-Based Trajectory Modeling (GBTM) [18].
[c]Global test: χ2 or Fisher's exact test for binary variables; analysis of variance for continuous variables.
[d]Body mass index is calculated as weight in kilograms divided by height in meters squared.
[e]Mini-Mental State Examination (MMSE) cut off point for cognitive impairment [11,12].
[f]Physical activity tertiles measured using the Physical Activity Scale for the Elderly [15].
[g]Balance score was based on 4 progressively difficult stands: feet side by side, semi-tandem, tandem, and 1-leg stand [17].
[h]Slow gait speed (m/s) is the lowest 25% based on time of lowest of 2 usual-paced 4-meter walks [17].
[i]Highest quartile (slowest performance) of time to complete 5 repeated chair stands [17].

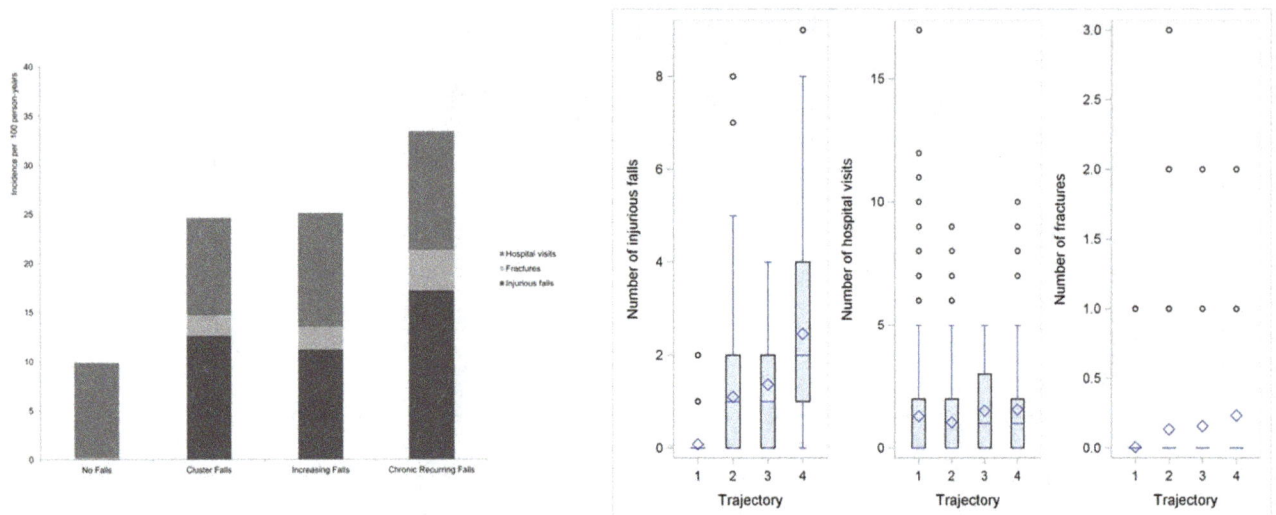

Figure 2. Clinical Outcomes according to Falls Trajectory group membership (The MOBILIZE Boston Study). A. Incidence Rate of Clinical Outcomes according to Falls Trajectory Group. **B.** Box plot showing Averages of Clinical Outcomes according to Falls Trajectory Group: *Trajectories*: 1 = No Falls; 2 = Cluster Falls; 3 = Increasing Falls; 4 = Chronic Recurring Falls. *Injurious Falls*: 2&4 p<0.001 (S); 3&4 p<0.001 (S); All others NS. *Hospital visits*: All are NS. *Fractures*: 1&2 p<0.001 (S), 1&3 p<0.001 (S), 1&4<0.0001, All others are NS.

trajectory group in which he or she was most likely to be, as determined by the group posterior probabilities from the final model. After using the "risk" command in Proc Traj software to identify predictors with beta coefficients and p values, we confirmed the findings and computed odds ratios using multinomial analyses. The outcome variable was falls trajectory group membership, and the testable predictors were sociodemographic characteristics, physiologic risk factors, health status, and amount of physical activity. The models were estimated using PROC LOGISTIC in SAS version 9.3. Partial R^2 was calculated for statistically significant predictors using R^2max values [23,24] and the Area Under the Curve was calculated for the model discrimination [25]. We assessed relevant clinical outcomes such as injurious falls, falls resulting in fractures, and hospital visits according to falls trajectories. All analyses were performed using SAS software, version 9.3 (SAS Institute Inc, Cary, North Carolina). A two-sided P value of less than 0.05 was considered indicative of statistical significance.

Results

Participants

Eight hundred nine individuals met study inclusion. Forty four of them older adults were missing data and therefore excluded from the analysis. **Table 1** summarizes the demographic and health characteristics of the study sample at baseline. Of the 765 older adults included in this study, 276 (36.1%) were male and 489 (63.9%) female, 156 (20.4%) were nonwhite, 245 (32.0%) met the PASE score of low intensity physical activity. On average, the cohort was 78.1±5.4 of age (range 64–97). Over five years, 90 (11.8%) older adults died during the follow-up period, with an incidence rate of 24 (95% CI 13–34) per 1,000 person-years.

Determining Falls Trajectories over 5 years

The BIC values and estimated proportions for the 3-, 4-, and 5-group GBTM models shown in **Table 2** were used to determine the best fit. A 6-group model was tested but failed to converge.

Consequently, the 4 group model was selected for each fall trajectory group. Additional diagnostic criteria for judging the adequacy of a GBTM demonstrated that the 4 group model performed well based on the Nagin criteria [18]. **Figure 1** illustrates each of the 4 trajectories along with the average raw group data at each point. The 4 distinct trajectories were: Cluster Falls (46.1%; 95CI, 40.0%–48.8%; n = 353) $P<0.001$, Increasing Falls (5.8%; 95CI, 3.7%–11.4%; n = 44) $P<0.001$, Chronic Recurring Falls (18.0%; 95CI, 12.7%–19.1%; n = 138) $P<0.001$, and No Falls (30.1%; 95CI, 28.8%–35.6%; n = 230) $P<0.001$. **Table 3** presents descriptive data for each falls trajectory group.

Coincident Clinical Outcomes of Falls Trajectories

Figure 2 panel A shows the distribution of the incidence of clinical outcomes namely injurious falls, fractures and hospital visits for each falls trajectory and summarized below. The average of clinical outcomes and incidence followed the same distribution in falls trajectories. The incidence of *Injurious Falls* was 172 (95% CI 111–237) per 1,000 person-years in Chronic Recurring Falls trajectory group, 126 (95% CI 98–169) per 1,000 person-years in Cluster Falls trajectory group, and 112 (95% CI 51–267) per 1,000 person-years in Increasing Falls trajectory group. The incidence of *Fractures* was 41 (95% CI 9–78) per 1,000 person-years in the Chronic Recurring Falls trajectory group, 21 (95% CI 7–38) per 1,000 person-years in the Cluster Falls trajectory group, 23 (95% CI 10–67) per 1,000 person-years in Increasing Falls trajectory group, and 2 per 1,000 person-years in No Falls trajectory group. The incidence of *Hospital visits* was 121 (95% CI 63–169) per 1,000 person-years in Chronic Recurring Falls trajectory group, 116 (95% CI 20–207) per 1,000 person-years in Increasing Falls trajectory group, 99 (95% CI 68–130) per 1,000 person-years in Cluster Falls trajectory group and 97 (95% CI 58–134) per 1,000 person-years in the No Falls trajectory group. **Figure 2** panel B shows that during the 5-year follow-up, the mean number of injurious falls was significantly higher in the "Chronic Recurring Falls" trajectory group. The mean number of fractures was also

Table 4. Adjusted Odds Ratios for every unit increase or Category Change in the Predictors of Falls Trajectory: Results from Multinomial Logistic Regressions at Baseline (n = 765[a]), The MOBILIZE Boston Study.

Predictor	Falls Trajectory Group[b]								
	Cluster Falls[1] (n = 353, 46.1%)			Increasing Falls[2] (n = 44, 5.8%)			Chronic Recurring Falls[3] (n = 138, 18.1%)		
	OR[c]	95CI	P Value[d]	OR[c]	95CI	P Value[d]	OR[c]	95CI	P Value[d]
Age, y	0.99	0.96, 1.04	0.94	1.01	0.88, 1.05	0.80	1.04	0.97, 1.12	0.21
Sex									
Male	1.00	Referent		1.00	Referent		1.00	Referent	
Women	1.31	0.88, 1.96	0.19	2.97	0.42, 2.87	0.10	1.85	0.92, 3.74	0.09
Race									
Nonwhite	1.00	Referent		1.00	Referent		1.00	Referent	
White Race	1.16	0.94, 1.43	0.17	1.07	0.67, 1.69	0.21	1.64	0.98, 2.67	0.06
Years of Education	1.02	0.99, 1.04	0.29	0.98	0.91, 1.05	0.49	1.04	0.99, 1.09	0.11
Body mass index, kg/m[e]	1.05	0.80, 1.37	0.73	1.04	0.56, 1.95	0.97	1.02	0.62, 1.68	0.94
Fell in past year	3.52	2.16, 6.34	<0.001	1.69	0.53, 5.38	0.16	3.82	2.34, 6.23	<0.001
Comorbidities ≥2	2.06	0.95, 3.14	0.08	2.52	0.89, 7.20	0.40	2.24	1.34, 5.32	0.015
Hypertension	0.70	0.55, 0.91	0.16	1.25	0.62, 2.53	0.80	0.85	0.40, 1.75	0.11
Stroke	0.83	0.46, 1.48	0.35	-	-	-	2.08	0.67, 6.45	0.20
Diabetes mellitus	0.69	0.40, 1.18	0.18	4.30	1.40, 13.3	<0.001	0.20	0.03, 1.27	0.08
Hyperlipidemia	1.19	0.84, 1.68	0.13	2.60	0.84, 8.06	0.32	2.05	0.98, 4.30	0.06
Congestive heart failure	1.24	0.56, 2.72	0.93	-	-	-	0.76	0.15, 3.91	0.75
Cognitive status[f]									
MMSE≥24	1.00	Referent		1.00	Referent		1.00	Referent	
MMSE<24	0.83	0.44, 1.58	0.57	2.82	1.34, 5.82	0.039	0.44	0.11, 1.66	0.21
CES-D Revised score[g]	1.03	1.01, 1.05	0.006	1.04	1.00, 1.07	0.013	1.07	1.03, 1.10	<0.001
Physical activity score[h]									
≥66	1.00	Referent		1.00	Referent		1.00	Referent	
<66	1.02	0.66, 1.37	0.92	1.23	0.70, 2.17	0.57	1.82	0.86, 3.87	0.12
Impaired balance, score <4 out 7[i]	1.29	0.84, 1.97	0.24	0.74	0.27, 2.00	0.26	1.94	0.91, 4.15	0.09
Fast gait speed, >0.78 m/s[j]	1.69	1.50, 2.56	0.012	0.84	0.21, 2.08	0.47	1.61	0.66, 3.85	0.29
Slow chair stands, >16.37 s[k]	1.18	0.65, 2.18	0.58	1.12	0.25, 5.26	0.75	1.04	0.52, 2.08	0.75

Abbreviations: 1, Model 1; 2, Model2; 3, Model3; OR, Odds Ratio; 95%CI, 95% Confidence Interval;

[a]Forty four of the 809 older adults were missing data and therefore excluded from the analysis;

[b]Estimated from Group-Based Trajectory Modeling (GBTM) [18].

[c]No Falls group was the reference category.

[d]Two-sided P value.

[e]Body mass index is calculated as weight in kilograms divided by height in meters squared;

[f]MMSE (Mini-Mental State Examination Scale) <24 [11,12], Cognitive impairment;

[g]CES-D, Center for Epidemiological Studies Depression Scale [16];

[h]Low physical activity, <66.01 PASE Score (using the Physical Activity Scale for the Elderly) [15];

[i]Balance score was based on 4 progressively difficult stands: feet side by side, semi-tandem, tandem, and 1-leg stand [17];

[j]Fast gait speed (m/s) is the highest 25% based on time of fastest of 2 usual-paced 4-meter walks [17];

[k]Highest quartile (slowest performance) of time to complete 5 repeated chair stands [17]. R^2max [23,24] (Model1: 0.32; Model2: 0.36; Model3: 0.57) AUC [25] (Model1: 0.80; Model2: 0.89; Model3: 0.92).

higher in the "Increasing Falls" and "Chronic Recurring Falls" trajectory groups compare to the "No falls Group".

Predictors of Falls Trajectories

Multinomial logistic regression revealed that specific baseline characteristics predicted membership within each of the three "faller" trajectory groups as compared to the no falls trajectory group are shown in **Table 4**. Predictors of the Cluster Falls trajectory were faster gait speed and falls in past year. Predictors of the Increasing Falls trajectory were Diabetes Mellitus (DM) and Cognitive Impairment. Predictors of Chronic Recurring Falls were two or more comorbid chronic conditions and falls in the past year. Symptoms of depression were predictive of all groups.

Discussion

In this 5-year prospective cohort study, we examined the course of falls in community-dwelling older adults. We found four clinically distinct trajectories of falls that we have labeled: cluster falls, increasing falls, chronic recurring falls, and no falls. We found that Diabetes mellitus, cognitive impairment, fast gait speed, falls in the past year at baseline, and multi-morbidity are predictors of these trajectories. Importantly, these trajectories were associated with adverse outcomes including injurious falls and fractures. Notably, people with chronic recurrent falls had the highest rate of injurious falls and fractures. There was a marginally significant increase in hospitalizations among those with increasing falls.

The number of falls that each participant reported each month was summated for each year over the 5 years study period and quantified as a "Falls Per Year of Aging" Score (FPYA Score). For each one year time interval, No Falls equaled FPYA 0, one fall equaled FPYA 1, two falls equaled FPYA 2 (recurrent falls), and three or more falls equaled FPYA 3 (high number of recurrent falls). These scores were distributed according the censored normal distribution and their modeling identified 4-groups.

The major utility of the 4-group solution is in the ability of these 4 groups to predict adverse outcomes. In addition, the 4-group trajectory solution identified some risk factors to target for interventions. These patterns of falls had a few distinguishing risk factors described above. Some of these are potentially modifiable, such as diabetes for increasing falls and comorbid conditions for Chronic recurring falls. The greater proportion of fast walkers in the cluster group may represent people who are less careful or have more acute condition rather than chronic diseases (e.g. these comorbity scores are lower than other fall groups). We believe that falls incidence declines in the chronic recurrent falls group beginning in year 4 because people who had recurrent falls had clinically adverse events like hospital visits or fractures which reduced their mobility and chance of falling. Recurrent falls over 3-years may signal the beginning of functional decline.

This study is unique in demonstrating that not all falls have the same clinical implications. As we have shown, some may occur in relatively short-lived clusters, perhaps from an acute illness or exposure to a new drug or environmental hazard; some may increase in frequency over time, possibly due to the progression of a disease or disability; and some may recur at a relatively high rate over time. Each of these presentations appears to have a distinct set of risk factors and in some circumstances different prognostic implications. For example, chronic recurrent falls seem to occur in people with multiple co-morbidities (multi-morbidity) [26,27] and

depressive symptoms, and, as might be expected, are associated with a relatively high rate of injuries and fractures.

Although a high incidence of falls has been reported in older populations [1], little is known about the progression of falls over a long period of time. To our knowledge there are no longitudinal studies that observed the trajectories of fallers. While some falls are isolated, non-recurring events, others may mark the beginning of a progressive down-hill course in which the injuries and fear associated with an initial fall may precipitate recurrences and spiraling functional decline. A previous study showed that illnesses and injuries leading to either hospitalization or restricted activity are strongly associated with the initial onset of disability [28]. Another study extended this earlier work by demonstrating that exposure to intervening illnesses and injuries are also associated with the subsequent course of disability [29]. Therefore, it is important to distinguish those falls that are likely to be isolated episodes from those that lead to further disability. A Cochrane review highlighted the difficulty identifying an appropriate group for preventive efforts as a result of this heterogeneity in the presentation and subsequent course of falls in older populations [7,8].

Our study has several limitations. 1) We used baseline clinical characteristics that were obtained up to 5 years before the falls occurred, so we were unable to identify risk factors at the time the falls. This limited our ability to determine whether cluster falls were due to acute illnesses, drugs, or environmental hazards, and whether other patterns followed the course of chronic diseases. 2) Some of our participants experienced falls before the study began. Thus, these falls were left censored in our analysis. It is therefore possible that some of our non-fallers experienced fall episodes before the study began. We performed secondary analyses, stratifying previous fallers by non-fallers and found similar patterns. Unfortunately, the sample sizes of these subgroups were too small to draw meaningful conclusions. 3) Finally, because our study participants were only from a Massachusetts geographic area within a 5-mile radius of the Institute for Aging Research, the cohort may not be generalizable. However, a comparison of the demographics of MBS study participants to the US Census showed comparable distributions by sex and racial group in the population aged 70 and older [9].

In summary, our study provides evidence suggesting four clinically distinct patterns of falls over five years among community-dwelling older adults. Each of these patterns has a distinct set of independent risk factors. Compared to all other groups, chronic recurring falls are associated with the highest rate of injuries. Older adults with recurrent falls should be targeted by health care professionals to identify their underlying cause and implement interventions to prevent subsequent injury.

Acknowledgments

The authors thank Thierry Dantoine, Hamid Siahmed, Denis Valleix, and Regional Council of Limousin from France for supporting Achille Tchalla, MOBILIZE Boston research team, Margaret Gagnon and study participants for their time, effort, and dedication.

Author Contributions

Conceived and designed the experiments: AT LAL. Performed the experiments: AT II LAL. Analyzed the data: AT ABD TGT DH BM LAL. Contributed reagents/materials/analysis tools: DH II ABD TGT LAL. Wrote the paper: AT ABD TGT LAL.

References

1. Tinetti ME, Speechley M (1989) Prevention of falls among the elderly. N Engl J Med 320: 1055–1059.

2. Lipsitz LA, Jonsson PV, Kelley MM, Koestner JS (1991) Causes and correlates of recurrent falls in ambulatory frail elderly. J Gerontol 46: M114–122.

3. Gorina Y, Hoyert D, Lentzner H, Goulding M (2005) Trends in causes of death among older persons in the United States. Aging Trends: 1–12.

4. Tinetti ME, Baker DI, King M, Gottschalk M, Murphy TE, et al. (2008) Effect of dissemination of evidence in reducing injuries from falls. N Engl J Med 359: 252–261.

5. Rubenstein LZ (2006) Falls in older people: epidemiology, risk factors and strategies for prevention. Age Ageing 35 Suppl 2: ii37–ii41.

6. Gates S, Fisher JD, Cooke MW, Carter YH, Lamb SE (2008) Multifactorial assessment and targeted intervention for preventing falls and injuries among older people in community and emergency care settings: systematic review and meta-analysis. BMJ 336: 130–133.

7. Gillespie LD, Robertson MC, Gillespie WJ, Sherrington C, Gates S, et al. (2012) Interventions for preventing falls in older people living in the community. Cochrane Database Syst Rev 9: CD007146.

8. Stevens JA, Corso PS, Finkelstein EA, Miller TR (2006) The costs of fatal and non-fatal falls among older adults. Inj Prev 12: 290–295.

9. Leveille SG, Kiel DP, Jones RN, Roman A, Hannan MT, et al. (2008) The MOBILIZE Boston Study: design and methods of a prospective cohort study of novel risk factors for falls in an older population. BMC Geriatr 8: 16.

10. Samelson EJ, Kelsey JL, Kiel DP, Roman AM, Cupples LA, et al. (2008) Issues in conducting epidemiologic research among elders: lessons from the MOBILIZE Boston Study. Am J Epidemiol 168: 1444–1451.

11. Escobar JI, Burnam A, Karno M, Forsythe A, Landsverk J, et al. (1986) Use of the Mini-Mental State Examination (MMSE) in a community population of mixed ethnicity. Cultural and linguistic artifacts. J Nerv Ment Dis 174: 607–614.

12. Folstein MF, Folstein SE, McHugh PR (1975) "Mini-mental state". A practical method for grading the cognitive state of patients for the clinician. J Psychiatr Res 12: 189–198.

13. (1987) The prevention of falls in later life. A report of the Kellogg International Work Group on the Prevention of Falls by the Elderly. Dan Med Bull 34 Suppl 4: 1–24.

14. Tinetti ME, Liu WL, Claus EB (1993) Predictors and prognosis of inability to get up after falls among elderly persons. JAMA 269: 65–70.

15. Washburn RA, Smith KW, Jette AM, Janney CA (1993) The Physical Activity Scale for the Elderly (PASE): development and evaluation. J Clin Epidemiol 46: 153–162.

16. Kohout FJ, Berkman LF, Evans DA, Cornoni-Huntley J (1993) Two shorter forms of the CES-D (Center for Epidemiological Studies Depression) depression symptoms index. J Aging Health 5: 179–193.

17. Guralnik JM, Ferrucci L, Simonsick EM, Salive ME, Wallace RB (1995) Lower-extremity function in persons over the age of 70 years as a predictor of subsequent disability. N Engl J Med 332: 556–561.

18. Nagin D (2005) Group-based modeling of development. Cambridge, Mass: Harvard University Press. x, 201 p. p.

19. Jones B ND, Roeder K, editor (2001) A SAS procedure based on mixture models for estimating developmental trajectories. 374–393 p.

20. Jones DJ, Runyan DK, Lewis T, Litrownik AJ, Black MM, et al. (2010) Trajectories of childhood sexual abuse and early adolescent HIV/AIDS risk behaviors: the role of other maltreatment, witnessed violence, and child gender. J Clin Child Adolesc Psychol 39: 667–680.

21. Nagin DS, Tremblay RE (2005) What has been learned from group-based trajectory modeling? Examples from physical aggression and other problem behaviors. Annals of the American Academy of Political and Social Science 602: 82–117.

22. Nagin DS, Odgers CL (2010) Group-Based Trajectory Modeling in Clinical Research. Annual Review of Clinical Psychology, Vol 6 6: 109–138.

23. Nagelkerke NJD (1991) A Note on a General Definition of the Coefficient of Determination. Biometrika 78: 691–692.

24. Cohen J, Cohen P, West S, L A (2003) Applied Multiple Regression/Correlation Analysis for the Behaviour Sciences; 3, editor.

25. Pepe MS (2003) The statistical evaluation of medical tests for classification and prediction. Oxford; New York: Oxford University Press. xvi, 302 p. p.

26. Marengoni A, Angleman S, Melis R, Mangialasche F, Karp A, et al. (2011) Aging with multimorbidity: a systematic review of the literature. Ageing Res Rev 10: 430–439.

27. Sibley KM, Voth J, Munce SE, Straus SE, Jaglal SB (2014) Chronic disease and falls in community-dwelling Canadians over 65 years old: a population-based study exploring associations with number and pattern of chronic conditions. BMC Geriatr 14: 22.

28. Gill TM, Allore HG, Holford TR, Guo Z (2004) Hospitalization, restricted activity, and the development of disability among older persons. JAMA 292: 2115–2124.

29. Gill TM, Allore HG, Gahbauer EA, Murphy TE (2010) Change in disability after hospitalization or restricted activity in older persons. JAMA 304: 1919–1928.

11

Boosting Long-Term Memory via Wakeful Rest: Intentional Rehearsal Is Not Necessary, Consolidation Is Sufficient

Michaela Dewar[1,2,3*¶], **Jessica Alber**[2¶], **Nelson Cowan**[2,4], **Sergio Della Sala**[2,3]

1 Department of Psychology, School of Life Sciences, Heriot-Watt University, Edinburgh, United Kingdom, 2 Human Cognitive Neuroscience, Department of Psychology, University of Edinburgh, United Kingdom, 3 Centre for Cognitive Ageing and Cognitive Epidemiology, Psychology, University of Edinburgh, Edinburgh, United Kingdom, 4 Department of Psychology, University of Missouri, Columbia, Missouri, United States of America

Abstract

People perform better on tests of delayed free recall if learning is followed immediately by a short wakeful rest than by a short period of sensory stimulation. Animal and human work suggests that wakeful resting provides optimal conditions for the consolidation of recently acquired memories. However, an alternative account cannot be ruled out, namely that wakeful resting provides optimal conditions for intentional rehearsal of recently acquired memories, thus driving superior memory. Here we utilised non-recallable words to examine whether wakeful rest boosts long-term memory, even when new memories could not be rehearsed intentionally during the wakeful rest delay. The probing of non-recallable words requires a recognition paradigm. Therefore, we first established, via Experiment 1, that the rest-induced boost in memory observed via free recall can be replicated in a recognition paradigm, using concrete nouns. In Experiment 2, participants heard 30 non-recallable non-words, presented as 'foreign names in a bridge club abroad' and then either rested wakefully or played a visual spot-the-difference game for 10 minutes. Retention was probed via recognition at two time points, 15 minutes and 7 days after presentation. As in Experiment 1, wakeful rest boosted recognition significantly, and this boost was maintained for at least 7 days. Our results indicate that the enhancement of memory via wakeful rest is *not* dependent upon intentional rehearsal of learned material during the rest period. We thus conclude that consolidation is *sufficient* for this rest-induced memory boost to emerge. We propose that wakeful resting allows for superior memory consolidation, resulting in stronger and/or more veridical representations of experienced events which can be detected via tests of free recall and recognition.

Editor: Howard Nusbaum, The University of Chicago, United States of America

Funding: This work was funded by Age UK (Grant 355; url: www.ageuk.org.uk/) as part of a Ph.D. studentship awarded to MD and SDS and held by JA, and by a Personal Research Fellowship (Grant number: 29400 R41255; url: www.ltsbfoundationforscotland.org.uk) awarded to MD by the Royal Society of Edinburgh and Lloyds/TSB Foundation for Scotland. The funders had no role in study design, data collection and analysis, decision to publish, or preparation of the manuscript.

Competing Interests: The authors have declared that no competing interests exist.

* Email: m.dewar@hw.ac.uk

¶ MD and JA are co-first authors on this work.

Introduction

A period of wakeful rest immediately after new learning boosts free recall of verbal material. Several studies show that both young and elderly people recall more newly learned verbal material after a 10-60-minute interval if this interval is filled with wakeful rest than with sensory stimulation [1–4]. A recent study showed that this memory enhancement via a brief wakeful rest is maintained for at least 7 days in healthy elderly people [2]. Here we investigate the cognitive basis of this memory boost.

Recent insights from human and animal neuroscience suggest that wakeful rest improves memory by enhancing memory consolidation [2,5–11]. Memory consolidation is defined as the automatic process by which memories strengthen over time [12]. Evidence for this consolidation process comes from animal work showing that, over time, new memories become less susceptible to the interfering effects of pharmacological manipulations [12–14]. In keeping with these animal findings, our work in humans shows

that new memories are retained better if post-learning cognitive tasks are delayed than if they take place immediately after learning, i.e. a temporal gradient of behavioural interference is observed [2,3].

Research in rodents suggests that consolidation is associated with the spontaneous reactivation of recent encoding-related neural activity, and that this reactivation occurs predominantly during states of relative immobility, such as sleep and wakeful rest [8,9,15,16]. Recent neuroimaging work in humans strengthens this consolidation hypothesis, revealing (i) reactivation of recent encoding-related neural activity during wakeful rest, and (ii) a direct link between the degree of such reactivation and performance on subsequent memory [10,11]. This work in animals and humans suggest that wakeful rest provides optimal conditions for consolidation of recently acquired memories, perhaps due to minimal encoding of novel interfering information [2,6,7].

However, an alternative account cannot be ruled out, namely that wakeful resting provides optimal conditions for *intentional rehearsal* of recently acquired memories, thus driving superior memory during wakeful rest delays, at least in humans. Intentional retrieval of learned material improves long-term retention of newly learned material [17,18], and this 'retrieval practice' effect is observed when participants rehearse material overtly or covertly [19]. Elaborative rehearsal, the intentional integration of newly acquired memory traces within an existing framework in long-term storage, also enhances long-term free recall and recognition memory [20–22].

Could intentional rehearsal be at the heart of the memory boost observed via post-learning wakeful rest? Several findings speak against this possibility: firstly, in the research on wakeful rest and memory, participants are not informed about the delayed recall test, thus reducing the motivation to intentionally rehearse the memoranda in order to augment test performance [1–3]. Secondly, during structured post-experimental debriefing, the majority of participants report that they did not think about test material during the wakeful rest period [2,3,11]. However, this evidence is derived indirectly rather than via controlled experiments, and therefore the intentional rehearsal hypothesis cannot be dismissed.

Here, we report two experiments, in which we explored whether wakeful resting boosts verbal long-term memory, even when new memories *cannot* be rehearsed *intentionally* during the rest interval. To this end, we aimed to use non-recallable non-words as our memoranda. The use of non-recallable words requires the application of a recognition paradigm. Therefore, our first experiment examined whether the rest-related boost in memory that is observed in free recall [1–3] is also observed in recognition when using common nouns. Our second experiment used a recognition paradigm to examine whether wakeful rest improves long-term recognition of non-words (e.g., *phiefnierds*) that could not be recalled freely.

Results indicating that even non-recallable stimuli can benefit from a post-learning interval of wakeful rest would refute the hypothesis that intentional rehearsal is necessary to achieve a long-lived memory benefit via wakeful rest.

Experiment 1

Methods

Ethics statement. Both experiments were approved by the University of Edinburgh's Psychology Research Ethics Committee (Ref: 187-1112/1; 190-1213/1). All participants provided their informed consent in writing prior to taking part in our research.

Participants. We tested healthy elderly people since we sought to follow up our previous findings involving this population [2]. Healthy elderly people constitute a growing portion of the population and often report age-related difficulties with memory [2]. Seventy healthy volunteers (21m/49f) were randomly divided into two groups, based on post-learning stimulation condition: *high sensory stimulation* (N = 36, mean age = 73 years, age range = 62–83 years; mean NART-predicted IQ = 119.29, range = 105.96–127.17, [23]; 8m/28f) and *minimal sensory stimulation* (N = 34, mean age = 71 years, age range = 61–87 years; mean NART-predicted IQ = 118.04, range = 106.74–125.81, [23]; 13m/21f).

Participants had no premorbid neurological or psychiatric history, and demonstrated normal scores on a thorough neuropsychological test battery, including the Addenbrooke's Cognitive Examination-Revised (ACE-R) [24]. The ACE-R is a widely-used screening test for cognitive impairment. We applied the conservative ACE-R cut-off of 88 to ensure that all of our participants were cognitively intact. The groups did not differ significantly in

age (p = .147), NART-predicted IQ (p = .245) or ACE-R scores (p = .204).

Design. Experiment 1 included two testing sessions, Session 1 and Session 2, which were separated by 7 days. We used a mixed design to examine retention of a list of words. There were two key manipulations: stimulation condition (high sensory stimulation vs. minimal sensory stimulation; between subjects) and retention interval (15 minutes vs. 7 days; within subjects).

Materials. A total of 30 unrelated, common nouns (e.g. platform, daylight, specialist) were grouped into two lists of 15 words each for memory testing. The words were selected from the MRC Psycholinguistic database and were matched for number of letters, syllables, familiarity, concreteness, imaginability and frequency (frequency was taken from the British National Corpus). One word list was used as the target list, the other as the foil list. The target and foil lists had a similar range in number of letters, syllables, familiarity, concreteness, and imaginability, but they did not overlap highly in terms of semantics or phonology, i.e. the foils were not highly similar to the targets.

30 picture pairs were employed as filler materials. The picture pairs were photographs of complex real-world scenes (e.g. landscapes, animals and people). They were manipulated so that the pictures in each pair differed in 2 subtle ways [2].

Procedure. Figure 1 illustrates the procedure of Experiment 1. In *Session 1*, participants were presented with the list of 15 target words. The words were presented aurally to participants at a rate of 1 word per second, with a 2-second interval between words. Participants were asked to try to remember as many words as possible, in any order, for an immediate recall test. This was followed by a 10-minute delay filled with either (i) high sensory stimulation or (ii) minimal sensory stimulation. Participants were not informed about subsequent delayed recall at this time.

Participants in the *high sensory stimulation group* completed 10 minutes of a spot-the-difference task, during which they were presented sequentially with 30 picture pairs on a laptop screen [2]. Their task was to identify and point to two differences between each picture pair within a 20-second time limit. Participants were instructed not to talk during the task, and care was taken to ensure that the spot-the-difference task was entirely visual: full instructions as well as a 1-minute practice trial were administered prior to Session 1 in order to minimalize verbalization during the delay. The spot-the-difference task was employed for two key reasons: firstly, it introduced new meaningful material and was cognitively demanding, thereby hampering word list *consolidation* [1–4,6]. Secondly, it was non-verbal and highly unlike the word lists, thereby minimising potential interference at *retrieval* between word list memories and filler task memories [1,2]. That is, the visual spot-the-difference task allowed us to examine the effect of sensory stimulation condition on word list consolidation specifically, without the potential confound of retrieval interference.

Participants in the *minimal sensory stimulation group* were instructed to rest quietly in a darkened testing room while the experimenter went to 'organize the next part of the study' [2,3]. To ensure minimal sensory stimulation, all equipment was turned off, and participants had no access to mobile phones, newspapers, etc.

In order to make sure that both groups engaged in identical activity prior to delayed recall, all participants completed a 5-minute spot-the-difference distractor task immediately after the 10-minute post-learning delay period [2]. Subsequent to this, participants were asked to recall orally as many of the 15 words as they could, in any order (15-minute delayed recall). To conclude Session 1, participants completed a structured post-experimental survey asking such questions (as applicable) as: 'did you expect to

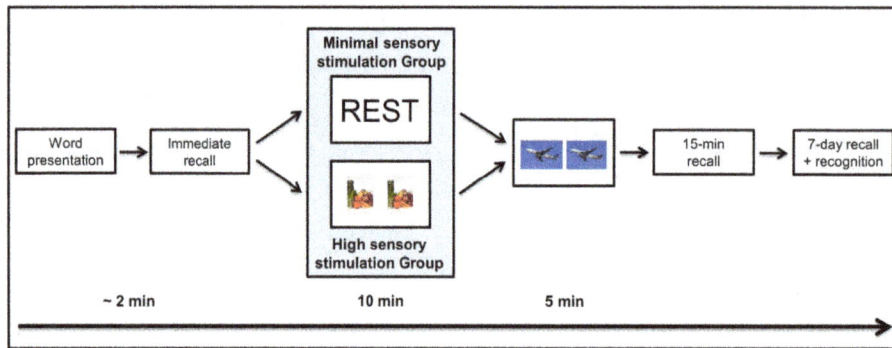

Figure 1. Participants were assigned randomly to the high sensory stimulation (N = 36) or minimal sensory stimulation (N = 34) group. In Session 1, all participants were presented with a list of 15 common nouns, which they were told to remember for subsequent immediate free recall. Following this, participants in the high sensory stimulation group completed a spot-the-difference task for 10 minutes, whereas participants in the minimal sensory stimulation group rested wakefully for 10 minutes. All participants then completed a 5-minute distractor task (spot-the-difference), which was succeeded by a surprise delayed recall test of the word list. In Session 2, which took place 7 days after Session 1, participants completed another surprise delayed free recall of the word list, as well a 30-item yes/no recognition test, including a remember/know paradigm.

be asked to remember the words again?' and 'did you think about the words during the wakeful rest delay?' Participants were not informed of the nature of Session 2 at this juncture.

At the beginning of *Session 2*, which occurred 7 days after Session 1, participants received a *free recall test*: they were asked again to recall orally as many of the 15 words as they could, in any order (7-day delayed recall). Upon completion of the 7-day free recall test, participants performed an untimed *recognition test*: this was a 30-item yes/no test, comprising the 15 target words and 15 foils. Target and foil words were presented orally in the same random order for each participant. Participants were asked whether the word was old (i.e. had been presented in Session 1) or new (i.e. had not been presented in Session 1). If they made an 'old' response, participants were asked to make a remember/know judgment [25,26]. Participants were instructed to respond 'remember' if their recognition of a word was accompanied by recollection of its occurrence a week earlier, and 'know' if a word 'rings a bell' but was not accompanied by any recollection of its occurrence a week earlier. They were given a number of examples prior to the remember/know test to ensure that they understood and were comfortable with the distinction between these two forms of memory. We applied the remember/know task to allow for a more fine-grained probing of the effect of wakeful rest on memory, in case this was not picked up adequately by a simple yes/no recognition test. The remember/know task is frequently used to differentiate between recollection (remember) and familiarity (know) [27–29], although there is a lively debate as to whether this apparent distinction between recollection and familiarity reflects separate memory processes (dual-trace theory) [27,29–32] or simply reflects variations in a continuous memory strength (single-process theory) [33,34].

At the end of *Session 2*, participants completed another post-experimental survey, asking whether they had thought about the words in the 7 days since Session 1, and whether they expected to be asked to recall the words again.

Scoring. For the *free recall test*, we computed the total number of words recalled correctly at (i) immediate recall, (ii) 15-minute delayed recall, and (iii) 7-day delayed recall. In order to discern how many words recalled at immediate recall were retained at 15-minute and at 7-day delayed recall, a percentage retention score was computed for each participant at 15-minute delayed recall and 7-day delayed recall [2,3,5,35–37]. Percentage

retention scores were calculated by dividing the number of words recalled at 15-minute and 7-day delayed recall by the number of words recalled at immediate recall, and multiplying this quotient by 100. All percentage retention scores were capped at 100%. Percentage retention scores control for individual differences and any between-group variation at immediate recall.

For the *recognition test*, hit rates were calculated by dividing the number of targets correctly identified by the total number of targets (/15). False alarm rates were calculated by dividing the number of foils incorrectly identified as targets by the total number of foils (/15). In order to measure recognition accuracy, d-prime (d') was calculated via the following equation: $d' = z(hit\ rate) - z(false\ alarm\ rate)$. None of the participants had a hit rate of 1, thus no corrections had to be made to hit rate scores during the computation of d'. 1 participant had a false alarm rate of 0, thus requiring correction for the computation of d'. In line with standard correction procedures, we corrected this score by adding half a false alarm to this score, i.e. (1/30), resulting in a corrected false alarm rate of 0.033. As a further measure of recognition accuracy, we calculated the correct response rate. This was computed by adding the number of targets correctly identified as targets (hits) and the number of foils correctly identified as foils (correct rejections) and dividing this number by the total number of targets and foils (/30).

Statistical analyses. The alpha level was set to .05 for all analyses, which were conducted in IBM SPSS Statistics 19. We compared the two sensory stimulation groups' immediate free recall via a one-way ANOVA. We analysed the free recall proportion retention data by carrying out a mixed model, repeated measures ANOVA with time as a within subjects factor (15 minutes vs. 7 days) and stimulation condition as a between subjects factor (high sensory stimulation vs. minimal sensory stimulation). Based on our previous findings [2], we ran two planned comparisons, using one-way ANOVAs, to examine whether minimal sensory stimulation improved proportion retention (i) after 15 minutes and (ii) after 7 days. We compared the sensory stimulation groups' 7-day recognition data via one-way ANOVAs. Furthermore, we ran repeated measures ANOVAs to compare within each group the proportion of hits 'remembered' and the proportion of hits 'known'. Lastly, we used Pearson's correlations to examine associations between 7-day free recall percentage retention and 7-day recognition performance.

Results

Immediate free recall. Immediate recall scores did not differ between the minimal sensory stimulation group (mean = 6.09, SEM = .218) and the high sensory stimulation group (mean = 6.06, SEM = .219), $(F(1, 68) = 0, p = .992)$. This indicates that baseline performance was matched for the stimulation condition groups.

Delayed free recall - Retention of word lists after (a) 15 minutes and (b) 7 days. Figure 2 shows that 15-minute wordlist retention was significantly higher in the minimal sensory stimulation group than in the high sensory stimulation group, $(F(1, 68) = 17.87, p < .001)$. Retention dropped over 7 days in both stimulation groups $(F(1, 68) = 138.488, p < .001, \eta_p^2 = .671)$. However, the superior retention in the minimal sensory stimulation group relative to the high sensory stimulation group was maintained at 7-day delayed recall, $(F(1, 68) = 12.957, p < .01)$, with no further additional benefit after 7 days, i.e. no significant time x group interaction $(F(1, 68) = 0, p = .991, \eta_p^2 = 0)$.

Table 1 shows all data for the yes/no *word recognition* test (15 targets and 15 foils) taking place *after 7 days*.

d′. d′ was significantly higher in the minimal sensory stimulation group than in the high sensory stimulation group, $(F(1, 68) = 5.694, p < .05)$.

Correct response rate. Correct response rate (hits + correct rejections/30) was significantly higher in the minimal sensory stimulation group than in the high sensory stimulation group $(F(1, 68) = 6.206, p < .05)$.

Hit rate and false alarm rate. Hit rate did not differ significantly between the high sensory stimulation group and the minimal sensory stimulation group $(F(1, 68) = .878, p = .352)$. However, false alarm rate was significantly higher in the high sensory stimulation group than in the minimal sensory stimulation group $(F(1, 68) = 4.477, p < .05)$.

Remember/Know. Figure 3 and Table 1 show that for hits, the proportion of 'remember' responses was significantly higher in the minimal sensory stimulation group than in the high sensory stimulation group $(F(1, 68) = 5.857, p < .05)$. Correspondingly, the proportion of 'know' responses was significantly lower in the minimal sensory stimulation than in the high sensory stimulation

group. Indeed, while in the minimal sensory stimulation group there was no significant difference in the proportion of 'remember' and 'know' responses $(F(1, 33) = .009, p = .927, \eta_p^2 = 0)$, in the high sensory stimulation group, the proportion of 'know' responses was significantly higher than the proportion of 'remember' responses $(F(1, 35) = 10.326, p < .01, \eta_p^2 = .228)$.

Associations between 7-day free recall and 7-day recognition performance (collapsed over both groups). Percentage retention at 7-day free recall correlated significantly and *positively* with d′ $(r = .322, p < .001)$, correct response rate $(r = .350, p < .01)$, and with proportion of hits 'remembered' $(r = .424, p < .001)$. Moreover, percentage retention at 7-day free recall correlated significantly and *negatively* with false alarm rate $(r = -.326, p < .01)$, and with proportion of hits known $(r = -.424, p < .001)$. However, percentage retention at 7-day free recall did not correlate significantly with hit rate $(r = .107, p = .377)$.

Post-experimental questionnaire. The questionnaire data revealed the following:

Expected recall - 1 participant in the high sensory stimulation group and 3 participants in the minimal sensory stimulation group reported that they had expected delayed recall in Session 1. Six participants in the high sensory stimulation group and 10 participants in the minimal sensory stimulation group reported that they had expected delayed recall in Session 2; *Delay activity and rehearsal* - four participants in the minimal sensory stimulation group reported thinking about the words during some of the wakeful rest period. The other participants reported mind-wandering. Ten of the participants in the high sensory stimulation group and 11 participants in the minimal sensory stimulation group reported thinking about the words during the 7-day interval (1–6 times).

We repeated the above analyses, including only those participants who did not report thinking about the words (during the wakeful rest period and/or between sessions) or expecting delayed recall (high sensory stimulation group N = 24, minimal sensory stimulation group N = 20). The results did not change, bar the group difference in 7-day hit rate (minimal sensory stimulation group mean = .697, SEM = .026; high sensory stimulation group mean = .608, SEM = .028), which became significant $(p < .05)$, and the correlations between percentage retention at 7-day free recall and (i) proportion of hits 'remembered' $(p = .1)$ and (ii) proportion of hits known $(p = .1)$, which no longer reached significance. See File S1, including Table S1 in File S1, for the results of all repeated analyses.

Comments. The results of Experiment 1 demonstrate that the memory enhancement via wakeful rest can be observed via recognition, thus (i) confirming the feasibility of this paradigm for Experiment 2, and (ii) opening novel avenues for the examination of the memory boost and its cognitive basis. The latter will be discussed further in the Discussion.

Experiment 2

The purpose of Experiment 2 was to examine whether a brief period of wakeful rest after new learning improves recognition memory, even for stimuli that cannot be rehearsed intentionally during the wakeful rest period. In everyday life people often learn new words that cannot be retrieved intentionally after a single exposure. For example, if one encountered someone with a foreign or unfamiliar name for the first time, one may not be able to recall their name freely. However, if the person's name was mentioned, one might recognize it as belonging to someone one has met before. Our paradigm was based on this scenario.

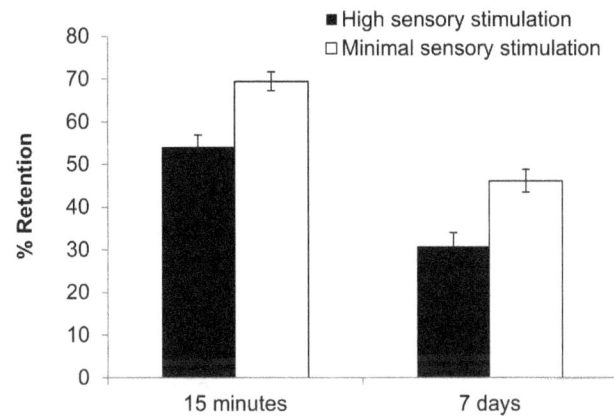

Figure 2. Mean percentage retention scores at 15-minute and 7-day delayed free recall ((Delayed/Immediate) x 100) in the high sensory stimulation and minimal sensory stimulation groups in Experiment 1. 15-minute retention was significantly higher in the minimal sensory stimulation group than in the high sensory stimulation group, and this benefit was maintained over 7 days. Error bars = standard error of the mean.

Table 1. Mean recognition performance (+ SEM) of the minimal sensory stimulation groups (wakeful rest delay) and the high sensory stimulation groups (spot-the-difference delay) in Experiment 1 and 2.

| | Experiment 2 (non-words) | | | | | | Experiment 1 (common nouns) | | |
| | 15 minutes | | | 7 days | | | 7 days | | |
	Minimal	High	p-value	Minimal	High	p-value	Minimal	High	p-value
Yes/No Test									
d'	1.209 (.091)	.696 (.103)	<.001	1.000 (.086)	.449 (.100)	<.001	1.032 (.084)	.757 (.078)	<.05
Correct response rate	.712 (.014)	.626 (.018)	<.001	.670 (.016)	.575 (.016)	<.001	.685 (.013)	.636 (.015)	<.05
Hit rate	.677 (.026)	.625 (.033)	.227	.553 (.036)	.469 (.034)	.094	.661 (.019)	.633 (.022)	.352
False alarm rate	.253 (.021)	.373 (.028)	<.005	.212 (.020)	.320 (.027)	<.005	.290 (.023)	.362 (.024)	<.05
Remember/Know									
Proportion Remember - Hits	.348 (.039)	.290 (.032)	.255	.304 (.039)	.273 (.034)	.55	.497 (.030)	.381 (.037)	<.05
Proportion Know - Hits	.652 (.039)	.710 (.032)	.255	.696 (.039)	.727 (.034)	.55	.503 (.030)	.619 (.037)	<.05
Proportion Remember - False alarms	.079 (.026)	.071 (.026)	.832	.130 (.047)	.070 (.042)	.392	.049 (.031)	.041 (.022)	.833
Proportion Know - False alarms	.921 (.026)	.929 (.026)	.832	.870 (.047)	.924 (.042)	.392	.951 (.031)	.959 (.022)	.833

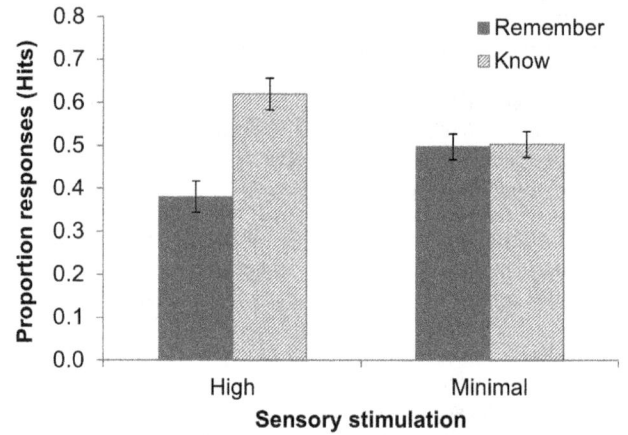

Figure 3. Proportion of 'remember' and 'know' responses for *hits* in the high sensory and minimal sensory stimulation groups after 7 days in Experiment 1. The proportion of 'remember' responses was higher in the minimal sensory stimulation than in the high sensory stimulation group. Error bars = standard error of the mean.

Methods

The procedure of Experiment 2 was aligned as closely as possible to that of Experiment 1, but used recognition testing instead of free recall at both the 15-min and 7-day time points. In contrast to Experiment 1, there was no immediate test in Experiment 2: a test of immediate recognition would have introduced new stimuli, i.e. the foils, as well as taking up several minutes, and this could have interfered with the early consolidation of the word list, thus reducing the effect of minimal sensory stimulation shown in tests of free recall. Moreover, in contrast to Experiment 1, the stimuli used in Experiment 2 were non-words.

Participants. As in Experiment 1, we tested healthy elderly people. Fifty-four healthy elderly adults (21m/33f) were randomly assigned to one of two stimulation condition groups, the *high sensory stimulation* group (N = 27, mean age = 72.22 years, age range = 61–89 years; NART-predicted IQ = 121.68, range = 112.98–127.02; 10m/17f) and the *minimal sensory stimulation* group (N = 27, mean age = 75.33 years, age range = 60–90 years; mean NART-predicted IQ = 120.9, range = 114.64–124.68; 11m/16f). As in Experiment 1, participants had no premorbid neurological or psychiatric history, and demonstrated normal scores on a thorough neuropsychological test battery, including the ACE-R [24], in which all participants scored ≥88 (high cut off). The groups did not differ significantly in age (p = .109), NART-predicted IQ (p = .268) or ACE-R scores (p = .349).

Design. Like Experiment 1, Experiment 2 included two testing sessions, Session 1 and Session 2, which were separated by 7 days. We used a mixed design to examine retention of a list of non-words. There were two key manipulations: stimulation condition (high sensory stimulation vs. minimal sensory stimulation; between subjects) and retention interval (15 minutes vs. 7 days; within subjects).

Materials. A total of 60 words were employed in this experiment, grouped into four lists of 15 words each. The four lists included the two lists used in Experiment 1 as well as two further lists. As in Experiment 1, the words were selected from the MRC Psycholinguistic database and were matched for number of letters, syllables, familiarity, concreteness, imaginability and frequency (frequency was taken from the British National Corpus). In order to obtain 60 non-recallable stimuli, each word was scrambled (e.g. Experiment 1 word 'junction' = Experiment 2 word 'toijcunn'). 30 of the scrambled non-words were used as targets, and the remaining 30 scrambled non-words were used as foils. Scrambled non-words had the same number of syllables as their English word counterparts to ensure consistency across experiments.

In order to avoid repetition of targets and foils in the 15-minute and 7-day tests, the target non-words were divided into two recognition tests, one for the 15-minute delay test, the other for the 7-day delay test: test A contained the target stimuli that had been presented in odd positions (word 1, word 3, word 5), and test B contained the target stimuli that had been presented in even positions (word 2, word 4, word 6). The order of tests A and B was counterbalanced across participants.

The 30 'spot-the-difference' picture pairs from Experiment 1 were also used in Experiment 2 during filled delay periods (see Experiment 1 Methods for details).

Pilot investigations. Prior to Experiment 2, two pilot investigations were conducted in order to ascertain (i) that our non-words could not be retrieved intentionally, but (ii) that they could be recognised well in a Yes/No recognition test.

In the first pilot investigation (N = 12), participants listened to each of the 60 non-words and were asked to state if the items were in any way semantically meaningful to them. A semantic connection was made by one participant to four of the non-words, and these four non-words were re-scrambled and re-piloted in order to ensure that no semantic connection was made to any of the non-words.

In the second pilot investigation (N = 12), participants were presented with the 30 target non-words aurally. Immediately after presentation, participants were asked to recall as many of the non-words as possible, in any order. None of the participants were able to freely recall any of the non-words accurately, thus indicating that our lists of words were indeed non-recallable. Immediately after the free recall phase, participants completed a recognition test with the 30 target non-words and 30 foils. Participants had a mean d′ score of 1.44, showing that they were able to recognize the target non-words immediately after presentation (mean hit rate = 0.73, mean false alarm rate = 0.21), and thus that recognition testing could be conducted over longer time intervals.

Procedure. Figure 4 illustrates the procedure of Experiment 2. In *Session 1* of Experiment 2, participants were presented with the 30 target non-words aurally. To provide context, the non-words were presented as peoples' names, and were paired with a face taken from the Glasgow Unfamiliar Face Database (15 faces were female, 15 male). The face/name pairs were used to simulate a real life situation, i.e. meeting someone new with a foreign name. The following instructions were provided to all participants prior to the experiment: 'I want you to imagine that you've moved to a new country and you've joined a bridge club. You're meeting the other club members for the first time, and they have names that sound foreign and unfamiliar to you. When you hear each name, you will see that person's face on the screen. I would like you to try to remember the club members' names. After you've heard all of the names, you are going to be asked to identify them from a longer list of names, some of which you have heard before, and some of which you have not heard before. Your task will be to tell me whether or not you've met that person at the bridge club. You probably won't recognize all of the names, but do your best. Do you have any questions?'

The 30 face/name pairs were presented in the same random order across participants. As was the case for words in Experiment 1, non-words were presented aurally for a duration of one second each, with two seconds between non-words. Faces remained on the computer screen for the two second gap between each non-word (for a cumulative total of 3 seconds) to ensure equal timings across experiments.

After the 30 target face/name pairs were presented, participants in the minimal sensory stimulation group had a 10-minute delay of wakeful rest (see Experiment 1), while participants in the high sensory stimulation group completed 10 minutes of the spot-the-difference task (see Experiment 1). As in Experiment 1, both groups completed 5 minutes of the spot-the-difference task immediately after the post-learning delay to ensure that both groups engaged in the same activity prior to delayed recognition testing.

15 minutes after name/face presentation, participants completed a yes/no recognition test (*15-minute recognition test*). As in Experiment 1, target and foil words were presented aurally in the same random order for each participant. Participants heard the non-word names only (without face presentation), and were asked

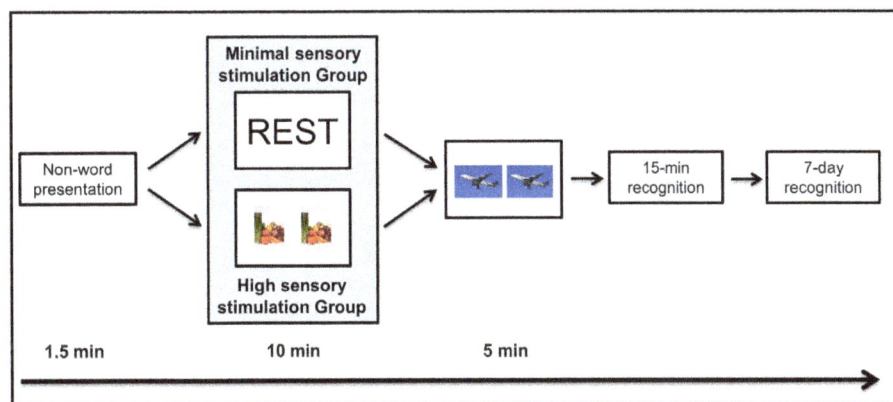

Figure 4. Participants were presented with 30 face/non-word name pairs at the beginning of Session 1, and instructed to try to remember as many non-word names as possible for subsequent recognition testing. Immediately after presentation, participants in the high sensory stimulation group completed a spot-the-difference task for 10 minutes, whereas participants in the minimal sensory stimulation group rested wakefully for 10 minutes. All participants then completed a 5-minute distractor task (spot-the-difference), which was succeeded by a 30-item (15 targets, 15 foils), yes/no non-word name recognition test, including a remember/know paradigm. 7 days later, participants completed a second and different 30-item (15 targets, 15 foils) yes/no non-word name recognition test, again including a remember/know paradigm.

whether they had heard the name 15 minutes before. If they made an 'old' response, participants were asked to make a remember/know judgment (see Experiment 1) [25,26]. Following the 15-minute recognition test, participants completed a post-experimental survey asking such questions as what they did during the wakeful rest delay (as applicable) and whether they thought about the non-words during the post-learning delay.

In *Session 2*, which occurred 7 days after Session 1, participants completed a second (and different) yes/no recognition test (*7-day recognition test*). Again, participants heard the non-word names, and were asked whether or not they heard the name 7 days before. If they made an 'old' response, a remember/know judgment was obtained as in Session 1.

Upon completion of the 7-day recognition test, participants were administered another post-experimental survey to ascertain whether they had thought about the non-word names or faces over the 7-day delay, and whether they expected to be asked about the names and/or faces again.

Scoring. As in Experiment 1, hit rates were calculated by dividing the number of targets correctly identified, by the total number of targets (/15). False alarm rates were calculated by dividing the number of foils incorrectly identified as targets, by the total number of foils (/15). These scores were used to calculate d-prime (d') using the same formula as in Experiment 1. None of the participants had a hit rate of 1 or false alarm rate of 0, thus no corrections had to be made during the computation of d'. As in Experiment 1, we also calculated the correct response rate as a further measure of recognition accuracy ((hits + correct rejections)/30).

Statistical analyses. As in Experiment 1, the alpha level was set to .05 for all analyses, which were conducted in IBM SPSS Statistics 19. For our recognition accuracy measures (d' and correct response rate) we carried out a mixed model, repeated measures ANOVA with within subjects factor time (15 minutes vs. 7 days) and between subjects factor group (high sensory stimulation vs. minimal sensory stimulation). Based on our previous findings [2], we ran two planned comparisons per recognition measure (d', correct response rate, hit rate, false alarm rate, proportion of hits remembered, proportion of hits known), using one-way ANOVAs, to examine whether minimal sensory stimulation improved recognition performance (i) after 15 minutes and (ii) after 7 days. For the recognition accuracy measures we ran an additional planned comparison, based on previous findings [2], to examine whether 7-day recognition performance in the minimal sensory stimulation condition was equal or superior to 15-min recognition performance in the sensory stimulation condition. Lastly, we ran repeated measures ANOVAs to compare within each group the proportion of hits 'remembered' and the proportion of hits 'known' after 15 minutes and after 7 days.

Results

Table 1 shows all data for the yes/no word recognition test (30 targets and 30 foils) after 15 minutes and after 7 days.

d' prime. As shown in Figure 5, the 15-minute d' score was significantly higher in the minimal sensory stimulation group than in the high sensory stimulation group, ($F(1, 52) = 13.810, p<.001$). In both groups the d' score dropped significantly over the 7-day delay ($F(1, 52) = 5.727, p<.05, \eta_p^2 = .099$). However, the superior d' score in the minimal sensory stimulation group relative to the high sensory stimulation group was maintained after 7 days ($F(1, 52) = 17.345, p<.001$) (see Figure 5 and Table 1), with no further additional benefit after 7 days, i.e. no significant group x time interaction ($F(1, 52) = 0.04, p = .841, \eta_p^2 = .001$, see Figure 5). As shown in Figure 5, *7-day* recognition (d') of non-words learned

prior to wakeful resting was higher than *15-minute* recognition (d') of non-words learned prior to the spot-the-difference task ($F(1, 52) = 5.080, p<.05$).

Correct response rate. The main results for the correct response rates paralleled those of d'prime, as shown in Table 1 and by the absence of a significant group x time interaction ($F(1, 52) = 0.08, p = .778, \eta_p^2 = .002$). Moreover, as for d', *7-day* correct response rate of non-words learned prior to wakeful resting was higher than *15-minute* correct response rate of non-words learned prior to the spot-the-difference task, and this difference was close to significance ($F(1, 52) = 3.473, p = .068$).

Hit rate and false alarm rate. As shown in Table 1, hit rate did not differ significantly between the high sensory stimulation group and the minimal sensory stimulation group after 15 minutes ($F(1, 52) = 1.497, p = .227$). After 7 days, a group difference emerged, although this did not reach significance ($F(1, 52) = 2.910, p = .094$). It should be noted however, that one participant in the high sensory stimulation group had a very high hit rate (0.9,>2.5 SD from group mean), coupled with a high false alarm rate (0.86), implying guessing. When this participant was removed from the analysis, the group difference in 7-day hit rate became significant ($F(1, 51) = 4.741, p<.05$). False alarm rate was significantly higher in the high sensory stimulation group than in the minimal sensory stimulation group after 15 minutes ($F(1, 52) = 11.819, p<.005$) and after 7 days ($F(1, 52) = 10.581, p<.005$). These results were unaffected when the aforementioned participant was removed from the analysis.

Remember/Know. There was no significant difference between the high sensory stimulation and minimal sensory stimulation group in the proportion of 'remember' responses for correctly identified targets, neither after 15 minutes ($F(1, 52) = 1.324, p = .255$) nor after 7 days ($F(1, 53) = .362, p = .550$). The same was true for 'know' responses. As shown in Table 1, in both groups there was a significantly lower proportion of 'remember' than 'know' responses after 15 minutes (minimal: $F(1,26) = 15.526, p<.01, \eta_p^2 = .374$; high: $F(1, 26) = 43.275, p<.001, \eta_p^2 = .625$) and after 7 days (minimal: $F(1,26) = 24.806, p<.001, \eta_p^2 = .488$; high: $F(1, 26) = 45.635, p<.001, \eta_p^2 = .637$).

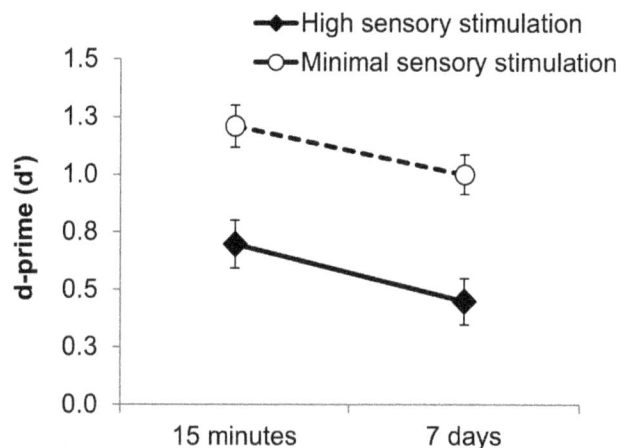

Figure 5. Mean d-prime (d)' scores for the high sensory and minimal sensory stimulation groups after 15 minutes and after 7 days in Experiment 2. The minimal sensory stimulation group showed superior recognition performance relative to the high sensory stimulation group in a paradigm employing non-recallable stimuli after 15 minutes, and this benefit was maintained for 7 days. Error bars = standard error of the mean.

Post-experimental questionnaire. The questionnaire data revealed the following: *Expected recall* - four participants in the high sensory stimulation group and 2 participants in the minimal sensory stimulation group reported that they had expected delayed recall in Session 2; *Delay activity and rehearsal* - no participants reported thinking about the words during the wakeful rest period. All participants reported mind-wandering. Moreover, no participants reported thinking about the words during the 7-day interval.

None of the results above changed when we repeated the analysis, including only those participants who did not report expecting delayed recall (high sensory stimulation group N = 23, minimal sensory stimulation group N = 25). See File S1, including Table S1 in File S1, for the results of all repeated analyses.

Discussion

Our aim was to establish, via a controlled study, whether intentional rehearsal is *necessary* in order for a brief wakeful rest to boost recently acquired memories [1–3]. Our results suggest that this is not the case. Using non-recallable non-words to minimise potential intentional rehearsal, we show that a brief wakeful rest after learning improved recognition (d′ and correct response rate) after 15 minutes, and that this benefit was maintained over at least 7 days. In fact, as Figure 5 shows, *7-day* recognition (d′) of non-words learned prior to wakeful resting was higher than *15-minute* recognition (d′) of non-words learned prior to the spot-the-difference task.

Our manipulation was successful as evinced by our pilot study, demonstrating that none of our non-words could be recalled freely, even though the recall test occurred immediately after list presentation. This result was corroborated by the finding that none of the Experiment 2 participants thought about the non-word material during the wakeful rest period. Our findings thus refute the hypothesis that intentional rehearsal is necessary in order for a period of wakeful rest to boost recently acquired memory traces. Indeed, our findings suggest that, like sleep, wakeful rest alone can improve memory, without the contribution of intentional and/or conscious repetition or elaboration of recently acquired memories.

What is the cognitive basis of this memory boost via rest?

Given the design of our paradigm it is unlikely that this rest-related memory enhancement could be accounted for by reduced interference at *retrieval* following the rest delay, as compared to following the spot-the-difference delay. Retrieval interference, i.e. the competition between similar memory traces at retrieval, would have been minimal in both conditions given that the photos presented during the spot-the-difference task were of a different modality than the wordlists, and participants completed the task in silence [2,3]. We acknowledge that some participants might have had an internal monologue while scanning the photos for differences, and that this could have produced a degree of verbal interference. However, the photos did not overlap semantically with any of the target words or foil words, certainly not with the non-words, all of which were deemed semantically meaningless by independent raters during piloting. Therefore, it is unlikely that any such internal monologue could have been sufficiently similar to the words/non-words to compete with subsequent word recall/recognition. Moreover, even if the spot-the-difference task had produced mild interference with retrieval, such interference should have been present in both groups, seeing as all participants completed a 5-minute distractor spot-the-difference task immediately before the 15-minute memory test (see Figures 1 and 4). However, the minimal sensory stimulation group outperformed

the high sensory stimulation group in both free recall and recognition testing despite these common factors.

Our paradigm also rules out the possibility that wakeful rest had a mere 'passive' effect on new memory traces. This 'passive' hypothesis, originating from the sleep/memory field [7,38], stipulates that wakeful rest passively protects new memories from new interfering information rather than actively promoting their consolidation [1,7]. Therefore, according to this hypothesis, the benefit of wakeful rest is transient, lasting only until participants are exposed to interfering new information [1,7]. Our findings are incompatible with this passive hypothesis. Specifically, the effect of wakeful rest was observed even though a 5-minute distractor task intervened between wakeful resting and 15-minute recall (see Figures 1 and 4), as observed also in related studies [2,3]. More importantly, as found previously [2], the effect of wakeful rest was sustained over 7 days, which were filled with much activity and interfering new information. These findings of a lasting benefit, following further activity and information, cannot be accounted for by a passive, transient hypothesis of wakeful resting.

However, our finding of a *lasting*, benefit of wakeful rest, as compared to a *non-similar* delay task, can be accounted for straightforwardly by memory consolidation. Memory consolidation strengthens new memories over time [12] and is associated with the *spontaneous* reactivation of recent encoding-related neural activity [8–11,15,16]. Research suggests that this spontaneous reactivation occurs predominantly during states of relative immobility, such as sleep and *wakeful rest* [8,9], perhaps due to the minimal amount of newly encoded information, which would otherwise hamper reactivation [2,6,7]. Therefore, it is hypothesised that periods of rest allow for more reactivations than do periods of sensory stimulation, thereby resulting in stronger memories [2,7]. Indeed, recent human fMRI work shows that the degree of reactivation during rest is associated positively with subsequent memory [10,11]. Our findings of a rest-related boost in free recall (Experiment 1) [2,3] and recognition (Experiment 1 and 2) align closely with these recent developments in the memory consolidation literature.

It is of note that in contrast to free recall percentage retention, hit rate was not increased significantly by wakeful rest in our study (although after 7 days the group difference approached significance, and was significant after removal of the high hit rate + high false alarm outlier in Experiment 2). This more subtle rest effect in hit rate is likely due to the reduced sensitivity of hit rate to variations in memory strength above the critical threshold for an 'Old' response. Indeed, the more-fine grained analysis of hits via remember/know responses in Experiment 1 revealed a higher proportion of 'remembered' hits in the minimal sensory stimulation group than in the high sensory stimulation group (see Table 1 and Figure 3). This finding, which parallels similar remember/know results after sleep [39], is in keeping with the view that wakeful rest allowed for stronger/richer memories to be formed (it is beyond the scope of this paper to arbitrate between single-process theory vs. dual-trace theory interpretations of this effect). We do not interpret the absence of a significant wakeful rest effect on remember/know responses in Experiment 2 since meaningless non-words could not be connected well to existing memory representations during encoding, thus reducing the likelihood of 'remember' responses. Indeed, several participants attempted to connect the non-words to an English word or name that they knew, but found it very difficult to do so.

False alarms were consistently lower in the minimal sensory stimulation group than in the high sensory stimulation group, at all delays and in both Experiments (see Table 1). This finding corroborates recent reports of reduced false alarms (i) in humans following sleep, using the Deese-Roediger-McDermott (DRM) task [40], and following a caffeine-filled consolidation delay-period [41], and (ii) in memory-impaired rodents, following reduced sensory stimulation [42,43]. The rest-induced reduction in false alarms observed here can be accounted for by superior memory consolidation, by means of the increased strength/quality bestowed on the target memory traces during wakeful resting: this increased strength/quality of the target memory traces could have allowed people to distinguish better whether or not a presented foil differed from one or more previous target memories, in particular where foils and targets overlapped to some degree. This interpretation of the reduced false alarms via rest is supported by the significant inverse correlation between false alarm rate and free recall percentage retention in Experiment 1, and by the 'recall-to-reject' literature, suggesting that sound/strong target memories are necessary for the correct rejection of foils [44,45].

It is of note that, as shown in previous work [2,3], the minimal sensory stimulation group was not completely immune to loss of word list material over the first 15 minutes. It is possible that the actual degree of benefit via wakeful rest was diminished in our study by the 5-minute distractor task that followed the 10-minute rest delay. However, a similar loss of word list material has been observed in a recent study, in which the rest delay (10 minutes) was followed immediately by the delayed recall test, without any intervening distractor task [3]. These findings suggest that some forgetting occurs, even over periods of minimal sensory stimulation. Given recent findings that autobiographical thinking can also interfere with word list consolidation [3], it is possible that the small drop in word list material during rest can be accounted for by this form of consolidation interference.

The present study and the previous free recall study [2] focused on healthy elderly people ($\geq$60 years). However, the effect of wakeful rest on memory is not restricted to elderly people, as evinced by the finding of a robust effect of wakeful rest on the retention of common nouns in young people [1,3]. This notwithstanding, the present recognition paradigm should be repeated in young people, in order to establish whether age affects the degree to which wakeful rest benefits recognition of common nouns and un-recallable non-words.

Our results indicate that the enhancement in memory via wakeful rest is *not* dependent upon intentional rehearsal of learned material during the rest period. We thus conclude that consolidation is *sufficient* for this rest-induced memory improvement to emerge. We propose that wakeful resting boosts memory consolidation, resulting in stronger and/or more veridical representations of experienced events, which can be detected both via tests of free recall and recognition, at least in healthy elderly people.

Supporting Information

File S1 Supporting Information for this article. This file includes a full report of all Experiment 1 and Experiment 2 analyses, including only those participants who did not report thinking about the words (during the wakeful rest period and/or between sessions) or expecting delayed recall. Group means and SEMs are provided in Table S1 at the end of this file.

Acknowledgments

We are extremely grateful to all participants who volunteered their time for this study. We also thank Professor John Wixted and two anonymous reviewers for their insightful and very constructive comments on an earlier version of our paper.

Author Contributions

Conceived and designed the experiments: MD JA SDS. Performed the experiments: JA. Analyzed the data: MD JA NC. Contributed reagents/materials/analysis tools: MD JA SDS NC. Wrote the paper: MD JA NC SDS.

References

1. Dewar MT, Cowan N, Della Sala S (2007) Forgetting due to retroactive interference: a fusion of Müller and Pilzecker's (1900) early insights into everyday forgetting and recent research on anterograde amnesia. Cortex 43: 616–634.
2. Dewar M, Alber J, Butler C, Cowan N, Della Sala S (2012) Brief wakeful resting boosts new memories over the long term. Psychol Sci 23: 955–960.
3. Craig M, Della Sala S, Dewar M (2014) Autobiographical thinking interferes with episodic memory consolidation. PLoS One 9: e93915.
4. Müller GE, Pilzecker A (1900) Experimentelle Beiträge zur Lehre vom Gedächtniss. Z Psychol 1: 1–300.
5. Dewar M, Garcia YF, Cowan N, Della Sala S (2009) Delaying interference enhances memory consolidation in amnesic patients. Neuropsychology 23: 627–634.
6. Wixted JT (2004) The psychology and neuroscience of forgetting. Annu Rev Psychol 55: 235–269.
7. Mednick SC, Cai DJ, Shuman T, Anagnostaras S, Wixted JT (2011) An opportunistic theory of cellular and systems consolidation. Trends Neurosci 34: 504–514.
8. Carr MF, Jadhav SP, Frank LM (2011) Hippocampal replay in the awake state: a potential substrate for memory consolidation and retrieval. Nat Neurosci 14: 147–153.
9. Foster DJ, Wilson MA (2006) Reverse replay of behavioural sequences in hippocampal place cells during the awake state. Nature 440: 680–683.
10. Deuker L, Olligs J, Fell J, Kranz TA, Mormann F, et al. (2013) Memory consolidation by replay of stimulus-specific neural activity. J Neurosci 33: 19373–19383.
11. Tambini A, Ketz N, Davachi L (2010) Enhanced brain correlations during rest are related to memory for recent experiences. Neuron 65: 280–290.
12. Dudai Y (2004) The neurobiology of consolidations, or, how stable is the engram? Annu Rev Psychol 55: 51–86.
13. Agranoff BW, Davis RE, Brink JJ (1966) Chemical studies on memory fixation in goldfish. Brain Res 1: 303–309.
14. Debiec J, LeDoux JE, Nader K (2002) Cellular and systems reconsolidation in the hippocampus. Neuron 36: 527–538.
15. O'Neill J, Pleydell-Bouverie B, Dupret D, Csicsvari J (2010) Play it again: reactivation of waking experience and memory. Trends Neurosci 33: 220–229.
16. Girardeau G, Benchenane K, Wiener SI, Buzsáki G, Zugaro MB (2009) Selective suppression of hippocampal ripples impairs spatial memory. Nat Neurosci 12: 1222–1223.
17. Roediger HL, Karpicke JD (2006) Test-enhanced learning: taking memory tests improves long-term retention. Psychol Sci 17: 249–255.
18. Roediger HL, Butler AC (2011) The critical role of retrieval practice in long-term retention. Trends Cogn Sci 15: 20–27.
19. Smith MA, Roediger HL, Karpicke JD (2013) Covert retrieval practice benefits retention as much as overt retrieval practice. J Exp Psychol Learn Mem Cogn 39: 1712–1725.
20. Craik FIM, Watkins MJ (1973) The role of rehearsal in short-term memory. J Verbal Learning Verbal Behav 12: 599–607.
21. Gardiner JM, Gawlik B, Richardson-Klavehn A (1994) Maintenance rehearsal affects knowing, not remembering; elaborative rehearsal affects remembering, not knowing. Psychon Bull Rev 1: 107–110.
22. Woodward AE, Bjork RA, Jongeward RH (1973) Recall and recognition as a function of primary rehearsal. J Verbal Learning Verbal Behav 12: 608–617.
23. Nelson HE (1982) National Adult Reading Test (NART): Test Manual. Windsor: NFER-Nelson.
24. Mioshi E, Dawson K, Mitchell J, Arnold R, Hodges JR (2006) The Addenbrooke's Cognitive Examination Revised (ACE-R): a brief cognitive test battery for dementia screening. Int J Geriatr Psychiatry 21: 1078–1085.
25. Gardiner JM (1988) Functional aspects of recollective experience. Mem Cognit 16: 309–313.
26. Tulving E (1985) Memory and consciousness. Can Psychol 26: 1–12.
27. Diana RA, Yonelinas AP, Ranganath C (2007) Imaging recollection and familiarity in the medial temporal lobe: a three-component model. Trends Cogn Sci 11: 379–386.

28. Mayes A, Montaldi D, Migo E (2007) Associative memory and the medial temporal lobes. Trends Cogn Sci 11: 126–135.

29. Yonelinas A (2002) The nature of recollection and familiarity: a review of 30 years of research. J Mem Lang 46: 441–517.

30. Wixted JT (2007) Dual-process theory and signal-detection theory of recognition memory. Psychol Rev 114: 152–176.

31. Wixted JT, Mickes L (2010) A continuous dual-process model of remember/know judgments. Psychol Rev 117: 1025–1054.

32. Wixted JT, Stretch V (2004) In defense of the signal detection interpretation of remember/know judgments. Psychon Bull Rev 11: 616–641.

33. Dunn JC (2004) Remember-Know: A Matter of Confidence. Psychol Rev 111: 524–542.

34. Dunn JC (2008) The dimensionality of the remember-know task: a state-trace analysis. Psychol Rev 115: 426–446.

35. Cowan N, Beschin N, Della Sala S (2004) Verbal recall in amnesiacs under conditions of diminished retroactive interference. Brain 127: 825–834.

36. Della Sala S, Cowan N, Beschin N, Perini M (2005) Just lying there, remembering: Improving recall of prose in amnesic patients with mild cognitive impairment by minimising interference. Memory 13: 435–440.

37. Dewar M, Della Sala S, Beschin N, Cowan N (2010) Profound retroactive interference in anterograde amnesia: What interferes? Neuropsychology 24: 357–367.

38. Ellenbogen JM, Payne JD, Stickgold R (2006) The role of sleep in declarative memory consolidation: passive, permissive, active or none? Curr Opin Neurobiol 16: 716–722.

39. Drosopoulos S, Wagner U, Born J (2005) Sleep enhances explicit recollection in recognition memory. Learn Mem 12: 44–51.

40. Fenn KM, Gallo DA, Margoliash D, Roediger HL, Nusbaum HC (2009) Reduced false memory after sleep. Learn Mem 16: 509–513.

41. Borota D, Murray E, Keceli G, Chang A, Watabe JM, et al. (2014) Post-study caffeine administration enhances memory consolidation in humans. Nat Neurosci 17: 201–203.

42. McTighe SM, Cowell RA, Winters BD, Bussey TJ, Saksida LM (2010) Paradoxical false memory for objects after brain damage. Science 330: 1408–1410.

43. Romberg C, McTighe SM, Heath CJ, Whitcomb DJ, Cho K, et al. (2012) False recognition in a mouse model of Alzheimer's disease: rescue with sensory restriction and memantine. Brain 135: 2103–2114.

44. Molitor RJ, Ko PC, Hussey EP, Ally BA (2014) Memory-related eye movements challenge behavioral measures of pattern completion and pattern separation. Hippocampus 00: 1–7.

45. Gallo DA (2004) Using recall to reduce false recognition: diagnostic and disqualifying monitoring. J Exp Psychol Learn Mem Cogn 30: 120–128.

12

Is There a Benefit in Receiving Concurrent Chemoradiotherapy for Elderly Patients with Inoperable Thoracic Esophageal Squamous Cell Carcinoma?

Peng Zhang[1]⑤, Mian Xi[1]⑤, Lei Zhao[1], Jing-Xian Shen[2], Qiao-Qiao Li[1], Li-Ru He[1], Shi-Liang Liu[1], Meng-Zhong Liu[1]*

1 Sun Yat-sen University Cancer Center, State Key Laboratory of Oncology in South China, Collaborative Innovation Center for Cancer Medicine, Department of Radiation Oncology, Cancer Center, Sun Yat-sen University, Guangzhou, People's Republic of China, 2 Sun Yat-sen University Cancer Center, State Key Laboratory of Oncology in South China, Collaborative Innovation Center for Cancer Medicine, Imaging Diagnosis and Interventional Center, Cancer Center, Sun Yat-sen University, Guangzhou, People's Republic of China

Abstract

Background and purpose: The benefit of concurrent chemoradiotherapy (CCRT) in elderly patients with inoperable esophageal squamous cell carcinoma (SCC) is controversial. This study aimed to assess the efficiency and safety of CCRT in elderly thoracic esophageal cancer patients.

Methods and materials: Between January 2002 and December 2011, 128 patients aged 65 years or older treated with CCRT or radiotherapy (RT) alone for inoperable thoracic esophageal SCC were analyzed retrospectively (RT alone, n = 55; CCRT, n = 73).

Results: No treatment-related deaths occurred and no patients experienced any acute grade 4 non-hematologic toxicities. Patients treated with CCRT developed more severe acute toxicities than patients who received RT alone. The 3-year overall survival (OS) rate was 36.1% for CCRT compared with 28.5% following RT alone ($p = 0.008$). Multivariate analysis identified T stage and treatment modality as independent prognostic factors for survival. Further analysis revealed that survival was significantly better in the CCRT group than in the RT alone group for patients ≤ 72 years. Nevertheless, the CCRT group had a similar OS to the RT group for patients > 72 years.

Conclusion: Our results suggest that elderly patients with inoperable thoracic esophageal SCC could benefit from CCRT, without major toxicities. However, for patients older than 72 years, CCRT is not superior to RT alone in terms of survival benefit.

Editor: Andreas-Claudius Hoffmann, West German Cancer Center, Germany

Funding: This work was supported by the grant from the Sci-Tech Project Foundation of Guangdong Province (No.42012B031800287). Website: http://www.gdstc.gov.cn. PZ and MX received the funding. The funders provided help in data collection and analysis.

Competing Interests: The authors have declared that no competing interests exist.

* Email: liumengzhong@126.com

⑤ These authors contributed equally to this work.

Introduction

Esophageal cancer is remains a virulent disease, with a 5-year survival rate of only 17% [1]. The risk of esophageal cancer increases with age, with a mean age at diagnosis of 67 years [2]. The number of elderly patients with esophageal cancers is expected to increase in the near future as the number of elderly people increases.

Surgical resection is the preferred treatment for localized esophageal cancer patients. However, a recent population-based study showed that older patients have less intensive treatment of esophageal cancer including surgery [3]. In addition, the literature states that patients over the age of 70 have relatively high rates of postoperative morbidity and mortality, and 75 years of age is often considered the age limit for surgery [4,5].

For the medically or technically inoperable patients, concurrent chemoradiotherapy (CCRT) is the mainstay of treatment for locally advanced esophageal cancer. The Radiation Therapy Oncology Group (RTOG) trial 85-01 established the superiority of CCRT compared with radiotherapy (RT) alone in esophageal cancer patients. However, the acute toxicity of this regimen was substantial: sixty-four percent of patients treated with CCRT experienced severe or life threatening side effects and only 23% of patients enrolled were aged over 70 [6].

Few studies have focused on elderly patients; therefore, no standard treatment modality has been established for inoperable

Table 1. Patient characteristics.

Characteristic	All patients (n = 128)	Patients with CCRT (n = 73)	Patients with RT alone (n = 55)
Age (years)			
> 72	57 (44.5%)	25 (34.2%)	32 (58.2%)
≤ 72	71 (55.5%)	48 (65.8%)	23 (41.8%)
Sex			
Male	89 (69.5%)	57 (78.1%)	32 (58.2%)
Female	39 (30.5%)	16 (21.9%)	23 (41.8%)
Charlson score			
≥ 1	42 (32.8%)	23(31.5%)	19 (34.5%)
< 1	86 (67.2%)	50 (68.5%)	36 (65.5%)
Pathological grade			
Well differentiated	10 (7.8%)	6 (8.2%)	4 (7.3%)
Moderately differentiated	47 (36.7%)	28 (38.3%)	19 (34.6%)
Poorly/undifferentiated	45 (35.2%)	21 (28.8%)	24 (43.6%)
Unknown	26 (20.3%)	18 (24.7%)	8 (14.5%)
Location			
Upper third	38 (29.7%)	24 (32.9%)	14 (25.4%)
Middle third	69 (53.9%)	38 (52.1%)	31 (56.4%)
Lower third	21 (16.4%)	11 (15.0%)	10 (18.2%)
Primary tumor length			
≤ 5 cm	78 (60.9%)	42 (57.5%)	35 (63.6%)
> 5 cm	50 (39.1%)	31 (42.5%)	20 (36.4%)
T stage			
T1-T2	25 (19.5%)	18 (24.7%)	10 (18.2%)
T3-T4	103 (80.5%)	55 (75.3%)	45 (81.8%)
N stage			
N0	26 (20.3%)	14 (19.2%)	15 (27.3%)
N1	102 (79.7%)	59 (80.8%)	40 (72.7%)
M stage			
M0	78 (60.9%)	40 (54.8%)	38 (69.1%)
M1	50 (39.1%)	33 (45.2%)	17 (30.9%)
Radiation dose (Gy)			
< 60	49 (38.3%)	23 (31.5%)	26 (47.3%)
≥ 60	79 (61.7%)	50 (68.5%)	29 (52.7%)

Abbreviations: CCRT, concurrent chemoradiotherapy; RT, radiotherapy.

esophageal cancer in elderly patients. Several studies have reported the efficacy and toxicity of CCRT in elderly patients with inoperable esophageal cancer, but the results were controversial [7–10]. In addition, the published reports are mainly on small series of patients, making it difficult to carry out reliable analysis. Therefore, we reviewed our institutional experience to evaluate the efficiency and safety of CCRT compared with RT alone in elderly thoracic esophageal cancer patients. We defined an elderly population according to Social Security and Medicare regulations as persons aged 65 years or older.

Patients and Methods

Ethics statement

This study was approved by the institutional review board (IRBs) of Cancer Center, Sun Yat-sen University. Written informed consent was obtained from all the patients in accordance with the regulations of the IRBs.

Patient's inclusion

Esophageal cancer patients treated with RT at Sun Yat-Sen University Cancer Center between January 2002 and December 2011 were retrospectively reviewed. The inclusion criteria were (1) aged 65 years or older at the time of diagnosis; (2) Eastern Cooperative Oncology Group performance status of ≤ 2; (3) histologically conformed as thoracic esophageal squamous carcinoma (SCC); (4) unable or refusing to undergo surgical resection; (5) no prior therapy; (6) no history of concomitant or previous malignancy; (7) complete and retrievable clinical records.

Among 795 esophageal cancer patients treated with RT from 2002 to 2011, 128 patients who fulfilled the criteria were included.

Table 2. Acute toxicity.

CTC Grade	Patients with CCRT (n=73)					Patients with RT alone (n=55)				
	0	1	2	3	4	0	1	2	3	4
Anemia	15	26	27	5	0	12	23	19	1	0
Leukocytopenia	9	18	29	12	5	8	24	16	7	0
Thrombopenia	27	23	16	7	0	26	23	6	0	0
Gastrointestinal	26	16	16	15	0	13	19	20	3	0
Skin toxicity	16	26	28	3	0	17	24	13	1	0
Esophagitis	12	30	27	4	0	16	23	14	2	0
Pneumonitis	50	16	5	2	0	39	13	2	1	0

Abbreviations: CCRT, concurrent chemoradiotherapy; RT, radiotherapy.

Patient pretreatment characteristics

The pretreatment work-up included complete history collection, physical examination, computed tomography (CT) scans of the chest and abdomen, barium esophagography, endoscopy, endoscopic ultrasonography, and pulmonary function test. Bone scans were performed if clinically indicated. The 6th edition (2002) of the American Joint Committee on Cancer TNM staging system was used to classify tumors. The Charlson comorbidity index was used to perform analysis of this cohort's comorbidity burden [11].

Treatment details

The majority of patients (102 of 128) received three-dimensional conformal radiotherapy (3DCRT) and other 26 patients were treated with intensity-modulated radiotherapy (IMRT). Gross tumor volume (GTV) was defined as any visible primary tumor on the computerized imaging or endoscopy and included metastatic lymph nodes. Clinical target volume (CTV) was defined as the GTV with superoinferior 3-cm and lateral 2-cm margins. The planning target volume (PTV) was created by adding 1-cm in the superoinferior dimension and 0.8-cm radically to the CTV. Radiotherapy was delivered with 6–8 MV photons using a 1.8–2.0 Gy daily fraction and five fractions per week. The median prescription dose was 60 Gy (range, 46–70 Gy) to PTV in 25–35 fractions administered over 5–7 weeks.

Application of concurrent chemotherapy was performed after careful evaluation of organ function, performance status, and severity of comorbidities. Platinum-based chemotherapy combined with 5-fluorouracil (5-FU) or docetaxel was administered to 73 patients and the remaining 55 patients received RT alone. In the CCRT group, 33 patients received two cycles of docetaxel 60 mg/m^2 and cisplatin 75 mg/m^2 delivered on day 1 and 22 of RT with standard premedication [12]. Forty patients were treated with two cycles of 60 mg/m^2 of cisplatin administered on days 1 and 29 and 1000 mg/m^2 of 5-FU administered as a continuous intravenous infusion for 96 hours on days 1–4 and 29–32 [13]. Dose reduction of chemotherapy was considered if any grade 4 hematological toxicities occurred.

Evaluation of response and toxicity

Patients were followed up every three months by physical examination, chest and abdominal CT, barium esophagography, and endoscopy or endoscopic ultrasonography. The clinical tumor response was evaluated 6–8 weeks after completion of RT according to the Response Evaluation Criteria in Solid Tumors (RECIST ver. 1.1). A complete response (CR) was defined as no remnant disease on CT image and pathological CR on endoscopy. The National Cancer Institute Common Toxicity Criteria (version 3.0) was used to score treatment toxicity.

Statistical analysis

The cutoff date of the last follow-up was April 30, 2013 for the censored data analysis. The Kaplan–Meier method was used to calculate overall survival (OS) and progression-free survival (PFS) for each potential prognostic factor, which were measured from the time of diagnosis. The log-rank test was used to test the differences between groups. The χ^2 test was used to compare patients' treatment-related toxicities between subgroups. Cox regression was used to perform multivariate analyses. All statistical analysis was performed using SPSS 16.0 software (SPSS Inc., Chicago, IL, USA). A p value of <0.05 was considered statistically significant.

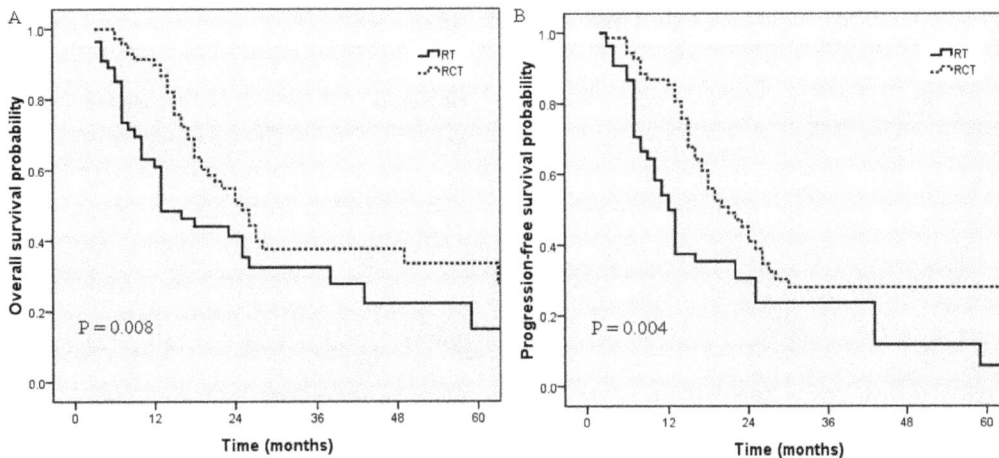

Figure 1. Overall survival (A) and progression-free survival (B) for the CCRT group and the RT alone group in the whole group of patients.

Results

Patients' characteristics

Clinical baseline characteristics are detailed in Table 1. The median age of the 128 patients was 72 years, ranging from 65 to 89 years. Twenty-eight patients (21.9%) had stage I/II disease and forty-nine patients (38.3%) had stage of III disease. Sixteen patients (12.5%) were diagnosed with stage IVa and the remaining 34 (26.6%) were diagnosed with stage IVb. Of the 34 stage IVb patients, except for one patient with liver metastasis and one with sacral bone metastasis, 32 had non-regional lymph nodal metastases. The Charlson score for the majority of patients was 0. Thirty patients (23.4%) had a Charlson score of 1, and 12 patients (9.4%) had a Charlson score $\geq$ 2. Twenty-three patients (18.0%) had chronic cardiovascular disease, 10 patients (7.8%) had chronic obstructive pulmonary disease, 17 patients (13.3%) had diabetes, and four patients (3.1%) had liver cirrhosis.

Tumor response and toxicity

All patients were evaluated for clinical tumor response. In the CCRT group (n = 73), CR was achieved in 17 (23.3%); partial response (PR) in 34 (46.6%); stable disease (SD) in 19 (26.0%); and progressive disease (PD) in 3 patients (4.1%), yielding an objective response rate of 67.1%. However, in the RT alone group (n = 55), the objective response rate declined to 47.3% (CR = 6 and PR = 20) and eight patients (14.5%) exhibited PD. A significant difference in response rate was observed between the two groups (p = 0.032).

All patients were evaluable for toxicity. As shown in Table 2, most treatment-related and documented acute toxicities were grade 1 and 2. No treatment-related deaths occurred and no patients experienced any acute grade 4 non-hematological toxicity. Most common grade 3 and 4 toxicities were leukopenia and gastrointestinal toxicity. Charlson score > 1 versus $\leq$ 1 did not influence the adverse events of grade 3–4 (p = 0.474). Acute grade 3–4 hematological toxicity was identified in 36.9% of the CCRT patients and 14.5% of the RT alone patients (p = 0.001). Patients treated with CCRT developed more grade $\geq$ 2 esophagitis and pneumonitis than patients who received RT alone (52.1% vs. 34.5%, p = 0.005).

Survival and prognostic analysis

The median follow-up period was 18.0 months (range, 3.0 to 89.0 months). During follow-up, 66 of the 128 patients (51.6%) relapsed and distant metastasis occurred in 33 patients (25.8%). Cancer was the cause of death in 64 patients (84.2%) among the patients who had died at the time of the current analysis (n = 76).

The 3-year OS and PFS rates for the whole group were 33.2% and 24.1%, respectively. The median OS of all patients was 16.0 months and the median PFS was 15.0 months. As shown in Fig.1, patients who received CCRT had a better OS compared with patients treated with RT alone (36.1% vs. 28.5% after 3 years, p = 0.008). The 3-year PFS rate of the CCRT group was also significantly higher than that for the RT alone group (27.2% vs. 16.3%, p = 0.004).

Sex, age, Charlson score, pathological grade, primary esophageal tumor location, tumor length, clinical T stage, clinical N stage, M stage, radiation dose and treatment modality were subjected to univariate analysis (Table 3). The results suggested that several variables were significantly associated with the OS: T stage (p<0.001), M stage (p = 0.012), tumor length (p = 0.039) and treatment modality (p = 0.008). The variables significantly associated with the PFS were: T stage (p = 0.007), M stage (p = 0.031) and treatment modality (p = 0.006).

To identify independent prognostic factors, the factors that were found to be significant on univariate analysis were subjected to multivariate analysis. Multivariate analysis revealed that clinical T stage (p = 0.002) and treatment modality (p = 0.002) were independent factors affecting OS and PFS in elderly esophageal SCC patients (Table 4).

Subgroup analysis

As the median age of the whole group was 72 years, we subdivided the elderly patients into two groups: > 72 years and $\leq$ 72 years. As shown in Fig. 2, for patients $\leq$ 72 years, OS and PFS were significantly better in the CCRT group than in the RT alone group (p = 0.003, 0.042). Median OS was 22.0 months in the CCRT group versus 13.0 months in the RT alone group. Nevertheless, for patients > 72 years, OS and PFS were similar in the two groups (p = 0.337, 0.363; Fig. 3).

Among patients who received CCRT, we further evaluated the efficacy of different chemotherapy regimens. Patients in the CCRT group were divided into two groups: those who received a

Table 3. Univariate analysis demonstrating factors associated with OS and PFS.

Factor	No.	OS p-value	PFS p-value
Sex		0.149	0.774
Male	89		
Female	39		
Age (years)		0.865	0.103
> 72	57		
≤ 72	71		
Charlson score		0.947	0.314
≥ 1	42		
< 1	86		
Pathological grade		0.847	0.683
Well differentiated	10		
Moderately differentiated	47		
Poorly/undifferentiated	45		
Unknown	26		
Location		0.325	0.634
Upper third	38		
Middle third	69		
Lower third	21		
Primary tumor length		0.039	0.169
≤ 5 cm	78		
> 5 cm	50		
T stage		0.000	0.007
T1-T2	25		
T3-T4	103		
N stage		0.804	0.359
N0	26		
N1	102		
M stage		0.012	0.041
M0	78		
M1	50		
Radiation dose (Gy)		0.056	0.226
< 60	49		
≥ 60	79		
Treatment modality		0.008	0.004
CCRT	73		
RT alone	55		

Abbreviations: OS, overall survival; PFS, progression-free survival; CCRT, concurrent chemoradiotherapy; RT, radiotherapy.

docetaxel combined regimen (n = 33) and those who received a 5-FU combined regimen (n = 40). The median OS periods were 21.0 and 17.0 months ($p = 0.013$), and the median PFS periods were 20.0 and 15.0 months ($p = 0.061$), respectively.

Discussion

Based on several clinical trials, CCRT has been the standard treatment for locally advanced esophageal cancer and is superior to RT alone [6]. However, very few studies have investigated CCRT in elderly patients [7–10]. The efficacy and toxicity of CCRT compared with RT alone for elderly patients have not been well documented previously. To clarify this issue, in the present study we compared the efficiency and safety of CCRT with RT alone in elderly patients with advanced thoracic esophageal SCC.

The surgical approach in elderly esophageal cancer patients remains a topic of debate because of the potentially higher rate of post-operative complications [14,15]. Several studies reported that CCRT was an effective treatment with no significant toxicity in elderly esophageal cancer patients [7–10,16–19]. However, Takeuchi et al. reported that an elderly patient group showed a significantly inferior median survival time compared with the nonelderly patient group (14.7 months $vs.$ 35.1 months, $P = 0.01$)

Table 4. Multivariate analysis of prognostic factors for patients with elderly esophageal SCC.

Endpoint	Variable	P^a	HR	95% CI for HR
OS	Tumor length	0.220	1.355	0.833–2.204
	T stage	0.002	3.139	1.546–6.371
	M stage	0.073	1.615	0.957–2.727
	Treatment modality	0.002	0.468	0.292–0.750
PFS	T stage	0.014	2.117	1.166–3.844
	M stage	0.032	1.668	1.044–2.665
	Treatment modality	0.001	0.480	0.308–0.747

Abbreviations: CI, confidence interval; HR, hazards ratio; OS, overall survival; PFS, progression-free survival; SCC, squamous cell carcinoma.
^{a}P values were calculated using an adjusted Cox proportional hazards model.

[20]. In the current study, patients who received CCRT had a 3-year OS of 37.6%, suggesting that CCRT is an effective treatment modality with a low incidence of severe toxicity for elderly patients.

Up to now, only two studies compared CCRT with RT alone in elderly esophageal cancer patients. Semrau et al. reported 51 patients aged ≥ 70 with inoperable esophageal cancer undergoing RT or CCRT, and revealed that patients treated with CCRT had a 2-year OS rate of 53.3% compared with 16.7% for RT patients ($P = 0.039$) [17]. In the study by Xu et al. [20], median OS for the CCRT group was 17 months, while it was 8 months in the RT group ($P = 0.013$). Consistent with previous reports, our study also revealed that CCRT had a higher response rate and an obvious survival benefit compared with RT alone, without a major increase in adverse events.

In the present study, 24 of 57 (42.1%) of patients aged older than 72 years received CCRT, whereas 49 of 71 (69.0%) of patients between 65 and 72 years received CCRT. Given this difference in treatment, we consider our analysis to be a comparison of the treatment outcomes between relatively none-lderly patients (65–72 years old) and elderly patients (> 72 years). In the subgroup analysis, CCRT has a survival benefit compared

with RT alone in patients between 65 and 72 years. Nevertheless, for patients > 72 years, OS and PFS were similar in the two groups. This may be partially explained by the poor life expectancy of patients older than 72 years. According to the Life Tables in 2010 in China, the average life expectancy was 74.8 years. The late toxicity of CCRT may be another reason. Marota et al reported that the 2-year cumulative incidence of late cardiopulmonary toxicities of Grade 3 or greater for patients 75 years or older was 29%, compared with 3% for younger patients, thus CCRT was not tolerated by patients older than 75 years [21].

Data on elderly patients who received RT alone are limited. Hishikawa et al. reported the survival within different age groups of esophageal cancer receiving external beam RT and brachy-therapy boost, and revealed that the 2-year OS rate of patients aged 70–79 years was 17.2%, which is similar to the patients aged 43–69 years (16.7%). Therefore, the study suggested that RT should be the first choice of treatment for patients > 80 years old [22]. Yamakava et al, reported on 40 cases aged ≥ 80 years treated with RT alone and concluded that RT is a safe and effective treatment for esophageal cancer in patients over 80 years old [23]. In our study, in terms of the limited survival benefit of CCRT over RT, treatment modality should be evaluated on an

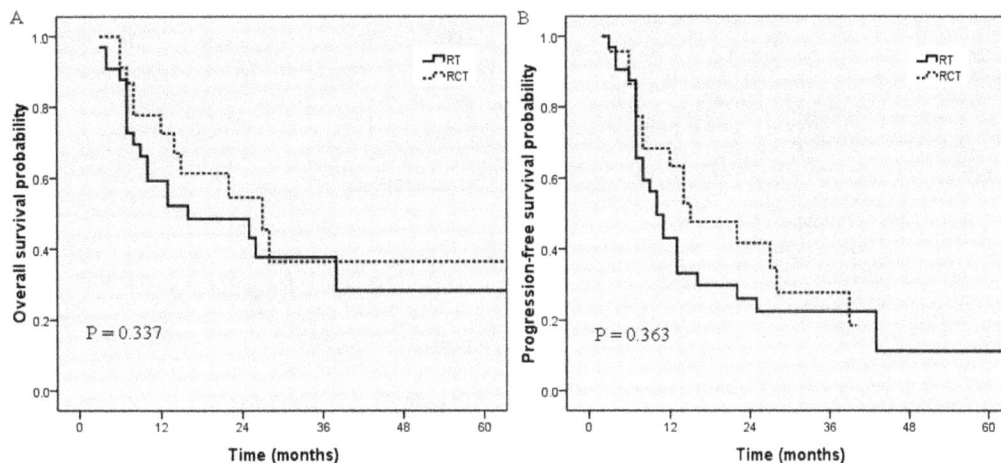

Figure 2. Overall survival (A) and progression-free survival (B) for the CCRT group and the RT alone group in patients older than 72 years.

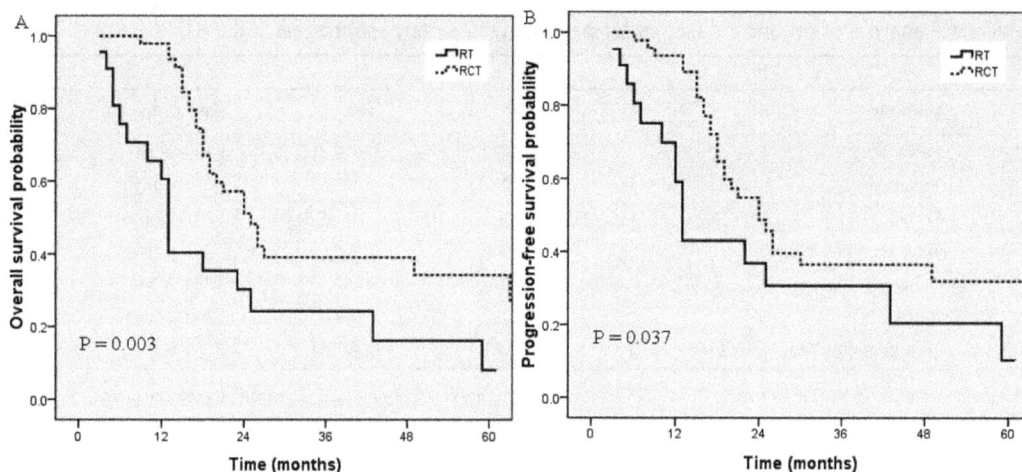

Figure 3. Overall survival (A) and progression-free survival (B) for the CCRT group and the RT alone group in patients between 65 and 72 years old.

individual basis in such cases and RT alone should be a reasonable option for patients in higher age groups.

Numerous studies on patients with advanced esophagogastric cancer suggested that cisplatin-based chemotherapy toxicities did not increase with age [24]. With regard to ≤ grade 3 side effects, it was possible to minimize and make tolerable such adverse events using previously described methods and careful close monitoring. Tougeron et al. reported that 4.6% of elderly patients who received combined chemoradiation experienced a grade 4 hematological toxicity [7]. In the CCRT group of our study, grade 4 hematological toxicities were observed in five patients (6.8%) only, suggesting that documented toxicities were not severe and supportive treatment was manageable. In addition, no treatment-related deaths occurred and no patients experienced any acute grade 4 non-hematologic toxicities. The incidence of severe acute toxicity in our cohort was lower than that reported in previous studies for non-elderly esophageal cancer patients [6,12]. Therefore, cisplatin-based CCRT is a safe treatment option for elderly esophageal SCC patients.

To improve survival for locally advanced esophageal cancer, taxane-based preoperative chemoradiotherapy schedules have been investigated in some exploratory trials. Wu et al compared the efficacy and feasibility of neoadjuvant chemoradiotherapy with docetaxel plus cisplatin or with cisplatin plus 5-FU for local advanced esophageal SCC, and showed that docetaxel plus cisplatin can be well tolerated and achieved a higher pathological complete response rate than cisplatin plus 5-FU (35.1% *vs.* 20.8%, $P = 0.048$) [25]. However, there has been no prospective randomized trial to validate the benefit of different concurrent chemotherapy regimens for definitive RT. Hsu et al retrospectively analyzed the effects of paclitaxel-based chemoradiation for esophageal SCC and showed improved local disease compared with the regimen of 5-FU and cisplatin [26]. In the CCRT group in our study, there was a survival advantage for patients who received the docetaxel combined regimen compared with those who received the 5-FU combined regimen; thus, a prospective study addressing this regimen is warranted.

Age as a prognostic factor is still debated and several studies did not show any prognostic significance for age [27,28]. Semrau et al. compared 152 patients aged < 70 years treated with the definitive CCRT protocol and 51 patients aged ≥ 70 with esophageal

cancer, and concluded that there was no significant difference in OS in the two groups; however, PFS showed a significant difference in favor of the ≥ 70 years group [17]. However, Takeuchi et al. demonstrated inferior survival in the elderly patient group compared with the non-elderly group. He attributed this to a lower response, a higher mortality from complications, and a lower compliance in the elderly group [20]. Our results showed that age has no bearing on the survival of elderly patients. This may be partially because our study did not include patients treated with best supportive care or endo-esophageal stenting only. The selected population may represent a favorable group of patients suffering from advanced esophageal cancer.

The prognostic value of comorbidity is far from conclusive. Tougeron et al. reported that a Charlson score ≤ 2 is an independent prognostic factor associated with better survival for elderly patients [16]. However, several studies showed that moderate to severe comorbidity are not predictive of survival [8,18]. In our study, a Charlson score ≥ 1 vs. <1 did not influence the incidence of adverse events. No significant association was found between the Charlson comorbidity index and OS or PFS; this may be attributed to the patients' selection bias.

The current study is limited by its retrospective design and the heterogeneity of the concurrent chemotherapy regimens. Considering all the aspects in the study, large-scale prospective clinical trials for elderly esophageal cancer patients are required in the future.

Conclusions

Elderly patients older than 65 years with inoperable thoracic esophageal SCC could benefit from CCRT without major toxicities. However, for patients older than 72 years, CCRT is not superior to RT alone in terms of survival benefit. Further prospective studies are warranted to confirm the results.

Author Contributions

Conceived and designed the experiments: PZ MX MZL. Performed the experiments: PZ MX LZ JXS QQL. Analyzed the data: QQL LRH SLL. Contributed reagents/materials/analysis tools: PZ MX QQL SLL. Contributed to the writing of the manuscript: PZ MX MZL.

References

1. Siegel R, Naishadham D, Jemal A (2013) Cancer Statistics, 2013. CA Cancer J Clin 63: 11–30.
2. Enzinger PC, Mayer RJ (2003) Esophageal cancer. N Engl J Med 349: 2241–2252.
3. Steyerberg EW, Neville B, Weeks JC, Earle CC (2007) Referral patterns, treatment choices, and outcomes in locoregional esophageal cancer: population-based analysis of elderly patients. J Clin Oncol 25: 2389–2396.
4. Kinugasa S, Tachibana M, Yoshimura H, Dhar DK, Shibakita M, et al. (2001) Esophageal resection in elderly esophageal carcinoma patients: improvement in postoperative complications. Ann Thorac Surg 71: 414–418.
5. Law S, Wong KH, Kwok KF, Chu KM, Wong J (2004) Predictive factors for postoperative pulmonary complications and mortality after esophagectomy for cancer. Ann Surg 240: 791–800.
6. Herskovic A, Martz K, al-Sarraf M, Leichman L, Brindle J, et al. (1992) Combined chemotherapy and radiotherapy compared with radiotherapy alone in patients with cancer of the esophagus. N Engl J Med 326: 1593–1598.
7. Tougeron D, Di Fiore F, Thureau S, Berbera N, Iwanicki-Caron I, et al. (2008) Safety and outcome of definitive chemoradiotherapy in elderly patients with oesophageal cancer. Br J Cancer 99: 1586–1592.
8. Anderson SE, Minsky BD, Bains M, Hummer A, Kelsen D, et al. (2007) Combined modality chemoradiation in elderly oesophageal cancer patients. Br J Cancer 96: 1823–1827.
9. Nallapareddy S, Wilding GE, Yang G, Iyer R, Javle M (2005) Chemoradiation is a tolerable therapy for older adults with esophageal cancer. Anticancer Res 25: 3055–3060.
10. Mak RH, Mamon HJ, Ryan DP, Miyamoto DT, Ancukiewicz M, et al. (2010) Toxicity and outcomes after chemoradiation for esophageal cancer in patients age 75 or older. Dis Esophagus 23: 316–323.
11. Reid BC, Alberg AJ, Klassen AC, Samet JM, Rozier RG, et al. (2001) Comorbidity and survival of elderly head and neck carcinoma patients. Cancer 92: 2109–2116.
12. Li QQ, Liu MZ, Hu YH, Liu H, He ZY, et al. (2010) Definitive concomitant chemoradiotherapy with docetaxel and cisplatin in squamous esophageal carcinoma. Dis Esophagus 23: 253–259.
13. Liu H, Lu L, Zhu Q, Hao Y, Mo Y, et al. (2011) Cervical nodal metastases of unresectable thoracic esophageal squamous cell carcinoma Characteristics of long-term survivors after concurrent chemoradiotherapy. Radiother Oncol 99: 181–186.
14. Sabel MS, Smith JL, Nava HR, Mollen K, Douglass HO, et al. (2002) Esophageal resection for carcinoma in patients older than 70 years. Ann Surg Oncol 9: 210–214.
15. Gockel I, Sultanov FS, Domeyer M, Goenner U, Junginger T (2007) Developments in esophageal surgery for adenocarcinoma: a comparison of two decades. BMC Cancer 7: 114.
16. Tougeron D, Hamidou H, Scotté M, Di Fiore F, Antonietti M, et al. (2010) Esophageal cancer in the elderly: an analysis of the factors associated with treatment decisions and outcomes. BMC Cancer 10: 510.
17. Semrau R, Herzog SL, Vallböhmer D, Kocher M, Hölscher A, et al. (2012) Radiotherapy in elderly patients with inoperable esophageal cancer. Is there a benefit? Strahlenther Onkol 188: 226–232.
18. Go SI, Sup Lee W, Hee Kang M, Song HN, Jin Kim M, et al. (2012) Response to concurrent chemoradiotherapy as a prognostic marker in elderly patients with locally advanced esophageal cancer. Tumori 98: 225–232.
19. Xu HY, Du ZD, Zhou L, Yu M, Ding ZY, et al. (2014) Safety and efficacy of radiation and chemoradiation in patients over 70 years old with inoperable esophageal squamous cell carcinoma. Oncol Lett 7: 260–266.
20. Takeuchi S, Ohtsu A, Doi T, Kojima T, Minashi K, et al. (2007) A retrospective study of definitive chemoradiotherapy for elderly patients with esophageal cancer. Am J Clin Oncol 30: 607–611.
21. Morota M, Gomi K, Kozuka T, Chin K, Matsuura M, et al. (2009) Late toxicity after definitive concurrent chemoradiotherapy for thoracic esophageal carcinoma. Int J Radiat Oncol Biol Phys 75: 122–128.
22. Hishikawa Y, Kurisu K, Taniguchi M, Kamikonya N, Miura T (1991) Radiotherapy for carcinoma of the esophagus in patients aged eighty or older. Int J Radiat Oncol Biol Phys 20: 685–688.
23. Yamakawa M, Shiojima K, Takahashi M, Saito Y, Matsumoto H, et al. (1994) Radiation therapy for esophageal cancer in patients over 80 years old. Int J Radiat Oncol Biol Phys 30: 1225–1232.
24. Trumper M, Ross PJ, Cunningham D, Norman AR, Hawkins R, et al. (2006) Efficacy and tolerability of chemotherapy in elderly patients with advanced oesophago-gastric cancer: A pooled analysis of three clinical trials. Eur J Cancer 42: 827–834.
25. Wu S, Chen MY, Luo JC, Wei L, Chen Z (2012) Comparison between docetaxel plus cisplatin and cisplatin plus fluorouracil in the neoadjuvant chemotherapy for local advanced esophageal squamous cell carcinoma. Zhonghua Zhong Liu Za Zhi 34: 873–876.
26. Hsu FM, Lin CC, Lee JM, Chang YL, Hsu CH, et al. (2008) Improved local control by surgery and paclitaxel-based chemoradiation for esophageal squamous cell carcinoma: results of a retrospective non-randomized study. J Surg Oncol 98: 34–41.
27. Lagarde SM, ten Kate FJ, Reitsma JB, Busch OR, van Lanschot JJ (2006) Prognostic factors in adenocarcinoma of the esophagus or gastroesophageal junction. J Clin Oncol 24: 4347–4355.
28. Eloubeidi MA, Desmond R, Arguedas MR, Reed CE, Wilcox CM (2002) Prognostic factors for the survival of patients with esophageal carcinoma in the U.S.: the importance of tumor length and lymph node status. Cancer 95: 1434–1443.

13

Impact of the Non-Contributory Social Pension Program *70 y más* on Older Adults' Mental Well-Being

Aarón Salinas-Rodríguez[1], Ma. Del Pilar Torres-Pereda[2], Betty Manrique-Espinoza[1]*, Karla Moreno-Tamayo[1], Martha María Téllez-Rojo Solís[1]

1 Center for Evaluation Research and Surveys, National Institute of Public Health, Cuernavaca, Mexico, 2 Center for Health Systems Research, National Institute of Public Health, Cuernavaca, Mexico

Abstract

Background: In 2007, a non-contributory pension program was launched in rural areas of Mexico. The program consisted in a non-conditional cash transfer of US$40 monthly to all older adults (OA) aged 70 and over. We evaluate the effect of the program on mental well-being of its beneficiaries.

Methods and Findings: Quantitative and qualitative methods were used. For the quantitative component, we used the selection criteria established by the program (age and locality size) to form the Intervention (OA aged 70–74 residing in rural localities, <2500 inhabitants) and Control groups (OA aged 70–74, in localities with 2501–2700 inhabitants). Baseline data collection was conducted in 2007 where 5,465 OA were interviewed. The follow-up survey was conducted in 2008, and it was possible to interview 5,270 OA, with a response rate of 96%. A difference-in-difference linear probability model with individual fixed effect was used to estimate the impact of the program on mental well-being indicators. In 2009 a qualitative component was designed to explore possible causal pathways of such effect.

Results: After a year of exposure, the program had a significant effect on reduction of depressive symptoms ($\beta = -0.06$, $CI_{95\%}$ -0.12; -0.01) and an increase in empowerment indicators: OA participated in important household decisions ($\beta = 0.09$, $CI_{95\%}$ $0.03;0.15$); and OA participated in household decisions pertaining to expenses ($\beta = 0.11$, $CI_{95\%}$ $0.05;0.18$). Qualitative analysis found a strong trend showing a reduction of sadness, and feeling of increasing empowerment.

Conclusions: These results suggest that a non-conditional transfer in older ages have an impact beyond the economic sphere, impacting even the mental well-being. This effect could be explained because the pension produces feelings of safety and welfare. It is recommendable that governments should invest efforts towards universalizing the non-contributory pension programs in order to ensure a basic income for the elderly.

Editor: Jerson Laks, Federal University of Rio de Janeiro, Brazil

Funding: This project has been funded in part by the Mexican Ministry of Social Development and by the International Initiative for Impact Evaluation, Inc. (3ie), through the Global Development Network (GDN) in partial fulfillment of the requirements of grant OW31229 issued under Open window 3. The contents of this publication do not represent the official position of the Mexican Ministry of Social Development. The views expressed in this article are not necessarily those of 3ie or its members, or of GDN. The elaboration of this study results required additional work by the authors. The Mexican Ministry of Social Development's Website is: http://www.sedesol.gob.mx/. The International Initiative for Impact Evaluation, Inc. Website is: http://www.3ieimpact.org/en/about/3ie-affiliates/3ie-members/. The funders had no role in study design, data collection and analysis, decision to publish, or preparation of the manuscript.

Competing Interests: The authors have declared that no competing interests exist.

* Email: bmanrique@insp.mx

Introduction

One of the most important demographic challenges expected for low and middle-income countries in the 21st century will be the increase of the number of older adults (OA) and the pressure this will have on social security systems, available medical assistance, and service demand for elderly care. Moreover, estimates of health problems and disability suggest OA in these countries are aging with more functional limitations and worse health conditions than OA in developed countries [1].

Aging process in low and middle-income countries is characterized by the presence of poverty and inequality. In these countries, poverty among OA (60 years and over) is higher than that for the entire population [2]. Because of this, old age could be a stage of life characterized by the reduction of formal work activities that in turns leads to a decrease in income and, consequentially, economic insecurity. Income insecurity in old age may have a negative effect on the welfare of the elderly and can often cause the impoverishment of the household.

Poverty in old age is also an important problem in low and middle-income countries. Studies in 15 low-income countries in sub-Saharan Africa report households with an elderly individual had higher levels of poverty that general population [3]. In particular, Latin America rates of poverty among the elderly range from 9.8% in Chile to 69.9% in Honduras [4]. More recent data from a study by CEPAL in 2008 reveals that in nine of 15 countries surveyed, more than 30% of the OA are poor. In Mexico, the incidence of poverty among the elderly population is about 30% [5].

In terms of income distribution, Latin America is considered the world's most imbalanced region [2]. Inequality is reflected in a significant number of socioeconomic dimensions, including access to social protection systems, in which Latin America's largest concern is its low coverage [2]. Economic insecurity affects OA living in poverty, but especially to those who formerly worked in the informal sector or were unpaid workers. Globally, it is estimated that four out of five elderly individuals have no pension or retirement, which forces the elderly to continue working and/or to depend on informal social support networks to subsist [6].

The majority of uninsured and retired individuals lives and works in low and middle-income countries. In Latin America, over 30% of the OA do not report retirement, pension, or employment income [5]. Many of them also do not participate in pension plans since they are unpaid caregivers, unemployed, or are employees in agriculture or in the informal work sector [7]. According to data from the survey CEPAL 2010 in Mexico, only about a quarter of OA receive benefits from the social security system through a social or retirement pension. In the richest quintile of the population, the coverage reaches 50%; however, in the poorest quintile, this number does not even reach 3% [8].

Non-contributory social pensions

The rapid growth of the OA population in low and middle-income countries and the low coverage of social security reinforce the need to adapt social protection systems at a faster rate than the developed countries did [2]. One example is the implementation of social pensions for the elderly in order to reduce poverty. Currently, there is documented experience in countries like Nepal, Lesotho, Brazil, and South Africa, which are among the 80 countries that have established social pensions in the world. Of these, 47 are low- and middle-income countries, such as Mexico [6].

The most distinctive characteristics of noncontributory social pensions are that they are designed to be accessible as a right to all those who meet the requirements of the program and that the grant conditions are unrelated to work experience or the history of the market [9]. Noncontributory pension programs provide cash benefits relatively uniformly in a targeted or categorical manner to reduce the risks of old age and disability. In some countries, these programs also focus on reducing the risks of disease, as well as on providing a way to access other benefits of the social protection system (e.g. family allocations). In general, these programs provide modest and relatively uniform benefits [10], and it is considered that these programs are useful tools for women and individuals from the informal sector of the economy, who have benefited less by the contributory retirement system [7].

The results from the evaluation studies suggest that noncontributory social pension programs have had a major impact in reducing poverty in old age, as well as the incidence of extreme poverty, and a positive effect on reducing indigence [10]. Reports from Brazil and South Africa, two countries with the highest noncontributory pension programs, report that these programs not only are efficient vehicles to reduce poverty, but also have an influence on the magnitude rather than simply the incidence of poverty. Households with a noncontributory pension beneficiary have greater financial stability and are less likely to experience a decline in their living standards. Also, receiving the pension is associated with investments in human, physical, and social capital,

in addition to being able to combat gender inequality [4,11–16]. Also there has been some evidence about the effect of pensions on subjective well-being [17–19]. However, evaluations mainly have focused on studying the effect of these programs on income and poverty, and still little is known about their effects on other facets of OA life, such as physical health and mental health.

Given the currently gap in the evaluation literature regarding the impact of economic transfer programs on the OA in other areas more than just economic effects, our objective was to estimate the impact of the non-contributory pension program 70 y más on mental well-being of its beneficiaries.

The Program 70 y más

Implemented nationally throughout Mexico, Program 70 y más was aimed at improving the living conditions among adults aged 70 years and older by boosting their social protection through policy mechanisms. Centered on two components, 70 y más pursues a twofold objective: (1) to raise the income of the elderly and (2) to improve the social protection of the elderly. At the start of the program in 2007, the program had enrolled a total of one million beneficiaries and had a total annual budget of 6,250 million Mexican pesos (approximately US$595 million). In 2009 the number of beneficiaries had grown to 1.8 million, and the total budget had more than doubled to 13,000 million Mexican pesos (US$1,400 million) [8]. For the most recent data from 2014, the number of beneficiaries will be 3.9 million, with a total budget of 45,200 million Mexican pesos (US$3,476 million) [20].

Under the first program objective, OA receive a direct unconditional cash transfer of 500 Mexican pesos (approximately US$40) every month, which can be collected every two months. At the start of the program in 2007, the established eligibility criteria included being 70 years and over and residing in a locality with 2,500 or less inhabitants (rural localities). It should be noted that our evaluation is based on the two eligibility criteria and does not account for the fact that the program expanded the eligibility criteria to those residing in a locality up to 30,000 inhabitants after 2011 [21]. Today, and with a new government, the program has expanded even until some poor urban localities (>2500 inhabitants) and reduced the age range (≥65 years) of its beneficiaries.

The second program objective related to health-oriented social participation and social protection actions was late to start, and during the period of this evaluation, it only had enrolled a very small percentage of beneficiaries. For that reason, this work will focus on evaluating the impact of the program's cash transfer feature only.

Methods

Ethics Statement

The Research and Ethics Committees of Mexico's National Institute of Public Health approved the original study. Participants received a detailed explanation of the procedures and signed an informed consent declaration before data collection occurred.

The estimated impact of 70 y más was derived from both quantitative and qualitative analyses of data. Both components (quantitative and qualitative) of the study are briefly presented in the next paragraphs.

Quantitative component

In 2007, at the start of the program, 70 y más established two eligibility criteria: (1) beneficiaries had to be 70 years old and over and (2) had to reside in localities of 2,500 or less inhabitants. We used these eligibility criteria to design our impact evaluation study and to identify the group exposed to the program (70–74 years of age, in localities with 2,500 or less inhabitants) and to establish three control groups: Group 1 (aged 65–69, in localities with 2,500 or less inhabitants); Group 2 (aged 70–74, in localities with 2,501–2,700 inhabitants), and Group 3 (aged 65–69, in localities with 2,501–2,700 inhabitants). Details about intervention and control group selection can be found in Appendix S1 in File S1.

Sample size, power calculations, and surveys. Sample size was determined according to 35 indicators related to household characteristics, household expenditures, health conditions of the OA, and use of healthcare services. Sample size was calculated using unilateral statistical tests with a 95% confidence level and a power of 80%. Additionally, the sample size calculation accounted for several scenarios based on the effect of the program, including expected effects of 1, 2, 3, 4, 5, 10, 15, and 20 percentage points for each of the 35 indicators proposed. The results of the analysis revealed that a sample size of 1,500 elderly per evaluation group would suffice to detect program effects of up to 4 or 5 percentage points in all of the variables.

The baseline survey was conducted in October-December 2007 among a total of 516 localities in seven states of Mexico. Out of the targeted 6,000 interviews of OA, 5,465 OA (a 91% response rate) were interviewed during baseline. The follow-up survey was conducted in November-December 2008, and it was possible to locate and interview 5,270 OA, or 96% of the OA interviewed at baseline.

Inclusion criteria for the present study sample were those subjects with information on both measurements: baseline and follow up. Figure 1 shows the sample included for the impact analysis of the *70 y más* program. As can be seen from the size of the originally estimated sample (6,000 elderly), 5,465 OA were interviewed at baseline, and 5,270 of these were interviewed during follow-up. The final analytical sample was defined based on the common rule from studies on OA that only mentally apt individuals or their caregivers (defined as the people who provide assistance to the OA in their basic and daily activities) can respond to survey questions. By this definition, caregivers can actually answer all questions related to the OA (e.g. demographics, labor, socioeconomic) except for the ones related to perception. For instance, a caregiver should not answer a question which requests information on the OA's emotions. Thus, any survey questions where the OA have to express their feelings or emotions are not answered by caregivers. Thus, of the 5,270 observations existing in both baseline and follow-up (Figure 1), 802 had cognitive impairment in either baseline or follow-up, and including those who had the caregivers respond to all sections with the exception of the sections on mental health, the final sample for the mental health indicators were 4,468 OA.

OA were interviewed at home by standardized personnel working for the National Institute of Public Health. Both at baseline and follow-up, data collected featured the following characteristics: socio-demographic, education, lifestyles, physical and mental health, nutrition and use of health services.

Measures

As impact indicators of mental well-being we used the following measurements:

Depressive symptoms. Within the framework of research on OA depression, the Geriatric Depression Scale is one of the most commonly used instruments. Developed by Sheikh and Yesavage, the scale has been validated in numerous countries and contexts [22,23]. Currently, it is the most frequently used instrument for measuring depression among the OA, including those residing in poor or marginalized conditions. Depressive symptoms (DS) were assessed using the Geriatric Depression Scale

(GDS) 15 items version. We defined a dummy variable equal to 1 if the older adult showed significant DS (GDS ≥6) and 0 otherwise.

Empowerment. One of the most immediate and likely effects of the program *70 y más* relates to the autonomy and empowerment of the elderly. To incorporate these two dimensions into our evaluation, we applied the World Health Organization (WHO) recommendation on active aging [24]. Specifically, the capacity of OA to participate in household decision making was used as the basic indicator for gauging the extent to which OA were empowered. This gave rise to two indicator variables (dummies): the first was equivalent to one where the older adult declared that he participated in important (non-economic) household decisions; the second was equivalent to one where the older adult declared that he participated in household decisions pertaining to expenses.

Statistical analysis. Assuming that our evaluation design succeeded in replicating the environmental conditions of the program and its beneficiaries, it was only necessary to carry out a simple comparison between the average of any indicator of interest for the intervention group and the average of that same indicator for the control group to estimate the program effect. However, this assumption can bias the results greatly, since it is possible that not all observable and unobservable differences between the intervention and control groups will have been removed by our design.

For this reason, we took advantage of the differences-in-differences (DD) model to estimate the program effect. Instead of analyzing the differences between the variables across treatment and control, this model allows us to analyze the differences in change between treatment and control groups by accounting for two types of potential differences between the groups: (1) the differences that existed prior to the intervention (i.e. at baseline or pre-intervention) between treatment and control groups, and (2) the differences arising from unobserved factors at the local level that do not change between baseline and follow-up data collection, which in this case is 2007 and 2008. The DD model is then based on the assumption that in the absence of the program, the change observed in the intervention group would have been the same as the change observed in the control group, or more succinctly, the trends of both groups would be equal. If there were differences between the groups for unobserved characteristics that vary over time and these were associated with program exposure, the DD model would generate biased estimates of the program effect. However, it is expected that the DD model removes a large proportion of the possible causes of bias in its estimates.

The general DD linear probability model for estimating the impact of the program is specified as follows:

$$Y_{ijt} = \beta_0 + \beta_1 T_{ijt} + \beta_2 P_{ij} + \beta_3 \left(T_{ijt} * P_{ij} \right) + \beta X + \mu_i + \varepsilon_{ijt}$$

Where Y_{ijt} is an outcome variable for individual i who lives in locality j at time t. T_{ijt} is an indicator variable that takes a value of 1 if the measurement of individual i is in the post-intervention survey (2008) or 0 if it is in the baseline survey (2007). P_{ij} represents an indicator variable that takes the value of 1 if individual i belongs to the intervention group or 0 if he or she belongs to the control group 1, while the term $(T_{ijt}*P_{ij})$ represents the estimate of the program impact, X it's a time-varying covariates vector, μ_i represents a fixed effect at individual level, and ε_{ijt} is the error term.

The DD model permits the identification of the treatment effect under the assumption that the change in the treated group in the absence of the program would have been the same as the observed change in the control group. When applying this model, the DD

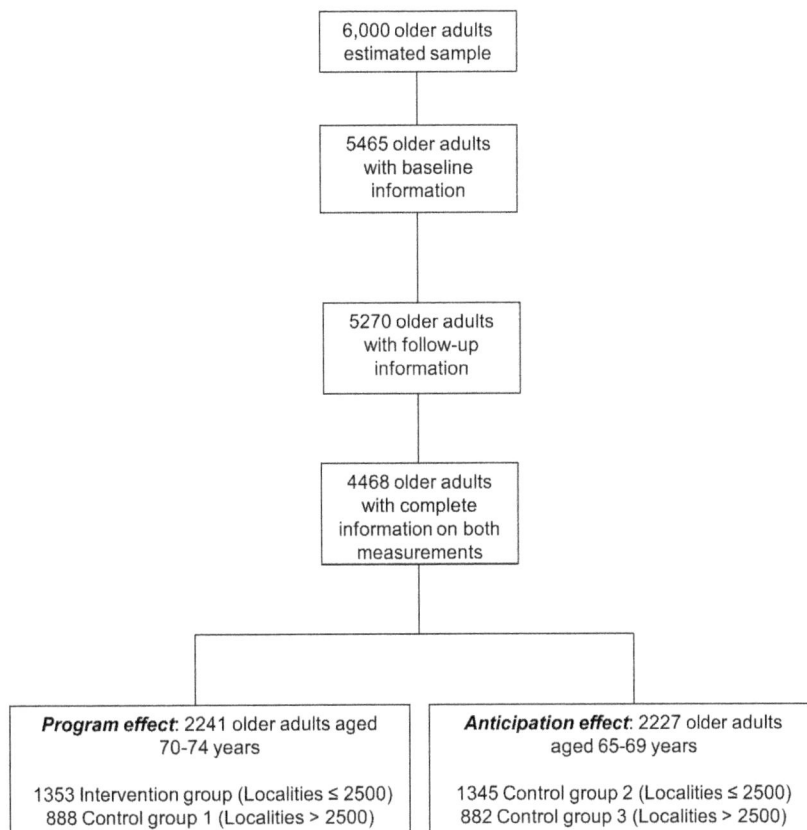

Figure 1. Analytic sample definition.

model already controls for fixed characteristics over time, thus, only time-varying covariates will be used, both individual/ household and locality levels. Differences were considered statistically significant if $p<0.05$, and considered marginally significant if $0.05<p<0.10$. All analyses were performed using STATA 13.1.

We also conducted additional analyses to complement the DD models (with fixed effects) in combination with propensity score matching as a strategy to verify the robustness of our results, and we verified the assumption of parallelism regarding the DD models. The results of these analyses and their rationale are presented in the Appendix S2 in File S1. Finally, we conducted an alternative analysis to test the robustness of our results, moving the older adults aged 69, and who were in the control group at baseline, to the intervention group.

Qualitative component

The qualitative study was conducted in January-February 2009 and was based on the data collected during the baseline measurement of the quantitative component. The objectives and research questions were established in accordance with the quantitative component in order to utilize the qualitative exploration to generate a complementary and expanded triangulation of the results.

The qualitative sample was purposively selected with maximum variation criteria to achieve maximum representation of the different subgroups observed [25]. While no established formula exists for defining the number of cases that should be selected for each minimum sample unit, other large-scale evaluation studies [26] have selected a minimum number of three cases per minimal

sample unit, to achieve a so-called theoretical or data saturation [27–29].

We included OA that have been captured in the quantitative baseline survey. Four localities were selected in two of the seven participating states at baseline. To select the participating states, certain criteria were used on structural characteristics that could determine the experience of the beneficiaries with respect to the program. Selected states shared the same levels of deprivation, migratory rates, and indigenous population proportion. For the selection of localities, the difficulty of accessing health services and the ethnicity composition of its inhabitants were also considered so that the perceived experience of the program could be determined by those characteristics. Sampling scheme for qualitative component can be found in Appendix S1 in File S1.

Data collection. Total sample consisted of: 129 semi-structured face to face interviews: 99 program beneficiaries; 16 potential beneficiaries; and 6 suspended OA beneficiaries; 8 interviews with local key actors (two per locality interviewed in public places like parks or schools), and 4 observations from support delivery, one in each selected locality. No refusals were faced during fieldwork.

Interview guide had four sections, self-perception of mental and physical health, use of program's transfer and decision taking over the money, self-perception of social network (family, friends and community) and evaluation of perceived impact of the program. Interview guide was piloted with 5 OA in a non-selected locality.

The fieldwork was conducted in February-April 2009 by a team of five female cultural anthropologists (two of them with M.A.) who lived in the study sites during data collection. In those localities where OA only spoke indigenous language three female

Table 1. Baseline characteristics by study group.

	Program effects			Anticipation effects		
	Intervention (70–74 years)	Control group 1 (70–74 years)	p-value[1]	Control group 2 (65–69 years)	Control group 3 (65–69 years)	p-value[1]
	n = 1353	n = 888		n = 1345	n = 882	
Outcomes						
Depressive symptoms	0.25 [0.01]	0.25 [0.01]	0.655	0.24 [0.01]	0.28 [0.02]	0.042
OA participates in household decisions	0.72 [0.01]	0.74 [0.01]	0.268	0.76 [0.01]	0.80 [0.01]	0.025
OA participates in household spending decisions	0.69 [0.01]	0.72 [0.02]	0.201	0.74 [0.01]	0.76 [0.01]	0.143
Individual covariates						
Time-stationary						
Sex (female)	0.50 [0.01]	0.64 [0.02]	<0.001	0.43 [0.01]	0.46 [0.02]	0.206
Literacy	0.33 [0.01]	0.37 [0.02]	0.047	0.36 [0.01]	0.41 [0.02]	0.019
Indigenous	0.35 [0.01]	0.30 [0.02]	0.018	0.37 [0.01]	0.33 [0.02]	0.052
Time-varying						
Age	72.52 [0.04]	72.57 [0.05]	0.446	67.43 [0.04]	67.54 [0.05]	0.078
OA living alone	0.04 [0.01]	0.13 [0.01]	<0.001	0.03 [0.00]	0.09 [0.01]	<0.001
OA having paid job	0.36 [0.01]	0.31 [0.02]	0.007	0.48 [0.01]	0.47 [0.02]	0.930
OA head of household	0.65 [0.01]	0.73 [0.01]	<0.001	0.72 [0.01]	0.79 [0.01]	<0.001
Number of co-moribidities[2]	0.84 [0.03]	0.89 [0.04]	0.300	0.72 [0.03]	0.73 [0.03]	0.845
Functional dependence	0.28 [0.01]	0.30 [0.02]	0.304	0.24 [0.01]	0.25 [0.01]	0.677
Marital status (married/cohabitating)	0.65 [0.01]	0.46[0.02]	<0.001	0.67 [0.01]	0.60 [0.02]	0.001
Household covariates						
Household size (# of equivalent adults)	5.16 [0.08]	3.67 [0.09]	<0.001	5.56 [0.08]	4.22 [0.09]	<0.001
Asset index	0.19 [0.03]	−0.14 [0.04]	<0.001	0.13 [0.03]	−0.17 [0.04]	<0.001
Enrolled in Oportunidades program	0.68 [0.01]	0.76 [0.02]	<0.001	0.68 [0.01]	0.82 [0.01]	<0.001
Locality covariates						
Financial services (Bank or saving popular services)	0.07 [0.01]	0.30 [0.02]	<0.001	0.07 [0.01]	0.30 [0.02]	<0.001
Basic services (electricity, water, sewer, garbage collection)	0.79 [0.01]	0.76 [0.02]	0.170	0.79 [0.01]	0.76 [0.02]	0.170
Educational infrastructure (primary and secondary schools)	0.03 [0.01]	0.37 [0.02]	<0.001	0.03 [0.01]	0.37 [0.02]	<0.001
Health services (any hospital, clinic or office doctor)	0.82 [0.01]	0.91 [0.01]	<0.001	0.82 [0.01]	0.91[0.01]	<0.001
Basic trade services (selling food and household goods)	0.69 [0.01]	0.79 [0.01]	<0.001	0.69 [0.01]	0.79[0.01]	<0.001
Basic communication services (telephone or telegraph)	0.41 [0.01]	0.65 [0.02]	<0.001	0.41[0.01]	0.65 [0.02]	<0.001
Any incident in the locality in the last four years (droughts, floods, frosts, fires, plagues, earthquakes, hurricanes)	0.61 [0.01]	0.54 [0.02]	0.002	0.61[0.01]	0.54 [0.02]	0.002

OA: Older adult.
Standard error in brackets.
[1]p-value for a t-test or z-proportion test.
[2]Hypertension, diabetes, dyslipidemia, myocardial infarction, angina pectoris, heart disease, stroke, chronic lung disease, osteoporosis, and cancer.

indigenous translators helped in order to translate questions and answers for the interviews. All team members were previously trained and have extensively experience doing fieldwork. All interviews and observations were audio-recorded, previous signed of the informed consent, and totally transcribed along with the ethnographic notes, and recorded in field diaries. Notes from the field diaries underwent content analysis [28,30] together with the interview transcripts in order to achieve data triangulation [30,31].

Analysis. The information generated by the qualitative component of the study consists of ethnographic data composed of selected excerpts from the transcripts collected from semi-structured interviews [32], non-participant observations [33], and fieldwork diaries [28].

The interviews were coded by all team doing fieldwork using pre-defined analytical codes, and live or empirical codes using the program NVivo 2. A content analysis [30] was conducted in order to find meaningful content and recurrent themes in the interviews and observations through deduction and inference [30]. Participants did not provide feedback on the findings. Aside from a preliminary analysis, the content analysis provided a deeper look at the central findings and common themes across one or more groups of individuals, as well as anything that may have reflected an exception or extraordinary perspective, which can help to explain the realities experienced by the individuals interviewed or observed. Major and minor themes where identified, but for the means of this paper, only major or central themes are reported. The validity of the final inferences of the qualitative analysis was confirmed through two types of methodological triangulation of data: (1) data triangulation, due to different voices and tools, and (2) analytical triangulation, result of different social scientists independently analyzing the same ethnographic data [28,31,34]. For this analysis, we extracted fragments of the transcripts from participant interviews. Codes used for the present analysis were self-perception of health (physical and mental), perceived health impact, decision making and use of money and perceived impact on social relationships (family and community). The excerpts that sustain the results presented were chosen among others that show similar patterns, because they were particularly emblematic. Hence, those testimonials used to illustrate our findings were chosen, because they articulately describe similar individual, social, and structural characteristics expressed in the interviews that are representative not only of this individual, but also of many other individuals as well.

Additionally, by using triangulation, the internal validity of the data was achieved. By stating the limitations of the qualitative data implicit in the variation of the characteristics of the participants involved in the qualitative exploration (e.g. men and women belonging to indigenous and mixed communities in two states of the country), we sought to create reflexivity to reduce selection bias.

Results

The quantitative baseline findings can be found in Table 1. For the outcomes variables, significant differences were not observed. In more detail, we observed that prevalence of depressive symptoms were not different across the study groups (25%), being the prevalence of these symptoms similar to the levels found in rural populations. On the other hand, for empowerment indicators, a relatively homogenous distribution was found in the comparison groups, and a high proportion of elderly claim that they contribute to decisions related to spending the household income, as well as to other types of decisions related to household organization. Regarding the covariates (at individual, household and locality levels) we found significant differences in almost of them.

The findings for the depressive symptoms indicator show the program had a significant overall effect on them. The negative value of the associated coefficient (-0.063, $p<0.05$, Table 2) reflect the fact that the program contributes primarily to greater feelings of safety and welfare associated with decreased depressive symptoms among the OA.

We also found a strong trend, shared by the vast majority of participants, regarding the reduction of sadness, and feeling of increasing empowerment. According to their words OA experienced a reduction or a relief of poverty and the stress related with having no income at all for most and an increased sense of security and well-being from receiving a regular income that they could consider their own and on which they can decide what to do with. In the following testimonials, we can see how a non-indigenous woman expresses her sadness as 'shame' when not having money

and when being sick and having to look for money within her networks. In the second testimony below, we see how an indigenous man declares being happy, since he has something to eat.

Q. …and about the program, how do you feel? Do you feel that your health has changed anything since you had the program?
R. *Now I eat better, now I have 'a cent' to buy at least a piece of meat, something like that… some bread. Before it was not like this, we couldn't buy anything because we did not have money (laughter), and now yes, now we have this. I do feel better.*
Q. And about how you feel, do you feel any change?
R. *No, I feel happy (laughter). I do, maybe there is a person who is not happy, but I do feel happy.*
Q. And do you think that how you feel is related somehow to the program, or is it because you are indeed a happy kind of person anyway?
R. *Well, indeed I did not feel sad, I was ashamed because the money was not enough to buy needed things, and then, when I got sick, I used to have to beg for money. But now, at least we have some money. If I get sick at least I have to buy medicine that [the health services] don't have. (SanBe, Non-indigenous man)*
On the other hand, the indigenous man expresses his joy at receiving the program:
Q. Please ask him how he feels now that he is receiving the program? How does he feel about getting [the support], does he feel comfortable, quiet, or does he feel bad or stressed, how does he feel?
Translator R. (Laughter) He says that when he receives the support he feels happy and brings some meat and more things. When he is home, he meets my godmother [elder's wife], close together, happy because they receive the support.
Q. And now, finally I only wanted to ask if he feels that after receiving this money has something changed in his health and mood?
Translator R. He feels better because before that support, he had no support, but since he already has support he feels better, more comfortable. But before, he says he did not, because sometimes he had no money to buy a little something for the kitchen. Well now he feels better because he already has the support. (Ahitic, Indigenous man)

Many of OA declared that pension was their only source of income at the moment. Moreover, because of the conditions in rural areas, which can also be characteristically peasantry, where most of the beneficiaries had lived their entire lives, receiving a stable and fixed monetary income was declared by OA, especially women, to be an event which had never before been experienced. This suggests that there was a significant perceived impact for these beneficiaries.

In empowerment, the overall effect of the program was significant for: *participates in household decision making* ($p<0.01$, Table 2) and *makes decisions on household spending* ($p<0.01$, Table 2). Specifically, receiving a pension boosted the percentage of OA participating in decision making at home by 9%. Likewise, the percentage of OA participating in decisions regarding household expenses rose by 10% in the intervention group. Results therefore indicate that, in general, the Program

Table 2. Overall effect on mental well-being indicators: Depressive symptoms and empowerment.

Effect	Depressive symptoms (GDS≥6)	Participates in making household decisions	Participates in household spending decisions
Intervention	−0.063** [0.031]	0.097*** [0.031]	0.116*** [0.033]
Anticipation	0.053* [0.029]	0.047 [0.029]	0.076*** [0.028]
Sensitivity analysis			
Intervention£	−0.057** [0.028]	0.085*** [0.030]	0.095*** [0.032]

£Moving older adults (aged 69) from control group at baseline to the intervention group.
GDS: Geriatric Depression Scale.
Linear probability models with fixed effect at individual level, adjusted for time-varying covariates in Table 1.
Standard errors in brackets.
*p<0.10; **p<0.05; *** p<0.01.

exerted a significant impact on the empowerment level of *70 y más* beneficiary OA.

Sharing their money with their household constituted an important action for the beneficiaries because by contributing for the household income they felt empower to give their opinion regarding household's decision. Thus, it can be inferred from the transcripts of the OA, that the practices and their significance in the communities can explain and make sense of the context at which we have arrived through our statistical findings on mental health and empowerment. The elderly consistently claimed that the money was not taken away by their families and that they themselves decided how and on what to use it. Several speeches support the fact that OA decide to share their money with their families and contribute as well to the wellbeing of their households. Here is a non-indigenous man talking about it:

Q. So, for example, do [your daughters] tell you how to spend your money?
R. No, no, nothing like that. They don't even ask me or tell me what to do with my money… I know I have to help them. But they don't take away anything from me, I have the money, I keep it. Anyway I give them money because I know they don't have, because they are poor and they don't have enough money for medicine for example, neither for transport.
Q. Ok…
R. But they are not telling me what to do, they don't tell me 'now you have money give it to us', no. It is clear, the money is mine and I do decide about it. (SanBe, Non-indigenous man)

Having one's own resources also gives a sense of economic independence for OA who in many cases are financially dependent on their children, whose own families demand the majority of their resources. For many women, the money they receive through the program *70 y más* is the first economic transaction of their entire lives, which has very revealing impact implications on autonomy, and empowerment. These women expressed in the semi structured interviews how the money gave both parts, themselves and their children, a kind of relief, feeling better for not only reduce the economic burden in their children, but gaining independence in terms of how to spend their own money.

In these interviews a man and a woman express their economic independence from their networks and children.

R. I, what I have left, I keep it [for savings] and… when I'm sick, well, not telling anyone to borrow me money. (SanBe, Non-indigenous woman)
Q. and how do you feel now that you have the Program?
R. Oh! It is a great help, because I don't have to ask my children anymore for help.
Q. And about them, how do you feel they feel about this?
R. I believe that they are ok with this. I say it because they do not worry anymore. They are not thinking that they have to help me. (SanBe, Non-indigenous man)

So then, by being able to offer to their household financial support to purchase food, OA creates reciprocity among they and their families obtaining acknowledgement from the household members and are empowering themselves to decide on issues that concern their lives, as well as the collective life of the household. In general, the diverse elements described around the noncontributory pensions contribute in different ways through complex social mechanisms to 'reduce suffering', 'give themselves value', 'increase happiness', as well as to improve the emotional health.

In the narrative of this indigenous woman reciprocity and empowerment are feelings expressed in relation to the program:

T. Mmm… She says that she feels good with the 70 y más program. She feels that it has helped her. She says she feels more important with this money, mainly in relation to her family because with this money she can help her daughter a little bit. She also says that she helps her daughter in embroideries; when her daughter cannot finish them, she helps her.
Q. And could you ask her what the most important thing is that she feels she gives her family?
T. She says that she cannot give them more than sharing her food. She says she always cooks for her grandchildren because they help her, too. When [her grandchildren] come, they give her some 1000 pesos, or they bring some [soda beverage] or some clothes. She says that it is because that she always prepares some food for them. That is all of what she gives them. (Ahitic, Indigenous woman)

Anticipation Effects

A possible effect of the program *70 y más*, given its eligibility criteria, is that OA a little younger than 70 years old and residing in localities with less than 2,500 inhabitants could modify some of their habits and behaviors related to income, and at the same time, they may be able to modify some dietary habits or some of their social, family-related, or personal expectations, particularly in terms of their emotional health. Although it has been referred to as different names in the literature, this process can be designated as the anticipation effect.

An advantage of our evaluation design is that we can identify the presence, or absence, of a potential anticipation effect and its magnitude. These reflect not only the extent the program would have on impacting future beneficiaries, but also a generalized idea of the real magnitude of the program effect. In order to estimate the anticipation effect, the same specification of our models described earlier was used with the inclusion of OA aged 65 to 69 years old from control groups 2 and 3. Table 1 shows the descriptive results comparing both groups with significant difference for almost all covariates.

For depressive symptoms (Table 2) we observed a significant effect of the program, with a negative coefficient associated (implying a decrease in depressive symptoms) and a positive coefficient for the anticipation effect, which means that in absence of the program there must be an increase of depressive symptoms, which in turn indicate that the estimated program effect could be even larger. As for the empowerment indicators (Table 2), significant effects (with positive coefficients) of both the program and anticipation were detected. For all these indicators, the magnitude of the anticipation effect is lower compared with the program effect.

Sensitivity analysis

Results of the analysis that included OA aged 69 (and who were in the control group at baseline) in the intervention group are in the sensitivity analysis panel of Table 2. As can be seen, the program effect remains significant for all indicators analyzed, although its magnitude is slightly smaller.

For the mental well-being outcomes using DD model estimates combined with the propensity score matching algorithms the results can be found in Table 3. Results obtained with the DD model were not modified by the matching models, with similar levels of significance and magnitude of the coefficients. For the analysis to test the parallelism assumption of DD models, results from comparing the alternative control groups appear to support the assumption of parallelism since just one coefficient is significant, whilst in the analyses with a series of alternative indicators was observed that the coefficients are statistically equal

to zero, suggestive of evidence in favor of the assumption for parallelism (Tables S4 and S5 in File S1).

Discussion

In our analysis context, we hypothesized that the program 70 y más could have an impact, related to the economic transfer, on the analyzed mental well-being indicators, because the transfer can be seen as a component of the SES among OA beneficiaries. The most conclusive result found in our analyses was the effect of the program on the presence of depressive symptoms, which can be interpreted from the OA transcripts. This is a very important finding, since of all mental health problems experienced by OA, the most important based on prevalence is depression. This issue is even more pressing because depression is associated with increased mortality and suicide, as well as morbidity, in terms of functional dependence [35–39]. So, if program has a significant effect on depressive symptoms, it is possible that it will also have an indirect effect on the mortality and disability of OA, an effect that can only be measured in the long term.

This same argument could be generalized as follows. If non-contributory pensions have a positive effect on economic and well-being indicators [11,15,16], then it is possible that also contribute to a healthy and active aging [24], which in turn will impact on the health status of older adults, and will decrease disability and mortality in this age group.

A significant effect was also observed for the OA empowerment, measured through the decision making at home and decision making on household expenditure, which can be found in the literature related to empowerment [40,41]. It is important to note that the effect seems to be more important for women (taking into account the qualitative testimonials), perhaps because for many of them this is the first time they have their own income, which could particularly favored a strong empowerment process. In addition women are more often widows, so paying third parts for work can make them a stronger feeling of empowerment and decision making.

Following a constructivist interpretative framework [42], understood as the collective generation of reality and transmission of modulating experiences, it can be deduced from the qualitative data that when receiving the pension, OA perceive the amount of money as their own and that it comes constantly (e.g. they know it reliably comes every two months), and this perception results in a feeling of a reduction of stress or sadness normally caused by poverty and uncertainty or total lack of income. This reduction of stress is meant to be a feeling of safety and welfare.

Table 3. Overall effect on mental health indicators.

	Depressive symptoms (GDS≥6)	Participates in making household decisions	Participates in household spending decisions
All sample	−0.063**[0.031]	0.097*** [0.031]	0.116*** [0.033]
Matched sample			
Caliper[1]	−0.067* [0.034]	0.110*** [0.035]	0.119*** [0.037]
Kernel-based[2]	−0.062**[0.031]	0.101*** [0.032]	0.110*** [0.033]

Alternative strategies of estimation
GDS: Geriatric Depression Scale.
[1]Caliper algorithm with a specified distance of 0.0005 and one-to-one merge (713 units in intervention and control groups).
[2]Using epanechnikov kernel, and one-to-one matching (875 units in intervention and control groups).
Linear probability models with fixed effect at individual level, adjusted for time-varying covariates in Table 1.
Standard errors in brackets.
*p<0.10; **p<0.05; *** p<0.01.

The interviews with OA help us to understand the mechanisms behind income appropriation and decision making within the household. Furthermore, the results presented here indicate that social mechanisms are at play under which the beneficiaries experience an effect from the pension that redefines the meaning of money in their lives. Thus, besides meaning a perceived reduction of poverty, the pension the OA receive has a positive effect on self-determination and decision making at both the individual and household levels. This decision-making power is translated into economic autonomy, self-sense of value, feeling of reciprocity and worth and the reduction of economic dependence on their children.

In turn, OA share or redistribute the income they receive across their household as found in the study by Marquez-Serrano [43]. In doing so, they regain the power to give their opinion on household matters, which in turn revitalizes their social networks through reciprocity and the sense of being recognized and not being a burden for their families. The resulting effects of these feelings have been previously identified in the literature on OA social networks [44–48], and are expressed by the OA participating in the present evaluation as *'no longer suffering'*, *'feeling valuable'*, and *'being happy'*.

Despite the beneficial aspect that is associated with increasing levels of decision making, it is also possible that there is a downside. For example, it is possible that older adults perceive the decision as a burden, as they lack strong social networks. While this is something that could not be analyzed in this study, it is important that future research will address this issue.

A central finding of the study was related to the use of the pension. The fact that OA make their own decisions on how and on what to spend their money is a key element linked to the feelings of empowerment described earlier. Decision making and the effects of decisions make up the key mechanisms that largely explain the feelings of reduced sadness, which can be associated with depressive symptoms.

Regarding anticipation effects it can be argued that since empowerment is associated with a higher income among OA, it is possible that in households where an OA is about to receive the *70 y más* program pension, the family dynamics can begin to change towards greater respect and consideration for the potential OA beneficiary, because they anticipate an economic transfer and along with it, potential economic benefits for all household members derived from the OA's decision to share their new income. However, it is important to emphasize that family dynamics may also be modified in an undesired manner. For example, it is possible that household members starting to treat the OA better knowing that in the short term could take the pension money. This is an issue that also must be analyzed in future research.

Beyond this discussion, presence of anticipation effects implies that the program's impact would be even greater, since the absence of expectations of becoming a *70 y más* beneficiary would not have had a modification to empowerment. In fact, and in our estimates, the difference observed between beneficiaries and non-beneficiaries would be larger.

Using matching techniques in our analysis confirms the robustness of our results regarding the significant effect that the *70 y más* program has on various indicators of mental well-being in OA residing in rural areas of Mexico.

We have mentioned that a great body of evidence on non-contributory pension's impact has mainly focused on socio economic indicators. This is an important flaw because research indicates that in old age health mental problems are highly prevalent among OA. Due to its devastating consequences, mental health represents an important public health issue [49].

Even so, some studies have analyzed the effect of non-contributory pension on OA's health status. A first set of studies demonstrated that the South African pension improved the self-report health status of its beneficiaries and the co-residing members of the household [50], whereas other showed that pensions are associated with the social well-being and quality of life [17,19]. In other study, using a quasi-experimental design, was evaluated the short-term effect (6 months) of a non-contributory social pension introduced in urban localities in Mexican State of Yucatan on a range of indicators including health. Despite of having found significant effects on labor supply, food availability, medical consumption, and memory, they did not find effect on depressed mood (dysphoria) [51].

Several limitations can be noted in our study. First, given we used a discontinuity regression approach to form our comparison groups, our estimate of the *70 y más* impact is a local estimator; this means that the observed effects are valid only for OA aged 70–74. So it is still pending analyze the impact of the program in older ages. Second, since *70 y más* started in rural localities, our analytical sample is also restricted to rural areas of Mexico, so nothing is known about the program's effect in urban areas where the program also operates nowadays. Third, we just had a short time of the exposure to pension (11 or 12 months), so our impact estimate reflects only an immediate effect, and it is important to determine the medium and long terms effects of the program. And fourth, the qualitative component of the study does not have a baseline measure and only took into account OA beneficiaries of *70 y más*. Even and when there is a debate about the relevance of using a control group from a constructivist point of view, the study could be have more robust results if qualitative component had been included a control group and/or a baseline measurement.

Finally, some of our results showed that if an intervention were implemented to increase the income and the SES of OA, some mental health outcomes may change, just as proposed in the literature [52,53]. For now, and in the short term, it is reasonable to think that this effect is almost exclusively attributable to the economic transfer and the strong sense of solidarity and sharing behind the social mechanisms described that could be observed in the short term through the qualitative component. Perhaps in the medium and long terms, it will be possible to identify other psychosocial or behavioral factors that contribute to explaining the effects observed.

Supporting Information

File S1 This file contains Appendix S1, Appendix S2, Table S1, Table S2, Table S3, Table S4 and Table S5. Appendix S1, Intervention and control group selection and Sampling scheme for qualitative component. Appendix S2, Propensity score matching and Parallelism assumption of DD model. Table S1, Probit regression to predict enrollment in *70 y más* program. Table S2, Results of matching using caliper algorithm. Table S3, Results of matching using kernel algorithm. Table S4, Testing the parallelism assumption: alternative control groups. Table S5, Testing the parallelism assumption: alternative outcomes.

Author Contributions

Conceived and designed the experiments: ASR BME MMTRS MPTP. Analyzed the data: ASR MPTP KMT. Wrote the paper: ASR BME MPTP KMT. Commented on the document before approving it: ASR BME KMT MMTRS MPTP.

References

1. Albala C, Lebrao ML, Leon Diaz EM, Ham-Chande R, Hennis AJ, et al. (2005) [The Health, Well-Being, and Aging ("SABE") survey: methodology applied and profile of the study population]. Rev Panam Salud Publica 17: 307–322.

2. Bertranou FM (2006) Envejecimiento, empleo y protección social en América Latina. Santiago, Chile: Oficina Internacional del Trabajo.

3. Kakwani N, Subbarao K (2005) Ageing and poverty in Africa and the role of social pensions. Brazil: United Nations Development Programme, International Poverty Center.

4. Barrientos A, Gorman M, Heslop A (2003) Old Age Poverty in Developing Countries: Contributions and Dependence in Later Life. World Development 31: 555–570.

5. CEPAL (2010) El envejecimiento y las personas de edad: Indicadores para América Latina y el Caribe. Separata.

6. HelpAge International. Why social pensions? Available: http://www.pension-watch.net/pensions/about-social-pensions/about-social-pensions/why-social-pensions/. Accessed 2014 Jan 30.

7. Willmore L (2007) Universal Pensions for Developing Countries. World Development 35: 24–51.

8. Rubio GM, Garfias F (2010) Análisis comparativo sobre los programas para adultos mayores en México. Serie Políticas Sociales N° 161. CEPAL.

9. Grushka C (2004) Seguridad económica en la vejez, Calidad de vida en la vejez. Conceptos e indicadores para el seguimiento de políticas y programas. CELADE, División de Población de la CEPAL, Mimeo.

10. Bertranou F, Solorio C, van Ginneken W (2002) La protección social a través de las pensiones no contributivas y asistenciales en América Latina. In: Bertranou F, Solorio C, van Ginneken W, editors. Pensiones no contributivas y asistenciales: Argentina, Brasil, Chile, Costa Rica y Uruguay. Santiago, Chile: Oficina Internacional del Trabajo.

11. Barrientos A (2008) Cash transfers for older people reduce poverty and inequality. In: Bebbington A, de Haan A, Dani A, Walton M, editors. Institutional Pathways to Equity: Addressing Inequality Traps. Washington DC: The World Bank. pp. 169–192.

12. Edmonds EV, Mammen K, Miller DL (2005) Rearranging the family? Income support and elderly living arrengments in a low-income country. Journal of Human Resources, University of Wisconsin Press 40: 186–207.

13. Case A, Deaton A (1998) Large Cash Transfers to the Elderly in South Africa. Economic Journal Royal Economic Society 108: 1330–1361.

14. Carvalho Filho IE (2008) Old-age benefits and retirement decisions of rural elderly in Brazil. J Dev Econ 86: 129–146.

15. Escobar-Loza F, Martinez-Wilde S, Mendizábal-Córdova J (2013) El impacto de la renta dignidad: política de redistribución del ingreso, consumo y reducción de la pobreza en hogares con personas adultas mayores. Bolivia: Unidad de Análisis de Políticas Sociales y Económicas del Ministerio de Planificación del Desarrollo, Representación en Bolivia del Fondo de Población de las Naciones Unidas & HelpAge International.

16. Kassouf AL, Rodrigues de Oliveira P (2012) Impact Evalutaion of the Brazilian Non-contributory Pension Program Beneficio de Prestaçao Continuada (BPC) on Family Welfare. (Working Paper No.2012-12). Available: http://www.pep-net.org/programs/pieri/working-papers/. Accessed 2014 Feb 04.

17. Møller V, Devey R (2003) Trends in living conditions and satisfaction among poorer older South Africans: objective and subjective indicators of quality of life in the October Household Survey. Development Southern Africa 20: 457–476.

18. Case A, Menendez A (2007) Does money empower the elderly? Evidence from the Agincourt demographic surveillance site, South Africa. Scand J Public Health Suppl 69: 157–164.

19. Schatz E, Gomez-Olive X, Ralston M, Menken J, Tollman S (2012) The impact of pensions on health and wellbeing in rural South Africa: does gender matter? Soc Sci Med 75: 1864–1873.

20. Sedesol (2013) Reglas de Operación del Programa Pension para Adultos Mayores, 65 y más para el Ejercicio Fiscal 2014. Diario Oficial, diciembre 2013. Available: http://www.normateca.sedesol.gob.mx/work/models/NORMATECA/Normateca/Reglas_Operacion/2014/rop_adultos_mayores.pdf. Accessed 2014 Jan 17.

21. Sedesol (2009) Reglas de Operación del Programa 70 y más para el Ejercicio Fiscal 2010. Diario Oficial, diciembre 2009. Available: http://dof.gob.mx/nota_detalle.php?codigo=5126475&fecha=28/12/2009. Accessed 2014 Jan 17.

22. Yesavage JA, Brink TL, Rose TL, Lum O, Huang V, et al. (1982) Development and validation of a geriatric depression screening scale: a preliminary report. J Psychiatr Res 17: 37–49.

23. Sheikh JI, Yesavage JA, Brooks JO 3rd, Friedman L, Gratzinger P, et al. (1991) Proposed factor structure of the Geriatric Depression Scale. Int Psychogeriatr 3: 23–28.

24. WHO (2002) Active Ageing: A Policy Framework. Second United Nations World Assembly on Ageing, Madrid, Spain. Available: http://whqlibdoc.who.int/hq/2002/WHO_NMH_NPH_02.8.pdf.Accessed 2014 Feb 05.

25. Teddlie C, Yu F (2007) Mixed Methods Sampling: A Typology With Examples. Journal of Mixed Methods Research 1: 77–100.

26. González de la Rocha M (2005) México: Oportunidades y capital social. In: Arriagada I, editor. Aprender de la experiencia El capital social en la superación de la pobreza. Santiago de Chile: CEPAL/Coperatzione Italiana.

27. Guest G, Bunce A, Johnson L (2006) How Many Interviews Are Enough?: An Experiment with Data Saturation and Variability. Field Methods 18: 59–82.

28. Patton M (2002) Qualitative Research & Evaluation Methods: Sage Publicac-tions, Thousand Oaks.

29. Abma T (2006) Patients as partners in a health research agenda setting: the feasibility of a participatory methodology. Eval Health Prof 29: 424–439.

30. Minayo C (2002) La etapa de análisis en los estudios cualitativos. In: Mercado F, Gastaldo D, Calderón C, editors. Investigación cualitativa en salud en Iberoamérica. Guadalajara, México: Universidad de Guadalajara/Centro universitario de Ciencias de la Salud. pp. 239–270.

31. Massey A (1999) Methodological triangulation, or how to get lost without being found out. In: Massey A, Walford G, editors. Explorations in Methodology (Studies in Educational Ethnography). Bingley/US: Emerald Group Publishing Limited. pp. 183–197.

32. Bernard H (1994) Research Methods in Anthropology: Qualitative and Quantitative Approaches. Thousand Oaks/US: SAGE Publications Inc.

33. Mack N, Woodsong C, MacQueen K, Guest G, Namey E (2005) Qualitative research methods: a data collector's field guide. Research Triangle Park, North Carolina, Family Health International, UNAIDS.

34. Denzin NK, Lincoln YS (1994) Handbook of qualitative research. New York: University of Chicago Press.

35. Chapman DP, Perry GS (2008) Depression as a major component of public health for older adults. Prev Chronic Dis 5: A22.

36. Cho HJ, Lavretsky H, Olmstead R, Levin M, Oxman MN, et al. (2010) Prior depression history and deterioration of physical health in community-dwelling older adults–a prospective cohort study. Am J Geriatr Psychiatry 18: 442–451.

37. Fiske A, Wetherell JL, Gatz M (2009) Depression in older adults. Annu Rev Clin Psychol 5: 363–389.

38. Mezuk B, Eaton WW, Golden SH (2008) Depression and osteoporosis: epidemiology and potential mediating pathways. Osteoporos Int 19: 1–12.

39. Schulz R, Beach SR, Ives DG, Martire LM, Ariyo AA, et al. (2000) Association between depression and mortality in older adults: the Cardiovascular Health Study. Arch Intern Med 160: 1761–1768.

40. Mayo M, Craig G (1995) Community participation and empowerment. A reader in participation and development. London: Zed Books.

41. Rowlands J (1997) Empoderamiento y mujeres rurales en Honduras: un modelo para el desarrollo. In: León M, editor. Poder y empoderamiento de las mujeres. Santa Fe de Bogotá, Colombia: Facultad de Ciencias Humanas, Tercer Mundo. pp. 213–245.

42. Connell Szasz M (2001) Between Indian and White Worlds. The Cultural Broker. Norman, Oklahoma: University of Oklahoma Press.

43. Márquez-Serrano M, Kageyama-Escobar M, Pelcastre-Villafuerte B, Ruelas-González G, Rueda-Neria C (2007) Diagnóstico de las condiciones de vida y bienestar del adulto mayor y evaluación del programa pensión Guerrero para vivir mejor. Guerrero: Instituto Nacional de Salud Pública.

44. Bebbington A (2005) Estrategias de vida y estrategias de intervención: el capital social y los programas de superación de la pobreza. In: Arriagada I, editor. Aprender de la experiencia El capital social en la superación de la pobreza. Santiago de Chile: CEPAL/Coperatzione Italiana.

45. Durston J (2005) Superación de la pobreza, capital social y clientelismos sociales. In: Arriagada I, editor. Aprender de la experiencia El capital social en la superación de la pobreza. Santiago de Chile: CEPAL/Coperatzione Italiana.

46. Jáuregui-Ortiz B, Poblete-Trujillo E, Salgado de Snyder V (2006) El papel de la red familiar y social en el proceso de envejecimiento en cuatro ciudades de México. In: Salgado de Snyder V, Wong R, editors. Envejecimiento, pobreza y salud en población urbana un estudio en cuatro ciudades de México. pp. 85–96.

47. Kessler G, Roggi M (2005) Programas de superación de la pobreza y capital social: la experiencia argentina. In: Arriagada I, editor. Aprender de la experiencia El capital social en la superación de la pobreza. Santiago de Chile: CEPAL/Coperatzione Italiana.

48. Puga D, Rosero-Bixby L, Glaser K, Castro T (2007) Red social y salud del adulto mayor en perspectiva comparada: Costa Rica, España e Inglaterra. Población y Salud Mesoamérica.

49. Kinsella K, He W (2009) An Aging World: 2008. Washington, DC: U.S. Census Bureau, International Population Reports, P95/09-1, U.S. Government Printing Office.

50. Case A (2004) Does money protect health status? Evidence from South African Pensions. In: Wise DA, editor. Perspectives on the Economics of Aging: University of Chicago Press.

51. Aguila E, Kapteyn A, Robles R, Vargas O, Weidmer B (2011) Experimental Analysis of the Health and Well-being Effects of a Non-contributory Social Security Program. RAND Corporation.

52. Dohrenwend BP, Levav I, Shrout PE, Schwartz S, Naveh G, et al. (1992) Socioeconomic status and psychiatric disorders: the causation-selection issue. Science 255: 946–952.

53. Hudson CG (2005) Socioeconomic status and mental illness: tests of the social causation and selection hypotheses. Am J Orthopsychiatry 75: 3–18.

14

Sexuality and Affection among Elderly German Men and Women in Long-Term Relationships: Results of a Prospective Population-Based Study

Britta Müller[1]*, Christoph A. Nienaber[2], Olaf Reis[3], Peter Kropp[1], Wolfgang Meyer[4]

1 Institute of Medical Psychology and Medical Sociology, Medical Faculty, University of Rostock, Rostock, Germany, 2 Medical Center Rostock, Department of Cardiology and Angiology, Rostock University Hospital, University of Rostock, Rostock, Germany, 3 Clinic for Child and Adolescent Psychiatry, Rostock University Hospital, University of Rostock, Rostock, Germany, 4 Queen Mary University of London, Barts and the London School of Medicine and Dentistry, London, United Kingdom

Abstract

Satisfaction with sexual activity i.e. sexual satisfaction and the importance of sexuality and affection were analysed using data from the German "Interdisciplinary Longitudinal Study of Adult Development" (ILSE). At three measurement points, 1993–1995, 1997–1998, and 2004–2006 i.e. subjects' ages of 63, 67, and 74 years, participants' reports about their affection and sexual activity were collected. The sample of completed records used for this study consisted of 194 urban non-institutionalised participants, 68% male, all living with partners. Median levels of sexual satisfaction were reported, fluctuating between the measurement points of ages 63 to 74. Between baseline, first and second follow-up no differences were found in levels of sexual satisfaction, though at measurement points age 63 and 67 women were more satisfied than men. When measured at age 74, affection was given a higher priority than sexual activity. Although men and women reported similar priorities, sexual activity and affection were more important for men than for women. Satisfaction within the relationship can be predicted by the importance of affection, but not by that of sexual activity. Our results confirm the thesis of the 'second language of sexuality': for humans in their later years affection seems to be more important than for younger individuals.

Editor: Cheryl McCormick, Brock University, Canada

Funding: The study was funded by the German Federal Ministry for Families, Senior Citizens, Women and Youth (AZ 314-1722-102/16; AZ 301-1720-295/2), the Ministry for Science, Research and Art Baden-Württemberg, and the University of Rostock (FORUN 989020; 889048). The funders had no role in study design, data collection and analysis, decision to publish, or preparation of the manuscript.

Competing Interests: The authors have declared that no competing interests exist.

* Email: britta.mueller@med.uni-rostock.de

Introduction

Cultural attitudes and concerns about sexuality vary between countries and even more so between Western ones and those of the developing world. In the former, sexuality and affection have long been looked at from a biomedical point of view [1]. Findings about the negative influences of hormonal disturbances, severe illness or side-effects of medication seem to support the idea that the need for intimacy and sexual activity in older age is not so important. This is reflected in the "deficit model of ageing".

Due to recent demographic changes, particularly with old age becoming a prolonged period of life spent in partnerships, the situation of the elderly and their perception of their health and partnerships became the subject of in-depth studies. Among elderly couples sexual activity and affection have an important impact on their physical and psychological well-being [2].

Recent studies of elderly couples in western societies focus almost exclusively on their sexuality and their perception of it. Affection has rarely been looked at. The findings with regards to sexuality concentrate on sexual intercourse, because of the assumption that most of the sexually active couples prefer this form of sexual activity [3]. Studies using representative samples from the US population showed that among people aged 65–74 partnered sexual activity is more frequent among married men

and women compared to those living on their own [4]. Among persons with a spouse or in another intimate relationship, men are more likely to be sexually active than women. However, this gender disparity is considerably greater in persons living without a partner [3,5].

Also the decline in sexual activity over the course of life is more pronounced in single persons than in people with partner. The earliest signs of decline in sexual activity in couples can be found between the 5th (aged 41–50) and 6th (aged 51–60) decade of their lives. In this phase a reduction both in percentage of sexually active couples and the frequency of intercourse in active couples could be demonstrated [6]. This decline is closely related to physical and hormonal changes that can result in functional impairments. Further, social standards and attitudes to sexual activity in the post-reproductive phase have to be considered [7,8,9]. Beckman et al. [10] demonstrated, analysing data of four birth cohorts of 70-year-old Swedish men and women, that later birth cohorts reported higher frequencies of sexual intercourse, fewer sexual dysfunctions and higher rates of satisfaction with sexual activity than those from earlier birth cohorts. These results apply to both unmarried and married persons [10]. The second decline occurs between the 8th (aged 71–80) and 9th (81–90) decade [6]. In developed countries in this phase of life chronic diseases with effects on sexual functioning are widespread, for example hypertension and diabetes [5,11,12,13]. Findings suggest that the risk of sexual impairment is greater in men than in women [5,14,15]. Further, stressful psychosocial situations seem to be more frequent between the 8th and 9th decade of life, when periods of care delivered by one partner with subsequent lower levels of sexual involvement become more likely [16].

Other than knowledge about sexual activity, very little is known about the intra- individual changes of satisfaction with sexual activity in individuals over 60 years old living with a partner. There are only a few studies, mostly showing inconsistent results. In the population-based longitudinal 'Olmsted Study of Urinary Symptoms and Health Status among Men' people between the ages of 40 and 79 were studied. It was demonstrated that men with a regular partner at the beginning of the study period (baseline) experienced a bigger decline than men without a partner. This is most likely due to higher baseline levels for men with a regular partner [13]. However, there are no corresponding longitudinal population-based studies of females in this regard. Heiman et al. [17], utilising a cross-sectional design, studied sexual satisfaction in couples in the USA, Brazil, Germany, Japan and Spain, participants aged between 39 and 70 years. Their results suggest a positive association between satisfaction with sexual activity and length of relationship in men; in women this association is even more pronounced. The results of Heiman et al. [17] were based on people living in a partnership between 1 and 50 years duration. However, the authors did not state whether sexual satisfaction increased with longer durations of relationships i.e. 40 years plus.

The findings do not indicate a decline in satisfaction with sexual activity of men and women; however no indication with regard to stability versus decline was made. Heiman et al. [17] showed gender differences regarding sexual satisfaction in relationships existing for 40 years and longer: satisfaction with sexual activity was greater in women than in men.

Recent studies regarding physical contact in older age focus mainly on sexual acts. Little is known about day-to-day intimacy of couples [18], though it has been used to predict the perception of sexual activity: Heiman et al. [17] reported that touching and caressing by partners, kissing and cuddling in men and woman could be used as a predictor for satisfaction with sexual activity. Waite et al. [3] studied the extent of nonsexual intimate contacts in relationships based on data of the National Social Life, Health, and Ageing Project-NSHAP. The results show that 95.6% of men and 95.8% of women living with a spouse and aged 57-64 hug or hold the partner once a month or more. Within the ageing process the corresponding percentages decreased little: in men aged to 75–85 to 90.4%; in women to 90.0%. The item 'once a month or more', however seems to be only a general criterion without proof that these interactions are part of day-to-day living.

In our study we considered intimacy as a special way of expressing affection short of actual intercourse i.e. nonsexual intimate interaction. These expressions of affection include a wide variety of activities such as greeting the partner with an embrace, a kiss, a pat on the back, a cuddle, hug or a caress [3]. Though

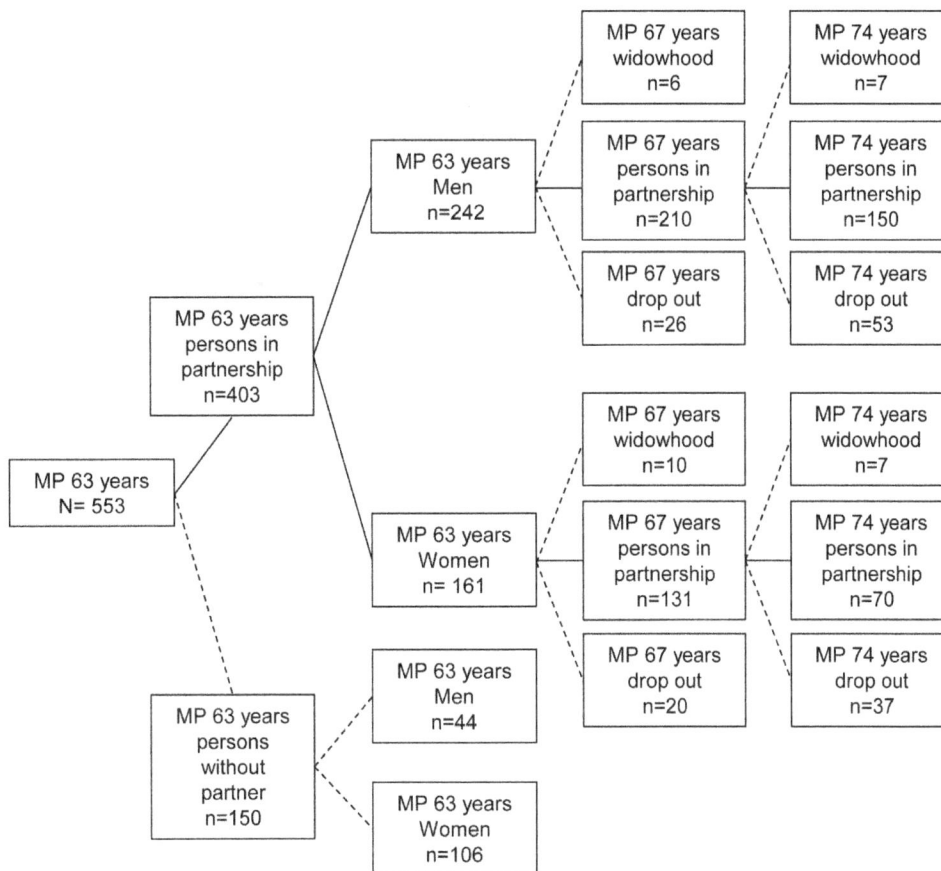

Figure 1. Selection process of the sub-samples at MP 63 years, MP 67 years, and 74 years. Persons who lived in relationship are shown with a solid line. Persons who dropped out or became a widow/widower are shown with a broken line.

Table 1. Characteristics of Sample.

		Men $n=132$	Women $n=62$
Average age (M, SD)	Baseline (1993–1995)	62.8 (0.9)	62.9 (0.9)
	First follow up (1997–1998)	66.8 (0.9)	66.7 (1.0)
	Second follow up (2004–2006)	74.1 (0.9)	74.0 (0.9)
Average duration of the current relationship MP 74 years (M, SD)		46.4 (8.0)	48.0 (8.0)
Duration of current relationship MP 74 years (n, %)	21 to under 30 years	10 (7.6)	4 (6.5)
	30 to under 40 years	8 (6.1)	5 (8.1)
	40 to under 50 years	56 (42.4)	15 (24.2)
	50 and more years	58 (43.9)	38 (61.3)
Number of marriages MP 74 years (n, %)	1	114 (86.4)	54 (87.1)
	2	15 (11.4)	8 (12.9)
	3	3 (2.3)	0
Average duration of education in years (M, SD)		14.1 (2.6)	13.1 (3.1)
Duration of education (n, %)	8 to 9 years	3 (2.3)	11 (17.7)
	10 to 15 years	90 (68.2)	36 (58.1)
	16 to 18 years	39 (29.5)	15 (24.2)
Occupation (n, %)	Higher-grade professionals	58 (43.9)	13 (21.0)
	Lower-grade professionals	16 (12.1)	15 (24.2)
	Routine non-manual employees	7 (5.3)	10 (16.1)
	Self-employed, artists	8 (6.1)	3 (4.8)
	Employed technicians; supervisors	10 (7.6)	2 (3.2)
	Skilled manual workers	29 (22.0)	5 (8.1)
	Semi-skilled/unskilled manual workers	4 (3.0)	14 (22.6)
Retirement (n, %)	Baseline (1994–1995)	100 (75.8)	59 (95.2)
	First follow up (1997–1998)	132 (100.0)	62 (100.0)
Physical health (M, SD)[a]	Baseline (1994–1995)	2.3 (0.8)	2.4 (0.9)
	First follow up (1997–1998)	2.5 (0.7)	2.6 (0.7)
	Second follow up (2004–2006)	2.5 (0.8)	2.5 (0.7)

[a]Assessment of physical health by a physician based on the history, physical assessment and blood tests using a six-point-scale: 1 = very good, 2 = good, 3 = satisfactory, 4 = sufficient, 5 = poor, 6 = very poor.
M: mean; SD: standard deviation.

sexual activity is often related to affection, the latter can also be found in day-to-day life without sexual activity.

The purpose of this paper was to describe the subjective experiences of sexual activity and affection among men and women in Germany, born 1930–1932 and living in long-term relationships. The sample was based on the data of the German 'Interdisciplinary Longitudinal Study of Adult Development' (ILSE), a multicenter cohort survey of a population-based urban sample.

Our assumption was that the process of ageing modifies social interactions and behaviours and the following become more important than sexual activity: physical closeness, being in an intimate relationship, belonging together and being cared for. To start with we analysed the development of satisfaction with sexual activity from ages 63 to 74. We then studied how affection and sexual activity were perceived by participants aged 74 years. Thirdly we tested the influence of person- and relationship-related items on the satisfaction with the partnership.

Four hypotheses were tested:

1. Satisfaction with sexual activity in long-term relationships does not decrease with age

2. Women living with a spouse are sexually more satisfied than men with a spouse

3. In long-term relationships affection is given a higher importance than sexual activity

4. The importance of both sexual activity and affection predicts satisfaction with the relationship

Methods

Ethics Statement

The study was examined, positively voted and approved by the Ethics Committee of the Faculty of Medicine, Heidelberg University, and the Ethics Committee of the Faculty of Medicine, Rostock University. Written informed consent was obtained from the participants.

Sample

The data used for this study were part of the pool of the German "Interdisciplinary Longitudinal Study of Adult Development" (ILSE). The study was funded by the German Federal Ministry of Family, Senior Citizens, Women and Youth

(BMFSFJ), the Baden-Württemberg Ministry of Science, Research and Art (MWA) and the University of Rostock. ILSE, an ongoing multicenter cohort study, commenced in 1993, aimed at identifying individual, social and economic determinants of a healthy, ageing population. Inter- and intra-individual differences and changes occurring from middle to higher adult age are studied, as well as the influences of environmental factors, behavioral aspects, life-events, health behaviors and mental and physical health on well-being.

ILSE utilises a biographical approach analysing the effects of the participants' perception of biographical key situations on performance and adaptation in later life. The design is based on the assumption that there are gender, cohort as well as systemic social influences. Two cohorts, pre-war born participants i.e. born 1930–32 and post-war born participants i.e. born 1950–52 were studied. Both lived through their childhood and adolescence in very different times of German history and went through their developments confronted with important historical events. Further, samples were drawn from West Germany (region of Heidelberg) and East Germany (regions of Leipzig and Rostock) thus enabling to study the effects of different political systems on processes of ageing.

Participants were identified by using their postal addresses, randomly chosen from the official government registry after implementation of the stratification criteria sex and cohort membership. As a result 1106 participants were recruited for ILSE, both cohorts comprised of 553 persons. Men (52%) and East Germans (55%) were slightly over represented. So far the sample has been analysed at 3 measurement points at which the participants were tested by multidisciplinary teams of medical doctors, psychologists, sociologists and sports scientists.

Because the experience of sexuality in old age was a topic long neglected by research, it is worthy of a secondary data analysis. For this study data of the earlier birth cohort born 1930–1932 were used. This cohort was studied at three measurement points: first measurement point 1993–1995 i.e. baseline, average age 63; N = 553; second measurement point 1997–1998 i.e. first follow-up, average age 67, response-rate = 89.9%, N = 497; third measurement point 2004–2006 i.e. second follow-up, average age 74, response-rate based on the baseline: 65.1%; N = 360. Only participants living in a relationship at all three measurement points and having provided a complete set of data about their sexual activity and affection at all three measurement points, were included in our study. At the first measurement point i.e. MP 63 years 74% of 553 participants were living in a relationship (Figure 1), 60% of those were male. At the second measurement point i.e. MP 67 years 341 persons still lived in a relationship, 62% of those were male. At the third measurement point i.e. MP 74 years 220 participants were in a relationship, 68% of those were male. 42% of the persons who had dropped out had died. A further 28% could not continue to participate because of ill health. The dropout analysis revealed that participants available at all three measurement points had better health at MP 63 (according to doctors' assessments), better subjective health (according to their own assessments), better cognitive abilities and were less depressed than those who dropped out at the first or second measurement point.

Of 220 persons who lived in a relationship at MP 63, 67 and 74 years, we acquired complete data sets of 132 men and 62 women. This sample of 194 persons was studied. The proportion of men and women in our sample living in a relationship was representative of the German population [19,20]. On average our female participants had male partners who were one year and nine months older. Looking at male participants, their female partners were on average three years and one month younger. So, being widowed is a less likely event for men than for women. All of the 194 participants had heterosexual partners and were married (Table 1). Most of the participants were living in long-term relationships. The averaged duration of the relationships was longer for women than for men, $U = 3236$, $p = .019$, $r = .17$. 87% of women and 86% of men were in their first marriage. Being married was not a criterion for participation. It can, however, be understood as an expression of social norms in the analysed cohort, for example the wish to legitimise a relationship by marriage. In addition, new relationships are less likely to be started by widowed women in advanced age [21]. In our sample of 194 participants we found differences between men and women regarding vocational training and occupation, which are typical for this generation. Men reported attending primary and secondary school and vocational training longer than women, $U = 3216$, $p = .014$, $r = -.18$. Their doctors 'assessments of participants' health were good overall and at none of the measurement points differed between men and women (see Table 1).

Measures

Data about 'sexuality and affection' were collected by a semi-structured interview. This was conducted to evaluate the participants' current situation of life regarding health, housing, finance, job, partnership and social networks. Further, data were gathered about the participants' subjective perception and individual summary of their lives so far and perspectives for the future. In addition, a detailed biography was obtained at the first point of measurement. That included details about how the participants perceived learning about sexuality in their adolescence, their first erotic encounters and sexual activity, and their sexuality in the first years of their relationship. In addition, from the second measurement point onwards they were asked about any changes in their life situation.

On average a semi-structured interview took one and a half hours. Interview techniques were honed extensively in training sessions of several days duration. Furthermore a concomitant quality control was implemented. All interviewers underwent a video-based certification process that required them to achieve at least 80% of the targets of an independently certified standard training [22].

The data regarding sexuality and affection described in our study were part of the interview part 'relationship'. Data relating to satisfaction with sexual activity were collected at all three MP, however, the importance of sexual activity and the issue 'affection' was only explored at the MP 74 years. This was due to increased importance given to affection and sexual activity during the years the study ran. Our data about sexuality have to consider the different meaning of the word 'sexuality' in English and German: In the English language the term 'sexuality' is ambiguous although commonly used in research. Further, English speaking elderly people might be in a relationship they regard as sexual, i.e. in a marriage, but may not currently be sexually active. In the German language the word 'Sexualität', used in the study, refers more strongly to sexual activity than the English word 'sexuality'. When asked what our participants understood as 'Sexualität' they indicated sexual activity in the sense of sexual intercourse. In the following we therefore refer to sexuality as 'sexual activity'.

At MP 63 and MP 67 years the participants were encouraged to reflect on sexuality by the standardized question regarding sexuality was: 'I now would like to speak about sexuality. Could you tell me how this is like in your partnership?' Following that, the participants were asked to rate how content they were with

Table 2. Levels of satisfaction with sexual activity at MP 62, 66 and 74 years: total sample by gender.

Level of satisfaction with sexual activity[a]	M (SD) [95% CI]			U-Test[b] (Men-Women) z-value (p-value)
	Total N=194	Men n=132	Women n=62	
Baseline: MP 63 years	3.42 (1.08) [3.26;3.57]	3.29 (1.14) [3.09;3.48]	3.69 (0.88) [3.47;3.92]	−2.22 (.026*)
First follow up: MP 67 years	3.44 (1.06) [3.29;3.59]	3.34 (1.08) [3.16;3.53]	3.66 (1.01) [3.41;3.92]	−1.92 (.054)*
Second follow up: MP 74 years	3.52 (0.98) [3.38;3.66]	3.48 (1.01) [3.31;3.66]	3.60 (0.93) [3.36;3.83]	−.76 (.448)

[a]Level of satisfaction with sexual activity on a five-point-scale: 1 = very poor, 2 = poor, 3 = satisfactory, 4 = good, 5 = excellent.
[b]Results of Mann-Whitney-U-Test, 2-Tail-Sig.
*p<.05.
M: mean; SD: standard deviation.

sexuality in their relationship. Participants recorded their own answers by completing a 5 point Likert scale ('How satisfied are you with sexuality in your partnership? 1 = very poor; 2 = poor; 3 = satisfactory; 4 = good; 5 = excellent').

At MP 73 years first the issue 'affection' was examined. Since we expected participants to know less about the concept of 'affection' compared to 'sexuality', verbal anchors for 'affection' were given in the standardized instruction: 'Now I would like to speak about mutual proximity and affection in your partnership, for example embracing, holding hands, cuddling or kissing. Could you tell me something about this in your partnership?' Answers contained very different behaviors, indicating that our participants understood the concept. For example everyday situations like guiding someone when walking were regarded as affection. Participants afterwards were asked to rate the importance of affection in their relationship and how satisfied they were with it. They recorded their answers in a 5 point Likert scale ('How important is intimacy and affection in your relationship?' 1 = not at all important; 2 = slightly

important; 3 = fairly important; 4 = quite important; 5 = very important; 'How satisfied are you with intimacy and affection in your relationship?' 1 = very poor; 2 = poor; 3 = satisfactory; 4 = good; 5 = excellent'). After that we shifted to the issue 'sexuality' with the following question: 'When you think about sexuality, could you tell me how this is like in your partnership?' In the same way as for the previous issue 'affection' the questions to importance of sexuality and satisfaction with sexuality followed. Again, a list with answers was handed to participants. At the end of the interview part 'affection and sexuality' satisfaction with the relationship was rated by participants on a five-point Likert scale (1 = very poor; 2 = poor; 3 = satisfactory; 4 = good; 5 = excellent).

Statistical analysis

In order to analyse the mean differences t-tests were used (Student's t-test; t-test for independent samples). Furthermore a repeated measurement analysis of variance and a multiple linear

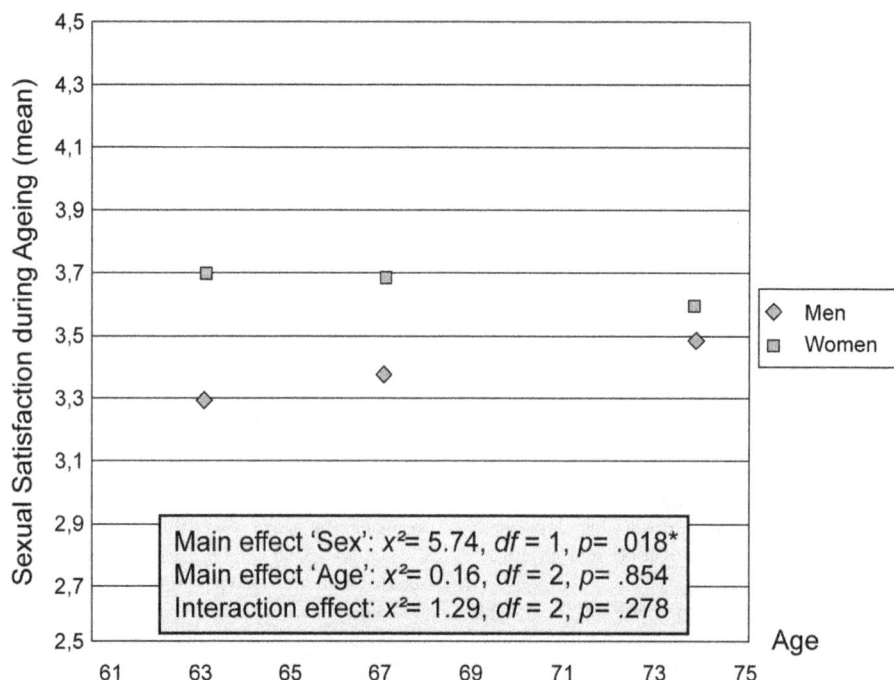

Figure 2. **Satisfaction with sexual activity during ageing: mean-values, differentiated by gender.** In the box are the results of the nonparametric repeated measures analysis of variance (Kruskal-Wallis-Test; Friedmann-Test). *p<.05.

Table 3. Levels of satisfaction with sexual activity: results of the analysis of differences between the measurement points (MP).

Wilcoxon-Test[a]; z-value (p-value)			
Measurement points (MP)	Total N = 194	Men n = 132	Women n = 62
MP 63–74 years	−1.10 (.270)	−1.63 (.102)	−.61 (.539)
MP 63–67 years	−.43 (.664)	−.67 (.502)	−.28 (.782)
MP 67–74 years	−.96 (.337)	−1.44 (.150)	−.57 (.57)

[a]Results of Wilcoxon-Matched-Pairs-Signed-Rank-Test; 2-Tail-Sig.

regression model were applied. The level of significance was set at p<0.05.

The data set for the study is available as a supplementary file for this publication (Table S1).

Results

Satisfaction with sexual activity

During the observational period of 12 years satisfaction with sexual activity ranked at a median level between 'satisfactory' (3.0) and 'good' (4.0) (see Table 2). Differences between men and women were found x^2 (1) = 5.74, p = .018 (see Figure 2) at baseline and first follow-up, none was seen at second follow-up. Women were more satisfied then men at MP 63 years (mean = 3.69, SD = .88 vs. mean = 3.29, SD = 1.14, p = .026) and at MP 67 years (mean = 3.66, SD = 1.01 vs. mean = 3.34, SD = 1.08, p = .054) (see Table 2). We did not find any differences of satisfaction with sexual activity between the three measurement points, neither in the total sub-sample nor in groups of either gender (Figure 2 and Table 3). Although levels of satisfaction between men and women became similar during the process of ageing, there was no significant age by sex interaction effect x^2(2) = 1.29, p = .278 (see Figure 2).

Sexual activity and affection

With the beginning of the eighth decade of life sexual activity and affection ranked differently (see Table 4). Affection had a higher priority (mean = 4.21; SD = .77) than sexual activity (mean = 3.23; SD = 1.04). Although men and women had the same ranking, they differed regarding the level of importance: for men, sexual activity and affection were more important (sexual activity: mean = 3.50, SD = .95; affection: mean = 4.32, SD = .68) than for women (sexual activity: mean = 2.66, SD = .99; affection: mean = 3.98, SD = .90) (see Table 4). This difference became particularly evident when the answering options "very important" and

"quite important" were collapsed into one; 60.6% of male participants reported that sexual activity would be important versus only 27.4% of women. However, for 90.9% of men and 80.6% of women affection played an important role in their life (see Figure 3).

Satisfaction with the relationship

We found high levels of satisfaction with the relationship at age 74 years with a mean between 'good' (4.0) and 'excellent' (5.0) (mean = 4.42; SD = .70). Men (mean = 4.45, SD = .74) and women (mean = 4.34, SD = .60) showed similar levels. The Mann-Whitney-Test did not indicate differences between men and women, U = 3489, p = .061, r = −.13. A multiple regression analysis was conducted using the following predictor variables: level of education, physical health, duration of relationship, importance of sexual activity and importance of affection. The dependent variable was satisfaction with the relationship. Regarding the total sample the model produced R^2 = .16, which was statistically significant, F (5,188) = 8.32, p<.001. The explained variation within the group of women with R^2 = .30, F (5.56) = 6.20, p<.001 was higher than that of men, R^2 = .11, F (5,126) = 4.09, p = .002. Satisfaction with the relationship were predicted by the importance of affection in the total sample, B = 0.39, t = 5.69, p<.001, among men, B = 0.44, t = 4.28, p<.001 and among women, B = 0.33, t = 4.12, p<.001. Neither women nor men showed a relation between importance of sexual activity and satisfaction with the relationship. The results of the regression analysis are shown in Table 5.

Discussion

The ILSE study covered a surveillance period of 12 years. The participants, born between 1930 and 1932 and in good mental and physical health, were examined at the measurement points aged 63, 67 and 74 years. The satisfaction with sexual activity among

Table 4. Importance of sexual activity and affection at MP 74 years (second follow up); total sample by gender.

Importance of...	M (SD) [95% CI]			U-Test[c] (Men-Women) z-value (p-value)
	Total N = 194	Men n = 132	Women n = 62	
sexual activity[a]	3.23 (1.04) [3.08; 3.38]	3.50 (0.95) [3.34; 3.66]	2.66 (0.99) [2.41; 2.91]	−5.12 (<.001***)
affection[b]	4.21 (0.77) [4.10; 4.32]	4.32 (0.68) [4.20; 4.44]	3.98 (0.90) [3.76; 4.20]	−2.48 (.013*)

[a]Importance of sexual activity on a five-point-scale: 1 = not important at all, 2 = hardly important, 3 = fairly important, 4 = quite important, 5 = very important.
[b]Importance of affection on a five-point-scale: 1 = not important at all, 2 = hardly important, 3 = fairly important, 4 = quite important, 5 = very important.
[c]Results of Mann-Whitney-U-Test, 2-Tail-Sig.
*p<.05;
***p<.001.
M: mean; SD: standard deviation.

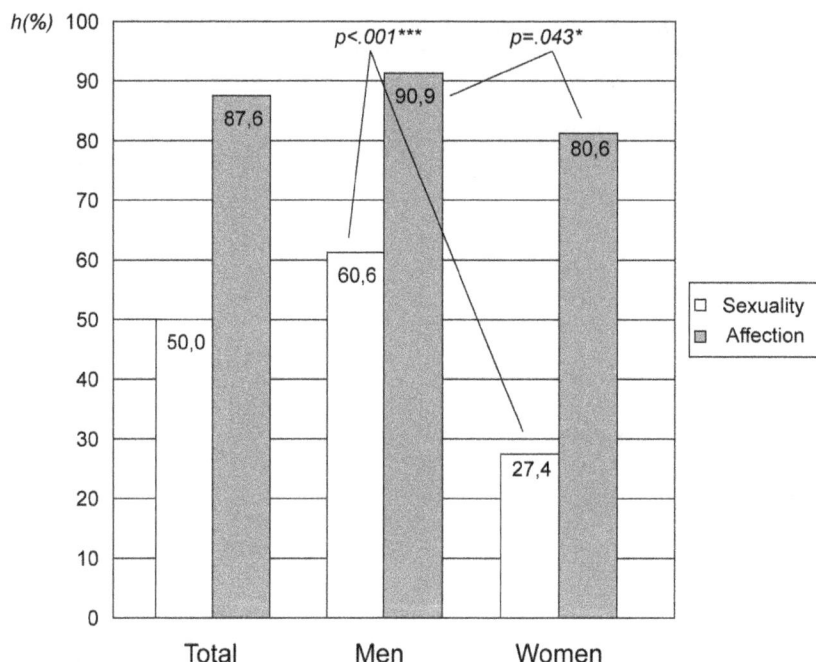

Figure 3. Percentage of elderly in the group MP 74 years to whom sexuality and affection is important. Summary of the relative frequencies 'level 4' (quite important) and 'level 5' (very important). Results of Pearson's Chi-Squared-Test. ***p<.001.

men and women remained stable during the study period. We regarded hypothesis 1 as confirmed. This finding is particularly interesting because there are consistent data in the literature showing decreases in sexual function with aging [3,4,12,13,14]. Married couples experience the first impact on sexual activity between the fifth and sixth decade of life [6]. ILSE started at age 63, when participants had already adapted to the first change. We suppose that psychological adaptation processes according to the theory of Rothermund and Brandstädter about coping with deficits and losses in later life may play an important role for achieving stability [23]. The model of selective optimization with compensation (SOC) provides a framework to understand the specific mechanisms in the processes of coping [24]. We assume that at baseline of ILSE individual coping strategies – as a reaction to sexual changes experienced - had already started, thus resulting in a good level of satisfaction. The participants' conditions for this adaptation process seemed favourable. They were in the so-called 'third age', characterised not only by good health and sufficient social, cognitive and physical activities, but also by high levels of cortical plasticity [25]. Further, a long period of cohabitation influences the way of coping with age-related physical and functional changes. Both previous relationships and partners' experiences during their lives determine perception and the reaction to it. It seems that particularly couples looking back on long-term relationships - like those of the ILSE-sample - could cope better with changes of sexual activity with age. A large number of years living together reflect both the maturity of the relationships and good choice of their partner. This could lead to mutual acceptance and feelings of worth within the relationship, something that could well alleviate negative experiences caused by physical and functional changes. Spouses are potential sources of emotional support especially when it comes to changes in sexuality. Familiarity and profound closeness built up over many years enables them to react favourably to changes and actively regain a fulfilling sexuality. In that sense the gap between

satisfaction and activity is smaller among couples than among individuals without partners.

At measurement points 63 and 67 years satisfaction with sexuality was less in men than in women. However, at measurement point 74 years there were no longer gender-related differences. Hypothesis 2 can only be partially verified. Similar results with regard to satisfaction in women were described in a cross-sectional study of couples by Heiman et al [17]. We could speculate that possible processes of coping are probably moderated by gender and may explain the differences found here. The literature states that changes in female sexual functioning start earlier in life than those of men [26,27,28,29,30]. Furthermore, findings show that changes in sexual functioning are perceived as stronger and more stressful by men than women [3,31,32]. We can therefore assume that the emotional adaptation to the perception of changes in sexuality needs a longer period in men than in women.

Regarding hypothesis 3, we demonstrated that for older individuals affection is more important than sexual activity. 61% of 74 years old men stated that sexual activity is an important factor in their relationship, whilst only 27% of women said so. This corresponds to the findings of Waite et al. [3], but in addition to available results we found that affection is regarded as more important than sexual activity: 91% of men and 81% of women stated that affection was an important or very important part of their lives. Though no data were collected about a 'second language of sexuality' [33], which refers to elderly people experiencing a stronger emotional sexuality than younger persons and to the growing importance of various kinds of affection become more important in later life [34], this theory could help explain our findings. Affection in old age can be seen as an expression of strong intimacy and profound closeness. During their lives spouses have acquired the capacity to identify specific needs of their partner and react accordingly. Furthermore the importance of affection could be a reflection of the finiteness of life,

Table 5. Summary of a multiple regression analysis to predict Satisfaction with relationship at MP 74 years.

Predictors	Total sample N=194			Men n=132			Women n=62		
	B	SE	β	B	SE	β	B	SE	β
Years of education	−0.01	0.02	−.03	−0.01	0.02	−.01	−0.02	0.02	−.09
Physical health	−0.06	0.07	−.06	−0.05	0.08	−.05	−0.10	0.10	−.11
Duration of relationship	−0.01	0.01	−.10	−0.01	0.01	−.04	−0.02	0.01	.24*
Importance of sexual activity	−0.06	0.05	−.09	−0.11	0.07	−.14	0.03	0.07	.05
Importance of affection	0.39	0.07	.43***	0.44	0.10	.40***	0.33	0.08	.50***
constant	3.61			3.31			4.30		
R²	.16			.11			.30		

B = regression coefficient; SE = standard error; β = standardized beta weight.
*p<.05;
***p<.001.

particularly in the context of the relationship. We showed that both sexual activity and affection were more important for men than for women in long-term relationships. This effect of gender is well described [2,35,36,37,38]. The percentage of participants stating that sexual activity is important goes down with age both in men and in women. For men, however, it has been described that the importance plateaus after an initial decline, whilst the decline for women is constant [3]. Our findings demonstrate that the gender effect regarding the importance of sexual activity is not solely dependent on the higher risk of widowhood in women based on higher male mortality rates in contrast to female mortality rates. Also attitudes to and beliefs about sexuality in old age differ between men and women in long-term relationships [3].

Following the fourth hypothesis, we examined how satisfied participants were with their relationships. We found high levels of satisfaction in older age. Longitudinal studies show that compared to middle age adults, satisfaction with relationships is more pronounced in old age [39,40,41]. This can be explained by the 'socioemotional selectivity theory': Older couples demonstrate more positive effective communication than middle-aged couples. In other words, over the years they have developed an ability to control the emergence of negative affects [42]. The regression analyses of predictors for satisfaction in relationships showed that neither education, physical health, nor the duration of the relationship could predict satisfaction. These results are consistent with the previous findings [17,43]. Hypothesis four, predicting an influence of sexual activity and affection, could only be verified in part: only the importance of affection predicted satisfaction with the relationship. No support was found for the importance of sexual activity as predictor. Heiman et al. [17] demonstrate that men aged 40 to 70 years react to gestures of intimacy with high satisfaction in their relationship whilst in women no such correlation was found. However, we demonstrated that for women in the group 74 years, satisfaction with their relationship can be predicted by the role of day-to-day intimacy. We can therefore conclude that satisfaction with the relationship among older people depends on their openness and willingness to exchange intimacies. Elderly people want to satisfy their growing needs for mutual physical closeness by pleasant intimate daily rituals like the daily good morning/goodnight kiss, holding hands etc, all of which relatively independent of 'with', 'instead' or 'despite' sexual activity. Individuals in stable and satisfactory relationships can use this 'second language' with more nuances than the unsatisfied elderly.

Limitations

Limitations are given by the specific protocol of exploration at MP 73 years. The sequence of the topics 'affection' and 'sexuality' and the different instructions to both may have affected the ratings, which slightly reduces comparability of both. Other limitations of our study are closely linked to the quantity and structure of the analysed sample. To study the course of satisfaction during the observation period of 12 years only subjects with complete data sets could be selected. Therefore the number of participants we could include in the study declined to194, which equates to 54% of all participants at the third measurement point. Death, separation or serious illness of a spouse were the most important reasons for non-responding. We therefore had to resort to a sub-sample of subjects almost exclusively living in long-term relationships. Our findings apply less to people living alone and mainly represent the elderly living in a relationship.

Acknowledgments

The authors would like to thank the participants of the "Interdisciplinary Longitudinal Study of Adult Development" (ILSE) for supplying the data and their support.

Author Contributions

Conceived and designed the experiments: BM. Performed the experiments: BM PK. Analyzed the data: BM OR. Contributed reagents/materials/analysis tools: PK CAN. Wrote the paper: BM WM.

References

1. DeLamater J (2012) Sexual Expression in Later Life: A Review and Synthesis. Journal of Sex Research 49: 125–141.

2. Fisher LL (2010) Sex, romance and relationship. AARP Survey of midlife and older adults. Washington DC: American Association for Retired Persons.

3. Waite LJ, Laumann EO, Das A, Schumm LP (2009) Sexuality: Measures of partnerships, practices, attitudes, and problems in the National Social Life, Health, and Aging Project. Journals of Gerontology: Social Sciences 64 B (Suppl.1): i56–i66.

4. Lindau ST, Gavrilova N (2010) Sex, health, and years of sexuality active life gained due to good health. Evidence from two US population based cross sectional surveys of ageing. British Medical Journal 340: 1–11, doi: 10.1136/bmj.c810.

5. Lindau ST, Schumm LP, Laumann EO, Levinson W, O'Muircheartaigh CA, et al. (2007) A national study of sexuality and health among older adults in the U.S. New England Journal of Medicine 357: 762–774.

6. Call V, Sprecher S, Schwartz P (1995) The incidence and frequency of marital sex in a national sample. Journal of Marriage and Family 57: 639–652.

7. Dillaway HE (in press) Reproductive history as social context: Exploring how woimen talk about menopause and sexuality at midlife. In: Carpenter L, DeLamater J, editors. Sex for life: From virginity to Viagra, how sexuality changes throughout our lives. New York: New York University Press.

8. Hinchliff S, Gott M (2011) Seeking Medical Help for Sexual Concerns in Mid- and Later Life: A Review of the Literature. Journal of Sex Research 48: 106–117.

9. Koch PB, Mansfield PK, Thurau D, Carey M (2005) "Feeling frumpy": The relationship between body image and sexual response changes in midlife women. Journal of Sex Research 42: 215–223.

10. Beckman N, Waern M, Gustafson D (2008) Secular trends in self-reported sexual activity and satisfaction in Swedish 70 year olds: cross sectional survey of four populations, 1971–2001. British Medical Journal 337 (7662): 151–154, doi: 10.1136/bmj.a279.

11. Thompson WK, Charo L, Vahia IV, Depp C, Allison M, et al. (2011) Association between higher levels of sexual function, activity, and satisfaction and self-rated successful aging in older postmenopausal women. Journal of the American Geriatrics Society 59: 1503–1508.

12. Woloski-Wruble AC, Oliel Y, Leefsma M, Hochner-Celnikier D (2010) Sexual activities, sexual and life satisfaction and successful aging in women. Journal of Sexual Medicine 7: 2401–2410.

13. Gades NM, Jacobson DJ, McGree ME, Sauver JL, Lieber MM, et al. (2009) Longitudinal evaluation of sexual function in a male cohort: the Olmsted County Study of Urinary Symptoms and Health Status among Men. Journal of Sexual Medicine 6(9): 2455–2466.

14. Moreira ED, Glasser DB, King R, Duarte F, Gingell C & the Global Study of Sexual Attitudes, and Behaviors Invesatigators Group (2008) Sexual difficulties and help-seeking among mature adults in Australia: Results from the Global Study of Sexual Attitudes and Behaviors. Sexual Health 5: 227–234.

15. Howard JR, O'Neill S, Travers C (2006) Factors affecting sexuality in older Australian women: Sexual interest, sexual arousal, relationships, and sexuell distress in older Australian women. Climacteric 9: 355–367.

16. Burgess EO (2004) Sexuality in midlife and later life coples. In: Harvey J, Wenzel A, Sprecher S, editors. The handbook of sexuality in close relationships. Mahwah NJ: Lawrence Erlbaum Associates Inc. pp. 437–454.

17. Heiman JR, Long JS, Smith SN, Fisher WA, Sand MS, et al. (2011) Sexual Satisfaction and Relationship Happiness in Midlife and Older Couples in Five Countries. Archives of Sexual Behavior 40: 741–753.

18. Clark LH (2006) Older Women and Sexuality: Experiences in Marital Relationships across the Life Course. Canadian Journal on Aging/La Revue canadienne du vieillissement 25: 129–140.

19. Bundesamt S (2011) Focus on the Elderly in Germany and the EU. Bonn.

20. Bomsdorf E (1993) Generationensterbetafeln für die Geburtsjahrgänge 1923 bis 1993: Modellrechnungen für die Bundesrepublik Deutschland. Köln: Verlag Josef Eul.

21. Höpflinger F (1987) Wandel der Familienbildung in Westeuropa. Frankfurt a.M.: Campus-Verlag.

22. Kruse A, Schmitt M, Wahl HW (2008) Interdisziplinäre Längsschnittstudie des Erwachsenenalters (ILSE)–Abschlussbericht anlässlich der Fertigstellung des dritten Messzeitpunkts. Heidelberg.

23. Rothermund K, Brandstädter J (2003) Coping with deficits and losses in later life: from compensatory action to accommodation. Psychology and aging 18(4): 896.

24. Müller B, Kropp P (2012) Freizeit im höheren Lebensalter: ein Bereich aktiver Lebensgestaltung. Befunde aus der Interdisziplinären Längsschnittstudie des Erwachsenenalters (ILSE). In: Kumlehn M, Kubik A, editors. Konstrukte gelingenden Alterns. Stuttgart: Kohlhammer. pp. 207–228.

25. Baltes PB, Freund AM (2003) Human strengths as the orchestration of wisdom and selective optimization with compensation. In: Aspinwall LG, Staudinger UM, editors. A psychology of human strengths: Perspectives on an emerging field. Washington, DC: American Psychological Association. pp. 23–35.

26. Avis NE, Zhao X, Johannes CB, Ory M, Brockwell S, et al. (2005) Correlates of sexual function among multi-ethnic middle-aged women: results from the Study of Women's Health Across the Nation (SWAN). Menopause 12(4): 385–398.

27. Gallicchio L, Schilling C, Miller SR, Zacur H, Flaws JA (2007) Correlates of depressive symptoms among women undergoing the menopausal transition. Journal of psychosomatic research 63(3): 263–268.

28. Leiblum SR, Koochaki PE, Rodenberg CA, Barton IP, Rosen RC (2006) Hypoactive sexual desire disorder in postmenopausal women: US results from the Women's International Study of Health and Sexuality (WISHeS). Menopause 13(1): 46–56.

29. Braun M, Wassmer G, Klotz T, Reifenrath B, Mathers M, et al. (2000) Epidemiology of erectile dysfunction: results of the 'Cologne Male Survey'. International journal of impotence research 12(6): 305–311.

30. Rosen R, Altwein J, Boyle P, Kirby RS, Lukacs B, et al. (2003) Lower urinary tract symptoms and male sexual dysfunction: the multinational survey of the aging male (MSAM-7). European urology 44(6): 637–649.

31. Edwards JN, Booth A (1994) Sexuality, marriage, and well being: The middle years. In: Rossi AS, editor. Sexuality across the life course. Chicago: University of Chicago Press. pp. 233–259.

32. Laumann EO, Nicolosi A, Glasser DB, Paik A, Gingell C, et al. (2004) Sexual problems among women and men aged 40–80 y: prevalence and correlates identified in the Global Study of Sexual Attitudes and Behaviors. International Journal of Impotence Research 17(1): 39–57.

33. Butler RN, Lewis MI (1996) Alte Liebe rostet nicht. Über den Umgang mit Sexualität im Alter. Bern: Hans Huber.

34. Fooken I (2006) Sexualität und Partnerschaft. In: Oswald WD, Lehr U, Sieber C, Kornhuber J, editors. Gerontologie. Medizinische, psychologische und sozialwissenschaftliche Grundbegriffe. Stuttgart: Kohlhammer. pp. 328–332.

35. Waite L, Das A (2010) Families, social life, and well-being at older ages. Demography 47(1): 87–109.

36. Laumann EO, Paik A, Glasser DB, Kang JH, Wang T, et al. (2006) A cross-national study of subjective sexual well-being among older men and women: Findings from the Global Study of Sexual Attitudes and Sexual Behaviors. Archives of Sexual Behavior 35: 145–161.

37. DeLamater J, Moorman SM (2007) Sexual behaviour in later life. Journal of Aging and Health 19: 921–945.

38. Hyde Z, Flicker L, Hankey GJ, Almeida OP, McCaul KA, et al. (2010) Prevalence of sexual activity and associated factors in men aged 75 to 95 years: a cohort study. Annals of Internal Medicine 153: 693–702.

39. Harper JM, Sandberg JG (2009) Depression and communication processes in later life marriages. Aging & Mental Health 13(4): 546–556.

40. Henry NJ, Berg CA, Smith TW, Florsheim P (2007) Positive and negative characteristics of marital interaction and their association with marital satisfaction in middle-aged and older couples. Psychology and Aging 22(3): 428.

41. Carstensen LL, Gottman JM, Levenson RW (1995) Emotional behavior in long-term marriage. Psychology and Aging 10(1): 140.

42. Carstensen LL, Fung HH, Charles ST (2003) Socioemotional selectivity theory and the regulation of emotion in the second half of life. Motivation and Emotion 27(2): 103–123.

43. Walker R, Isherwood L, Burton C, Kitwe-Magambo K, Luszcz M (2013) Marital Satisfaction among Older Couples: The Role of Satisfaction with Social Networks and Psychological Well-Being. The International Journal of Aging and Human Development 76(2): 123–139.

15

Potentially Inappropriate Medication Use in Older Patients in Swiss Managed Care Plans: Prevalence, Determinants and Association with Hospitalization

Oliver Reich[1]*, Thomas Rosemann[2], Roland Rapold[1], Eva Blozik[3], Oliver Senn[2]

1 Department of Health Sciences, Helsana Group, Zurich, Switzerland, **2** Institute of General Practice and Health Services Research, University Hospital, Zurich, Switzerland, **3** Department of Primary Medical Care, University Medical Center Hamburg-Eppendorf, Hamburg, Germany

Abstract

Objectives: To describe the prevalence and determinants of potentially inappropriate medication (PIM) use and association with hospitalizations in an elderly managed care population in Switzerland.

Methods: Using health care claims data of four health insurers for a sample of managed care patients 65 years of age and older to compare persons on PIM with persons not on PIM. Beers' 2012 and PRISCUS criteria were used to determine the potential inappropriateness of prescribed medications. The sample included 16'490 elderly patients on PIM and 33'178 patients not on PIM in the time period of January 1, 2008 through December 31, 2012. Prevalence estimates are standardized to the population of Switzerland. Associations between PIM and hospitalizations were examined by multivariate Cox regression analyses controlling for possible confounding variables.

Results: The estimated prevalence of PIM use in our managed care sample was 22.5%. Logistic regression analysis showed that number of different medications used in the previous year, total costs in the previous year and hospitalization in the previous year all significantly increased the likelihood of receiving PIM. Multiple Cox regression analysis revealed that those on cumulative levels of PIM use acted significantly as a factor related to greater hospitalization rates: the adjusted HR was 1.13 (95% CI 1.07–1.19) for 1 PIM, 1.27 (95% CI 1.19–1.35) for 2 PIM, 1.35 (95% CI 1.22–1.50) for 3 PIM, and 1.63 (95% CI 1.40–1.90) for more than 3 PIM compared to no PIM use.

Conclusions: The prevalence of PIM in managed care health plans are widely found but seem to be much lower than rates of non-managed care plans. Furthermore, our study revealed a significant association with adverse outcomes in terms of hospitalizations. These findings stress the need for further development of interventions to decrease drug-related problems and manage patients with multiple chronic conditions.

Editor: Terence J. Quinn, University of Glasgow, United Kingdom

Funding: This work was supported by an unconditional grant from the Swiss Academy of Medical Sciences (SAMS), Basel, Switzerland. The funders had no role in study design, data collection and analysis, decision to publish, or preparation of the manuscript.

Competing Interests: The authors have declared that no competing interests exist.

* Email: oliver.reich@helsana.ch

Background

Prescribing potentially inappropriate medications (PIM) can lead to adverse drug events (ADE), significant morbidity and mortality, and may increase health care expenditures [1–5].

The elderly are at particular risk for inappropriate drug prescription. Many of the older persons suffer from chronic conditions that necessitate the use of multiple drugs [6]. In particular, the use of multiple medication increases the risk of prescribing PIM for elderly [7–9]. The physiologic changes in pharmacokinetics and pharmacodynamics in old age go together with polypharmacy and PIM and contribute to a higher risk of ADEs [10]. In Switzerland, people of 65 years of age or older account for 17.2% of the total population and it is estimated that this percentage will increase to 24% by 2030 [11]. Hence, the prevention and recognition of drug-related problems in the elderly represents an area of concern in the delivery of medical care and will be a principal challenge in clinical practice in the upcoming years.

A number of studies of the elderly in various settings have presented data indicating potentially inappropriate drug prescribing, with prevalences of up to 28% in community-dwelling elderly and up to 40% in nursing home residents, and have shown that a large proportion of hospital admissions and mortality are a result of ADEs [12 21]. A high prevalence of potentially inadequate medication (PIM) use in the community-dwelling older population in Switzerland has been recently reported [22]. Little is known about medication-related problems in a managed care setting. There are only a few studies, which used different approaches to estimate the prevalence or association of PIM on different outcomes in managed care populations in the U.S. [4,23–25]. However, the prevalence and determinants of potentially inappropriate medication use and the impact of these on various adverse outcomes in the elderly managed care population have not been previously evaluated in Switzerland. In 2014 nearly 58% of the Swiss population were enrolled in managed care models illustrating the increasing significance of integrated health provision in Switzerland [26]. Social health insurance is compulsory for the population in Switzerland. Basic insurance allows the insured person the freedom of choice of doctors in the outpatient sector and unlimited access to physicians. Alternative forms of insurance exist with the option of restrained choice of medical providers granting policyholders discounts on the basic premium if they agree to sign up to managed care models and only consult certain providers. Reich et al. have described the main forms of managed care models found in Switzerland in detail [27].

This study used population-based claims data to evaluate prescribing for older adults in managed care health plans and defined potentially inappropriate medications using the updated 2012 Beers criteria [28] and the PRISCUS list [29]. The objectives of this study were to determine the prevalence and determinants of PIM use and the hospitalizations associated with incident PIM use in older patients in managed care health plans in Switzerland.

Methods

Study design, sample and data source

The database of this study included health care claims data from four statutory health and accident insurance companies in Switzerland (Helsana Group) during a 5-year study period, from January 1, 2008, until December 31, 2012. The study population was extracted from a dataset of circa 1.2 million persons (year 2012) with mandatory health insurance across Switzerland, which provides an approximate representativeness to the general population (proportion of 15 percent of 8.04 million inhabitants). All health care invoices submitted to Helsana for reimbursement were considered. Since the recorded insurance claims cover almost all health care invoices, these data are highly reliable. We estimate that 2–3% of all claims invoices are paid directly by the patient (e.g. due to high deductibles chosen) and not reimbursed by the health insurer. We conducted a retrospective claims data analysis, identifying 239,075 community-dwelling individuals age 65 and older (Switzerland: 1.31 million elderly). All elderly persons (49,668 individuals) enrolled in a managed care plan at individual incident PIM date during the study period were finally included in our study. We built our PIM definition on preliminary work performed [22] and used the updated Beers criteria [28] and the PRISCUS list [29] to identify and measure PIM use. Each drug prescription provided a unique identifier for the individual as an incident PIM date. In order to focus our analysis on incident PIM use, individuals who received any PIM prescription medication in the year before their individual incident PIM date were excluded from the sample.

Statistical analysis

The prevalence rates of PIM use in the community-dwelling elderly population were calculated per age group. This was done for the Beers criteria and the PRISCUS list separately and in combination. All rates were adjusted for differences between the Helsana sample and the Swiss general population using census data from the Swiss Federal Office of Statistics [30]. In order to compare our rates in a managed care population with prior research findings (in the general population), we applied the PRISCUS list and actual Beers criteria as well as the old Beers definition to our prevalence rates [31]. Furthermore, the Beers criteria is the most widely used internationally and the PRISCUS list for the northern neighbor Germany to assess medication

therapy adequacy in the elderly [20]. Other and newer geriatric PIM criteria have been devised and validated such as the STOPP/START criteria [32]. The STOPP/START criteria, however, requires clinical information on diagnosis (e.g. chronic obstructive pulmonary disease, glaucoma), which is unfortunately not available in our claims data and therefore cannot be applied in this study.

We calculated descriptive statistics to illustrate characteristics of the study population by comparing persons on PIM with persons not on PIM. Differences between the two groups were assessed by the two-sample Wilcoxon-test and chi-squared test. Concurrent PIM use was defined as number of PIM prescriptions within individual incidence year. To control for differences in health status among the sample we considered pharmacy based cost groups (PCG) [33]. PCGs are widely used to control for confounding by chronic diseases when clinical diagnosis information is lacking [34–36]. We entered the number of different chronic diseases per individual into the analyses as a numerical variable.

Logistic regression analysis was performed to identify the determinants for PIM exposure, where PIM usage (0 or 1) was the dependent variable and the independent variables included age, gender, deductible chosen, number of different drugs taken, number of chronic diseases, total costs in the previous year and acute hospital admission in the previous year.

In addition, for the analysis of the time until the occurrence of an adverse event (all-cause acute hospital admissions within 1 year of individual incident prescription in days after initial PIM prescription), we used hazard ratios (HR) as effect measures and their 95% confidence intervals (CIs), calculated by means of Cox proportional hazards regression models. We applied a multivariate Cox regression model to adjust for morbidity and other potential confounders. Possible interactions between covariates (e.g. number of concurrent PIM use*number of different medication previous year; number of concurrent PIM use*number of different chronic conditions) were assessed. Including these interactions resulted in increased hazard ratios for the main effects of PIM exposure. The interaction term was marginally below 1, accounting for a reduction of the effect of concurrent PIM in combination with the other interaction variable. This first increase in the estimates with subsequent reduction due to interactions are much more cumbersome to interpret with no effect on the conclusion. Therefore we decided to use the reported model without interaction variables. A two-sided p-value <0.05 was considered significant. All statistical analyses performed using R, version 2.14.2.

Ethics

In compliance with the Swiss Federal Law on data protection, all data were anonymized and de-identified to protect the privacy of patients, physicians, and hospitals. Because the data were retrospective, pre-existing, and de-identified, this study was exempted from ethics committee approval.

Results

Based on reimbursement data and adjusted for differences between Helsana enrollees and the total population in Switzerland in terms of age, gender, and canton of residence, 22.5% of the community-dwelling population aged more than 65 years in managed care models received at least one medication which is potentially inappropriate according to the updated 2012 Beers criteria or PRISCUS list. Figure 1 shows the proportion of individuals per age group and gender who were prescribed a PIM.

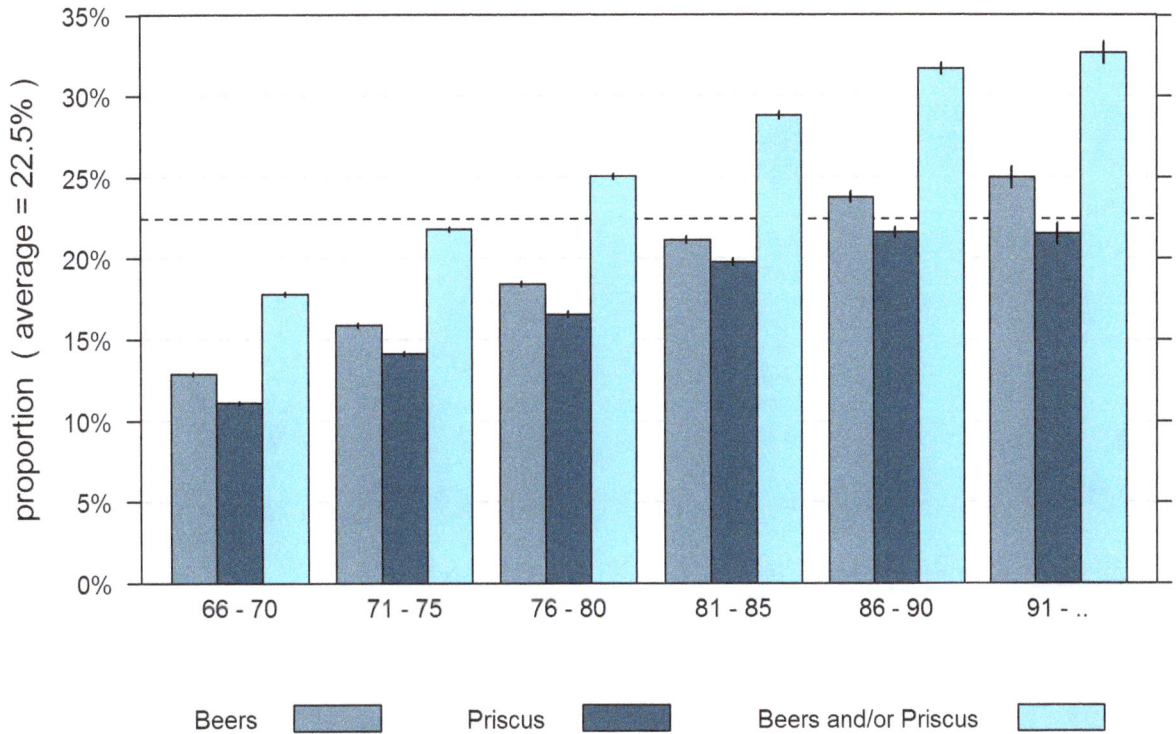

Figure 1. Proportion of persons in managed care models aged more than 65 years receiving PIM with 95 % confidence interval; years 2008-2012 (standardised for Swiss population); new Beers criteria.

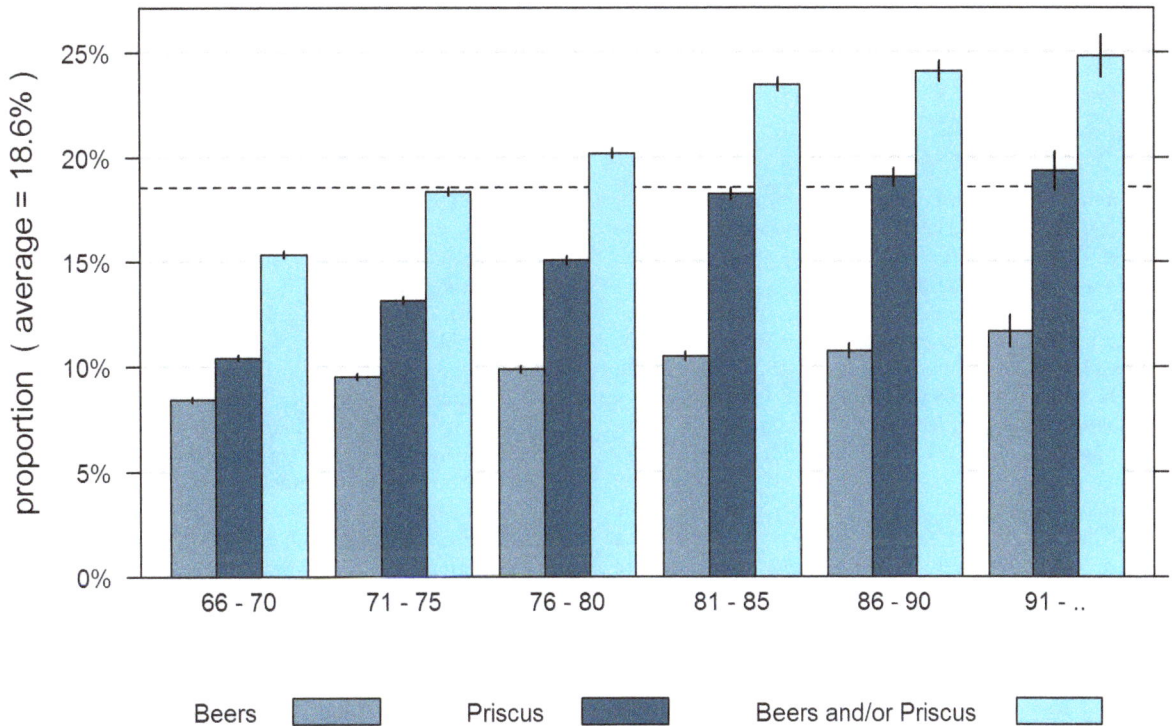

Figure 2. Proportion of persons in managed care models aged more than 65 years receiving PIM with 95% confidence interval; years 2008–2010 (standardised for Swiss population); old Beers criteria.

Table 1. Characteristics and hospitalizations in elderly Swiss managed care patients with potentially inappropriate medication (PIM) use versus non-PIM use, years 2008–2012.

Variables	PIM use (n = 16'490)	Non-PIM use (n = 33'178)	Total (n = 49'668)	p-Value[a]
Gender [no. (%)]				<0.001
Female	7'798 (47.3%)	14'449 (43.5%)	22'247 (44.8%)	
Male	8'692 (52.7%	18'729 (56.5%)	27'421 (55.2%)	
Age [mean ±SD]	74.3 (6.3)	74.8 (6.6)	74.6 (6.5)	<0.001
Deductible [no. (%)]				<0.001
Low (CHF 300, 500)	14'120 (85.6%)	27'786 (83.7%)	41'906 (84.4%)	
High (>CHF 500)	2'370 (14.4%)	5'392 (16.3%)	7'762 (15.6%)	
No. of different medication used [mean ±SD]	11.8 (7.1)	9.2 (7.8)	10.1 (7.7)	<0.001
No. of chronic diseases [mean ±SD]	3.5 (1.8)	2.9 (2.2)	3.1 (2.1)	<0.001
Total costs previous year [mean, median, ±SD]	5'736; 2'972 (9'162)	5'540; 2'673 (9'264)	5'605; 2'779 (9'231)	<0.001
Hospitalization previous year [no. (%)]	3'572 (21.7%)	5'687 (17.1%)	9'259 (18.6%)	0.787
≤2 days	1'153 (7.0%)	1'786 (5.4%)	2'939 (5.9%)	
>2 days	2'772 (16.8%)	4'422 (13.3%)	7'194 (14.5%)	
No. of concurrent PIM (within incidence year) [no. (%)]				<0.001
0	0 (0%)	33'178 (100%)	33'178 (66.8%)	
1	11'004 (66.7%)	0 (0%)	11'004 (22.2%)	
2	3'964 (24.0%)	0 (0%)	3'964 (8.0%)	
3	1'109 (6.7%)	0 (0%)	1'109 (2.2%)	
>3	413 (2.5%)	0 (0%)	413 (0.8%)	
Hospitalizations within 1 year[no. (%)]	4'211 (25.5%)	6'216 (18.7%)	10'427 (21.0%)	<0.001

[a]Two-sample Wilcoxon-tests for age, no. of different medication used, no. of chronic diseases, total costs previous year; ×2-tests for comparing difference between the two groups PIM use and Non-PIM use.

The effect of the revised Beers criteria on the prevalence of PIM is depicted in figure 2 showing a lower overall prevalence of PIM use of 18.6% in this standardized managed care plan population according to the 2003 Beers criteria.

Descriptive statistics for the incident PIM cases are displayed in table 1. The number of managed care insured who were newly prescribed a PIM during the study period was 16,490. Significant differences between those prescribed and those not prescribed a PIM were found for sex, age, deductible class, number of different medication used, number of chronic conditions, total costs previous year, and number of concurrent PIM. However, the variable hospitalization in the previous year was not found to be related to be different between the two groups (p = 0.787). During the study period, the observed overall incidence of adverse outcome as in hospitalizations was 21% for the whole study population. The rate for individuals in the PIM-group was 25.5% compared with 18.7% in the Non-PIM use group (p<0.001).

Applying multivariate logistic regression analysis, the factors that exhibited significant associations with PIM prescriptions included the following (table 2): age 81–85 years (OR 0.86; 95% CI 0.78–0.94), age 86–90 years (OR 0.68; 95% CI 0.60–0.78), age 91+ years (OR 0.73; 95% CI 0.57–0.93), 1–4 different medication used previous year (OR 1.82; 95% CI 1.53–2.15), 5–10 different medication used previous year (OR 2.14; 95% CI 1.76–2.59), 11–20 different medication used previous year (OR 1.94; 95% CI 1.57–2.39), number of chronic diseases (OR 0.34–0.86), total costs previous year (OR 1.99–2.71) and hospitalization previous year (OR 1.5; 95% CI 1.35–1.67). However, the variables of gender and deductible class lost their significance in this analysis.

Table 3 presents the proportional hazard model for hospitalization within one year after incident PIM use. The analysis revealed that potentially inappropriate medication use was significantly associated with hospitalization. The adjusted hazard ratios (HR) for those on cumulative levels of PIM use were: 1.13 (95% CI 1.07–1.19) for 1 PIM, 1.27 (95% CI 1.19–1.35) for 2 PIM, 1.35 (95% CI 1.22–1.50) for 3 PIM, and 1.63 (95% CI 1.40–1.90) for more than 3 PIM compared to no PIM use. Increasing age, as well as polypharmacy and having high costs in the previous year increased the hazard ratio, whereas females and the variable high deductible class had a decreased HR for hospitalization. The variables number of chronic disease and hospitalization in the previous year had no significant association with hospitalization. In addition, figure 3 displays a Kaplan-Meier curve comparing persons receiving PIM and time to first hospitalization and persons without PIM-prescription and time to first hospitalization.

Table 2. Results of multivariate logistic regression analysis of determinants for PIM exposure in elderly managed care patients in Switzerland, years 2008–2012.

Independent variables	Odds ratio	95% CI	p-Value
Gender			
Male			
Female	0.95	0.90–1.01	0.092
Age			
...65–70 years	1.00 (reference)		
...71–75 years	0.95	0.88–1.02	0.180
...76–80 years	1.01	0.93–1.10	0.745
...81–85 years	0.86	0.78–0.94	0.002 **
...86–90 years	0.68	0.60–0.78	0.000 ***
...91+ years	0.73	0.57–0.93	0.012 *
Deductible			
Low (CHF 300, 500)	1.00 (reference)		
High (>CHF 500)	1.02	0.94–1.11	0.656
No. of different medication used previous year			
None	1.00 (reference)		
...1–4	1.82	1.53–2.15	0.000 ***
5–10	2.14	1.76–2.59	0.000 ***
11–20	1.94	1.57–2.39	0.000 ***
21+	1.04	0.81–1.33	0.778
No. of chronic diseases			
None	1.00 (reference)		
1	0.86	0.74–0.98	0.030 *
2	0.76	0.66–0.88	0.000 ***
3	0.71	0.61–0.83	0.000 ***
4–6	0.54	0.46–0.63	0.000 ***
7+	0.34	0.27–0.42	0.000 ***
Total costs previous year			
None	1.00 (reference)		
Group 1	1.99	1.73–2.28	0.000 ***
Group 2	2.54	2.18–2.95	0.000 ***
Group 3	2.36	2.02–2.76	0.000 ***
Group 4	2.71	2.31–3.19	0.000 ***
Group 5	2.57	2.18–3.03	0.000 ***
Group 6	2.59	2.17–3.09	0.000 ***
Group 7	2.24	1.86–2.71	0.000 ***
Group 8	2.31	1.87–2.85	0.000 ***
Group 9	2.30	1.81–2.92	0.000 ***
Hospitalization previous year			
No	1.00 (reference)		
Yes	1.50	1.35–1.67	0.000 ***

Discussion

Our study revealed a standardised PIM prevalence rate of 22.5% in elderly managed care patients according to the updated Beers criteria and PRISCUS list. This finding is in concordance with earlier studies with a large proportion of the non-managed care population with inappropriate medications [37–40]. For example, Blozik et al. [22] reported a high prevalence of PIM use

of 21.1% for the community-dwelling elderly residents in Switzerland recently. The PIM criteria adopted in this mentioned study is however different to our research and the interpretation of the results have to be done with caution. Siebert et al. compared the application of selected PIM criteria in clinical routine and found the PRISCUS list was less sensitive than the application of STOPP criteria [41]. Bearing this in mind, our finding is therefore most probably underestimated and this suggests a much higher

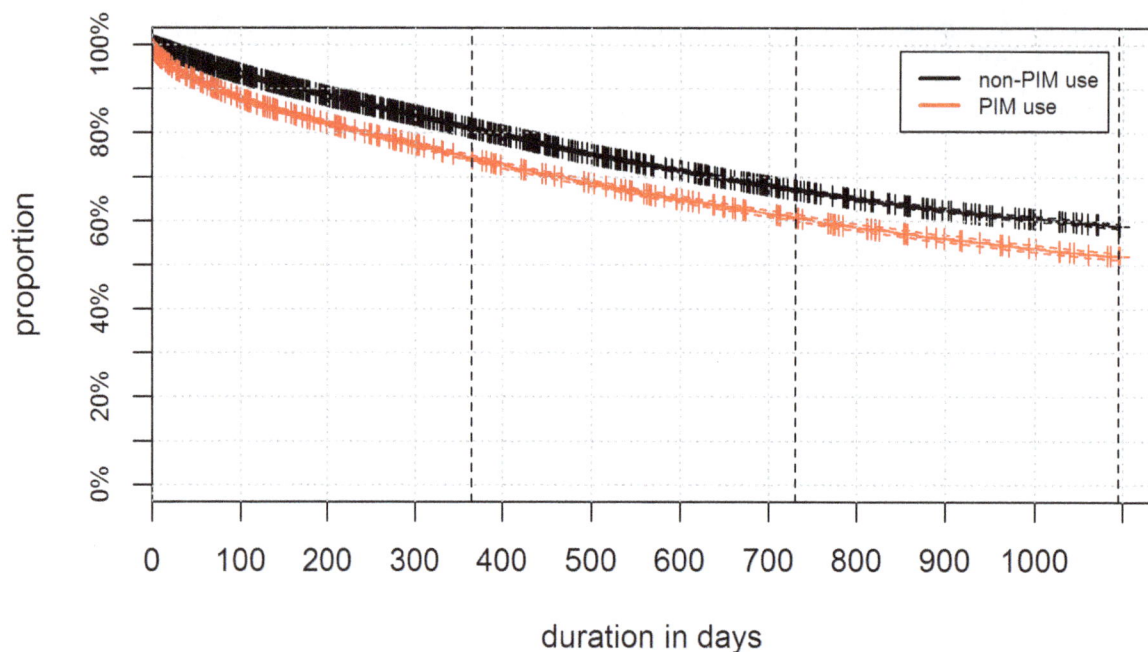

Figure 3. Kaplan-Meier curve comparing persons in managed care models aged more than 65 years receiving PIM and time to first hospitalization and persons without PIM-prescription and time to first hospitalization in Switzerland, years 2008–2012.

rate of prescription of PIM. The Swiss study of Blozik et al. used the 2003 Beers criteria to determine the overall prevalence rate, whereas our study is based on the updated 2012 Beers criteria. In the course of updating the Beers list, three additional medications have been included (glyburide, megestrol, and sliding-scale insulin) and, as the mentioned authors already assumed in their paper, this enhancement would lead to higher PIM prevalence rates. In order to be able to compare the two prevalence rates correctly, we applied the old Beers definition to our managed care sample and found a prevalence rate for PIM of 18.6%, which is significantly lower to the rate reported by Blozik et al.. It seems there does appear to be some greater risk awareness in prescribing potentially inappropriate medications in managed care plans compared to the general fee-for-service delivery models in Switzerland. Moreover, the significantly lower PIM prevalence rate might be due to the fact that managed care systems allow for improving care coordination. Previous research reveals the importance of care coordination [42] and indicates the great potential for continuous cost containment by applying managed care models [27]. However, prevalence rates from other study results (based on older or different PIM definitions and with much smaller patient samples) also examining persons in managed care plans in the United States are significantly higher than our rate (24.2–29%) [23–25], revealing the general difficulty of international comparisons in the different health care settings.

In our study, it appears that the probability of patients receiving potentially inappropriate medication is significantly associated with polypharmacy, total costs in the previous year and hospitalization in the previous year. Moreover, the multivariate analysis indicates that older persons and the persons with chronic diseases possess a lower probability for PIM exposure. Our study is supported by previous studies that have found that especially polypharmacy and female sex are important determinants for an increased likelihood of receiving a PIM prescription [38,43–45]. In contrast to our study, however, Lin et al. [37] found a significant association between two further risk factors, advanced age and

number of chronic diseases, and the likelihood of receiving inappropriate medications. An explanation for this may be the fact that their study was based on the inclusion of only elderly patients with a chronic disease who received long-term (3-month) prescriptions and using the Beers' 2002 criteria, thus, making it difficult to make a proper comparison. We suggest that within the Swiss managed care setting, physicians might be more cautious about avoiding PIM for older elders with chronic diseases and might put more emphasis on what to prescribe and on coordinating the respective medication for the treatment of the chronic diseases. Based on our findings and in line with previous research conducted [46–47], it seems to be important to reduce the number of medications prescribed in order to improve the safety of medication use in elderly managed care patients.

The last study objective was to examine the harmful impact of PIM exposure in the managed care population, since little evidence exists regarding adverse events such as hospitalizations. Therefore, all-cause acute hospital admissions within 1 year of individual incident prescription (in days after initial PIM prescription) was used as outcome, controlling for morbidity and other possible confounders. There was significant and increasing association between the number of concurrent PIM use and hospitalizations. Those on a PIM had significantly higher risk of a hospitalization than those not on an inappropriate medication. This result is consistent with findings from other studies [5,37,39,48–52]. Several other factors such as advanced age, high number of different medications and total costs in the previous year were also found to be associated with more frequent hospitalizations. Additional research is necessary to prove causation and the results of this study cannot assess the appropriateness of drug prescribing. Nevertheless, focusing on the identification of PIM use can play an important role in risk management improvement efforts within the medical practice.

This study is one of few investigating the outcome of hospitalizations of PIM use in an older managed care population, and to our knowledge the only national study to provide a

Table 3. Results of Cox regression analysis for determinants and adverse outcome hospitalization in elderly managed care patients in Switzerland, years 2008–2012.

Independent variables	Hospitalization		
	Hazard ratio	95% CI	p-Value
No of concurrent PIM use			
0	1.00 (reference)		
1	1.13	1.07–1.19	0.000 ***
2	1.27	1.19–1.35	0.000 ***
3	1.35	1.22–1.50	0.000 ***
>3	1.63	1.40–1.90	0.000 ***
Gender			
Male	1.00 (reference)		
Female	0.89	0.85–0.93	0.000 ***
Age			
...65–70 years	1.00 (reference)		
...71–75 years	1.09	1.03–1.16	0.004 **
...76–80 years	1.21	1.13–1.28	0.000 ***
...81–85 years	1.34	1.25–1.43	0.000 ***
...86–90 years	1.50	1.37–1.64	0.000 ***
...91+ years	1.68	1.44–1.96	0.000 ***
Deductible			
Low (CHF 300, 500)	1.00 (reference)		
High (>CHF 500)	0.91	0.85–0.98	0.013 *
No. of different medication used			
previous year			
None	1.00 (reference)		
...1–4	1.15	0.98–1.35	0.083
5–10	1.24	1.04–1.48	0.018 *
11–20	1.42	1.18–1.70	0.000 ***
21+	1.56	1.27–1.91	0.000 ***
No. of chronic diseases			
None	1.00 (reference)		
1	0.94	0.83–1.05	0.267
2	0.97	0.86–1.09	0.563
3	0.91	0.80–1.03	0.137
4–6	1.00	0.89–1.14	0.955
7+	1.10	0.94–1.29	0.225
Total costs previous year			
...None	1.00 (reference)		
Group 1	1.23	1.08–1.41	0.003 **
Group 2	1.40	1.22–1.61	0.000 ***
Group 3	1.43	1.24–1.65	0.000 ***
Group 4	1.43	1.24–1.66	0.000 ***
Group 5	1.56	1.35–1.81	0.000 ***
Group 6	1.75	1.50–2.03	0.000 ***
Group 7	1.83	1.56–2.13	0.000 ***
Group 8	1.88	1.60–2.22	0.000 ***
Group 9	1.88	1.57–2.25	0.000 ***
Hospitalization previous year			
No	1.00 (reference)		
Yes	1.01	0.94–1.08	0.778

comprehensive overview about the situation of PIM prevalence in this specific health plan type in Switzerland. Although our data set is extremely broad and comprehensive, there are a number of limitations that influence the conclusions that can be drawn. First, our study was limited to a managed care population that may not be generalizable to other populations. Second, detailed clinical information on the patients were not available. However, drug-based diagnoses are a valid proxy for medical diagnoses and widely used in epidemiological and outcomes research to control for various chronic conditions. Third, using information from claims data restricted our ability to guarantee that the medications were genuinely taken by the individual patient and not dispensed in the garbage for example. Lastly, the information in our claims data may be slightly underrepresented as about 3% of the used claims invoices were paid directly by the patients and not by the health insurer.

In conclusion, the prevalence of PIM use is substantially lower in Swiss managed care populations compared to the general fee-for-service health delivery, which could signify better performance in drug prescription. The probability of harmful outcome as in hospitalizations occurring in patients with PIM exposure was much higher than in those not receiving PIM.

Our research suggests that managed health care plans in Switzerland offer a powerful model for improving medication prescriptions. These plans have found a way to engage the right set of physicians around the objective of delivering optimal and coordinated health care. Coordinated care helps ensure that patients, especially the chronically ill, get the right care at the right time, with the goal of avoiding unnecessary duplication of services and preventing adverse outcomes. Our research demonstrates that managed care plans potentially deliver more appropriate poly-pharmacy care than uncoordinated medicine and thus do a better job of improving health care value.

Author Contributions

Conceived and designed the experiments: OR TR OS. Performed the experiments: RR. Analyzed the data: RR OR. Contributed reagents/materials/analysis tools: EB OR RR. Wrote the paper: OR TR OS.

References

1. Fick DM, Mion LC, Beers MH, Waller JL (2008) Health outcomes associated with potentially inappropriate medication use in older adults. Res Nurs Health 31(1): 42–51.
2. Zuckerman IH, Langenberg P, Baumgarten M (2006) Inappropriate drug use and risk of transition to nursing homes among community dwelling older adults. Med Care 44(8): 722–730.
3. Fu AZ, Jian JZ, Reeves JH, Fincham JE, Liu GG, et al. (2007) Potentially inappropriate medication use and healthcare expenditures in the US community-dwelling elderly. Med Care 45(5): 472–476.
4. Stockl KM, Le L, Zhang S, Harada ASM (2010) Clinical and Economic Outcomes Associated With Potentially Inappropriate Prescribing in the Elderly. Am J Manag Care 16(1): e1–e10.
5. Jano E, Aparasu RR (2007) Healthcare Outcomes Associated with Beers' Criteria: A Systematic Review. Ann Pharmacoth 41(3): 438–447.
6. Huber CA, Schneeweiss S, Signorell A, Reich O (2013) Improved prediction of medical expenditures and health care utilization using an updated chronic disease score and claims data. J Clin Epidemiol 66(10): 1118–1127.
7. Cannon KT, Choi MM, Zuniga MA (2006) Potentially inappropriate medication use in elderly patients receiving home health care: a retrospective data analysis. Am J Geriatr Pharmacother 4(2): 134–143.
8. Tamura BK, Bell CL, Inaba M, Masaki KH (2012) Outcomes of polypharmacy in nursing home residents. Clin Geriatr Med 28(2): 217–236.
9. Hilmer SN, Gnjidic D (2009) The effects of polypharmacy in older adults. Clin Pharmacol Ther 85(1): 86–88.
10. McLean AJ, Le Couteur DG (2004) Aging Biology and Geriatric Clinical Pharmacology. Pharmacol Rev 56(2): 163–184.
11. Federal Statistical Office (2010) Szenarien zur Bevölkerungsentwicklung der Schweiz 2010–2060. Neuchâtel: Federal Statistical Office. 27 p.
12. Barry PJ, Gallagher P, Ryan C (2008) Inappropriate prescribing in geriatric patients. Curr Psychiatry Rep 10: 37–43.
13. Rothberg MB, Pekow PS, Liu F, Korc-Grodzicki B, Brennan MJ, et al. (2008) Potentially inappropriate medication use in hospitalized elders. J Hosp Med 3: 91–102.
14. Aparasu RR, Mort JR (2000) Inappropriate prescribing for the elderly: Beers criteria-based review. Ann Pharmacother 34: 338–346.
15. Giron MST, Wang HX, Bernsten C (2001) The appropriateness of drug use in an older nondemented and demented population. J Am Geriatr Soc 49 (3): 277–283.
16. Hanlon JT, Schmader KE, Coult C (2002) Use of inappropriate prescription drugs by older people. J Am Geriatr Soc 50(1): 26–34.
17. Liu GG, Christensen DB (2002) The continuing challenge of inappropriate prescribing in the elderly: an update of the evidence. J Am Pharm Assoc 42(6): 847–857.
18. Cahir C, Fahey T, Teeling M, Teljeur C, Feely J, et al. (2010) Potentially inappropriate prescribing and cost outcomes for older people: a national population study. Br J Clin Pharmacol 69: 543–552.
19. Tragni E, Casula M, Pieri V, Favato G, Marcobelli A, et al. (2013) Prevalence of the Prescription of Potentially Interacting Drugs. PLoS ONE 8(10): e78827. doi:10.1371/journal.pone.0078827.
20. Sichieri K, Baldacin Rodrigues AR, Takahashi JA, Secoli SR, Cuce Nobre MR, et al. (2013) Mortality Associated with the Use of Inappropriate Drugs According Beers Criteria: a Systematic Review. Adv Pharmacol Pharm 1: 74–84.
21. Galvin R, Moriarty F, Cousins G, Cahir C, Motterlini N, et al. (2014) Prevalence of potentially inappropriate prescribing and prescribing omissions in older Irish adults: findings from The Irish Longitudinal Study on Ageing study (TILDA). Eur J Clin Pharmacol 70(5): 599–606.
22. Blozik E, Rapold R, von Overbeck J, Reich O (2013) Polypharmacy and potentially inappropriate medication in the adult, community-dwelling population in Switzerland. Drugs Aging 30(7): 561–568.
23. Fick DM, Waller JL, Maclean JR (2001) Potentially inappropriate medication use in a Medicare managed care population: association with higher costs and utilization. J Manag Care Pharmacy (5)7: 407–413.
24. Simon SR, Chan KA, Soumerai SB, Wagner AK, Andrade SE, et al. (2005) Potentially inappropriate medication use by elderly persons in U.S. Health Maintenance Organizations, 2000–2001. J Am Geriatr Soc 53(2): 227–232.
25. Barnett MJ, Perry PJ, Langstaff JD, Kaboli PJ (2006) Comparison of Rates of Potentially Inappropriate Medication Use According to the Zhan Criteria for VA Versus Private Sector Medicare HMOs. J Managed Care Pharm 12(5): 362–370.
26. Federal Office of Public Health FOPH (2013) Statistik der obligatorischen Krankenversicherung 2012 [Statistics of compulsory health insurance 2012]. Berne: Federal Office of Public Health; [cited 2014 Feb 17]. Available from: http://www.bag.admin.ch/themen/krankenversicherung/01156/index.html?lang=de[in German].
27. Reich O, Rapold R, Flatscher-Thöni M (2012) An empirical investigation of the efficiency effects of integrated care models in Switzerland. Int J Integr Care 12:e2.
28. American Geriatrics Society 2012 Beers Criteria Update Expert Panel (2012) American Geriatrics Society updated Beers Criteria for potentially inappropriate medication use in older adults. J Am Geriatr Soc 60(4): 616–631.
29. Holt S, Schmiedl S, Thurmann PA (2010) Potentially inappropriate medications in the elderly: the PRISCUS list. Dtsch Arztebl Int. 107(31–32): 543–551.
30. Swiss Federal Office of Statistics SFOS (2013) Ständige Wohnbevölkerung nach Geschlecht und Staatsangehörigkeitskategorie, am Ende des Jahres 2000–2013 [Population size and population composition at the end of the year 2000–2013]. Berne: Swiss Federal Office of Statistics. [cited 2013 Nov 29]. Available from: http://www.bfs.admin.ch/bfs/portal/de/index/themen/01/02/blank/key/bevoelkerungsstand/02.html [in German].
31. Fick DM, Cooper JW, Wade WE, Waller JL, et al. (2003) Updating the Beers criteria for potentially inappropriate medication use in older adults: results of a US consensus panel of experts. Arch Intern Med. 163(22): 2716–2724.
32. O'Mahony D, Gallagher P, Ryan C, Byrne S, Hamilton H, et al. (2010) STOPP & START criteria: A new approach to detecting potentially inappropriate prescribing in old age. Eur Geriatr Med 1: 45–51.
33. Huber C, Szucs TD, Rapold R, Reich O (2013) Identifying patients with chronic conditions using pharmacy data in Switzerland: an updated mapping approach to the classification of medications. BMC Public Health 13: 1030.
34. Cossman RE, Cossman JS, James WL, Blanchard T, Thomas R, et al. (2010) Correlating pharmaceutical data with a national health survey as a proxy for estimating rural population health. Popul Health Metr 8: 25.
35. O'Shea M, Teeling M, Bennett K (2013) The prevalence and ingredient cost of chronic comorbidity in the Irish elderly population with medication treated type 2 diabetes: a retrospective cross-sectional study using a national pharmacy claims database. BMC Health Serv Res 13: 23.

36. Chini F, Pezzotti P, Orzella L, Borgia P, Guasticchi G (2011) Can we use the pharmacy data to estimate the prevalence of chronic conditions? a comparison of multiple data sources. BMC Public Health 11: 688.

37. Lin HY, Liao CC, Cheng SH, Wang PC, Hsueh YS (2008) Association of Potentially Inappropriate Medication Use with Adverse Outcomes in Ambulatory Elderly Patients with Chronic Diseases. Experience in a Taiwanese Medical Setting. Drugs Aging 25(1): 49–59.

38. Schubert I, Küpper-Nybelen J, Ihle P, Thürmann P (2013) Prescribing potentially inappropriate medication (PIM) in Germany's elderly as indicated by the PRISCUS list. An analysis based on regional claims data. Pharmacoepidemiol Drug Saf 22(7): 719–727.

39. Klarin I, Wimo A, Fastbom J (2005) The Association of Inappropriate Drug Use with Hospitalisation and Mortality. A Population-Based Study of the Very Old. Drugs Aging 22(1): 69–82.

40. Opondo D, Eslami E, Visscher S, de Rooij SE, Verheij R, et al. (2012) Inappropriateness of Medication Prescriptions to Elderly Patients in the Primary Care Setting: A Systematic Review. PLoS One 7(8):e43617.

41. Siebert S, Elkeles B, Hempel G, Kruse J, Smollich M (2013) Die PRISCUS-Liste im klinischen Test. Praktikabilität und Vergleich mit internationalen PIM-Listen. [The PRISCUS list in clinical routine. Practicability and comparison to international PIM lists]. Z Gerontol Geriatr 46(1): 35–47. [Article in German].

42. Bodenheimer T (2008) Coordinating care—a perilous journey through the health care system. New Engl J Med 358(10): 1064–1071.

43. Goltz L, Kullak-Ublick GA, Kirch W (2012) Potentially inappropriate prescribing for elderly oupatients in Germany: a retrospective claims data analysis. Int J Clin Pharmacol Ther 50(3): 185–194.

44. Oliveira MG, Amorim WW, de Jesus SR, Rodrigues VA, Passos LC (2012) Factors associated with potentially inappropriate medication use by the elderly in the Brazilian primary care setting. Int J Clin Pharm 34(4): 626–632.

45. Harugeri A, Joseph J, Parthasarathi G, Ramesh M, Guido S (2010) Potentially inappropriate medication use in elderly patients: a study of prevalence and predictors in two teaching hospitals. J Postgrad Med 56(3):186–191.

46. Maio V, Yuen EJ, Novielli K, Smith KD, Louis DZ (2006) Potentially inappropriate medication prescribing for elderly outpatients in Emilia Romagna, Italy: a population-based cohort study. Drugs Aging 23(11):915–924.

47. Vieira de Lima T, Garbin C, Garbin A, Sumida D, Saliba O (2013) Potentially inappropriate medications used by the elderly: Prevelence and risk factors in Brazilian care homes. BMC Geriatrics 13: 52.

48. Price SD, Holman SDJ, Sanfilippo FM, Emery JD (2014) Association Between Potentially Inappropriate Medications From the Beers Criteria and the Risk of Unplanned Hospitalization in Elderly Patients. Ann Pharmacother DOI: 10.1177/1060028013504904.

49. Ruggiero C, Dell'Aquila G, Gasperini B, Onder G, Lattanzio F, et al. (2010) Potentially Inappropriate Drug Prescriptions and Risk of Hospitalization among Older, Italian, Nursing Home Residents. The ULISSE Project. Drugs Aging 27(9): 747–758.

50. Lau DT, Kasper JD, Potter DEB, Lyles A, Bennett RG (2005) Hospitalization and Death Associated with PIM Prescription Among Elderly Nursing Home Residents. Arch Intern Med 165: 68–74.

51. Dedhiya SD, Hancock E, Craig BA, Doebbeling CC, Thomas J (2010) Incident Use and Outcomes Associated With Potentially Inappropriate Medication Use in Older Adults. Am J Geriatr Pharmacother 8(6): 562–570.

52. Albert SM, Colombi A, Hanlon J (2010) Potentially Inappropriate Medications and Risk of Hospitalization in Retirees. Drugs Aging 27(5): 407–415.

16

A Nation-Wide Study of Prevalence and Risk Factors for Fecal Impaction in Nursing Homes

Enrique Rey[1]*, Marta Barcelo[1], Maria Jose Jiménez Cebrián[2,3], Angel Alvarez-Sanchez[1], Manuel Diaz-Rubio[1], Alberto Lopez Rocha[3]

1 Division of Digestive Diseases, Hospital Clinico San Carlos, Universidad Complutense, Instituto de Investigacion Sanitaria San Carlos (IdISSC), Madrid, Spain, 2 Centro Valdeluz, Madrid, Spain, 3 Spanish Society of Nursing Homes Physicians (Sociedad Española de Medicos de Residencias – SEMER), Madrid, Spain

Abstract

Background: There are no existing studies that provide data regarding the epidemiology of, and risk factors for, fecal impaction, either in the general population or in any sub-group of people.

Objective: Estimate the prevalence of and factors associated with fecal impaction on a representative sample of the institutionalized elderly population.

Design: Two-phase study. Phase 1: pilot study validating the methodology in which all residents of a single nursing home participated. Phase 2: national multi-center cross-sectional study.

Setting: 34 randomly selected nursing homes.

Measurements: The presence of fecal impaction and associated factors were evaluated using three different tools: data collected from medical records; a self-completion questionnaire filled out by the subjects or a proxy; and a rectal examination.

Subjects: Older subjects living in nursing homes.

Results: The prevalence of chronic constipation was 70.7% (95%CI: 67.3–74.1%), of which 95.9% of patients were properly diagnosed and 43.1% were properly controlled. The prevalence of FI according to patient history was 47.3% (43.6–51.0%) and 6.6% (4.7–8.5%) according to rectal examination. Controlled constipation (OR: 9.8 [5.2–18.4]) and uncontrolled constipation (OR: 37.21 [19.7–70.1]), the number of medications (OR: 1.2 [1.1–1.3]), reduced functional capacity (OR: 0.98 [0.97–0.99]) and the occasional use of NSAIDs were independent risk factors for fecal impaction.

Conclusions: Constipation affects more than 70% of people living in nursing homes. Although it is properly diagnosed in more than 95% of cases, the disease is only controlled in less than 50%. Constipation, especially when not controlled, is the most significant risk factor leading to fecal impaction, which is prevalent in almost 50% of this population.

Editor: Antony Bayer, Cardiff University, United Kingdom

Funding: This project was funded by an unrestricted grant from Norgive Iberia. The funders has no role in study desing, data collection and analysis, decision to publish, or preparation of the manuscript.

Competing Interests: One of the authors are employed by a commercial company (Centro Valdeluz).

* Email: rey.enrique.spain@gmail.com

Background

The increase in life expectancy has led to a rise in the proportion of older people living in developed countries; in Europe, 17.1% of the population were over 65 years-old in 2008 and this is expected to rise to 23.5% in 2030 [1]. Older people require more assistance and care, which may be delivered at home, however sometimes a nursing home is necessary. In the USA, there were 17,000 nursing homes and 1.5 million residents in 2004 [2]. The need of long term care facilities has grown; according to a report from the Organisation for Economic Co-operation and Development (OECD), between 2000 and 2009 the number of beds in nursing homes grew in most countries, reaching an average of 44 per 1,000 inhabitants over 65 and this is expected to continue to grow [3].

Constipation is a condition characterized by infrequent or difficult defecation, and is one of the most common medical problems in institutionalized people. It is estimated to affect up to 80% of this population [4–6], given the multiple concurrent risk factors for constipation such as immobility, multiple medications, co-morbidity, and cognitive decline. The high prevalence of constipation in institutionalized elderly patients results in not only a reduced quality of life [7,8] and high economic burden [9–11], but it is also associated with the potentially serious complication of fecal impaction [12–14].

Table 1. Comparison between the pilot sample and the general sample.

	Pilot Sample (N = 199)	General Sample (N = 488)
Age		
≤80 years old	32 (16.1%)	130 (26.6%)
81–90 years old	113 (56.8%)	246 (50.4%)
>90 years old	54 (27.1%)	112 (23%)*
Gender [female N (%)]	144 (72.4%)	336 (68.9%)
Marital status [widow; N (%)]	127 (63.8%)	265 (56.5%)
Educational level [primary or less; N (%)]	139 (69.8%)	400 (81.9%)*
Time of stay in nursing home		
<1 year	8 (4%)	11 (2.3%)
1–10 years	76 (38.4%)	91 (18.8%)
>10 years	114 (57.6%)	382 (78.9%)*
Cognitive and Functional Status		
Functional disability (Barthel Index; score)	64.5±28.8 (0–100)	61.3±31.3 (0–100)
Cognitive impairment (Folstein Test; score)	23.0±8.4 (0–35)	22.1±8.6 (0–35)
Nutritional Status		
Body Mass Index (kg/m^2)	24.1±4.5 (14.9–43.3)	25.7±4.5 (14.7–41.5)*
Modified Ward Index (score)	5.5±5.7 (0–22)	3.6±4.9 (0–24)*
Fibre intake (g/day)	10.6±3.6 (3.9–21.9)	9.1±3.6 (2.5–24.4)*
Liquids intake (l/day)	1.5±0.3 (0.8–2.2)	1.6±0.5 (0.4–3.5)
Physical activity		
Immobility [bed-chair; N (%)]	56 (28.1%)	135 (28.7%)
Moderate or more [>60 min/day; N (%)]	31 (15.6%)	52 (12%)
Metodologic		
Needed proxy for completing [N (%)]	160 (80.4%)	384 (81.4%)
Understood every question [N (%)]	142 (71.4%)	364 (77.6%)
Co-Morbidity		
Diabetes [N (%)]	57 (28.6%)	129 (26.4%)
Thyroid disease [N (%)]	22 (11.1%)	55 (11.3%)
High blood pressure [N (%)]	132 (66.3%)	270 (55.3%)*
Cardiovascular diseases [N (%)]	100 (50.3%)	174 (35.6%)*
Respiratory diseases [N (%)]	50 (25.1%)	125 (25.6%)
Parkinson's disease [N (%)]	10 (5.0%)	36 (7.3%)
Stroke [N (%)]	37 (18.6%)	111 (23.1%)
Other Neurological diseases [N (%)]	78 (39.2%)	208 (42.6%)
Osteoarthritis [N (%)]	117 (58.8%)	302 (61.9%)
Renal/urinary disease [N (%)]	35 (17.6%)	66 (13.5%)
Depression [N (%)]	59 (29.6%)	200 (41.0%)*
Other psychiatric diseases [N (%)]	2 (1%)	44 (9.0%)*
Abdominal/abdominal wall Surgery [N (%)]	39 (19.6%)	110 (22.5%)
Number of Co-morbidities per subject	2.84±1.32 (0–7)	2.97±1.55 (0–8)
Drugs		
Antihypertensive drugs [N (%)]	147 (73.9%)	256 (52.4%)*
SSRIs [N (%)]	69 (34.7%)	176 (36.1%)
Tryciclic antidepressant drugs [N (%)]	7 (3.5%)	12 (2.5%)
Benzodiazepines [N (%)]	63 (31.7%)	130 (26.3%)
Hypolipemic drugs [N (%)]	53 (26.6%)	117 (24.0%)
PPIs [N (%)]	131 (65.8%)	277 (56.8%)
Calcium channel blockers [N (%)]	27 (13.6%)	53 (10.9%)
Nitrates [N (%)]	11 (5.5%)	48 (9.8%)
NSAIDs [N (%)]	26 (13.1%)	53 (10.9%)

Table 1. Cont.

	Pilot Sample (N = 199)	General Sample (N = 488)
ASA [N (%)]	68 (34.2%)	155 (31.8%)
Opiates [N (%)]	37 (18.6%)	25 (5.1%)*
Diuretics [N (%)]	84 (42.2%)	174 (35.6%)
Hypnotic drugs [N (%)]	52 (26.6%)	102 (20.9%)
Number of drugs per subject	4.56±2.29 (0–12)	4.02±2.20 (0–12)
Constipation		
Medical Diagnosis [N (%)]	119 (59.8%)	319 (65.4%)
Rome III Criteria [N (%)]	74 (37.2%)	183 (40.0%)
Regular laxatives		
Regular use of laxatives [N (%)]	114 (57.3%)	321 (65.8%)*
Regular use of enemas [N (%)]	4 (2.0%)	13 (2.7%)
Fecal Impaction		
Recurrent fecal impaction	62 (31.1%)	136 (27.8%)
Fecal impaction according to rectal examination	9 (4.5%)	35 (7.2%)

*p<0.05.

Although a definition of fecal impaction is elusive [15], it usually refers to the accumulation of hard feces in the rectum and colon that the subject cannot evacuate alone. There are no existing studies that provide data regarding the prevalence, incidence or risk factors for fecal impaction, either in the general population or in any subgroup of people. However, indirect data suggest that it is highly prevalent among institutionalized elderly patients, with 20% of those with fecal incontinence being diagnosed with the condition within a year [16], a prevalence of 25% in those with urinary dysfunction [17], 55% in those with diarrhea [18], and a description of stercoral ulcers (caused by fecal impaction) in autopsies of 1.3–5.7% of this population [19].

The following are considered risk factors for fecal impaction: certain medications including stimulant laxatives, immobility, neurological diseases such as Parkinson's or dementia, low fiber intake, chronic kidney failure, diabetes, or the existence of a malign neoplasm in any location [20], but there are no specific studies to support this.

The objective of this study is to estimate the prevalence of fecal impaction in a representative sample of the elderly institutionalized population, and to evaluate the risk factors associated with experiencing fecal impaction.

Materials and Methods

Design and population

The study was performed in two phases. The first phase consisted of a pilot study to validate the methodology, in which all residents of a single nursing home were invited to participate; the results of the validation have been published previously [21]. Once the first phase was complete and the methods were validated, the second phase was carried out: this was a national multi-center cross-sectional study. For the second phase, 34 nursing homes were selected at random from the SEMER (Sociedad Española de Médicos de Residencias [Spanish Society of Nursing Home Physicians]) members list, geographically proportional to the only estimation of the Spanish nursing home population [22]. For that purpose, physicians associated with the SEMER at the time of the study were classified into three geographical areas and chosen randomly by an officer (not related to SEMER) according to a prior specified geographical quota. When the physician either worked in the same nursing home of a previously selected physician, or was not reached (contact information not updated or impossibility to contact him/her directly after three calls on different days), an alternative physician was chosen in the same way.

Each nursing home physician was invited to include 25 residents in the study. Given that it was not possible to obtain lists of residents to form a purely random sample (due to national data protection laws), the residents of each nursing home were selected semi-randomly in accordance with pre-defined quotas according to the initial of the resident's surname and their year of birth (even/odd).

Ethical aspects

The study was approved by the Clinical Research Ethics Committee at Hospital Clinico San Carlos, and all of the study's participants or their legal representatives signed an informed consent document prior to their participation.

Protocol

The data gathering protocol included:

Clinical records abstraction. Clinical history (medical and nursing) data were gathered for each resident using a closed form that collected data on specific co-morbidities (detailed in Table 1), habitual or occasional use of several medications (detailed in Table 1), and the diagnosis of constipation. Specifically, data were gathered on diagnoses of fecal impaction in the last year, as well as its frequency and the treatment options used to resolve it.

Subject reported information. Each participating resident completed, with the help of a proxy if necessary, a questionnaire that included the items on abdominal and defecatory symptoms from the Rome III [23] questionnaire and on nutritional information, using the Spanish version of the Ward questionnaire [24]. For the analysis, the Ward score was modified, eliminating the item regarding the need for help with cooking, since there is a central dining room at each nursing home and none of the subjects cook for him or herself.

In addition, information was also collected on some lifestyle habits (liquid intake, fiber intake, physical exercise) with an ad-hoc questionnaire. All subjects were asked to record the average number of glasses or cups of liquid (including water, soda, soup, etc.) they drank daily during the morning, lunch, evening, dinner, and night. The daily intake of liquids was calculated as the sum of these amounts, estimating 0.2 liters per glass/cup. Fiber intake was calculated with a simplified food frequency questionnaire, including six questions referring to the usual weekly intake of fruits (1 question), vegetables (2 questions), cereals (1 question), legumes (1 question), and nuts (1 question). Answers were categorized as less than one ration weekly, 1 to 3 rations weekly, 3 to 6 rations weekly, one ration daily, and 2 or more rations daily. For the analyses, these categories were summarized as 0.5, 2, 4.5, 7 and 14 rations weekly, respectively. Total fiber intake was calculated assuming 2.5 g per ration of fruits, 3.5 g for vegetables, 1 g for cereals, 3 g for legumes and 1.5 g for nuts, and expressed as grams daily. To estimate physical activity, subjects were asked to describe their usual physical activity under one of the following items: "practice sports regularly", "walk long distances", "walk short distances (around my house)", "do not walk anywhere, or just a little bit", and classified for the analysis in three categories.

Objective measurements. All patients were evaluated in terms of functional capacity using the Barthel test [25] and cognitive capacity using the Lobo version of the Folstein mini-mental state exam [26,27]. Folstein's test is a widely used method to detect cognitive impairment. It is a questionnaire that evaluates temporal and spatial orientation, attention span, concentration and memory, capacity for abstraction (calculation), language ability, and visuospatial perception and ability to follow basic instructions. Validated Spanish Lobo's version provides a score ranging 0–35; 25 points or more indicates normal cognitive ability, 20 to 24 points a mild cognitive impairment, 15 to 19 a moderate impairment and 14 or less a severe cognitive impairment. Barthel's Index is a generic measure assessing the level of functional capacity independence) of the subjects for some basic activities of daily living, Each activity is evaluated by the physician with different prespecified scores according to the capacity of the examined subject to carry out these activities. The overall score ranges between 0 (completely dependent) to 100 points (completely independent). A score of 100 means complete functional capacity (independence), 90 to 99 good functional capacity (low dependence), 60 to 90 moderate functional capacity (moderate dependence), 20 to 60 low functional capacity (severe dependence), and 0 to 20 implies complete dependence.

In addition, the physician conducted a rectal examination (within two weeks of completion of the self-reported questionnaires), on all residents except those who did not consent to it. The physician was required to categorize the characteristics of the feces into one of the following categories: absence of feces, soft feces, non-impacted hard feces, and impacted feces. All physicians were provided with an information leaflet on the technique for carrying out a rectal examination and on the categorization to be used.

Definitions

A resident was considered to experience chronic constipation when he or she was diagnosed by the physician with constipation or, having not been diagnosed with chronic constipation in their clinical history, he or she complained of sufficient symptoms to meet the Rome III criteria for chronic constipation on the intestinal symptoms questionnaire. Constipation was further categorized as "uncontrolled constipation" when, on the Rome III intestinal symptoms questionnaire, the resident complained of sufficient symptoms to meet the Rome III criteria for chronic constipation, and as "controlled constipation" when the resident did not report sufficient symptoms to meet Rome III criteria despite having being diagnosed with constipation.

Fecal impaction was defined as the existence of a hard mass of feces in the rectum which the subject was unable expel. To estimate annual prevalence of fecal impaction we defined it as the medical diagnosis of fecal impaction as registered in the medical or nurse record of the subject in the last year, with recurring impaction being defined as a record of at least two episodes in the last year. Fecal impaction was defined on the rectal examination when the physician described the feces as hard and impacted. We applied these two definitions in the same population. Since fecal impaction is an intermittent event, the first definition was intended to estimate the annual prevalence of fecal impaction while the diagnosis through rectal examination was intended to estimate how many subjects are impacted at the same time.

Fecal incontinence was defined as the involuntary loss of liquid or solid stools occurring at least once monthly according to responses to a self-report questionnaire.

Analysis

Prevalences are reported as relative frequency accompanied by their 95% confidence interval. Quantitative variables are expressed as mean (standard deviation). Univariate analysis was used to evaluate possible risk factors associated with fecal impaction, and the factors associated with fecal impaction in that univariate analysis were subsequently included in a multivariate logistic regression (forward stepwise). Missing data were treated as missing.

Sample size

The sample size was set at 863 subjects, which allowed for the estimation of a prevalence of 10% with 2% precision.

Table 2. Association between the laxative treatment used and the constipation control level.

	N*	Controlled Constipation (N = 201)	Uncontrolled Constipation (N = 257)
No laxatives	23	6 (3%)	17 (6.6%)
Laxatives only occasionally	26	9 (4.5%)	17 (6.6%)
Bulk-forming laxatives	51	31 (15.4%)	20 (7.8%)
Osmotic laxatives**	293	128 (63.7%)	165 (64.2%)
Other laxatives or combinations	65	27 (13.4%)	38 (14.8%)

*28 subjects without symptomatic data to classify constipation control;
**260 (88.7%) were using lactulose and 33 (11.3%) were using PEG.

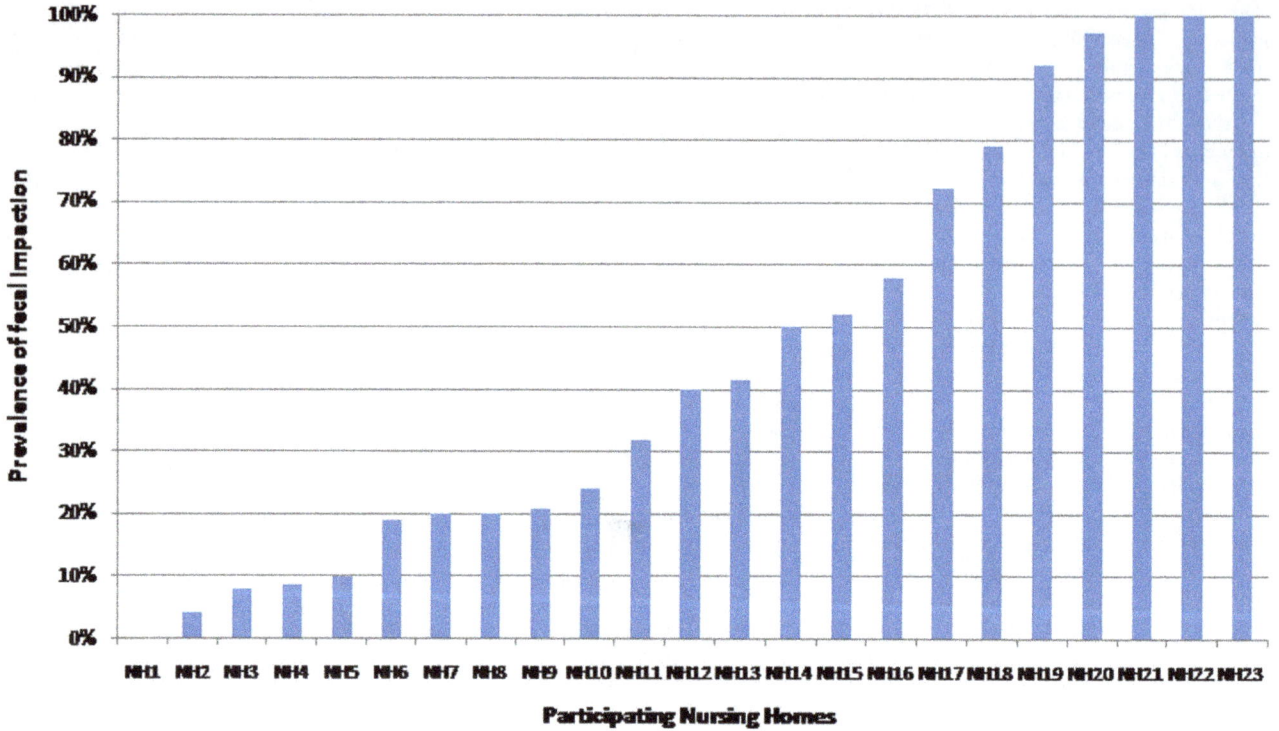

Figure 1. Annual prevalence of fecal impaction across the participating nursing hours.

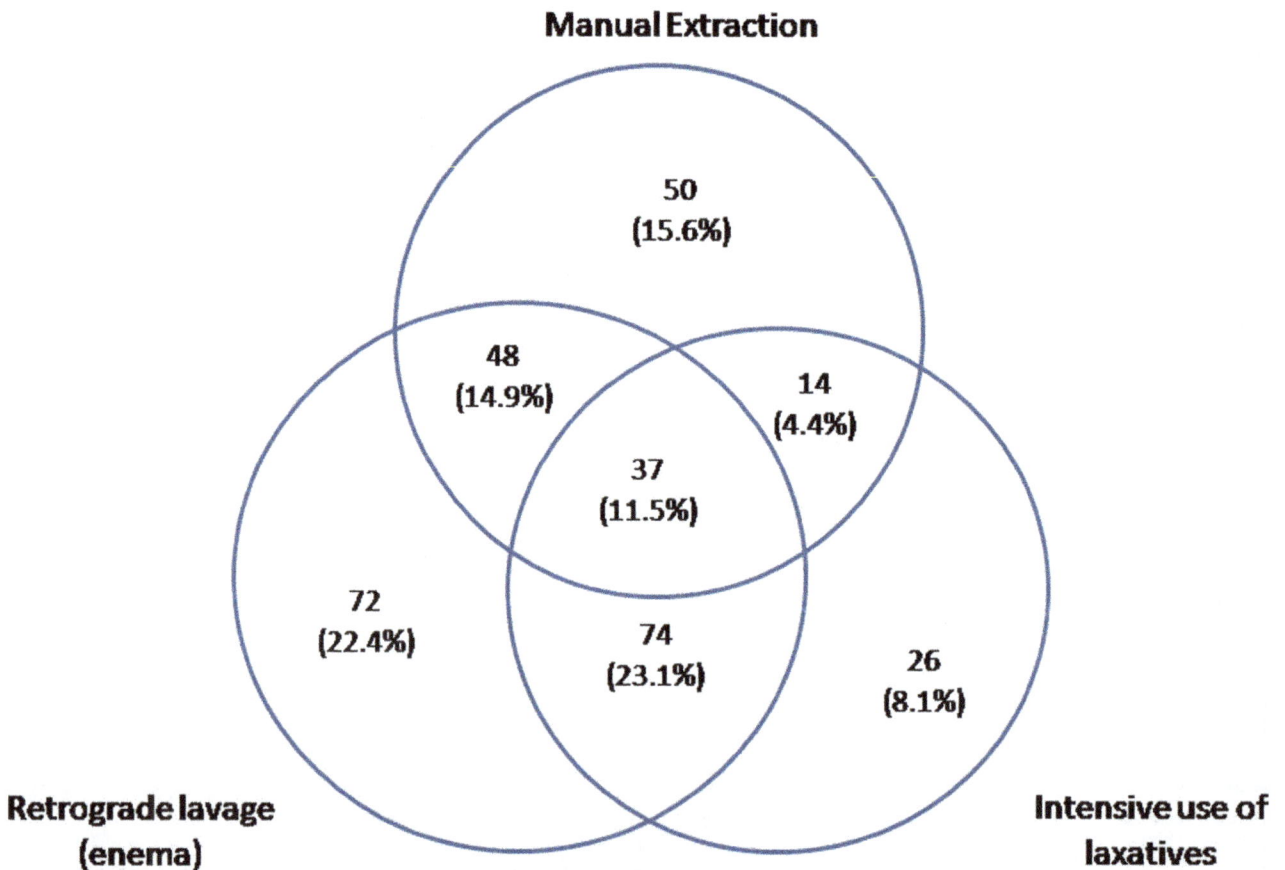

Figure 2. Methods used to solve fecal impaction in the population studied.

Table 3. Fecal Impaction and control of chronic constipation.

	Faecal impaction (medical records)	OR*	Faecal impaction (rectal examination)	OR*
No Constipation	15 (7.5%)	1	1 (0.5%)	1
Controlled constipation	96 (47.8%)	11.1 (6.1–20.1)	5 (2.5%)	4.9 (0.5–42.7)
Uncontrolled constipation	196 (76.3%)	39.2 (21.5–71.6)	35 (13.6%)	30.7 (4.2–226.4)

*adjusted by age and gender.

Results

Response rate

80% (N = 199) of the residents of a nursing home participated in the pilot study, and 21 of the 34 (61.7%; N = 488) invited nursing homes participated in the second phase, with an average of 25 subjects per site. There were no differences between the characteristics of the nursing homes that participated and those that did not. The participating nursing homes had capacity for 3302 residents (average: 157, range: 40–236) and 5 homes had a quality certificate issued because of the quality of their services. The 13 sites not participating had a total of 1736 residents (average: 134; range: 16–233) and one had a services quality certificate.

There were no relevant differences between the samples from the pilot study and from the general study, either in terms of the participants' socio-demographic, cognitive or functional traits, or in their medical characteristics (co-morbidities, use of medications), or in the prevalence of constipation, impaction, or the degree of control over constipation (Table 1). The proportion of subjects needing a proxy to complete a questionnaire was the same in both samples (80.4% vs 81.4%). We therefore believe that the general sample is representative of the nursing home population in Spain, and the samples were pooled for the final analysis, yielding a sample size of 687 subjects for analysis.

Prevalence of chronic constipation

The prevalence of chronic constipation was 70.7% (95%CI: 67.3–74.1%). In total, 466 subjects were diagnosed with constipation (67.8%; 95%CI: 64.3–71.3%) and 20 (2.9%; 95%CI: 1.7–4.2%) had symptoms of constipation sufficient to meet the Rome III criteria, although they had not been diagnosed with constipation in their medical history.

Of the residents with chronic constipation that filled out the symptoms questionnaire properly (N = 458), 201 (43.1%) were adequately controlled and 257 (52.9%) were not adequately controlled.

Prevalence of laxative consumption

63.3% (95%CI: 59.7–66.9%) of the subjects took laxatives on a regular basis. 53 (7.7%; 95%CI: 5.7–9.7%) subjects took bulk-producing laxatives, 313 (45.6%; 95%CI: 41.8–49.3%) took osmotic laxatives and 69 (10.0%; 95%CI: 7.8–12.3%) took other laxatives or combinations of laxatives. (Table 2) shows the relationship between the laxative guidelines followed and the control of constipation.

Prevalence of fecal impaction

According to their medical history, 325 subjects had experienced at least one episode of fecal impaction during the last year, which represents an annual prevalence of fecal impaction of 47.3% (95%CI: 43.6–51.0%). Variability of the prevalence of fecal impaction among participating nursing homes is shown in Figure 1. Of those with fecal impaction, 127 (18.5%) had experienced a single episode, 173 (25.2%) had experienced more than one episode but less than one per month, and 25 (3.6%) had experienced at least one episode per month. The prevalence of recurring fecal impaction was therefore 28.8% (95%CI: 25.4–32.2%).

Of the 665 (96.8%) residents that underwent rectal examination, 169 had non-impacted hard feces and 44 had impacted hard feces in the rectum, representing a prevalence of 6.6% (95%CI: 4.7–8.5%).

Methods to solve fecal impaction

Manual extraction was used in 151 persons, retrograde lavage was used in 236, and intensive use of laxatives in 155. Figure 2 shows how these therapeutic resources were used in the sample.

Chronic constipation and fecal impaction

The prevalence of fecal impaction, both according to the patient's medical history and present on rectal examination, was clearly related to constipation and the lack of adequate control of this (p<0.001; chi-squared test) (Table 3).

Fecal impaction and fecal incontinence

Prevalence of fecal incontinence was 16.4% (59 of 359) among those without history of fecal impaction and 28.2% (88 of 312) among those with history of fecal impaction (p<0.001; chi-2).

Factors associated with fecal impaction

In the univariate analysis, multiple factors (Table 4) were associated with the risk of having experienced fecal impaction in accordance with the diagnosis gathered from the medical history.

When the variables associated with fecal impaction in the univariate analysis were included in a final multivariate logistic regression model (forward stepwise), the factors independently associated with fecal impaction were controlled constipation (OR: 9.8 [5.2–18.4]) and uncontrolled constipation (OR: 37.21 [19.7–70.1]), the number of medications (OR: 1.2 [1.1–1.3]), reduced functional capacity (OR: 0.98 [0.97–0.99]) and the occasional use of NSAIDs (OR: 2.3 [1.2-4-5]) (Table 4).

Factors associated with fecal impaction in the rectal examination

In the univariate analysis, multiple factors (Table 5) were associated with the risk of having impacted feces in the rectum during the rectal examination.

Applying a multivariate model, without including constipation in its codification, because the existence of a single case in the reference category (no constipation) made calculations impossible, and including, in its place, two categories: (1) no constipation or

Table 4. Factors associated to Fecal Impaction.

	N	No Impaction	Impaction	OR not adjusted	OR adjusted*
Age (years)		83.6 (8.5)	85.1 (7.8)	**1.02 (1.00–1.04)**	
Gender					
Male	207	125 (60.4%)	82 (39.6%)	1	
Female	480	237 (49.4%)	243 (50.6%)	**1.56 (1.12–2.18)**	
Body Mass Index (kg/m2)		25.8 (4.4)	24.7 (4.5)	**0.94 (0.91–0.98)**	
Time of staying in nursing home (months)		38.4 (47.5)	43.9 (41.3)	1.00 (1.00–1.01)	
Functional Status (Barthel Index; score)		68.7 (29.0)	55.1 (30.7)	**0.99 (0.98–0.99)**	**0.98 (0.97–0.99)**
Cognitive Status (Folstein Test; score)		22.0 (8.9)	22.8 (8.2)	1.01 (0.99–1.03)	
Modified Ward Index (score)		3.3 (4.6)	5.2 (5.7)	**1.07 (1.04–1.11)**	
Fiber intake (g/day)		9.8 (3.9)	9.3 (3.3)	0.97 (0.93–1.01)	
Liquids intake (l/day)		1.6 (0.5)	1.5 (0.4)	0.90 (0.64–1.27)	
Physical activity					
Sport or long walks	71	53 (74.6%)	18 (25.4%)	1	
Light or moderate	407	230 (56.5%)	177 (43.5%)	**2.27 (1.28–4.00)**	
Minimum	191	76 (39.8%)	115 (60.2%)	**4.46 (2.43–8.18)**	
Number of co-morbidities		2.7+/−1.4	3.2+−1.5	**1.23 (1.11–1.36)**	
Diabetes					
No	501	256 (51.1%)	245 (48.9%)		
Yes	186	106 (57.0%)	80 (43.0%)	0.79 (0.56–1.11)	
Thyroid					
No	610	328 (53.8%)	282 (46.2%)		
Yes	77	34 (44.2%)	43 (55.8%)	1.47 (0.91–2.37)	
High blood pressure					
No	285	173 (60.7%)	112 (39.3%)		
Yes	402	189 (47.0%)	213 (53.0%)	**1.74 (1.28–2.37)**	
Cardiovascular diseases					
No	413	231 (55.9%)	182 (44.1%)		
Yes	274	131 (47.8%)	143 (52.2%)	**1.39 (1.02–1.88)**	
Respiratory diseases					
No	512	286 (55.9%)	226 (44.1%)		
Yes	175	76 (43.4%)	99 (56.6%)	**1.65 (1.17–2.33)**	
Parkinson's disease					
No	641	340 (53.0%)	301 (47.0%)		
Yes	46	22 (47.8%)	24 (52.2%)	1.23 (0.68–2.24)	
Stroke					
No	539	288 (53.4%)	251 (46.6%)		
Yes	148	74 (50.0%)	74 (50.0%)	1.15 (0.80–1.65)	
Other Neurological diseases					
No	400	212 (53.0%)	188 (47.0%)		
Yes	287	150 (52.3%)	137 (47.7%)	1.03 (0.76–1.40)	
Osteoarthritis					
No	268	168 (62.7%)	100 (37.3%)		
Yes	419	194 (46.3%)	225 (53.7%)	**1.95 (1.42–2.67)**	
Renal/Urinary diseases					
No	586	314 (53.6%)	272 (46.4%)		
Yes	101	48 (47.5%)	53 (52.5%)	1.27 (0.84–1.95)	
Constipation					
No	201	186 (92.5%)	15 (7.5%)	1	
Controlled	201	105 (52.2%)	96 (47.8%)	**11.33 (6.26–20.54)**	**9.8 (5.2–18.4)**
Uncontrolled	257	61 (23.7%)	196 (76.3%)	**39.84 (21.88–72.56)**	**37.21 (19.7–70.4)**

Table 4. Cont.

	N	No Impaction	Impaction	OR not adjusted	OR adjusted*
Depression					
No	428	242 (56.5%)	186 (43.5%)		
Yes	259	120 (46.3%)	139 (53.7%)	**1.51 (1.11–2.06)**	
Psychiatric-Other					
No	641	330 (51.5%)	311 (48.5%)		
Yes	46	32 (69.6%)	14 (30.4%)	**0.46 (0.24–0.89)**	
Abdominal Surgery					
No	548	292 (53.3%)	256 (46.7%)		
Yes	139	70 (50.4%)	69 (49.6%)	1.12 (0.77–1.63)	
Number of drugs		3.6+/−2.1	4.8+/−2.2	**1.29 (1.20–1.39)**	**1.2 (1.1–1.3)**
Antihypertensive					
No	281	168 (59.8%)	113 (40.2%)	1	
Regular	403	193 (47.9%)	210 (52.1%)	**1.62 (1.19–2.20)**	
Occasional	3	1 (33.3%)	2 (66.7%)	2.97 (0.27–33.18)	
SSRIs					
No	441	249 (56.5%)	192 (43.5%)	1	
Regular	245	113 (46.1%)	132 (53.9%)	**1.51 (1.11–2.07)**	
Occasional	1	0 (0.0%)	1 (100.0%)		
Tricyclic Antidepressant					
No	668	352 (52.7%)	316 (47.3%)	1	
Regular	19	10 (52.6%)	9 (47.4%)	1.00 (0.40–2.50)	
Benzodiazepine					
No	488	267 (54.7%)	221 (45.3%)	1	
Regular	193	94 (48.7%)	99 (51.3%)	1.27 (0.91–1.78)	
Occasional	6	1 (16.7%)	5 (83.3%)	6.04 (0.70–52.09)	
Hypolipemics					
No	515	276 (53.6%)	239 (46.4%)	1	
Regular	170	85 (50.0%)	85 (50.0%)	1.15 (0.82–1.63)	
Occasional	2	1 (50.0%)	1 (50.0%)	1.15 (0.07–18.56)	
PPIs					
No	258	159 (61.6%)	99 (38.4%)	1	
Regular	408	198 (48.5%)	210 (51.5%)	**1.70 (1.24–2.34)**	
Occasional	21	5 (23.8%)	16 (76.2%)	**5.14 (1.83–14.47)**	
Antacids					
No	655	350 (53.4%)	305 (46.6%)	1	
Regular	25	9 (36.0%)	16 (64.0%)	2.04 (0.89–4.68)	
Occasional	7	3 (42.9%)	4 (57.1%)	1.53 (0.34–6.89)	
Calcium channel blockers					
No	607	322 (53.0%)	285 (47.0%)	1	
Regular	80	40 (50.0%)	40 (50.0%)	1.13 (0.71–1.80)	
Nitrates					
No	627	346 (55.2%)	281 (44.8%)	1	
Regular	59	15 (25.4%)	44 (74.6%)	**3.61 (1.97–6.63)**	
Occasional	1	1 (100.0%)	0 (0.0%)		
NSAID					
No	517	297 (57.4%)	220 (42.6%)	1	
Regular	79	32 (40.5%)	47 (59.5%)	**1.98 (1.22–3.21)**	**1.7 (0.9–3.2)**
Occasional	91	33 (36.3%)	58 (63.7%)	**2.37 (1.50–3.76)**	**2.3 (1.2–4.5)**
ASA					

Table 4. Cont.

	N	No Impaction	Impaction	OR not adjusted	OR adjusted*
No	463	269 (58.1%)	194 (41.9%)	1	
Regular	223	93 (41.7%)	130 (58.3%)	**1.94 (1.40–2.68)**	
Occasional	1	0 (0.0%)	1 (100.0%)		
Opiates					
No	620	342 (55.2%)	278 (44.8%)	1	
Regular	62	18 (29.0%)	44 (71.0%)	**3.01 (1.70–5.32)**	
Occasional	5	2 (40.0%)	3 (60.0%)	1.85 (0.31–11.12)	
Antidiarrheals					
No	672	350 (52.1%)	322 (47.9%)	1	
Regular	5	4 (80.0%)	1 (20.0%)	0.27 (0.03–2.44)	
Occasional	10	8 (80.0%)	2 (20.0%)	0.27 (0.06–1.29)	
Anticholinergics					
No	628	332 (52.9%)	296 (47.1%)	1	
Habitual	59	30 (50.8%)	29 (49.2%)	1.08 (0.64–1.85)	
Diuretics					
No	406	236 (58.1%)	170 (41.9%)	1	
Regular	258	116 (45.0%)	142 (55.0%)	**1.70 (1.24–2.33)**	
Occasional	23	10 (43.5%)	13 (56.5%)	1.80 (0.77–4.21)	
Phenothiazines					
No	650	334 (51.4%)	316 (48.6%)	1	
Regular	37	28 (75.7%)	9 (24.3%)	**0.34 (0.16–0.73)**	
Hypnotics					
No	507	272 (53.6%)	235 (46.4%)	1	
Regular	155	80 (51.6%)	75 (48.4%)	1.09 (0.76–1.56)	
Occasional	25	10 (40.0%)	15 (60.0%)	1.74 (0.77–3.94)	

Nagelkerke $R^2 = 0.49$.

controlled constipation, (2) uncontrolled constipation, the factors independently associated with having impacted feces in the rectum during the rectal examination were the lack of control of constipation (OR: 11.84 [3.87–36.24]), the number of medications (OR: 1.26 [1.02–1.56]), reduced functional capacity (OR: 0.98 [0.97–0.99]), risk of malnutrition (OR: 1.14 [1.02–1.22]), the habitual use of ASA (OR: 3.12 [1.24–7.87]) and the occasional use of diuretics (OR: 18.94 [3.69–97.15]) (Table 6).

Discussion

This is the first study specifically designed to evaluate the prevalence of both constipation and fecal impaction in a sample representative of the nursing home population. The data available up until now came from studies that were not specifically designed for this objective, and were obtained from a single nursing home, which limits its interpretation in terms of representation, given the variation in standards of care and human and material resources among institutions.

Institutionalized elderly patients represent a very specific population, given that they can be expected to suffer constipation more frequently than the non-institutionalized elderly population due to the high prevalence of known risk factors for it [4,6,28–30], but they are under constant nursing and medical supervision. Our study provides information on the prevalence of the conditions studied, as well as on the outcome of care, and the known or supposed therapeutic and preventive measures taken against these.

Our study confirms that constipation in the nursing home population is very highly prevalent, affecting more than 70% of said population. Although there are no other studies on prevalence with which we can compare our results, this figure is similar to the one obtained in studies providing indirect data on the prevalence of constipation, such as the use of laxatives on at least an occasional basis by 93% of the residents of nursing homes [31], the daily use of laxatives by 50–74% of institutionalized persons [4–6,32], or the fact that more than 50% of institutionalized patients complain of straining or difficulty passing feces in more than 25% of bowel movements [33].

Moreover, in spite of the fact that constipation is well-known and is diagnosed correctly (95.9% of patients with constipation were correctly diagnosed in the study sample), treatment efforts to control it are generally insufficient, as shown by the fact that more than 50% of patients diagnosed with constipation continue to meet the Rome III criteria for constipation, in spite of the treatment prescribed by their physicians, and in spite of being surrounded by constant care. It may suggest that laxatives are less effective in this population; an alternative explanation is that the effectiveness of laxatives is not checked after prescription. Future studies should be focused on this relevant matter, since control of constipation is the main objective of treatment.

Table 5. Factors associated to Fecal Impaction in rectal examination.

	N	No Impaction	Impaction	OR not adjusted
Age (years)	687	84.2 (8.2)	86,3 (7.3)	1.04 (0.99–1.08)
Gender				
Male	207	195 (94.2%)	12 (5.8%)	1
Female	480	448 (93.3%)	32 (6.7%)	1.16 (0.59–2.30)
Body Mass Index (kg/m²)	643	25.2 (4.5)	26.0 (4.2)	1.04 (0.97–1.11)
Time of staying in nursing home (months)	682	40.3 (45.0)	50.6 (39.9)	**1.00 (1.00–1.01)**
Functional Status (Barthel Index; score)	642	63.3 (30.3)	46,4 (30.5)	**0.98 (0.97–0.99)**
Cognitive Status (Folstein Test; score)	673	22.3 (8.6)	23.6 (7.0)	1.02 (0.98–1.06)
Modified Ward Index (score)	687	3.9 (5.2)	7.8 (5.0)	**1.12 (1.07–1.17)**
Fibre intake (g/day)	665	9.6 (3.6)	8.3 (4.2)	**0.89 (0.80–0.98)**
Liquids intake (l/day)	664	1.6 (0.4)	1.3 (0.5)	**0.29 (0.13–0.63)**
Physical activity				
Sport or long walks	71	70 (98.6%)	1 (1.4%)	1
Light or moderate	407	378 (92.9%)	29 (7.1%)	5.37 (0.72–40.07)
Minimal	191	179 (93.7%)	12 (6.3%)	4.69 (0.60–36.77)
Number of co-morbidities	687	2.8 (1.4)	4.3 (18.8)	**1.77 (1.46–2.15)**
Diabetes				
No	501	476 (95.0%)	25 (5.0%)	1
Yes	186	167 (89.8%)	19 (10.2%)	**2.17 (1.16–4.04)**
Thyroid diseases				
No	610	575 (94.3%)	35 (5.7%)	1
Yes	77	68 (88.3%)	9 (11.7%)	**2.17 (1.00–4.72)**
High blood pressure				
No	285	274 (96.1%)	11 (3.9%)	1
Yes	402	369 (91.8%)	33 (8.2%)	**2.23 (1.11–4.49)**
Cardiovascular diseases				
No	413	399 (96.6%)	14 (3.4%)	1
Yes	274	244 (89.1%)	30 (10.9%)	**3.50 (1.82–6.74)**
Respiratory diseases				
No	512	496 (96.9%)	16 (3.1%)	1
Yes	175	147 (84.0%)	28 (16.0%)	**5.90 (3.11–11.21)**
Parkinson's Disease				
No	641	598 (93.3%)	43 (6,7%)	1
Yes	46	45 (97.8%)	1 (2.2%)	0.31 (0.04–2.30)
Stroke				
No	539	506 (93.9%)	33 (6.1%)	1
Yes	148	137 (92.6%)	11 (7.4%)	1.23 (0.61–2.50)
Other Neurological diseases				
No	400	372 (93.0%)	28 (7.0%)	1
Yes	287	271 (94.4%)	16 (5.6%)	0.78 (0.42–1.48)
Osteoarthritis				
No	268	259 (96.6%)	9 (3.4%)	1
Yes	419	384 (91.6%)	35 (8.4%)	**2.62 (1.24–5.55)**
Renal/Urinary Diseases				
No	586	551 (94.0%)	35 (6.0%)	1
Yes	101	92 (91.1%)	9 (8.9%)	1.54 (0.72–3.31)
Constipation				
No	201	200 (99.5%)	1 (0.5%)	1
Controlled	201	196 (97.5%)	5 (2.5%)	**5.10 (0.59–44.07)**
Uncontrolled	257	222 (86.4%)	35 (13.6%)	**31.53 (4.28–232.27)**

Table 5. Cont.

	N	No Impaction	Impaction	OR not adjusted
Anxiety Disorder				
No	492	469 (95.3%)	23 (4.7%)	1
Yes	195	174 (89.2%)	21 (10.8%)	**2.46 (1.33–4.56)**
Depression				
No	428	411 (96.0%)	17 (4.0%)	1
Yes	259	232 (89.6%)	27 (10.4%)	**2.81 (1.50–5.27)**
Other Psychiatric diseases				
No	641	600 (93.6%)	41 (6.4%)	1
Yes	46	43 (93.5%)	3 (6.5%)	1.02 (0.30–3.43)
Abdominal Surgery				
No	548	508 (92.7%)	40 (7.3%)	1
Yes	139	135 (97.1%)	4 (2.9%)	0.38 (0.13–1.07)
Number of drugs	687	4.0 (2.2)	6.2 (2.1)	**1.46 (1.28–1.67)**
Antihypertensive				
No	281	272 (96.8%)	9 (3.2%)	1
Regular	403	368 (91.3%)	35 (8.7%)	**2.87 (1.36–6.08)**
Occasional	3	3 (100.0%)	0 (0.0%)	
SSRIs				
No	441	422 (95.7%)	19 (4.3%)	1
Regular	245	220 (89.8%)	25 (10.2%)	**2.52 (1.36–4.68)**
Occasional	1	1 (100.0%)	0 (0.0%)	
Tricyclic Antidepressant				
No	668	625 (93.6%)	43 (6.4%)	1
Regular	19	18 (94.7%)	1 (5.3%)	0.81 (0.11–6.19)
Benzodiazepines				
No	488	460 (94.3%)	28 (5.7%)	1
Regular	193	177 (91.7%)	16 (8.3%)	1.49 (0.78–2.81)
Occasional	6	6 (100.0%)	0 (0.0%)	
Hypolipemics				
No	515	486 (94.4%)	29 (5.6%)	1
Regular	170	155 (91.2%)	15 (8.8%)	1.62 (0.85–3.10)
Occasional	2	2 (100.0%)	0 (0.0%)	
PPIs				
No	258	240 (93.0%)	18 (7.0%)	1
Regular	408	385 (94.4%)	23 (5.6%)	0.80 (0.42–1.51)
Occasional	21	18 (85.7%)	3 (14.3%)	2.22 (0.60–8.26)
Antiacids				
No	655	616 (94.0%)	39 (6.0%)	1
Regular	25	22 (88.0%)	3 (12.0%)	2.15 (0.62–7.51)
Occasional	7	5 (71.4%)	2 (28.6%)	**6.32 (1.19–33,61)**
Calcium channel blockers				
No	607	573 (94.4%)	34 (5.6%)	1
Regular	80	70 (87.5%)	10 (12.5%)	**2.41 (1.14–5.08)**
Nitrates				
No	627	595 (94.9%)	32 (5.1%)	1
Regular	59	47 (79.7%)	12 (20.3%)	**4.75 (2.29–9.82)**
NSAID				
No	517	492 (95.2%)	25 (4.8%)	1
Regular	79	68 (86.1%)	11 (13.9%)	**3.18 (1.50–6.76)**

Table 5. Cont.

	N	No Impaction	Impaction	OR not adjusted
Occasional	91	83 (91.2%)	8 (8.8%)	1.90 (0.83–4.35)
ASA				
No	463	449 (97.0%)	14 (3.0%)	1
Regular	223	193 (86.5%)	30 (13.5%)	**4.99 (2.59–9.61)**
Opiates				
No	620	581 (93.7%)	39 (6.3%)	1
Regular	62	59 (95.2%)	3 (4.8%)	0.76 (0.23–2.53)
Occasional	5	3 (60.0%)	2 (40.0%)	**9.93 (1.61–61.19)**
Antidiarrheals				
No	672	628 (93.5%)	44 (6.5%)	1
Regular	5	5 (100.0%)	0 (0.0%)	
Occasional	10	10 (100.0%)	0 (0.0%)	
Anticholinergics				
No	628	586 (93.3%)	42 (6.7%)	1
Regular	59	57 (96.6%)	2 (3.4%)	0.49 (0.12–2.08)
Diuretics				
No	406	396 (97.5%)	10 (2.5%)	1
Regular	258	230 (89.1%)	28 (10.9%)	**4.82 (2.30–10.11)**
Occasional	23	17 (73.9%)	6 (26.1%)	**13.98 (4.55–42.94)**
Phenothiazines				
No	650	607 (93.4%)	43 (6.6%)	1
Regular	37	36 (97.3%)	1 (2.7%)	0.39 (0.05–2.93)
Hypnotics				
No	507	474 (93.5%)	33 (6.5%)	1
Regular	155	147 (94.8%)	8 (5.2%)	0.78 (0.35–1.73)
Occasional	25	22 (88.0%)	3 (12.0%)	1.96 (0.56–6.88)

Our study provides, for the first time, figures on the prevalence of fecal impaction in the institutionalized population, revealing the enormous magnitude of the problem and its high recurrence rate. Around 50% of residents experienced fecal impaction at least once a year, 30% experienced recurring bouts, and 6.6% were impacted at any given time when a rectal examination was performed. This occurred despite them living in institutions that guarantee daily healthcare and that provide medical supervision, in many cases with procedures submitted for external evaluation and certification. Our figures for recurring fecal impaction align greatly with those obtained in a 1975 study, in which it was revealed that 39% of patients with fecal impaction had a prior history of impaction [34]. The fact that almost 40 years later the prevalence of recurring fecal impaction has not dropped to any

Table 6. Multivariate Model: factors associated with fecal impaction in rectal examination.

	P	OR adjusted*
Number of drugs	0,03	1.26 (1.02–1.56)
Functional Status (Barthel score)	0.02	0.98 (0.97–0.99)
Modified Ward index	<0.001	1.14 (1.02–1.22)
Uncontrolled constipation	<0.001	11.84 (3.87–36.24)
ASA	0.01	3.12 (1.24–7.87)
Diuretics		
No		
Regular	0.08	2.48 (0.90–6.81)
Occasional	<0.001	18.94 (3.69–97.15)

Nagelkerke R2 = 0.42.

significant extent clearly demonstrates that the measures currently being taken to prevent its occurrence are insufficient.

Of all the factors associated with fecal impaction, our study confirms that constipation is the most significant individual factor associated with the occurrence of fecal impaction. Moreover, the results reinforce the idea that the main risk factor, specifically, is the inability to control constipation, in spite of treatment. Other factors, such as a lack of activity, the risk of malnutrition, and medications taken, are additional factors that contribute to fecal impaction in a population with a high incidence of constipation.

Of all of the identified risk factors for fecal impaction, there is one that has not previously been described in the literature: the occasional use of NSAIDs. Although this is not one of the factors most strongly associated with fecal impaction, it is relevant due to the high prevalence of NSAID use in the institutionalized elderly population. Although we know that the use of NSAIDs is a risk factor for constipation in the general population [35], our study shows that it is also a risk factor for experiencing fecal impaction that is independent of the risk for constipation.

The fact that our study does not show an association with certain factors that have been related to fecal impaction in other studies, such as neurological co-morbidities [13], or low liquid intake [20], not even in the univariate analysis, is probably related to the nursing home healthcare staff's knowledge of these risk factors for constipation, and their thus paying special attention to them in these patients.

A notable limitation of our study is the semi-random selection of the patients at each nursing home, imposed by the data protection laws, which made it impossible for us to access the patient registry for each nursing home. Although some bias in the selection of the subjects may exist in some centers, it would have occurred in both directions towards the most well and the most unwell. Overall, we believe that the consequences of this limitation are minimal, since we were able to compare the semi-randomness at a single nursing home with 80% of the residents included with random selection of nursing homes. The nursing homes included in the study are representative of all of the nursing homes in Spain, in accordance with the nursing home physician's census from the SEMER. Moreover, the response rate was lower than expected, which allowed us to reach the pre-established sample size: nevertheless,

the sample size reached allows for at least 4% accuracy for the prevalence of 47% observed for impaction.

The objectivity of the self-reported measures by this population may be considered another possible limitation to our study. Although the instruments used have been previously validated for this purpose, the study was controlled by categorizing the patients according to the degree of cognitive decline, and by including only the medically defined data as an outcome for the analysis. Although 100% self-reporting would be desirable, it is impossible in this population without the aid of a proxy. In fact, more than 80% needed a proxy to complete the questionnaire mainly for two reasons: functional limitation (visual or motor impairment), and cognitive limitations for self-completing the questionnaire. More than 70% of the participants were able to fully understand the questions included in the questionnaire; some required a proxy due to reading or writing difficulties. The remainder of subjects required a proxy for completing the questionnaire due to cognitive impairment, but in these subjects the usual caregiver is likely to provide more reliable answers than the subject. The pilot study was designed in part to address this limitation by evaluating if the project was affordable.

Another limitation that should be acknowledged is that estimates of food, fluid and fiber intake are approximate, but a more accurate measure, such as a 3-day diary, was unaffordable; in the pilot study we tested that approach and it was not possible to obtain complete and reliable information.

The final conclusions of our study from a practical and clinical point of view are that fecal impaction is a problem of significant magnitude and that constipation is the most relevant associated factor. In an environment of constant medical care such as a nursing home, particular attention should be paid to ensuring that treatment for constipation is effective, regardless of the patient's capacities, habits, medical characteristics, or co-treatments.

Author Contributions

Conceived and designed the experiments: ER MB. Performed the experiments: MJJC MB ER. Analyzed the data: ER MDR. Wrote the paper: ER MB MJJC AAS MDR ALR.

References

1. Konstantinos Giannakouris (2010) Regional population projections EURO-POP2008: Most EU regions face older population profile in 2030. Eurostat. Statistic in focus. http://epp.eurostat.ec.europa.eu/portal/page/portal/product_details/publication?p_product_code=KS-SF-10-001.

2. Jones AL, Dwyer LL, Bercovitz AR, Stahan G (2009) The National Nursing Home Survey: 2004 overview. National Center for Health Statistics Vital Health Stat;13(167). http://www.cdc.gov/nchs/data/nnhsd/nursinghomefacilities2006.pdf

3. OECD (2011) "Long-term care beds in institutions and hospitals", in Health at a Glance 2011: OECD Indicators, OECD Publishing. http://dx.doi.org/10.1787/health_glance-2011-72-en.

4. Primrose WR, Capewell AE, Simpson GK, Smith RG (1987) Prescribing patterns observed in registered nursing homes and long-stay geriatric wards. Age Ageing January;16(1):25–8.

5. Kinnunen O (1991) Study of constipation in a geriatric hospital, day hospital, old people's home and at home. Aging (Milano) June;3(2):161–70.

6. Harari D, Gurwitz JH, Avorn J, Choodnovskiy I, Minaker KL (1994) Constipation: assessment and management in an institutionalized elderly population. J Am GeriatrSoc September;42(9):947–52.

7. O'Keefe EA, Talley NJ, Tangalos EG, Zinsmeister AR (1992) A bowel symptom questionnaire for the elderly. J Gerontol July;47(4):M116–M121.

8. Glia A, Lindberg G (1997) Quality of life in patients with different types of functional constipation. Scand J Gastroenterol November;32(11):1083–9.

9. Singh G, Lingala V, Wang H, Vadhavkar S, Kahler KH, et al. (2007) Use of health care resources and cost of care for adults with constipation. Clin Gastroenterol Hepatol September;5(9):1053–8.

10. Rao SS (2007) Constipation: evaluation and treatment of colonic and anorectal motility disorders. GastroenterolClin North Am September;36(3):687–711, x.

11. Dennison C, Prasad M, Lloyd A, Bhattacharyya SK, Dhawan R, et al. (2005) The health-related quality of life and economic burden of constipation. Pharmacoeconomics;23(5):461–76.

12. Kimberly BS (2007) Constipation in the elderly: implication in skilled nursing facilities. Director;15(3):20–3.

13. Gallagher P, O'Mahony D (2009) Constipation in old age. Best Pract Res ClinGastroenterol;23(6):875–87.

14. De Lillo AR, Rose S (2000) Functional bowel disorders in the geriatric patient: constipation, fecal impaction, and fecal incontinence. Am J Gastroenterol April;95(4):901–5.

15. Creason N, Sparks D (2000) Fecal impaction: a review. NursDiagn January;11(1):15–23.

16. Chassagne P, Landrin I, Neveu C, Czernichow P, Bouaniche M, et al. (1999) Fecal incontinence in the institutionalized elderly: incidence, risk factors, and prognosis. Am J Med February;106(2):185–90.

17. Starer P, Likourezos A, Dumapit G (2000) The association of fecal impaction and urinary retention in elderly nursing home patients. Arch GerontolGeriatr January;30(1):47–54.

18. Kinnunen O, Jauhonen P, Salokannel J, Kivela SL (1989) Diarrhea and fecal impaction in elderly long-stay patients. Z Gerontol November;22(6):321–3.

19. Lal S, Brown GN (1967) Some unusual complications of fecal impaction. Am J Proctol June;18(3):226–31.

20. Wrenn K (1989) Fecal impaction. N Engl J Med September 7;321(10):658–62.

21. Barcelo M, Jimenez-Cebrian MJ, Diaz-Rubio M, Rocha AL, Rey E (2013) Validation of a questionnaire for assessing fecal impaction in the elderly: impact of cognitive impairment, and using a proxy. BMC Geriatr;13:24.

22. Equipo Portal Mayores (2010) Estadisticas sobre residencias: distribucion de centros y plazas residenciales por provincia. Datos de octubre. Informes Portal

Mayores Núm 104 Pág: 19 p.ISSN: 1885–6780. Available: http://envejecimiento.csic.es/documentacion/biblioteca/registro.htm?id = 57572.

23. Morgan DR, Squella FE, Pena E, Mearin F, Rey E, et al. (2010) Multinational validation of the Spanish Rome III Adult diagnostic questionnaire: comparable sensitivity and specificity to English instrument (abstract). Gastroenterology;138(Suppl 1):S386.

24. Morillas J, Garcia-Talavera N, Martin-Pozuelo G, Reina AB, Zafrilla P (2006) [Detection of hyponutrition risk in non-institutionalised elderly]. NutrHosp November;21(6):650–6.

25. Mahoney FI, Barthel DW (1965) Functional evaluation: the Barthel index. Md State Med J February;14:61–5.

26. Lobo A, Ezquerra J, Gomez BF, Sala JM, Seva DA (1979) [Cognocitive mini-test (a simple practical test to detect intellectual changes in medical patients)]. Actas Luso EspNeurolPsiquiatrCienc Afines May;7(3):189–202.

27. Folstein MF, Folstein SE, McHugh PR (1975) "Mini-mental state". A practical method for grading the cognitive state of patients for the clinician. J Psychiatr Res November;12(3):189–98.

28. Bouras EP, Tangalos EG (2009) Chronic constipation in the elderly. GastroenterolClin North Am September;38(3):463–80.

29. Coyne KS, Cash B, Kopp Z, Gelhorn H, Milsom I, et al. (2011) The prevalence of chronic constipation and faecal incontinence among men and women with symptoms of overactive bladder. BJU Int Jan;107(2):254–61.

30. Talley NJ (2004) Definitions, epidemiology, and impact of chronic constipation. Rev GastroenterolDisord;4Suppl 2:S3–S10.

31. Frank L, Schmier J, Kleinman L, Siddique R, Beck C, et al. (2002) Time and economic cost of constipation care in nursing homes. J Am Med Dir Assoc July;3(4):215–23.

32. Wigzell FW (1969) The health of nonagenarians. GerontolClin (Basel) ;11(3):137–44.

33. Marfil C, Davies GJ, Dettmar PW (2005) Laxative use and its relationship with straining in a London elderly population: free-living versus institutionalised. J Nutr Health Aging ;9(3):185–7.

34. Gurll N, Steer M (1975) Diagnostic and therapeutic considerations for fecal impaction. Dis Colon Rectum September;18(6):507–11.

35. Chang JY, Locke GR, Schleck CD, Zinsmeister AR, Talley NJ (2007) Risk factors for chronic constipation and a possible role of analgesics. Neurogastroenterol Motil November;19(11):905–11.

17

Nutritional Status in Community-Dwelling Elderly in France in Urban and Rural Areas

Marion J. Torres[1,2,3]*, **Béatrice Dorigny**[3], **Mirjam Kuhn**[4], **Claudine Berr**[5], **Pascale Barberger-Gateau**[1,2], **Luc Letenneur**[1,2]

1 Univ. Bordeaux, ISPED, Centre INSERM U897-Epidémiologie-Biostatistique, F-33000, Bordeaux, France, 2 INSERM, ISPED, Centre INSERM U897-Epidémiologie-Biostatistique, F-33000, Bordeaux, France, 3 Nutricia Advanced Medical Nutrition, Danone Research, Saint-Ouen, France, 4 Nutricia Research, Advanced Medical Nutrition, Utrecht, Netherlands, 5 INSERM, U1061, Neuropsychiatrie: recherche épidémiologique et clinique, Université Montpellier I, Hôpital La Colombière, F-34093, Montpellier, France

Abstract

Malnutrition is a frequent condition in elderly people, especially in nursing homes and geriatric wards. Its frequency is less well known among elderly living at home. The objective of this study was to describe the nutritional status evaluated by the Mini Nutritional Assessment (MNA) of elderly community-dwellers living in rural and urban areas in France and to investigate its associated factors.

Methods: Subjects aged 65 years and over from the Approche Multidisciplinaire Intégrée (AMI) cohort (692 subjects living in a rural area) and the Three-City (3C) cohort (8,691 subjects living in three large urban zones) were included. A proxy version of the MNA was reconstructed using available data from the AMI cohort. Sensitivity and specificity were used to evaluate the agreement between the proxy version and the standard version in AMI. The proxy MNA was computed in both cohorts to evaluate the frequency of poor nutritional status. Factors associated with this state were investigated in each cohort separately.

Results: In the rural sample, 38.0% were females and the mean age was 75.5 years. In the urban sample, 60.3% were females and the mean age was 74.1 years. Among subjects in living in the rural sample, 7.4% were in poor nutritional status while the proportion was 18.5% in the urban sample. Female gender, older age, being widowed, a low educational level, low income, low body mass index, being demented, having a depressive symptomatology, a loss of autonomy and an intake of more than 3 drugs appeared to be independently associated with poor nutritional status.

Conclusion: Poor nutritional status was commonly observed among elderly people living at home in both rural and urban areas. The associated factors should be further considered for targeting particularly vulnerable individuals.

Editor: Alberico Catapano, University of Milan, Italy

Funding: The 3C Study is conducted under a partnership agreement between the Institut National de la Santé et de la Recherche Médicale (INSERM), the Victor Segalen – Bordeaux II University and the Sanofi-Synthélabo Company. The Fondation pour la Recherche Médicale funded the preparation and initiation of the study. The 3C Study is also supported by the Caisse Nationale Maladie des Travailleurs Salariés, Direction Générale de la Santé, Conseils Régionaux of Aquitaine, Languedoc-Roussillon and Bourgogne, Fondation de France, Ministry of Research-INSERM Programme 'Cohortes et collections de données biologiques', Mutuelle Générale de l'Education Nationale, Institut de la longévité, Conseil Général de la Côte d'or. The authors thank the Génopôle of Lille, the Laboratory of Biochemistry of the University Hospital of Dijon (Prof. Gambert) and Montpellier (Prof. Descomps), the Neuroradiology Departments of the University Hospitals of Bordeaux (Prof. Caillé), Dijon (Prof. Krausé) and Montpellier (Prof. Bonafé), the University Hospital Gui de Chauliac in Montpellier, the Council of Dijon and the Conseil Général of Côte d'Or. The 3C Study supports are listed on the Study website (www.three-city-study.com). The AMI project was funded by AGRICA (CAMARCA, CRCCA, CCPMA PREVOYANCE, CPCEA, AGRI PREVOYANCE), la Mutualité Sociale Agricole (MSA) de Gironde, la Caisse Centrale de la Mutualité Sociale Agricole (CCMSA). The authors declare that the funders of the cohorts and the commercial company that finance some authors of this paper had no role in study design, data collection and analysis, decision to publish, or preparation of the manuscript.

Competing Interests: The authors have received funding from a commercial source (Sanofi-Synthélabo Company) and some authors are employed by a commercial company (Nutricia).

* Email: Marion.Torres@isped.u-bordeaux2.fr

Introduction

Worldwide, the proportion of elderly people is constantly increasing. According to the United Nations, in 2025, it is estimated that the population aged 60 years or older will be 1.2 billion and 2 billion in 2050 (representing about 22% of the world population) [1]. The risk of developing a chronic condition such as malnutrition increases with age [2]. According to the French National Authority for Health, malnutrition is caused by an imbalance between intake and the body's requirements. This imbalance causes tissue loss, in particular muscle tissue loss, with harmful functional consequences [3]. The potential risk factors of malnutrition are multiple: reduced food intake due to loss of appetite, episodes of fasting, poor dentition, swallowing difficulties, inability to eat independently, digestive disorders, chronic diseases and depression [3,4]. Poor nutritional status is associated with higher risks of morbidity and mortality in elderly people [5] causing economic consequences for society [6].

The prevalence estimates of malnutrition in elderly are highly variable due to the use of different tools and different settings. In particular, there are few studies on malnutrition in community-dwelling elderly based on validated tools [5]. Moreover, individual characteristics that may influence the nutritional status of elderly community dwellers are poorly understood, such as living in rural or urban areas in the same country, which may influence lifestyle and food availability [7]. To determine nutritional status, the Mini-Nutritional Assessment (MNA) is one of the most recognised screening instruments and is used all around the world, especially in elderly people [3,8,9]. Since its first publication in 1996 [9], the MNA has been translated into more than twenty languages, including French. It has been validated with high sensitivity, specificity and reliability. It is an easy and cheap way to detect malnourished people or those at risk of malnutrition. The objective of this study was to describe the nutritional status of elderly community-dwellers, living in rural and urban areas in France, based on the MNA items, and to investigate its associated factors, notably socio-demographic factors, in order to better target individuals at risk [10].

Methods

Population and samples

For the current cross-sectional analysis, we used the baseline data of two French cohorts of elderly people aged 65 years and over: The AMI (Approche Multidisciplinaire Intégrée) cohort and Three-City (3C) Study.

Between 1999–2000, 9,294 elderly community-dwellers were included in the 3C cohort study, chosen from the electoral rolls of 3 large French cities and their suburbs: Bordeaux (n = 2,104), Dijon (n = 4,931) and Montpellier (n = 2,259). The aim of 3C is to study the vascular risk factors of dementia; its methodology was described previously [11].

In 2007, AMI included 1,002 subjects living in rural areas in Gironde, an administrative area in southwest France, randomly recruited from the reimbursement database of the unique French Farmer Health Insurance System. At baseline, 961 of these individuals were living at home. All had worked in the field of agriculture for at least 20 years. The aim of AMI is to study health and aging in elderly farmers living in rural areas. Details on this cohort have been published previously [12].

For 3C, the protocol was approved by the Consultative Committee for the Protection of Persons participating in Biomedical Research of the Kremlin-Bicêtre University Hospital (Paris). AMI was approved by the Ethics Committee of the University Hospital of Bordeaux according to the principles of the Declaration of Helsinki. All participants signed a written consent.

In both cohorts, data on socio-demographics, lifestyle, neuro-psychological testing, physical examination, blood sampling, symptoms and complaints, medical history and food intake were collected at baseline.

Mini Nutritional Assessment

The MNA is an 18-item questionnaire divided into four parts as described in Table 1 [9]: anthropometric measurements (i.e.,

weight, height, mid-arm circumference, calf circumference, and weight loss during the past 3 months); global assessments (six questions related to lifestyle, medication, and mobility); dietary questionnaire (eight questions related to number of meals, food and fluid intake, and autonomy of feeding); and subjective assessment (self-perception of health and nutrition). The aim of this tool is to identify elderly at risk of malnutrition or those who already are malnourished. A two-step procedure is applied to classify the subjects [13]. The first part of the questionnaire (items A to F) is administered and a score greater than 11 indicates a normal nutritional status. The second part of the questionnaire (item G to R) is administered to subjects with a score equal to or lower than 11. If the total score is greater or equal to 24, subjects are considered to have a normal nutritional status. A score between 17 and 23.5 indicates a risk of malnutrition and a score lower than 17 indicates a malnourished person. Due to the small number of subjects classified in the "malnutrition" category, the variable was dichotomised: "malnutrition" was collapsed with "at risk of malnutrition" to identify people in "poor nutritional status" versus those with a "normal nutritional status."

Reconstruction of the Mini Nutritional Assessment using proxy items

The MNA was administered in its standard version in the AMI cohort but was not included in the baseline questionnaire of the 3C cohort, which started 7 years earlier. However, some items of the MNA were also available in the 3C questionnaire, and other items could be replaced by similar questions that will be called proxy items. In the AMI cohort, these proxy items were also available. Therefore, a proxy MNA was constructed in the AMI cohort in order to assess its agreement with the standard MNA on the same subjects. The correspondence between the items of the standard MNA and the proxy MNA is given in Table 1. For item A regarding quantity of food intake, we used a question of the Center for Epidemiologic Studies Depression Scale (CES-D) [14] which is a scale used to identify depressive symptomatology. For item E on neurophysiological problems, we used the clinical diagnosis of dementia given by a neurologist combined with the score on the Mini Mental State Examination [15] to assess the severity of dementia (10 to 20 for a moderate dementia and 0 to 9 for a severe dementia). The CES-D scale was used to assess depressive symptomatology with a score superior or equal to 17 for men and superior or equal to 23 for women [16]. Item G on independency, was replaced by the Activity of Daily Living (ADL) scale developed by Katz [17] and subjects were considered independent if none of the ADL items was altered. Items about dairy products, fruits and vegetables consumption (items K and L) were replaced by the information obtained from a Food Frequency Questionnaire (FFQ) [18]. Item N about mode of feeding was replaced by a question from the ADL scale. In the construction of the proxy MNA, a lack of sensitivity was observed in the screening part of the questionnaire. Indeed, several subjects who scored 11 or less with the standard MNA and were therefore considered at risk of malnutrition, scored 12 with the proxy MNA and were classified as normal. In order to increase the sensitivity of the proxy MNA, the cut-off of the screening score was modified to 12 points or less for identifying individuals possibly at risk of malnutrition.

All the data needed to compute the proxy MNA were available for 692 subjects in AMI and 8,691 subjects in 3C.

Socio-demographic information

Socio-demographic information included age (in 3 categories: <75 years, between 75 and 84 years and 85 years and older),

Table 1. Correspondence between the items of the standard MNA and the proxy MNA in the AMI cohort.

Standard MNA	Proxy MNA
Item A: Has food intake declined over the past 3 months due to loss of appetite, digestive problems, chewing or swallowing difficulties?	**Item 2 of CESD: During the past week, I did not want to eat, my appetite was poor**
0) Severe decrease in food intake	0) Frequently, all the time
1) Moderate decrease in food intake	1) Never or very rarely, Occasionally
2) No decrease in food intake	2) Often
Item B: Weight loss during the last 3 months	**No proxy, same item.**
Item C: Mobility	**Restriction of mobility**
0) Bed or chair bound	0) Confined to bed
1) Able to get out of bed/chair but does not go out	1) Confined to home
2) Goes out	2) Confinement in close proximity, Confined to the quarter, Simple difficulty to use transport, No restrictions
Item D: Has suffered psychological stress or acute disease in the past 3 months?	**No proxy, same item.**
Item E: Neuropsychological problems	**Diagnosis of dementia, MMSE and CESD**
0) Severe dementia or depression	0) Diagnosis of dementia and MMSE<10, Depressive symptomatology by the CES-D
1) Mild dementia	1) Diagnosis of dementia and $10 \geq MMSE \leq 20$ and CES-D negative
2) No psychological problems	2) Diagnosis of dementia and MMSE>20, CES-D negative
Item F: BMI	**No proxy, same item.**
Item G: Lives independently	**Scale of ADL of Katz**
0) No	0) Dependent on minimum one item
1) Yes	1) No dependence for each item
Item H: Takes more than 3 prescription drugs per day	**Listing of drugs taken according to the medical prescription**
0) No	0)≤ 3
1) Yes	1)>3
Item I: Pressure sores or skin ulcers	**No proxy, same item.**
Item J: How many full meals does the patient eat daily?	**No proxy, same item.**
Item K: Selected consumption markers for protein intake? At least one serving of dairy products per day, Two or more servings of legumes or eggs per week, Meat, fish or poultry every day	**FFQ for only dairy products, Do you eat dairy products per day?**
0) If 0 or 1 yes	0) No
0.5) If 2 yes	0.5) Yes but not $> = 2$ servings of legumes or eggs per week and not meat, fish or poultry every day
1) If 3 yes	1) Yes
	No proxy for legumes, eggs, meat, fish and poultry consumption, same item.
Item L: Consumes two or more servings of fruit or vegetables per day?	**FFQ: Do you eat fruits every day? Yes/No, How many times per day if yes, and per week if no? Same question with vegetables**
0) No	0) No
1) Yes	1) Yes, if they eat 1 fruit and 1 vegetable per day minimum or 2 fruits or 2 vegetables per day minimum
Item M: How much fluid is consumed per day?	**No proxy, same item.**
Item N: Mode of feeding	**Item 6 of ADL of Katz: Eating**
0) Unable to eat without assistance	0) Need help completely or artificial feeding
1) Self-fed with some difficulty	1) Need help to cook full meals
2) Self-fed without any problem	2) Need any help
Item O: Self view of nutritional status	**No proxy, same item.**
Item P: In comparison with other people of the same age, how does the patient consider his/her health status?	**No proxy, same item.**
Item Q: Mid-arm circumference in cm	**No proxy, same item.**
Item R: Calf circumference in cm	**No proxy, same item.**

Abbreviations: ADL = Activities Daily Living, BMI = Body Mass Index, CESD = Center for Epidemiologic Studies Depression Scale, FFQ = Food Frequency Questionnaire, MMSE = Mini Mental State Examination, MNA = Mini Nutritional Assessment.

gender, education (low level which represented no education or primary school only, medium level representing short secondary school: Certificate of Professional Aptitude (CAP) or the Diploma of Occupational Studies (BEP), and high level representing long secondary school: Baccalaureate degree or university), marital status (married, widowed and separated, single or other) and income (less than €750, €750 to €1,500, €1,500 to €2,250, more than €2,250 per month and refused to answer). In 3C, location (Bordeaux, Dijon or Montpellier) was also taken into account.

The autonomy of the subjects was assessed by the validated Katz ADL scale [17]. Individuals were considered to have a loss of autonomy when they presented at least one impairment in these five activities: bathing, dressing, toileting, transferring from bed to chair and eating.

Statistical methods

Quantitative and qualitative variables were compared respectively by student t-test or chi-square test. Sensitivity, specificity and agreement of the proxy MNA were calculated using the standard MNA as the gold standard. Sensitivity was defined as the proportion of individuals correctly classified as having an impaired nutritional status. Specificity was defined as the proportion of individuals classified correctly as not having an impaired nutritional status. Agreement was assessed by the AC1 statistic [19] that showed less dependency upon trait prevalence [20] than the Kappa coefficient [21].

The proportion of subjects with a malnutrition status was estimated in both cohorts using the proxy MNA. As the proxy MNA showed different sensitivity and specificity than the standard MNA, the apparent frequency estimate was adjusted using the Rogan-Gladen estimator [22]. Statistical tests were performed at the 0.05 level of significance using the SAS statistical package (version 9.3; SAS Institute Inc., Cary, NC, USA).

Results

Of the 961 subjects included in the AMI cohort and living at home, the standard MNA was available for 851 individuals. Excluded subjects had lower incomes, were more often demented (18% vs. 9%) and dependent for ADLs (11.0% vs. 5.0%). Among these 851 subjects, the proxy MNA was available for 692 individuals (81.3%). The 159 subjects with missing data in the proxy MNA were older, more often widowed, had a lower level of education, a lower income and were in poorer health.

The mean age of the 692 included subjects was 75.5 years (standard deviation (SD) 6.2). Participants were mainly males (62.0%), married (71.0%), had a low level of education (49.4% primary or less, 32.2% short secondary school) and half earned between 750 and 1,500 Euros per month (Table 2).

Of the 9,294 subjects included in the 3C cohort, 603 were excluded due to missing data in the proxy MNA. Excluded subjects were more frequently women (67.5% vs. 60.3%), older, widowed (35.4% vs. 45.8%), less educated (no education or primary school level: 35.2% vs. 25.6%), had lower income and were in poorer health. The 8,691 remaining subjects had a mean age of 74.1 years (SD 5.5), were mainly females (60.3%), married (59.9%), had a medium level of education (35.7% short secondary school, 38.8% long secondary school and over), and had a medium level of income (59.8% earned more than 1,500 Euros) (Table 2).

Among the 692 subjects of AMI, the standard MNA identified 51 subjects with a poor nutritional status (7.4%, CI 95% 5.4–9.3). Using the proxy MNA, 44 subjects (6.4%, CI 95% 4.6–8.2) were identified as having poor nutritional status. The inter-rater reliability measured by the kappa coefficient showed good

agreement ($\kappa = 0.81$) but was influenced by the low frequency of poor nutritional state; thus, instead we used the AC1 statistics that showed an excellent agreement with a value of 0.97. Using the standard MNA as the gold standard, the proxy MNA sensitivity was estimated to be 76.4% and the specificity to be 99.2%. Due to the imperfect characteristics of the proxy MNA, the Rogan-Gladen estimator was used and the corrected frequency of poor nutritional status was estimated to be 7.4%; hence, similar to that obtained with the standard MNA.

The proxy MNA was applied for the 8,691 subjects of the 3C cohort and 1,284 (14.8%) were identified as having poor nutritional status. The frequency of poor nutritional status using the Rogan-Gladen estimator was estimated to be 18.5%.

The characteristics associated with poor nutritional status were examined in each sample separately (Table 3). In AMI, older age, being widowed, a low BMI, being demented, having a depressive symptomatology, a loss of autonomy and an intake of more than 3 drugs appeared to be significantly associated with a poor nutritional status (p<0.05). In 3C, the similar trends were observed and female gender, a low education level and low income were also significantly associated with poor nutritional status in this cohort. In both cohorts, a low BMI was associated with poor nutritional status. However, poor nutritional status was also observed in overweight subjects (4.2% in AMI vs. 11.0% in 3C among individuals with a BMI greater than 25). The multivariate analyses included gender, marital status, level of education, level of income, BMI, depressive symptomatology (only in 3C), presence of dementia, loss of autonomy and intake of more than 3 drugs (Table 4). In AMI, low BMI, being demented and an intake of more than 3 drugs remained significantly associated with poor nutritional status. In 3C, female gender, marital status, BMI, depressive symptomatology, dementia, loss of autonomy and intake of more than 3 drugs remained significantly associated with poor nutritional status after controlling for other factors.

Discussion

The frequency of poor nutritional status in elderly subjects living at home was estimated in two distinct samples and showed marked differences. The frequency was 7.4% in the rural sample (AMI) and was 18.5% in the urban sample (3C). Although the definition of malnutrition varies across studies, our results were similar to other studies in the community with a prevalence ranging from 7% to 17% [23–26]. A recent meta-analysis showed a prevalence of 37.7% for elderly people at risk of malnutrition or as being malnourished as evaluated by the MNA in community-dwellers [2]. The lower prevalence observed in our subjects may reflect the fact that our subjects were younger and had a higher BMI.

One of the interests of our study was to compare estimates of nutritional status in rural and urban areas. The frequency of malnourished people appeared to be more than twice as high in the urban sample. The different estimates between the two samples may be explained by the different composition of the cohorts. The AMI sample included more males and more often married subjects than the 3C sample, both characteristics associated with a lower risk of poor nutritional status. The AMI subjects have higher BMI. By contrast, participants of the AMI sample had a lower educational level and a lower income, both factors associated with a higher risk of poor nutritional status. Despite the fact that people in rural areas could have a more limited accessibility to shops and less accessible services related to nutrition because of longer distance to cover, this could be offset by greater solidarity between people and socialisation that could lead to higher food intake [27]. Indeed, elderly people in rural

Table 2. Baseline description of the participants in the AMI and 3C cohorts.

	AMI (n = 692)	3C (n = 8,691)
	N (%)	N (%)
Gender		
Males	429 (62.0)	3,454 (39.7)
Females	263 (38.0)	5,237 (60.3)
Age		
65–74	346 (50.0)	5,155 (59.3)
75–84	295 (42.6)	3,141 (36.1)
≥85	51 (7.4)	395 (4.6)
Marital status		
Married	491 (71.0)	5,201 (59.9)
Widower	147 (21.2)	2,253 (25.9)
Single, divorced, separated or other	54 (7.8)	1,234 (14.2)
Education		
Low	342 (49.4)	2,219 (25.6)
Medium	223 (32.2)	3,098 (35.7)
High	127 (18.4)	3,365 (38.8)
Income (Euros)		
<750	64 (9.2)	458 (5.3)
750–1500	364 (52.6)	2,503 (28.8)
1500–2500	120 (17.3)	2,320 (26.7)
≥2500	46 (6.7)	2,874 (33.1)
Don't want to answer	98 (14.2)	536 (6.2)
BMI (kg/m²)		
≤21	15 (2.2)	916 (10.5)
21>BMI<25	155 (22.4)	3,234 (37.2)
25≥BMI<30	319 (46.1)	3,397 (39.1)
≥30	203 (29.3)	1,144 (13.2)
Depressive symptoms		
Yes	15 (2.2)	1,161 (13.4)
No	677 (97.8)	7,530 (86.6)
Dementia		
Yes	39 (5.6)	157 (1.8)
No	653 (94.4)	8,534 (98.2)
Loss of autonomy (ADL)		
Yes	17 (2.5)	78 (0.9)
No	675 (97.5)	8,598 (99.1)
Using> 3 drugs		
Yes	461 (66.9)	5,044 (58.0)
No	228 (33.1)	3,647 (42.0)

Abbreviations: 3C = Three-City study, ADL = Activities Daily Living, BMI = Body Mass Index.

areas were more likely to be obese than those in urban areas [7]. This was also found in our samples and a lower BMI was associated with poor nutritional status after controlling for others factors. Moreover, the AMI sample is not fully representative of people living in a rural area but rather of people who worked in the agricultural sector. They may continue to produce food (eggs, chicken, vegetables …) and have a more diverse diet leading to better nutritional status.

The factors associated with poor nutritional status were in agreement with most of the recent studies conducted on malnutrition showing that older age [26,28–30], gender (being female) [29–33], marital status (widowed) [28,34], lower education [28,35], lower income [5,31], low BMI [26,35], depressive symptoms [25], dementia [24,32], loss of autonomy [32,36] and polymedication [37] were associated with poorer nutritional status. In AMI, gender, marital status, level of education and income were not significantly associated with poor nutritional status,

Table 3. Frequency of poor nutritional status evaluated by the proxy MNA according to baseline characteristics in the AMI and in 3C cohorts.

	AMI		p-value[1]	3C		p-value[1]
	n	Poor nutritional status (n = 44, 6.4%)		n	Poor nutritional status (n = 1284, 14.8%)	
Gender			0.17			<0.0001
Males	429	23 (5.4%)		3,454	338 (9.8%)	
Females	263	21 (8.0%)		5,237	946 (18.1%)	
Age			0.01			<0.0001
65–74	346	13 (3.8%)		5,155	640 (12.4%)	
75–84	295	25 (8.5%)		3,141	542 (17.3%)	
≥85	51	6 (11.8%)		395	102 (25.8%)	
Marital status			0.02			<0.0001
Married	491	23 (4.7%)		5,201	601 (11.6%)	
Widower	147	16 (10.9%)		2,253	469 (20.8%)	
Single, divorced, separated or other	54	5 (9.3%)		1,234	213 (17.3%)	
Education			0.53			<0.0001
Low	342	25 (7.3%)		2,219	375 (16.9%)	
Medium	223	11 (4.9%)		3,098	482 (15.6%)	
High	127	8 (6.3%)		3,365	423 (12.6%)	
Income (Euros)			0.25			<0.0001
<750	64	7 (10.9%)		458	115 (25.1%)	
750–1500	364	26 (7.1%)		2,503	458 (18.3%)	
1500–2500	120	5 (4.2%)		2,320	297 (12.8%)	
≥2500	46	3 (6.5%)		2,874	318 (11.1%)	
Don't want to answer	98	3 (3.1%)		536	96 (17.9%)	
BMI (kg/m²)			<0.0001			<0.0001
≤21	15	8 (53.3%)		916	395 (43.1%)	
21>BMI<25	155	14 (9.0%)		3,234	391 (12.1%)	
25≥BMI<30	319	17 (5.3%)		3,397	335 (9.9%)	
≥30	203	5 (2.5%)		1,144	163 (14.2%)	
Depressive symptoms			<0.0001			<0.0001
Yes	15	15 (100.0%)		1,161	667 (57.4%)	
No	677	29 (4.3%)		7,530	617 (8.2%)	
Dementia			<0.0001			<0.0001
Yes	39	9 (23.1%)		157	58 (36.9%)	
No	653	35 (5.4%)		8,534	1,226 (14.4%)	
Loss of autonomy (ADL)			<0.01			<0.0001
Yes	17	4 (23.5%)		78	42 (53.9%)	
No	675	40 (5.9%)		8,598	1,242 (14.4%)	
Using> 3 drugs			<0.001			<0.0001
Yes	461	41 (8.9%)		5,044	1,043 (20.7%)	
No	228	3 (1.3%)		3,647	241 (6.6%)	

Abbreviations: 3C = Three-City study, ADL = Activities Daily Living, BMI = Body Mass Index, MNA = Mini Nutritional Assessment.
[1]Chi-square test.

probably due to a lack of power, but these factors showed the same trends as the 3C sample.

The prevalence of malnutrition among elderly people is lacking in many studies because investigators did not included a specific tool to measure it, such as the MNA. However, the information to complete the MNA questionnaire was available. An alternative way to solve this problem could be to replace the missing information with other similar available data, as is the case in this study. The use of proxy variables to reconstruct the MNA was feasible and led to good agreement with the original tool. However, the estimations of the frequency of poor nutritional status are potentially under-estimated. First, participants in this analysis were selected since only subjects with no missing data were included. Indeed, in the AMI sample, the standard MNA was

Table 4. Factors associated with poor nutritional status in AMI and 3C cohorts: multivariate logistic regression analysis.

	AMI (n = 689)		p-value[1]	3C (n = 8664)		p-value[1]
	OR	CI 95%		OR	CI 95%	
Gender			0.71			<0.0001
Males	1			1		
Females	0.86	0.38–1.93		1.46	1.22–1.75	
Age			0.50			0.82
65–74	1			1		
75–84	1.61	0.70–3.67		0.98	0.84–1.15	
≥85	1.14	0.31–4.20		1.09	0.79–1.50	
Marital status			0.51			<0.01
Married	1			1		
Widower	1.69	0.66–4.33		1.36	1.12–1.66	
Single, divorced, separated or other	1.59	0.44–5.72		1.18	0.92–1.50	
Education			0.06			0.17
Low	1			1		
Medium	0.40	0.17–0.99		0.89	0.73–1.07	
High	1.41	0.53–3.73		0.82	0.66–1.01	
Income (Euros)			0.21			0.39
<750	1			1		
750–1500	0.73	0.26–2.06		0.84	0.61–1.14	
1500–2500	0.47	0.11–1.99		0.73	0.52–1.03	
≥2500	1.29	0.24–6.99		0.72	0.50–1.04	
Don't want to answer	0.15	0.02–0.89		0.83	0.55–1.26	
BMI (kg/m^2)			<0.0001			<0.0001
≤21	23.09	5.10–104.46		9.11	7.39–11.23	
21>BMI<25	1			1		
25≥BMI<30	0.41	0.18–0.94		0.74	0.61–0.89	
≥30	0.16	0.05–0.50		0.96	0.75–1.22	
Depressive symptoms						<0.0001
No	NA		NA	1		
Yes	NA	NA		20.67	17.46–24.49	
Dementia			0.04			<0.0001
No	1			1		
Yes	3.04	1.08–8.57		3.42	2.22–5.28	
Loss of autonomy (ADL)			0.14			<0.0001
No	1			1		
Yes	3.38	0.68–16.74		6.94	3.91–12.31	
Using>3 drugs			<0.01			<0.0001
No	1			1		
Yes	10.40	2.59–41.69		3.52	2.95–4.20	

Abbreviations: 3C = Three-City study, ADL = Activities Daily Living, BMI = Body Mass Index, MNA = Mini Nutritional Assessment, NA = Not Available, OR = Odds Ratio.
[1]Multivariate logistic regression including all variables presented in this table.

available on 851 subjects for whom the frequency of poor nutritional status was estimated to 9%. When considering only subjects with no missing data to reconstruct the proxy MNA, 692 subjects were included, leading to a frequency of poor nutritional status measured with the standard MNA of 7.4%. Secondly, the proxy MNA lacks sensitivity as it was estimated to be 76.4%, leading to an underestimation of the frequency of poor nutritional status, although the frequency was corrected using the Rogan-Gladen estimator. The lack of sensitivity is mainly due to border effects since subjects considered as having a poor nutritional status according to the standard MNA were close to the threshold when using the proxy MNA. One item (E: neuropsychological problems) is particularly sensitive to misclassification. Indeed, 13.4% of the individuals were considered to be without neuropsychological problems with the proxy MNA (according to the diagnosis of dementia and the MMSE for dementia and CES-D for depressive symptomatology) although they were considered to have moderate neuropsychological problems according to the standard MNA. For this reason, we decided to use another cut-off in the first part of the proxy MNA (increasing the threshold to 12 points) in order to get further information in the second part of the questionnaire and better classify the subjects. In the second part of the questionnaire, no item showed high discordance, but again, a border effect was observed. Indeed, among the 12 subjects considered to have a normal nutritional status with the proxy MNA and considered to have a poor nutritional status with the standard MNA, 8 subjects had a proxy MNA score equal to 24 or 24.5.

In conclusion, poor nutritional status was not uncommon in elderly people living at home in rural or urban areas in southwest France. Practitioners should monitor the nutritional status of their patients in order to participate in the reduction of the prevalence of this disorder and its consequences. Several factors are associated with poor nutritional state and practitioners should be encouraged to develop screening strategies according to these characteristics, even among subjects with a high BMI.

Author Contributions

Conceived and designed the experiments: MJT LL. Performed the experiments: MJT LL. Analyzed the data: MJT LL. Contributed reagents/materials/analysis tools: MJT BD MK CB PBG LL. Contributed to the writing of the manuscript: MJT BD MK CB PBG LL.

References

1. United-Nations (2009) World Population Ageing, New York XXXV/XXXVI. Available: http://www.un.org/esa/population/publications/WPA2009/WPA2009_WorkingPaper.pdf. Accessed 16 June 2014.
2. Kaiser MJ, Bauer JM, Ramsch C, Uter W, Guigoz Y, et al. (2010) Frequency of malnutrition in older adults: a multinational perspective using the mini nutritional assessment. J Am Geriatr Soc 58: 1734–1738.
3. Raynaud-Simon A, Revel-Delhom C, Hebuterne X, French N, Health Program FHHA (2011) Clinical practice guidelines from the French Health High Authority: nutritional support strategy in protein-energy malnutrition in the elderly. Clin Nutr 30: 312–319.
4. Hickson M (2006) Malnutrition and ageing. Postgrad Med J 82: 2–8.
5. Chen CC, Schilling LS, Lyder CH (2001) A concept analysis of malnutrition in the elderly. J Adv Nurs 36: 131–142.
6. Loser C (2010) Malnutrition in hospital: the clinical and economic implications. Dtsch Arztebl Int 107: 911–917.
7. National Center for Health Statistics (2001) Health, United States, 2001 with urban and rural health chartbook. Hyattsville, MD: National Center for Health Statistics.
8. Vellas B, Villars H, Abellan G, Soto ME, Rolland Y, et al. (2006) Overview of the MNA—Its history and challenges. J Nutr Health Aging 10: 456–463; discussion 463–455.
9. Guigoz Y, Vellas B, Garry PJ (1996) Assessing the nutritional status of the elderly: The Mini Nutritional Assessment as part of the geriatric evaluation. Nutr Rev 54: S59–65.
10. Payette H, Shatenstein B (2005) Determinants of healthy eating in community-dwelling elderly people. Can J Public Health 96 Suppl 3: S27–31, S30–25.
11. 3C Study Group (2003) Vascular factors and risk of dementia: design of the Three-City Study and baseline characteristics of the study population. Neuroepidemiology 22: 316–325.
12. Peres K, Matharan F, Allard M, Amieva H, Baldi I, et al. (2012) Health and aging in elderly farmers: the AMI cohort. BMC public health 12: 558.
13. Guigoz Y, Lauque S, Vellas BJ (2002) Identifying the elderly at risk for malnutrition. The Mini Nutritional Assessment. Clin Geriatr Med 18: 737–757.
14. Roberts RE, Vernon SW (1983) The Center for Epidemiologic Studies Depression Scale: its use in a community sample. Am J Psychiatry 140: 41–46.
15. Folstein MF, Folstein SE, McHugh PR (1975) "Mini-mental state". A practical method for grading the cognitive state of patients for the clinician. J Psychiatr Res 12: 189–198.
16. Fuhrer R RF (1989) La version française de l'échelle CES-D (Center for Epidemiologic Studies–Depression Scale). Description et traduction de l'échelle d'auto-évaluation. (French version of the CES-D. Description and translation.). Psychiatr Psychobiol 4: 163–166.
17. Katz S, Ford AB, Moskowitz RW, Jackson BA, Jaffe MW (1963) Studies of Illness in the Aged. The Index of Adl: A Standardized Measure of Biological and Psychosocial Function. JAMA 185: 914–919.
18. Larrieu S, Letenneur L, Berr C, Dartigues JF, Ritchie K, et al. (2004) Sociodemographic differences in dietary habits in a population-based sample of elderly subjects: the 3C study. J Nutr Health Aging 8: 497–502.
19. Gwet KL (2008) Computing inter-rater reliability and its variance in the presence of high agreement. Br J Math Stat Psychol 61: 29–48.
20. Wongpakaran N, Wongpakaran T, Wedding D, Gwet KL (2013) A comparison of Cohen's Kappa and Gwet's AC1 when calculating inter-rater reliability coefficients: a study conducted with personality disorder samples. BMC Med Res Methodol 13: 61.
21. Cohen J (1960) A Coefficient of Agreement for Nominal Scales. Educ Psychol Meas 20: 37–46.
22. Rogan WJ, Gladen B (1978) Estimating prevalence from the results of a screening test. Am J Epidemiol 107: 71–76.
23. Johansson L, Sidenvall B, Malmberg B, Christensson L (2009) Who will become malnourished? A prospective study of factors associated with malnutrition in older persons living at home. J Nutr Health Aging 13: 855–861.
24. Johansson Y, Bachrach-Lindstrom M, Carstensen J, Ek AC (2009) Malnutrition in a home-living older population: prevalence, incidence and risk factors. A prospective study. J Clin Nurs 18: 1354–1364.
25. Iizaka S, Tadaka E, Sanada H (2008) Comprehensive assessment of nutritional status and associated factors in the healthy, community-dwelling elderly. Geriatr Gerontol Int 8: 24–31.
26. Salminen H, Saaf M, Johansson SE, Ringertz H, Strender LE (2006) Nutritional status, as determined by the Mini-Nutritional Assessment, and osteoporosis: a cross-sectional study of an elderly female population. Eur J Clin Nutr 60: 486–493.
27. Locher JL, Robinson CO, Roth DL, Ritchie CS, Burgio KL (2005) The effect of the presence of others on caloric intake in homebound older adults. J Gerontol A Biol Sci Med Sci 60: 1475–1478.
28. Aliabadi M, Kimiagar M, Ghayour-Mobarhan M, Shakeri MT, Nematy M, et al. (2008) Prevalence of malnutrition in free living elderly people in Iran: a cross-sectional study. Asia Pac J Clin Nutr 17: 285–289.
29. Cuervo M, Garcia A, Ansorena D, Sanchez-Villegas A, Martinez-Gonzalez M, et al. (2009) Nutritional assessment interpretation on 22,007 Spanish community-dwelling elders through the Mini Nutritional Assessment test. Public Health Nutr 12: 82–90.
30. Morillas J, Garcia-Talavera N, Martin-Pozuelo G, Reina AB, Zafrilla P (2006) Deteccion del riesgo de desnutricion en ancianos no institucionalizados (Detection of hyponutrition risk in non-institucionalised elderly). Nutr Hosp 21: 650–656.
31. Ferdous T, Kabir ZN, Wahlin A, Streatfield K, Cederholm T (2009) The multidimensional background of malnutrition among rural older individuals in Bangladesh—a challenge for the Millennium Development Goal. Public Health Nutr 12: 2270–2278.
32. Ulger Z, Halil M, Kalan I, Yavuz BB, Cankurtaran M, et al. (2010) Comprehensive assessment of malnutrition risk and related factors in a large group of community-dwelling older adults. Clin Nutr 29: 507–511.
33. Soini H, Routasalo P, Lagstrom H (2005) Nutritional status in cognitively intact older people receiving home care services—a pilot study. J Nutr Health Aging 9: 249–253.
34. Brownie S (2006) Why are elderly individuals at risk of nutritional deficiency? Int J Nurs Pract 12: 110–118.
35. Timpini A, Facchi E, Cossi S, Ghisla MK, Romanelli G, et al. (2011) Self-reported socio-economic status, social, physical and leisure activities and risk for malnutrition in late life: a cross-sectional population-based study. J Nutr Health Aging 15: 233–238.
36. Nykanen I, Lonnroos E, Kautiainen H, Sulkava R, Hartikainen S (2013) Nutritional screening in a population-based cohort of community-dwelling older people. Eur J Public Health 23: 405–409.
37. Pickering G (2004) Frail elderly, nutritional status and drugs. Arch Gerontol Geriatr 38: 174–180.

18

Interrelationship of Postoperative Delirium and Cognitive Impairment and Their Impact on the Functional Status in Older Patients Undergoing Orthopaedic Surgery: A Prospective Cohort Study

Chih-Kuang Liang[1,2,3], Chin-Liang Chu[1,3,4], Ming-Yueh Chou[1,3,5], Yu-Te Lin[1,2,3]*, Ti Lu[4], Chien-Jen Hsu[6], Liang-Kung Chen[3,7]*

1 Center for Geriatrics and Gerontology, Kaohsiung Veterans General Hospital, Kaohsiung, Taiwan, 2 Division of Neurology, Department of Medicine, Kaohsiung Veterans General Hospital Kaohsiung, Taiwan, 3 Aging and Health Research Center, National Yang Ming University, Taipei, Taiwan, 4 Department of Psychiatry, Kaohsiung Veterans General Hospital, Kaohsiung, Taiwan, 5 Department of Family Medicine, Kaohsiung Veterans General Hospital, Kaohsiung, Taiwan, 6 Department of Orthopaedics, Kaohsiung Veterans General Hospital, Kaohsiung, Taiwan, 7 Center for Geriatrics and Gerontology, Taipei Veterans General Hospital, Taipei, Taiwan

Abstract

Background: The impact of postoperative delirium on post-discharge functional status of older patients remains unclear, and little is known regarding the interrelationship between cognitive impairment and post-operative delirium. Therefore, the main purpose was to evaluate the post-discharge functional status of patients who experience delirium after undergoing orthopaedic surgery and the interrelationship of postoperative delirium with underlying cognitive impairment.

Method: This prospective cohort study, conducted at a tertiary care medical center from April 2011 to March 2012, enrolled all subjects aged over 60 years who were admitted for orthopaedic surgery. The baseline characteristics (age, gender, BMI, and living arrangement), surgery-related factors (ASA class, admission type, type of surgery, and length of hospital stay), results of geriatric assessment (postoperative delirium, cognition, depressive mood, comorbidity, pain, malnutrition, polypharmacy, ADL, and instrumental [I]ADL) and 1–12-month postoperative ADL and IADL functional status were collected for analysis.

Results: Overall, 9.1% of 232 patients (mean age: 74.7±7.8 years) experienced postoperative delirium, which was significantly associated with IADL decline at only 6 and 12 months postoperatively (RR: 6.22, 95% CI: 1.08–35.70 and RR: 12.54, 95% CI: 1.88–83.71, respectively). Delirium superimposed on cognitive impairment was a significant predictor for poor functional status at 6 and 12 months postoperatively (RR: 12.80, 95% CI: 1.65–99.40 for ADL at the 6th month, and RR: 7.96, 95% CI: 1.35–46.99 at the 12th month; RR: 13.68, 95% CI: 1.94–96.55 for IADL at the 6th month, and RR: 30.61, 95% CI: 2.94–318.54 at the 12th month, respectively).

Conclusion: Postoperative delirium is predictive of IADL decline in older patients undergoing orthopaedic surgery, and delirium superimposed on cognitive impairment is an independent risk factor for deterioration of ADL and IADL functional status. Early identification of cognitive function and to prevent delirium are needed to improve functional status following orthopaedic surgery.

Editor: Stephen D. Ginsberg, Nathan Kline Institute and New York University School of Medicine, United States of America

Funding: This work was supported by grants from the Veteran Affairs Commission of Taiwan. The funders had no role in study design, data collection and analysis, decision to publish, or preparation of the manuscript.

Competing Interests: The authors have declared that no competing interests exist.

* Email: ytlin@vghks.gov.tw (YTL); lkchen2@vghtpe.gov.tw (LKC)

Introduction

Delirium is an acute mental disorder that is characterized by rapid onset and a fluctuating course of consciousness disturbance and inattention, possibly leading to further adverse health consequences in the elderly population [1]. Although delirium is a well-recognized geriatric syndrome, it is often overlooked by clinicians and nurses [2,3]. The incidence of delirium following orthopaedic surgery has been reported to be 4–65%. Considerable variation is seen and is dependent on the type of procedure, with the reported incidence being 35–65% in patients undergoing operative treatment of a hip fracture and 9–15% in patients undergoing elective orthopaedic procedures [4,5]. Risk factors for the development of postoperative delirium in older patients include older age, cognitive impairment, depressed mood, poor baseline physical function, comorbid diseases, type of surgery, and institutionalization before admission [6–10]. Although delirium is a common geriatric syndrome, its etiopathogenesis remains unclear. However, preventive strategies focused on early identification and management of risk factors are believed to be superior to strategies that emphasize treatment of delirium after it occurs [10–13].

Delirium subsequent to surgery is associated with higher rates of in-hospital and long-term mortality [14–20], as well as longer hospital stay, longer intensive care unit stay, and higher chance of discharge to nursing facilities [14–16,21]. Although the adverse impact of postoperative delirium has been clearly identified, the impact of postoperative delirium on long-term functional status remains unclear. Dementia or cognitive impairment has been reported as an independent risk factor for delirium [10], and the overall incidence of new delirium was significantly higher among older patients with dementia than among older patients with no dementia [22]. Moreover, pre-fracture cognitive impairment and post-fracture delirium were also strongly associated with higher mortality rate and risk for institutionalization [23,24], and delirium might be an early indicator for post-discharge cognitive decline [25,26]. Although it can result in long-term cognitive decline, postoperative cognitive decline secondary to delirium does not occur in all patients [10]. To date, little is known regarding the interrelationship between delirium and cognitive impairment and their impact on adverse functional status in older patients. Therefore, the purpose of the present study was to evaluate the impact of postoperative delirium, in the presence of underlying cognitive impairment, on changes in the post-discharge functional status of patients who underwent orthopaedic surgery.

Methods

Study design

This prospective cohort study was conducted in a tertiary care medical center in Southern Taiwan. All subjects aged 60 years and older who were admitted for orthopaedic surgery during the period April 2011 to March 2012 were screened for this study. Patients were excluded for the following reasons: (1) medical conditions that prevented comprehensive geriatric assessment (CGA), or admission or transfer to an intensive care unit before enrollment, (2) inability to complete the comprehensive geriatric assessment (CGA), (3) inability to provide informed consent, (4) limited life expectancy less than 6 months such as in cancer and terminal stage heart failure cases, (5) delirium occurring before enrollment or surgery, and (6) incomplete data. The study protocol was approved by the Institutional Review Board of Kaohsiung Veterans General Hospital and written informed consents were obtained from all participants before the study started. During a one-year period, a total of 232 patients were enrolled with mean age of 74.7±7.8 years (range: 60–93). Among them, 28 (12.1%) patients were admitted to the hospital from the emergency department. The incidence of postoperative delirium was 9.1% (21/232).

Preoperative evaluation

Demographic data and surgery characteristics. Two research nurses interviewed all participants to collect the preoperative demographic data (including age, gender, educational level, living arrangement, and body mass index [BMI]), and data on other characteristics including admission type (emergency or elective surgery), type of surgery (including spinal decompression only, spinal surgery with instrumented fusion, total knee arthroplasty, other elective knee surgery, elective total hip arthroplasty [total hip replacement]/bipolar hemiarthroplasty, revision hip surgery, and open reduction and internal fixation [ORIF]/arthroplasty for hip fracture), ASA (American Society of Anesthesiologists) physical status, and length of hospital stay.

Comprehensive geriatric assessment (CGA). All participants were assessed by trained research nurses using the CGA before preceding the orthopaedic operation, and within the first 24 hours after hospital admission from the outpatient clinics or emergency department. The assessment covered visual and hearing impairments, polypharmacy (defined as currently using >4 prescription drugs for over 2 weeks), depressive symptoms (using the 15-item Chinese Geriatric Depression Scale) [27,28], nutritional status (as determined by the Mini Nutritional Assessment) [29], comorbidity (as evaluated by the Charlson's Comorbidity Index) [30], symptoms of pain (rated on a Visual Analogue Scale) [31], cognitive function (as assessed by the Chinese version of the Mini-Mental State Examination at admission) [32], the Activities of Daily Living (ADL, evaluated by the Barthel Index) [33], and the Lawton-Brody Instrumental ADL (IADL) [34].

Patients were screened for delirium daily by the primary care nurses in the orthopaedic wards after orthopaedic surgery using the Confusion Assessment Method (CAM) [35], and a senior psychiatrist would confirm the diagnosis if the patient was deemed to be confused. The research nurses obtained ADL and IADL scores by conducting telephone interviews of the participating patients or their primary caregivers at 1, 3, 6, and 12 months after hospital discharge.

Statistical analysis

Continuous data are expressed as means ± SD, and categorical data are expressed as percentages. Dichotomous and ordinal variables were compared in those with and without delirium using the Chi-square test or Fisher exact test, and continuous variables were compared using the independent Student t-test or Mann-Whitney U test when appropriate.

The independent Student t-test or Mann-Whitney U test were used to compare the ADL or IADL scores between groups based on delirium status at 1, 3, 6, and 12 months. The differences in mean ADL and IADL scores between those with and without delirium at different time points were evaluated using the Analysis of Covariance (ANCOVA) with the inclusion of baseline ADL or IADL scores as covariates. To compare functional changes at 1, 3, 6, and 12 months, ADL or IADL functional decline was defined as lower ADL or IADL score at follow-up than at baseline. Multivariable logistic regression analysis was performed to determine whether delirium was an independent predictor of ADL or IADL decline at follow-up. In this model, age, gender, admission type, type of surgery, hearing impairment, polypharmacy, cognitive impairment, depressive symptoms, BMI, high risk of malnutrition, Charlson's Comorbidity Index (CCI), symptoms of pain, ASA class, and hospital length of stay were entered as explanatory variables.

To evaluate the effect of cognitive problems on long-term functional status (ADL and IADL scores at 1, 3, 6, and 12 months follow-up), four categorical variables representing four groups were defined (no cognitive problem [group A]; cognitive impairment alone indicated by MMSE <24 [group B]; postoperative delirium superimposed on cognitive problems [group C], and delirium only [group D]). ANCOVA was used to compare the mean ADL and IADL scores between these four groups after adjusting for baseline ADL and IADL scores (the covariates). The independent effect of each categorical variable on ADL and IADL outcomes was assessed using multivariable logistic regression

Table 1. Demographic data, functional status, and surgery-related factors in 232 subjects with postoperative delirium or no delirium.

Variables	Total N=232 (% or mean ± SD)	Postoperative delirium N=21 (% or mean ± SD)	No delirium N=211 (% or mean ± SD)	p value
Age	74.7±7.8	81.3±5.2	74.1±7.7	<0.001
Educational level	5.8±4.7	6.4±4.6	5.7±4.7	0.522
Gender (male)	108(46.6%)	17(81.0%)	91(43.1%)	0.001
Admission route				0.149
Emergency room	28(12.1%)	5(23.8%)	23(10.9%)	
Outpatient clinic (elective)	204(87.9%)	16(76.2%)	188(89.1%)	
Living				0.035
Alone	32(13.8%)	1(4.8%)	31(14.7%)	
Institutionalized	10(4.3%)	3(14.3%)	7(3.3%)	
With relatives/friends	190(81.9%)	17(81.0%)	173(82.0%)	
BMI	26.5±4.3	23.7±3.2	26.8±4.2	0.001
Polypharmacy (Yes)	106(45.7%)	13(61.9%)	93(44.1%)	0.118
Psychotic drugs (Yes)	36(15.5%)	4(19.0%)	32(15.2%)	0.751
Visual impairment (Yes)	157(67.7%)	18(85.7%)	139(65.9%)	0.064
Hearing impairment (Yes)	38(16.4%)	8(38.1%)	30(14.2%)	0.010
ADL(BI) before admission	94.1±2.3	85.0±19.9	95.0±1.0	0.034
IADL before admission	5.7±1.4	4.4±1.9	5.8±1.3	0.004
Cognitive impairment at admission (MMSE <24)	91(39.2%)	16(76.2%)	75(35.5%)	<0.001
Presence of depressive symptoms (defined by GDS-15>=5)	19(8.2%)	1(4.8%)	18(8.5%)	1.000
Risk of malnutrition (screening by MNA)	19(8.2%)	7(33.3%)	12(5.7%)	<0.001
CCI	0.82±1.07	1.71±1.79	0.73±0.93	0.022
Pain VAS score	4.72±1.58	5.14±1.71	4.68±1.56	0.203
ASA				0.124
ASA 1 and 2	225(97.0%)	19(90.5%)	206(97.6%)	
ASA 3	7(3.0%)	2(9.5%)	5(2.4%)	
Length of hospital stay	8.45±4.46	8.42±4.63	8.76±2.221	0.736
Type of surgery				0.090
Elective spine surgery	60(25.9%)	7(11.7%)	53(88.3%)	
Elective knee surgery	100(43.1%)	6(6.0%)	94(94.0%)	
Elective hip arthroplasty	39(17.7%)	1(2.6%)	38(97.4%)	
ORIF/arthroplasty for hip fracture	33(13.4%)	7(21.2%)	26(78.8%)	

BMI: Body Mass Index; ADL: Activities of Daily Living; BI: Barthel Index; IADL: Instrumental Activities of Daily Living; MMSE: Mini-mental State Examination; GDS: Geriatric Depression Scale; MNA: Mini-nutritional Assessment; CCI: Charlson's Comorbidity Index; VAS: Visual Analogue Scale; ASA: American Society of Anesthesiologists physical status; ORIF: open reduction and internal fixation.
Elective Spine Surgery: Spinal decompression only and Spinal surgery with instrumented fusion.
Elective knee surgery: includes total knee replacement (N=92) and other elective knee surgery (N=8).
Elective hip arthroplasty: includes total hip replacement, bipolar hemiarthroplasty, and revision hip surgery.

analysis after controlling for age, gender, admission type, type of surgery, hearing impairment, polypharmacy, cognitive impairment, depressive symptoms, BMI, high risk of malnutrition, CCI, symptoms of pain, ASA class, and hospital length of stay and baseline IADL or ADL scores as covariates. For all tests, a P value (two-tailed) less than 0.05 was considered statistically significant. All statistical analyses were performed using IBM SPSS version 21 (SPSS Inc., Chicago, IL).

Results

The effect of delirium on functional status

Demographic characteristics of all 232 patients are summarized in Table 1. Fifty of the 232 patients were lost to follow up and therefore excluded from the evaluation of post-discharge functional status. The demographic characteristics of the excluded patients were similar to those of the enrolled patients except for age (77.0±8.7 years vs 74.1±7.4 years, p=0.018) and BMI (25.2±4.5 vs 26.7±4.1 kg/m^2, p=0.015). The number of patients who underwent spinal decompression only, spinal surgery with

Table 2. Comparing the ADL and IADL scores at baseline and 1, 3, 6, and 12 months of follow-up in groups with delirium.

	Time of follow-up (months)								
	Non-adjusted functional status (mean ± SE)					Adjusted baseline functional status by ANCOVA (mean ± SE)			
Outcomes variables	Baseline	1	3	6	12	1	3	6	12
ADL (BI) scores (mean ± SE)									
Delirium (N = 17)	85.9±4.81#	77.9±5.25#	79.4±5.62#	81.8±5.44#	81.8±5.86#	83.0±2.82#	84.5±2.77#	86.9±3.06#	86.4±3.18#
No delirium (N = 165)	95.6±0.80	93.2±0.93	94.9±0.89	95.2±1.00	95.6±0.99	92.7±0.88	94.4±0.87	94.6±0.96	95.2±1.00
IADL scores (mean ± SE)									
Delirium (N = 17)	4.4±0.40#	3.4±0.45#	3.4±0.47#	3.2±0.53#	2.9±0.53#	4.4±0.28#	4.4±0.28#	4.3±0.33#	4.0±0.33#
No delirium (N = 165)	5.8±0.09	5.3±0.11	5.6±0.11	5.6±0.12	5.7±0.12	5.2±0.09	5.5±0.09	5.5±0.10	5.6±0.10

#p<0.05 for comparing groups by delirium status. ANCOVA: Analysis of Covariance.

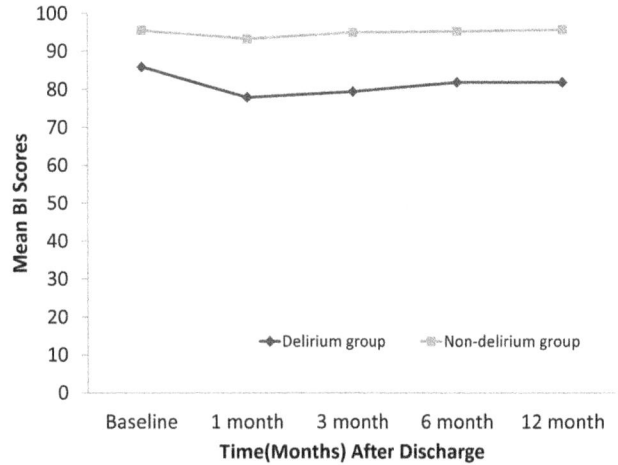

Figure 1. The trend of Barthel Index scores (ADL) (a) and IADL (b) for the delirium and no delirium groups.

instrumented fusion, total knee arthroplasty, other elective knee surgery, elective total hip replacement/bipolar hemiarthroplasty, revision hip surgery, and ORIF/arthroplasty for hip fracture was 7 (3.0%), 53 (22.8%), 92 (39.7%), 8 (3.4%), 31 (13.4%), 8 (3.4%), and 33 (14.2%), respectively. These procedures were grouped into four categories (elective spine surgery, elective knee surgery, elective hip arthroplasty, and ORIF/arthroplasty for hip fracture) for further analysis. Comparing the 50 patients lost to follow up with the 182 included patients, the delirium occurred in a similar proportion of both groups (8.0% [4/50] vs 9.3% [17/182]; data not shown), indicating that delirium did not increase the likelihood of loss to follow up.

At baseline, the 182 enrolled subjects (17 with delirium and 165 without delirium) had an ADL score of 85.9 (standard error [SE] = 4.81) vs 95.6 ([SE] = 0.80) and an IADL score of 4.4 ([SE] = 0.40) vs 5.8 ([SE] = 0.09; Table 2). Figure 1 shows the change in ADL and IADL scores over time after hospitalization for both groups. ADL and IADL scores were significantly different between those who developed post-operative delirium and those who did not. When controlling for baseline ADL, IADL scores remained significantly lower in patients who developed postoperative delirium than in those who did not. Table 3 shows the differences in ADL and IADL decline between the two groups at different follow-up times. Results of univariate logistic regression analysis identified delirium as a predictor of ADL decline at 6 and 12 months (p value: 0.036 vs 0.014), and IADL decline at 3, 6, and 12 months after surgery (p value: 0.033 vs 0.005 vs 0.001). In addition, multivariable logistic regression analysis identified delirium as a predictor of only IADL decline at 6 and 12 months (for IADL at 6 months, adjusted RR: 6.22, 95% CI:1.08–35.70, p value = 0.040; for IADL at 12 months, adjusted RR: 12.54, 95% CI: 1.88–83.71, p value = 0.009).

Impact of combined cognitive problems on functional status

The 182 included patients were divided into four groups based on delirium and cognitive status. The patients in group D (with delirium, but without baseline cognitive impairment) were excluded because of small sample size (N = 4). Baseline ADL and IADL scores were significantly different between patients with no cognitive problems (group A), and those with both baseline cognitive dysfunction and delirium (group C) or with baseline

Table 3. Analysis of the percentage of functional decline and the predicted effect on functional status in groups divided by delirium status using Chi-square test and multivariable logistic regression.

	Percentage of functional decline						Predicted effect on functional decline											
	ADL decline			IADL decline			RR of delirium for ADL decline						RR of delirium for IADL decline					
	Delirium	No delirium		Delirium	No delirium		Unadjusted			Adjusted			Unadjusted			Adjusted		
Follow-up times	N(%)	N(%)	p value	N(%)	N(%)	p value	RR	95% CI	p value	RR	95% CI	p value	RR	95% CI	p value	RR	95% CI	p value
1-month	8/17(47.1)	46/165(27.9)	0.099	6/13(46.2%)	59/165(35.8)	0.380	2.30	0.84–6.32	0.107	2.45	0.60–9.99	0.210	2.02	0.74–5.52	0.170	1.84	0.47–7.12	0.380
3-month	5/17(29.4)	25/165(15.2)	0.164	6/13(46.2%)	45/165(27.3)	0.164	2.33	0.76–7.20	0.141	1.85	0.36–9.68	0.465	3.00	1.09–8.25	0.033	2.75	0.66–11.47	0.164
6-month	6/15(40.0)	27/160(16.9)	0.040	7/13(53.8)	41/165(24.8)	0.040	3.28	1.08–9.99	0.036	3.68	0.64–21.18	0.144	4.32	1.55–12.08	0.005	6.22	1.08–35.70	0.040
12-month	7/17(41.2)	26/165(15.8)	0.017	8/13(61.5)	39/165(23.6)	0.009	3.74	1.31–10.72	0.014	3.55	0.70–17.91	0.125	5.92	2.06–17.06	0.001	12.54	1.88–83.71	0.009

Covariates after adjusting for ADL: age, gender, admission type, type of surgery, hearing impairment, polypharmacy, MMSE scores, GDS-15 scores, BMI, risk of malnutrition, CCI scores, ASA physical status, length of hospital stay, baseline IADL scores.

Covariates after adjusting for IADL: age, gender, admission type, type of surgery, hearing impairment, polypharmacy, MMSE scores, GDS-15 scores, BMI, risk of malnutrition, CCI scores, pain VAS scores, ASA physical status, length of hospital stay, baseline ADL scores.

Table 4. Comparing the ADL and IADL scores at baseline and 1, 3, 6, and 12 months of follow-up in groups divided on the basis of cognitive problems.

	Time of follow-up (months)								
	Non-adjusted functional status (mean ± SE)					Adjusted baseline functional status by ANCOVA (mean ± SE)			
Outcomes variables	Baseline	1	3	6	12	1	3	6	12
ADL (BI) scores (mean ± SE) [a,b]									
Non-cognitive problems (A), N = 109	97.2±0.71*,$	94.2±1.10*	95.8±1.05*	96.3±1.00*	96.8±0.89*	93.0±1.10*	94.5±1.08*	95.0±1.19*	95.6±1.24*
Cognitive impairment alone (B), N = 56	92.4±1.85$	91.3±1.68$	93.2±1.62#	92.9±2.19#	93.4±2.32#	92.6±1.53#	94.6±1.51#	94.4±1.66#	94.8±1.72#
Delirium superimposed on cognitive impairment (C), N = 13	87.3±5.36*	77.7±6.01*,#	78.5±6.76*,#	79.6±6.83*,#	79.2±7.42*,#	81.8±3.21*,#	82.7±3.16*,#	84.2±3.47*,#	83.3±3.61*,#
IADL scores (mean ± SE) [a,b]									
Non-cognitive problems (A), N = 109	6.1±0.09*,$	5.7±0.14*,$	5.8±0.13*,$	5.9±0.14*,$	6.0±0.14*,$	5.4±0.11*	5.5±0.11*	5.6±0.13*	5.7±0.13*
Cognitive impairment alone (B), N = 56	5.3±0.20#,$	4.7±0.20#,$	5.0±0.21#,$	5.0±0.22#,$	5.1±0.22#,$	5.0±0.15#	5.4±0.15#	5.3±0.18#	5.4±0.18#
Delirium superimposed on cognitive impairment (C), N = 13	4.3±0.47*,#	3.3±0.49*,#	3.2±0.51*,#	3.1±0.60*,#	2.7±0.58*,#	4.4±0.32*,#	4.4±0.32*,#	4.2±0.38*,#	3.7±0.38*,#

*p<0.05 for comparing C and A; #p<0.05 for comparing C and B; $p<0.05 for comparing A and B.

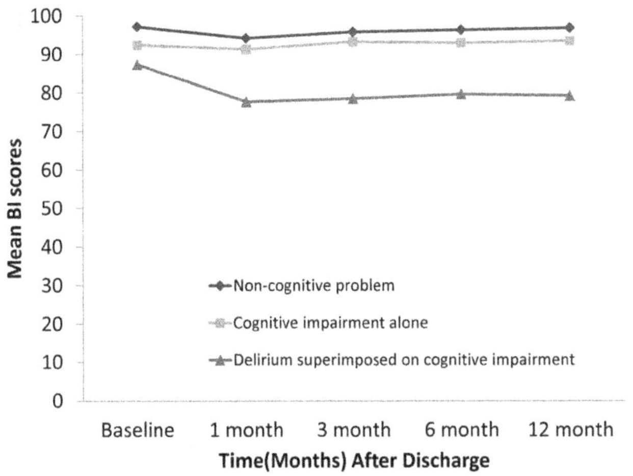

Figure 2. The trend of Barthel Index scores (ADL) (a) and IADL (b) for three groups corresponding to non-cognitive problem, cognitive impairment alone, and delirium superimposed on cognitive impairment.

cognitive dysfunction only (group B; Table 4). In terms of the decline in ADL and IADL scores at 1, 3, 6, and 12 months of follow up, ANCOVA (after adjustment for baseline ADL and IADL values) found significant ADL and IADL decline only in group C (Figure 2). After controlling for confounders (Table 5), multivariable logistic regression still showed the tendency for ADL and IADL to decline in patients in group C at 6 and 12 months (Adjusted RR for ADL at 6 months: 12.80, 95% CI: 1.65–99.40; Adjusted RR for ADL at 12 months: 7.96, 95% CI: 1.35–46.99; Adjusted RR for IADL at 6 months: 13.68, 95% CI: 1.94–96.55; Adjusted RR for IADL at 12 months: 30.61, 95% CI: 2.94–318.54).

Discussion

This prospective study investigated the effects of postoperative delirium on functional status (defined as decline in ADL and IADL scores) in patients who underwent orthopaedic surgery, and examined the interrelationship between underlying cognitive impairment and post-operative delirium. Postoperative delirium was an important predictor for poor IADL but not for poor ADL results. Moreover, delirium superimposed on cognitive problems was a stronger predictor of poor post-discharge functional status than cognitive impairment alone. The risk factors for the development of postoperative delirium identified in this study were in agreement with those identified by previous studies [6–10]. However, the incidence of postoperative delirium was lower in the present study than in previous studies, and the difference might be attributed to the higher percentage of elective surgery patients in our study (elective vs emergency surgery: 87.9% vs 12.1%). Moreover, patients in critical condition and unable to give their informed consent, such as some demented patients, were excluded from our study, thereby reducing the incidence of postoperative delirium.

Postoperative delirium had a strong adverse impact on IADL score after controlling for common geriatric problems, comorbidity, polypharmacy, and surgery-related conditions. A previous study reported that delirium had no significant effect on ADL score 6 months after surgery and attributed the relationship between delirium and mortality to some significant underlying medical problems [36]. An association between postoperative

Table 5. Multivariable logistic regression analysis of the predicted effect on functional status at the 6 and 12-month follow-up in groups divided on the basis of cognitive problems.

Independent variables	ADL decline at 6 months Unadjusted RR	95% CI	Adjusted RR	95% CI	ADL decline at 12 months Unadjusted RR	95% CI	Adjusted RR	95% CI	IADL decline at 6 months Unadjusted RR	95% CI	Adjusted RR	95% CI	IADL decline at 12 months Unadjusted RR	95% CI	Adjusted RR	95% CI
Cognitive impairment only (B) vs non-cognitive problem (A)	1.44	0.62–3.36	1.50	0.52–4.39	1.04	0.43–2.50	0.99	0.32–3.06	1.54	0.73–3.20	1.95	0.79–4.78	1.5	0.71–3.14	1.88	0.76–4.66
Delirium superimposed on cognitive impairment (C) vs non-cognitive problem (A)	6.75&	1.84–24.78	12.80*	1.65–99.40	6.31&	1.89–21.11	7.96*	1.35–46.99	4.13*	1.27–13.46	13.68&	1.94–96.55	5.98&	1.79–20.03	30.61&	2.94–318.54

*p<0.05, &p<0.01.
Covariates after adjusting for ADL: age, gender, admission type, type of surgery, hearing impairment, polypharmacy, GDS-15 scores, BMI, risk of malnutrition, CCI scores, pain VAS scores, ASA physical status, length of hospital stay, baseline IADL scores.
Covariates after adjusting for IADL: age, gender, admission type, type of surgery, hearing impairment, polypharmacy, GDS-15 scores, BMI, risk of malnutrition, CCI scores, pain VAS scores, ASA physical status, length of hospital stay, baseline ADL scores.

delirium and change in functional status at the time of hospital discharge and/or during follow up has also been shown in past studies [37–39]. However, the focus of most of these studies is short-term functional status. Although Vida et al. reported that delirium had an adverse effect on long-term IADL functional status 18 months after hospitalization, the effect disappeared after controlling for confounders [40]. In contrast to our results showing a relationship of postoperative delirium to IADL functional decline, those of Edelstein et al. demonstrated that decline in basic ADL but not IADL at 1-year follow-up was more likely in hip fracture surgery patients with postoperative delirium [41]. All the patients in the study by Edelstein et al. underwent hip fracture surgery, which has a greater impact on postoperative delirium and functional status than elective orthopaedic surgery. Furthermore, our study placed more emphasis on geriatric problems as confounders, e.g., malnutrition, polypharmacy, mood status, and symptoms of pain, which impact the risk of postoperative delirium as well as postoperative function. To the best of our knowledge, this is the first study to demonstrate the adverse impact of postoperative delirium on post-discharge ADL and IADL functional status after controlling for most geriatric problems considered as potential confounders. The adverse impact of postoperative delirium in this study was more profound on the IADL than ADL score. The baseline ADL scores for patients developing postoperative delirium and not developing postoperative delirium (85.9 ± 4.81 and 95.6 ± 0.80, respectively) indicated only mild impairment. It implied that the adverse effect of postoperative delirium might be reduced in robust elderly patients. Moreover, the predictive effect of delirium on IADL functional status was only noted 6 and 12 months after surgery. Therefore, factors other than delirium might have a greater effect on short-term functional status of elderly patients undergoing orthopaedic surgery.

Although delirium alone is not predictive for ADL decline during follow-up (after adjusting for confounders such as MMSE), delirium superimposed on cognitive impairment was significantly associated with ADL and IADL decline after surgery. In addition, postoperative delirium was more likely to develop in patients with severe cognitive impairment than in patients with moderate cognitive impairment (mean MMSE scores: group A 26.7 ± 1.8 vs group B 19.8 ± 3.8 vs group C 16.0 ± 4.2). Underlying cognitive impairment (MMSE score <24) alone was not associated with postoperative ADL and IADL decline. The effects of severe cognitive impairment and postoperative delirium were highly interactive. Recovery from postoperative functional impairment by elderly patients undergoing orthopaedic surgery was dependent on the cognitive ability to adhere to rehabilitation programs. Givens et al. reported that each additional cognitive or mood disorder was associated with a greater risk of poor functional status [42]. Therefore, the results of this current study not only confirm the need to identify patients at risk for postoperative delirium, but also the highly interactive nature of the effects of baseline cognitive impairment and superimposed delirium on both ADL and IADL decline.

Despite the effort put into it, this study has several limitations. First, 21.6% (50/232) of the study subjects did not complete follow-up interviews. It has been reported that patients who experience delirium are more likely to miss follow-up appointments [43]. Although the incidence of delirium and the demographic data were similar between patients who completed follow-up and those who did not, there may still be a high risk of systematic attrition bias. Followed-up patients may have poorer clinical outcomes, therefore, the impact of delirium on long-term functional status may be underestimated in these patients. Second, the incidence of postoperative delirium was lower in our study than in previously published studies. Though delirium in this study was detected by the CAM and confirmed by a senior psychiatrist, who avoided overestimation, underestimation was still possible because we excluded patients who were admitted or transferred to ICU or unable to give informed consent, e.g., demented patients. Third, although the baseline cognitive function (assessed on admission before orthopaedic surgery) may be influenced by fracture or pain and lead to overestimation of cognitive impairment, it was not a predictor of ADL and IADL decline in our studies. Fourth, use of a wide range of procedures (performed within a single anatomic region) will impact both the risk of delirium as well as postoperative functional status. Because there were few patients undergoing operations, such as spinal decompression only, other elective knee surgery, and revision hip surgery, we treated similar types of surgery as single covariates, grouping them into four categories (elective spine surgery, elective knee surgery, elective hip arthroplasty, and ORIF/arthroplasty for hip fracture). Further work is needed to investigate the link between postoperative delirium and functional status in patients undergoing orthopaedic surgery at single operative site.

In conclusion, this prospective study evaluated the impact of different cognitive factors on ADL and IADL decline in elderly people undergoing orthopaedic surgery, and it was noted that delirium superimposed on cognitive impairment strongly affects both long-term ADL and IADL functional status. Early identification of patients with baseline cognitive impairment and implementation of strategies to prevent delirium may reduce the likelihood of functional decline following orthopaedic surgery in older patients. Further study is needed to confirm this.

Acknowledgments

Our local Institutional Review Board approved the present study protocol. The study was supported by the Veteran Affairs Commission of Taiwan. All authors declare no conflicts of interest.

The authors would like to thank all staff in the Orthopaedic Department for their valuable assistance in collecting the delirium symptom data. We also wish to thank Mr. Zhao-Rong Li, Associate Professor, Department of Business Management, National Kaohsiung Normal University, for his statistical assistance.

Author Contributions

Conceived and designed the experiments: CKL CLC YTL LKC. Performed the experiments: CKL CLC MYC TL CJH. Analyzed the data: CKL CLC LKC. Contributed reagents/materials/analysis tools: CLC MYC TL CJH. Wrote the paper: CKL YTL LKC.

References

1. Inouye SK (2006) Delirium in older persons. N Engl J Med 354: 1157–1165.
2. Élie M, Rousseau F, Cole M, Primeau F, McCusker J, et al. (2000) Prevalence and detection of delirium in elderly emergency department patients. CMAJ 163(8): 977–981.
3. Inouye SK, Foreman MD, Mion LC, Katz KH, Cooney LM Jr (2001) Nurses' recognition of delirium and its symptoms: comparison of nurse and researcher ratings. Arch Intern Med 161(20): 2467–2473.
4. Rudolph JL, Marcantonio ER (2011) Review articles: postoperative delirium: acute change with long-term implications. Anesth Analg 112: 1202–1211.
5. Gustafson Y, Berggren D, Brännström B, Bucht G, Norberg A, et al. (1988) Acute confusional states in elderly patients treated for femoral neck fracture. J Am Geriatr Soc 36: 525–530.
6. Schor JD, Levkoff SE, Lipsitz LA, Reilly CH, Cleary PD, et al. (1992) Risk factors for delirium in hospitalized elderly. JAMA 267: 827–831.

7. Levkoff SE, Evans DA, Liptzin B, Cleary PD, Lipsitz LA, et al. (1992) Delirium. The occurrence and persistence of symptoms among elderly hospitalized patients. Arch Intern Med 152: 334–340.

8. Wu CH, Chang CI, Chen CY (2012) Overview of studies related to geriatric syndrome in Taiwan. J Clin Gerontol Geriatr 3: 14–20.

9. Pompei P, Foreman M, Rudberg MA, Inouye SK, Braund V, et al. (1994) Delirium in hospitalized older persons: outcomes and predictors. J Am Geriatr Soc 42: 809–815.

10. Sanders RD, Pandharipande PP, Davidson AJ, Ma D, Maze M (2011) Anticipating and managing postoperative delirium and cognitive decline in adults. BMJ 343: d4331.

11. Chu CL, Liang CK, Lin YT, Chow PC, Pan CC, et al. (2011) Biomarkers of delirium: Well evidenced or not? J Clin Gerontol Geriatr 2: 100–104.

12. Inouye SK, Bogardus ST Jr, Charpentier PA, Leo-Summers L, Acampora D, et al. (1999) A multicomponent intervention to prevent delirium in hospitalized older patients. N Engl J Med 340: 669–676.

13. Marcantonio ER, Flacker JM, Wright RJ, Resnick NM (2001) Reducing delirium after hip fracture: a randomized trial. J Am Geriatr Soc 49: 516–522.

14. Rudolph JL, Jones RN, Rasmussen LS, Silverstein JH, Inouye SK, et al. (2007) Independent vascular and cognitive risk factors for postoperative delirium. Am J Med 120: 807–813.

15. Norkiene I, Ringaitiene D, Misiuriene I, Samalavicius R, Bubulis R, et al. (2007) Incidence and precipitating factors of delirium after coronary artery bypass grafting. Scand Cardiovasc J 41: 180–185.

16. Marcantonio ER, Flacker JM, Michaels M, Resnick NM (2000) Delirium is independently associated with poor functional recovery after hip fracture. J Am Geriatr Soc 48: 618–624.

17. Robinson TN, Raeburn CD, Tran ZV, Angles EM, Brenner LA, et al. (2009) Postoperative delirium in the elderly: risk factors and outcomes. Ann Surg 249: 173–178.

18. Koster S, Hensens AG, van der Palen J (2009) The long-term cognitive and functional outcomes of postoperative delirium after cardiac surgery. Ann Thorac Surg 87: 1469–1474.

19. Gottesman RF, Grega MA, Bailey MM, Pham LD, Zeger SL, et al. (2010) Delirium after coronary artery bypass graft surgery and late mortality. Ann Neurol 67: 338–344.

20. Lundstrom M, Edlund A, Bucht G, Karlsson S, Gustafson Y (2003) Dementia after delirium in patients with femoral neck fractures. J Am Geriatr Soc 51: 1002–1006.

21. Witlox J, Eurelings LS, de Jonghe JF, Kalisvaart KJ, Eikelenboom P, et al. (2010) Delirium in elderly patients and the risk of postdischarge mortality, institutionalization, and dementia: a meta-analysis. JAMA 304: 443–451.

22. Fick DM, Steis MR, Waller JL, Inouye SK (2013) Delirium superimposed on dementia is associated with prolonged length of stay and poor outcomes in hospitalized older adults. J Hosp Med 8: 500–505.

23. Steiner JF, Kramer AM, Eilertsen TB Kowalsky JC (1997) Development and validation of a clinical prediction rule for prolonged nursing home residence after hip fracture. J Am Geriatr Soc 45: 1510–1514.

24. Holmes J, House A (2000) Psychiatric illness predicts poor outcome after surgery for hip fracture: A prospective cohort study. Psychol Med 30: 921–929.

25. Francis J, Kapoor WN (1992) Prognosis after hospital discharge of older medical patients with delirium. J Am Geriatr Soc 40: 601–606.

26. Koponen H, Stenbäck U, Mattila E, Soininen H, Reinikainen K, et al. (1989) Delirium among elderly persons admitted to a psychiatric hospital: clinical course during the acute stage and one-year follow-up. Acta Psychiatr Scand 79: 579–585.

27. Liao YC, Yeh TL, Ko HC, Luoh CM, Lu HF (1995) Geriatric depression scale (GDS) – a preliminary report of reliability and validity for Chinese version. Changhua Med J 1; 11–17. (in Chinese)

28. Nyunt MS, Fones C, Niti M, Ng TP (2009) Criterion-based validity and reliability of the Geriatric Depression Screening Scale (GDS-15) in a large validation sample of community-living Asian older adults. Aging Ment Health 13: 376–382.

29. Kaiser MJ, Bauer JM, Ramsch C, Uter W, Guigoz Y, et al. (2009) Validation of the Mini Nutritional Assessment Short-Form (MNA-SF): a practical tool for identification of nutritional status. J Nutr Health Aging 13: 782–788.

30. Charlson ME, Pompei P, Ales KL, MacKenzie CR (1987) A new method of classifying prognostic comorbidity in longitudinal studies: development and validation. J Chronic Dis 40: 373–383.

31. Huskisson EC (1974) Measurement of pain. Lancet 2(7889): 1127–1131.

32. Folstein MF, Folstein SE, McHugh PR (1975) Mini-mental status: a practical method for grading the cognitive state of patients for the clinical use. J Psychiatr Res 12: 189–198.

33. Collin C, Wade DT, Davies S, Horne V (1988) "The Barthel ADL Index: a reliability study." Int Disability Study 10: 61–63.

34. Lawton MP, Brody EM (1969) Assessment of older people: Self-maintaining and instrumental activities of daily living. The Gerontologist 9: 179–186.

35. Inouye SK, Van Dyck CH, Alessi CA, Balkin S, Siegal AP, et al. (1990) Clarifying confusion: the confusion assessment method. A new method for detection of delirium. Ann Intern Med 113: 941–948.

36. Francis J, Kapoor WN (1990) Delirium in hospitalized elderly. J Gen Intern Med 5: 65–79.

37. Inouye SK, Rushing JT, Foreman MD, Palmer RM, Pompei P (1998) Does delirium contribute to poor hospital outcomes? A three-site epidemiologic study. J Gen Intern Med 13: 234–242.

38. Marcantonio ER, Flacker JM, Michaels M, Resnick NM (2000) Delirium is independently associated with poor functional recovery after hip fracture. J Am Geriatr Soc 48: 618–624.

39. Quinlan N, Rudolph JL (2011) Postoperative delirium and functional decline after noncardiac surgery. J Am Geriatr Soc 59 Suppl 2: S301–304.

40. Vida S, Galbaud du Fort G, Kakuma R, Arsenault L, Platt RW, et al. (2006) An 18-month prospective cohort study of functional outcome of delirium in elderly patients: activities of daily living. Int Psychogeriatr 18: 681–700.

41. Edelstein DM, Aharonoff GB, Karp A, Capla EL, Zuckerman JD, et al. (2004) Effect of postoperative delirium on outcome after hip fracture. Clin Orthop Relat Res (422): 195–200.

42. Givens JL, Sanft TB, Marcantonio ER (2008) Functional recovery after hip fracture: the combined effects of depressive symptoms, cognitive impairment, and delirium. J Am Geriatr Soc 56: 1075–1079.

43. Rudolph JL, Marcantonio ER, Culley DJ, Silverstein JH, Rasmussen LS, et al. (2008) Delirium is associated with early postoperative cognitive dysfunction. Anaesthesia 63: 941–947.

19

Recipient-Related Risk Factors for Graft Failure and Death in Elderly Kidney Transplant Recipients

Xingqiang Lai[9], **Guodong Chen**[9], **Jiang Qiu, Changxi Wang, Lizhong Chen***

Organ Transplant Center, The First Affiliated Hospital, Sun Yat-sen University, Guangzhou, China

Abstract

Background: Elderly patients with end-stage renal disease have become the fastest growing population of kidney transplant candidates in recent years. However, the risk factors associated with long-term outcomes in these patients remain unclear.

Methods: We retrospectively analyzed 166 recipients aged 60 years or older who underwent primary deceased kidney transplantation between 2002 and 2013 in our center. The main outcomes included 1-, 3- and 5-year patient survival as well as overall and death-censored graft survival. The independent risk factors affecting graft and patient survival were analyzed using Cox regression analysis.

Results: The 1-, 3-, 5-year death-censored graft survival rates were 93.6%, 89.4% and 83.6%, respectively. Based on the Cox multivariate analysis, panel reactive antibody (PRA)>5% [hazard ratio (HR) 4.295, 95% confidence interval (CI) 1.321–13.97], delayed graft function (HR 4.744, 95% CI 1.611–13.973) and acute rejection (HR 4.971, 95% CI 1.516–16.301) were independent risk factors for graft failure. The 1-, 3-, 5-year patient survival rates were 84.8%, 82.1% and 77.1%, respectively. Longer dialysis time (HR 1.011 for 1-month increase, 95% CI 1.002–1.020), graft loss (HR 3.501, 95% CI 1.559–7.865) and low-dose ganciclovir prophylaxis (1.5 g/d for 3 months) (HR 3.173, 95% CI 1.063–9.473) were risk factors associated with patient death.

Conclusions: The five-year results show an excellent graft and patient survival in elderly kidney transplant recipients aged ≥ 60 years. PRA>5%, delayed graft function, and acute rejection are risk factors for graft failure, while longer duration of dialysis, graft loss and low-dose ganciclovir prophylaxis are risk factors for mortality in elderly recipients. These factors represent potential targets for interventions aimed at improving graft and patient survival in elderly recipients.

Editor: Stanislaw Stepkowski, University of Toledo, United States of America

Funding: This study was supported by the 5010 Clinical Research Project of Sun Yat-sen University (2007003) and the National Natural Science Fund Youth Science project (81302549). The funders had no role in study design, data collection and analysis, decision to publish, or preparation of the manuscript.

Competing Interests: The authors have declared that no competing interests exist.

* Email: clz@medmail.com.cn

9 These authors contributed equally to this work.

Introduction

Kidney transplantation is considered to be the best treatment option for patients with end-stage renal disease (ESRD), regardless of their age. Currently, the mean age of patients undergoing renal transplantation has increased. This trend is observed not only in western countries such as America but also in Asian countries. Patients ≥60 years with ESRD have become the fastest growing population of wait-listed individuals and kidney transplant candidates [1,2]. Over the last decade, both the absolute number and percent of transplants performed in patients aged ≥65 years have approximately doubled [1]. Previous studies have reported that elderly ESRD patients after kidney transplantation have lower mortality rates and improved quality of life compared with those who remain on dialysis treatment [3,4,5].

However, despite the known benefits of kidney transplantation over dialysis in the elderly patients, long-term outcomes of the recipients and their grafts are still limited [6]. Given the rapid increase in the number of senior renal transplant candidates combined with a growing shortage of donor kidneys, it is increasingly important to optimize the long-term outcomes in the elderly recipients. The characteristics of the elderly patients at transplantation may have an important impact on graft and patient survival. Published studies regarding the recipient factors that predict outcomes in elderly recipients are limited, especially in China. Accurately determining the possible predictors involved in graft and patient survival is crucial for improving long-term outcomes in elderly recipients.

Therefore, the aim of this study was to evaluate graft and patient survival in kidney transplant recipients aged ≥60 years and to determine the possible recipient-related risk factors associated with clinical outcome.

Patients and Methods

This retrospective cohort study was approved by the Institutional Review Board/Ethics Committee of The First Affiliated Hospital of Sun Yat-sen University, and all aspects of the study complied with the Helsinki Declaration of 1975. The Ethics Committee of The First Affiliated Hospital of Sun Yat-sen University specifically approved that not informed consent was required because all data were going to be analyzed anonymously. All of the organs were from donation after brain death (DBD) or donation after cardiac death (DCD), and all of the organ donors had provided informed written consent. No prisoner organs were used in this study.

All patients aged 60 years or older who underwent first-time kidney transplantation from deceased donors in our center between January 2002 and June 2013 were collected. We excluded patients who had received another organ besides the kidney. The recipient characteristics included age, gender, causes of ESRD, pre-transplant comorbidities [including diabetes mellitus, hypertension, coronary artery disease (CAD)], type and time on dialysis, and panel reactive antibody (PRA) level at transplantation. The induction agents, basic maintained immunosuppressive regimens, and regimens for cytomegalovirus (CMV) prophylaxis were also recorded. After surgery, the number and frequency of adverse events including delayed graft function (DGF), acute rejection (AR) and chronic rejection (CR) at any time, leucopenia, infectious events, graft loss and patient death, malignancy and other new onset diseases were recorded. The causes of graft failure and mortality were also recorded.

Patients received IL-2 receptor antagonist (IL2RA, including basiliximab or daclizumab) or rabbit anti-thymocyte globulin (rATG) as induction agents. The maintained immunosuppressive regimens consisted of cyclosporine or tacrolimus, mycophenolate mofetil (MMF) and prednisone. From 2002 to 2006, most of the recipients received a low-dose ganciclovir (1.5 g/d for 3 months) for CMV prophylaxis, whereas patients mainly received a high-dose ganciclovir (3.0 g/d for 3 months) since 2007. Sulfamethoxazole was administered orally for 3 months for Pneumocystis jirovecii pneumonia prophylaxis.

DGF was defined as the need for dialysis in the first week after transplantation. AR was diagnosed based on clinical manifestations such as fever, oliguria, and serum creatinine elevation of > 25% from the baseline value and was confirmed by a subsequent renal allograft biopsy. Biopsy-proven acute rejections (BPAR) included all acute rejections which were graded borderline or higher by Banff'97 criteria. CR was diagnosed by clinical findings with a decrease in kidney function and developing a gradual rise in serum creatinine, and was confirmed by renal allograft biopsy with histological features including thickening of the intima of arterioles and arteries, sclerosis of glomeruli, and tabular atrophy.

Statistical analysis

All data were analyzed by SPSS for Windows Version 19.0 (SPSS, Chicago, Illinois, USA). Continuous variables are expressed as counts and percentages, and categorical variables are expressed as the means with standard deviations (mean ± SD). Actuarial graft and patient survival were calculated using Kaplan–Meier analysis. To assess variables associated with transplant outcome, univariate and multivariate Cox proportional hazards regression models were employed. The association between outcomes and all co-variables were tested separately in univariate Cox analyses. To evaluate the potential independent risk factors for transplant outcomes, all variables associated with graft loss or patient death at a $P<0.2$ level in the univariate Cox analysis were

included in the final multivariate model. A P-value <0.05 was considered to indicate statistical significance.

Results

Patient characteristics

We collected data from 166 primary deceased kidney transplant recipients aged 60 or older between January 2002 and June 2013. The demographic and baseline characteristics of these elderly patients are shown in Table 1. The mean recipient age was 64.6 ± 3.8 years, and 109 (65.7%) recipients were male. The main cause of ESRD was chronic glomerulonephritis, followed by diabetes mellitus. Hypertension was the most prevalent comorbidity in these aged recipients. The mean duration of dialysis was 18.6 ± 22.1 months. Initial immunosuppressive induction therapy based on IL2RA was 68.1% and that based on rATG was 31.9%. At baseline, 56.6% and 43.4% of patients were on cyclosporine-based and tacrolimus-based immunosuppression, respectively; for CMV prophylaxis, 101 (60.8%) recipients received low-dose ganciclovir (1.5 g/d for 3 months), and 65 (39.2%) received high-dose ganciclovir (3.0 g/d for 3 months).

Graft and patient survival

The adverse events during the 5-year follow-up are shown in Table 2. The incidence of DGF, AR and chronic rejection (CR) was 9%, 16.9% and 8.3%, respectively. Infection was the most common adverse event in the elderly patients, with an incidence of 55.4%. The incidence of CMV infection was 17.5%, and most of which occurred in the first year post-transplantation. A total of 36 patients experienced graft loss and 29 patients died within 5-year follow-up. Overall and death-censored graft survival and patient survival are shown in Figure 1. The 1-, 3-, 5-year overall graft survival was 84.3%, 78% and 70.6%, respectively. However, when patient death was not considered as graft loss (death-censored), the 1-, 3-, 5-year graft survival reached 93.6%, 89.4% and 83.6%, respectively. Patient survival was 84.8% at 1 year, 82.1% at 3 year and 77.1% at 5 year. The causes of graft loss and patient death are shown in Table 3. The main causes of graft loss were patient death (52.8%) and AR (16.7%). Most of the patients died of infection (55.2%) and CAD (17.2%). In addition, among the infectious mortality, there were 11 deaths due to severe CMV disease.

Risk factors for graft loss

During a 5-year follow-up, there were 36 cases of graft loss in the cohort. More than half of the graft losses (52.8%) were due to patient death. Univariate analysis showed that longer dialysis time, PRA>5%, DGF and AR were risk factors for death-censored graft loss. Based on the Cox multivariate models, a PRA>5% [hazard ratio (HR) 4.295, 95% confidence interval (CI) 1.321–13.97], DGF (HR 4.744, 95% CI 1.611–13.973) and AR (HR 4.971, 95% CI 1.516–16.301) remained independent risk factors for death-censored graft loss, except for longer dialysis time (Table 4). The status of comorbidities, including diabetes mellitus, hypertension and CAD were not associated with shorter graft survival.

Risk factors for patient death

There were 29 deaths during the 5-year follow-up. The risk factors for patient death were shown in Table 5. Univariate analysis showed that longer dialysis time, AR, graft loss and low-dose ganciclovir prophylaxis were risk factors for patient death. However, when data was analysis by final Cox multivariate model, we found that longer dialysis time (HR 1.011 for 1-month increase, 95% CI 1.002–1.020), graft loss (HR 3.501, 95% CI 1.559–7.865) and low-dose ganciclovir prophylaxis (HR 3.173,

Table 1. Recipient baseline characteristics (N = 166).

Recipient age, yr (mean±SD)	64.6±3.8	Dialysis, n (%)	
Male recipients, n (%)	109 (65.7)	Nondialysis	46 (27.7)
Cause of ESRD, n (%)		Hemodialysis	87 (52.4)
Chronic glomerulonephritis	73 (44)	Peritoneal dialysis	33 (19.9)
Diabetes mellitus	51 (30.7)	Time on dialysis, months (mean±SD)	18.6±22.1
Hypertension	19 (11.4)	PRA>5%, n (%)	16 (9.6)
Obstructive nephropathy	7 (4.2)	IL2RA, n (%)	113 (68.1)
Polycystic kidney	6 (3.6)	rATG, n (%)	53 (31.9)
Others or unknown	10 (6)	Cyclosporine, n (%)	94 (56.6)
Comorbidities, n (%)		Tacrolimus, n (%)	72 (43.4)
Diabetes mellitus	70 (42.1)	Low-dose ganciclovir (1.5 g/d), n (%)	101 (60.8)
Hypertension	120 (72.3)	High-dose ganciclovir (3.0 g/d), n (%)	65 (39.2)
Coronary artery disease (CAD)	24 (14.5)		

95% CI 1.063–9.473) remained significant independent risk factors for mortality. AR, diabetes mellitus, hypertension, CAD, and DGF were not significantly associated with patient death.

Discussion

The rapid increase in elderly patients with ESRD has raised an important issue regarding the optimization of long-term outcomes in this population. Despite a higher percentage of cadaveric kidney donors being allocated to older patients, the short-term graft survival is excellent in the majority of these patients. However, longer-term graft survival in the elderly recipients is less than expected due to death with a functioning graft, which is the major cause of graft loss. Elderly renal transplant recipients are at

increased risk of graft loss and death compared with younger cohorts [7,8]. Considering the rapid growth of an aging ESRD population and the shortage of donor kidneys, identifying the possible risk factors of graft and patient survival in elderly recipients is crucial for improving their long-term outcome.

In this study, we retrospectively analyzed 166 cases of renal transplantation from deceased donors in recipients aged ≥60 years and identified the possible risk factors predicting poor clinical outcome. Consistent with previous studies, death with a functioning graft is the leading cause of graft loss in elderly patients, with a percentage of more than 50% [9]. When patient death was not considered as the cause of graft loss, the 1-, 3-, 5-year graft survival reached 93.6%, 89.4% and 83.6%, respectively. Similar to previous studies, a PRA>5% at the time of transplantation was

Table 2. Adverse events in 5-year follow-up.

Adverse events	n (%)
DGF	15 (9)
AR	28 (16.9)
CR	3 (8.3)
Leukopenia	9 (5.4)
All infections	92 (55.4)
Urinary tract	7 (4.2)
Probable bacterial or other	35 (21.1)
Confirmed bacterial	64 (38.6)
CMV	29 (17.5)
BK polyoma virus	1 (0.6)
Fungal	10 (6)
Liver impairment	39 (23.5)
New onset diabetes mellitus	18 (10.8)
Congestive heart failure	8 (4.8)
Cerebrovascular accident	4 (2.4)
Malignancy	9 (5.4)
Graft loss	36 (21.7)
Death	29 (17.5)

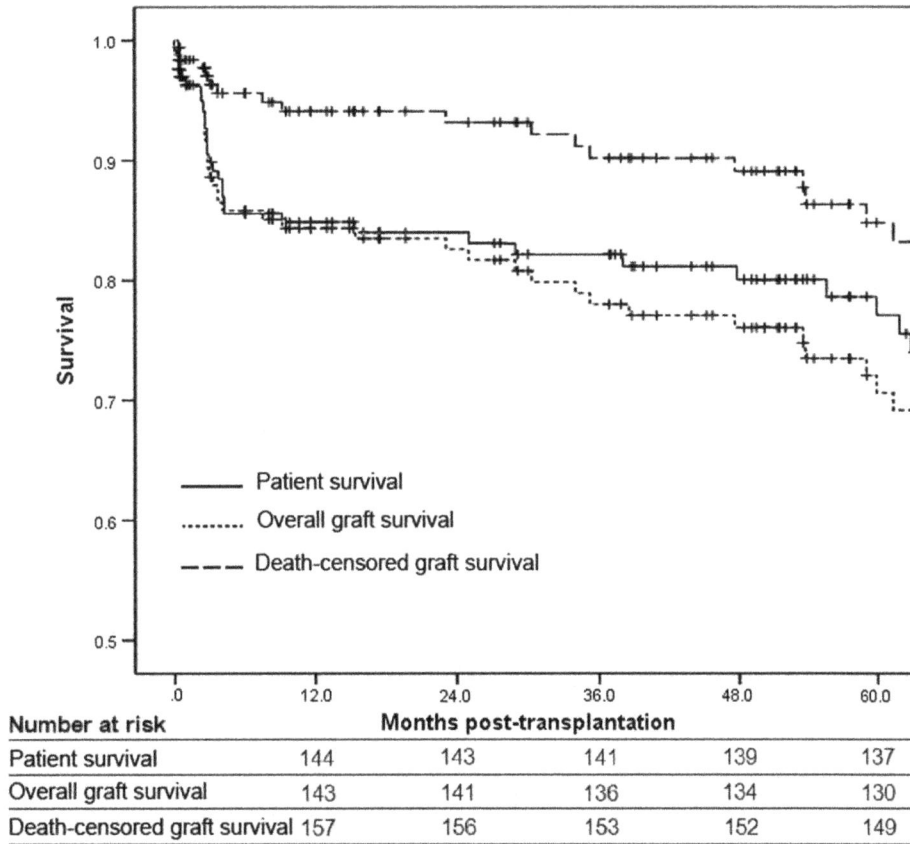

Figure 1. Patient survival, overall and death-censored graft survival.

a significant independent risk factor for graft loss in recipients aged ≥60 years. Heldal et al. [10] reported a PRA>5% as a risk factor for graft loss in patients aged ≥70 years, whereas Faravardeh et al. [11] demonstrated that a PRA>10% was a risk factor for graft failure in recipients aged ≥65 years.

In our study, we found that patients aged ≥60 years experienced a low incidence of AR episodes, which were similar to previous findings [12]. Although the incidence of AR was lower in the elderly transplant recipients, the impact of AR episodes was far more severe than in the young recipients [13]. We found that both DGF and AR were risk factors for graft loss in recipients aged

≥60 years. Heldal et al. [10] reported that DGF was an independent predictor for death-censored graft loss in the elderly recipients aged 60 years or older. Similarly, in the study by Faravardeh et al. [11], DGF and AR were risk factors for graft failure not only in younger recipients but also in elderly cohorts aged ≥65 years. In a multicenter case-control study in Spain, Moreso et al. [14] also confirmed that AR was an independent predictor of death-censored graft failure in adult renal transplant recipients. However, in another prospective multicenter study performed in Spain, the authors did not find any significant association between AR and allograft loss in neither recipients

Table 3. Causes of graft loss and mortality (5 years).

Graft loss (N = 36)	n (%)	Mortality (N = 29)	n (%)
Patient death	19 (52.8)	Infection	16 (55.2)
AR	6 (16.7)	CAD	5 (17.2)
CR	3 (8.3)	Cerebrovascular accident	2 (6.9)
Chronic allograft nephropathy	4 (11.1)	Malignancy	3 (10.3)
Recurrence	1 (2.8)	Liver disease	1 (3.5)
ARF	1 (2.8)	Hemorrhage	1 (3.5)
PNF	1 (2.8)	Unknown	1 (3.5)
Technical failure	1 (2.8)		

ARF, acute renal failure; PNF, primary no function.

Table 4. Risk factors for death-censored graft loss (5 years).

Variables	Univariate analysis			Cox multivariate analysis		
	HR	95% CI	P value	HR	95% CI	P value
Age (1-year increase)	1.059	0.95–1.179	0.3	—	—	—
Gender (male vs female)	1.255	0.464–3.397	0.655	—	—	—
Dialysis time (1-month increase)	1.013	1.001–1.026	0.028	1.014	0.999–1.029	0.061
Diabetes mellitus	0.624	0.231–1.691	0.354	—	—	—
Hypertension	2.016	0.458–8.866	0.353	—	—	—
CAD	0.638	0.146–2.795	0.551	—	—	—
PRA>5%	10.503	4.037–27.325	<0.001	4.295	1.321–13.97	0.015
Induction (IL2RA vs rATG)	0.553	0.156–1.959	0.359	—	—	—
Cyclosporin vs tacrolimus	2.05	0.778–5.396	0.146	1.322	0.495–3.534	0.577
DGF	5.908	2.059–16.954	0.001	4.744	1.611–13.973	0.005
AR	6.782	2.612–17.609	<0.001	4.971	1.516–16.301	0.008

HR, hazard ratio; CI, confidence interval.

aged ≥60 years nor in younger recipients [15]. Nevertheless, AR and DGF can result in functional and structural damage to the graft, which leads to late poor graft outcomes. Therefore, a decrease in the incidence of AR or DGF may result in an improvement of late graft outcome.

The literature on the association between duration of dialysis and transplant outcome is rich and at times inconsistent. Most of the studies reported that longer duration of dialysis was associated with poorer patient and graft outcome in kidney transplant recipients [16,17,18], whereas some other studies didn't find any association between dialysis duration and patient or graft survival [15]. In addition, there are also some studies reported that longer time on dialysis was independent risk factor only for patient death, but not for graft loss [9,19]. In the study by Faravardeh et al. [11], the authors reported that longer dialysis time was a risk factor for graft loss and mortality in recipients aged <50 years, but not in those aged ≥50 years. Therefore, the risk of transplant outcome associated with increased dialysis duration time may differ

between various countries and populations. In this retrospective study, we demonstrated that increased time on dialysis was an independent risk factor for patient death. Since the maintenance of dialysis status may accelerate cardiovascular changes, including vascular calcification, left ventricular hypertrophy and congestive heart failure [20], longer time on dialysis may result in an increased risk of death, especially in the elderly with a higher incidence of vascular complications. In the current study, we did not find longer duration of dialysis to be a significant independent risk factor for graft failure in multivariate Cox regression model. This finding may be explained by the fact that the elderly may differ somewhat from the younger population, since the incidence of acute rejection appears to steadily reduce with increased age [1]. In addition, the mean duration of pretransplant dialysis in our cohort is 18.6 months, which is relatively short compared to previous studies. Furthermore, the relatively small sample may somewhat weaken the impact of dialysis time on graft survival.

Table 5. Risk factors for patient death (5 years).

Variables	Univariate analysis			Cox multivariate analysis		
	HR	95% CI	P value	HR	95% CI	P value
Age (1-year increase)	1.068	0.974–1.171	0.16	1.081	0.985–1.186	0.1
Gender (male vs female)	1.243	0.577–2.675	0.579	—	—	—
Dialysis time (1-month increase)	1.013	1.004–1.022	0.004	1.011	1.002–1.020	0.02
Diabetes mellitus	0.713	0.336–1.51	0.377	—	—	—
Hypertension	0.924	0.393–2.171	0.856	—	—	—
CAD	1.412	0.574–3.47	0.452	—	—	—
Induction (IL2RA vs rATG)	0.438	0.166–1.155	0.095	1.627	0.38–6.966	0.512
CsA vs FK506	1.627	0.777–3.407	0.197	1.554	0.735–3.289	0.249
DGF	2.345	0.889–6.185	0.085	2.303	0.856–6.196	0.098
AR	3.595	1.697–7.617	0.001	1.91	0.715–5.101	0.197
Graft loss	4.571	2.073–10.081	<0.001	3.501	1.559–7.865	0.002
Ganciclovir (1.5 g/d vs 3 g/d)	3.947	1.366–11.401	0.011	3.173	1.063–9.473	0.039

Graft failure was a significant risk factor for mortality for patients aged ≥60 years in our study, which was confirmed in previous studies [11]. The increased death rate was partly due to the potential immediate complications of graft loss and longer-term worse survival of returning to dialysis.

CMV infection is a common problem in immunocompromised hosts and an important cause of morbidity and mortality in kidney transplant recipients [21]. Previous studies had demonstrated that CMV infection was associated with acute and chronic graft rejection [22], increased incidence of opportunistic infection [23], graft loss and decreased recipient survival [24]. Universal prophylaxis with effective antiviral agents is one of the possible approaches for prevention of CMV infection. In China, ganciclovir remains the preferred agent for prophylaxis and treatment of CMV infection due to its effectiveness and affordable price to most patients. The study by Ahmed and colleagues demonstrated that low-dose ganciclovir (1.0 g/d for 3 months) was as effective at decreasing the incidence of clinical CMV disease as high-dose ganciclovir (3.0 g/d for 3–6 months) in renal transplant recipients [25]. However, in the present study, we found that a low-dose ganciclovir (1.5 g/d for 3 months) was significantly associated with shorter patient survival in elderly recipients. This difference could be explained by the fact that the mean age of Ahmed's recipients was 46.1±2.2 years, which was much lower than those in our study. Elderly patients are thought to generate a less robust immune response due to a decreased immunogenicity with increased age [26] combined with more pre-transplant comorbidities, which may increase the overall risk of infectious death in elderly transplant recipients [27,28]. Low-dose ganciclovir may be not as effective as high-dose ganciclovir for CMV prophylaxis in elderly recipients. Therefore, it is important to widely use a high-dose ganciclovir to decrease the incidence of CMV infection in the more susceptible population such as the elderly renal transplant recipients.

CAD was one of the most common comorbidities and causes of death in elderly recipients. Faravardeh et al. [11] reported that CAD was a risk factor for mortality in both recipients aged ≥65 years and the younger cohort aged <50 years, while Heldal et al. [10] found that CAD increased mortality in transplant recipients up to 70 years but not in older recipients. However, in our study, we did not find CAD to be a risk factor for mortality in patients aged ≥60 years at transplantation, which was consistent with Doyle's finding [29]. The lower prevalence of CAD in the elderly recipients may be a likely explanation for our finding because

there were fewer patients with CAD in our cohort and this likely led to a loss of some power to detect the significance of this factor. This is not surprising, as China is known traditionally for low incidence of CAD and low plasma cholesterol levels due to the Chinese diet and lifestyle [30,31]. Although the incidence of CAD has increased in the last 2 decades, the incidence attained is still significantly lower than that in the Western countries [32]. Furthermore, the morbidity and mortality of CAD is much lower in south China compared with in the north [30]. Since all of the patients included were from south of China, it is reasonable that the number and proportion of CAD was low in our study. Similar to previous studies, we did not find an association between diabetes and patient survival [9,29,33]. We also did not find hypertension as a significant risk factor for graft failure or patient death.

Our study has certain limitations inherent in its retrospective nature because data were collected from patients transplanted from 2002 to June 2013. There were certain patients missing in the follow-up (10.5% of the overall cohort), which may reduce potential adverse effects of various risk factors that would be observed over a longer-term. In addition, the relatively small sample size might have less power to detect the effect of variables that have a smaller impact on the poor clinical outcome.

In conclusion, the transplant outcomes are excellent among recipients aged 60 years or older. We found that PRA>5%, DGF and AR were risk factors for graft failure, while longer time on dialysis, failed grafts and low-dose ganciclovir prophylaxis were risk factors for mortality in recipients aged ≥60 years. These factors represent potential targets for interventions aimed at improving graft and patient survival in elderly recipients. Therefore, reducing PRA level and decreasing the incidence of DGF and AR may result in longer graft survival, while shortening the duration of dialysis may lead to longer patient survival. In addition, high-dose ganciclovir prophylaxis should be widely used in elderly recipient to decrease the incidence of CMV infection. Nevertheless, further prospective, randomized and multicenter studies are needed to confirm these findings.

Author Contributions

Conceived and designed the experiments: XQL GDC. Performed the experiments: XQL GDC. Analyzed the data: XQL GDC. Contributed reagents/materials/analysis tools: GDC JQ CXW LZC. Wrote the paper: XQL GDC. Finalized the manuscript: XQL GDC. Read and approved the final manuscript: LZC.

References

1. Danovitch GM, Gill J, Bunnapradist S (2007) Immunosuppression of the elderly kidney transplant recipient. Transplantation 84: 285–291.
2. McCullough KP, Keith DS, Meyer KH, Stock PG, Brayman KL, et al. (2009) Kidney and pancreas transplantation in the United States, 1998–2007: access for patients with diabetes and end-stage renal disease. Am J Transplant 9: 894–906.
3. Wolfe RA, Ashby VB, Milford EL, Ojo AO, Ettenger RE, et al. (1999) Comparison of mortality in all patients on dialysis, patients on dialysis awaiting transplantation, and recipients of a first cadaveric transplant. N Engl J Med 341: 1725–1730.
4. Johnson DW, Herzig K, Purdie D, Brown AM, Rigby RJ, et al. (2000) A comparison of the effects of dialysis and renal transplantation on the survival of older uremic patients. Transplantation 69: 794–799.
5. Oniscu GC, Brown H, Forsythe JL (2004) How great is the survival advantage of transplantation over dialysis in elderly patients? Nephrol Dial Transplant 19: 945–951.
6. Meier-Kriesche HU, Schold JD, Srinivas TR, Kaplan B (2004) Lack of improvement in renal allograft survival despite a marked decrease in acute rejection rates over the most recent era. Am J Transplant 4: 378–383.
7. Roodnat JI, Zietse R, Mulder PG, Rischen-Vos J, van Gelder T, et al. (1999) The vanishing importance of age in renal transplantation. Transplantation 67: 576–580.

8. Meier-Kriesche H, Ojo AO, Arndorfer JA, Port FK, Magee JC, et al. (2001) Recipient age as an independent risk factor for chronic renal allograft failure. Transplant Proc 33: 1113–1114.
9. Cardinal H, Hebert MJ, Rahme E, Houde I, Baran D, et al. (2005) Modifiable factors predicting patient survival in elderly kidney transplant recipients. Kidney Int 68: 345–351.
10. Heldal K, Hartmann A, Leivestad T, Svendsen MV, Foss A, et al. (2009) Clinical outcomes in elderly kidney transplant recipients are related to acute rejection episodes rather than pretransplant comorbidity. Transplantation 87: 1045–1051.
11. Faravardeh A, Eickhoff M, Jackson S, Spong R, Kukla A, et al. (2013) Predictors of graft failure and death in elderly kidney transplant recipients. Transplantation 96: 1089–1096.
12. Patel SJ, Knight RJ, Suki WN, Abdellatif A, Duhart BJ, et al. (2011) Rabbit antithymocyte induction and dosing in deceased donor renal transplant recipients over 60 yr of age. Clin Transplant 25: E250–E256.
13. Meier-Kriesche HU, Srinivas TR, Kaplan B (2001) Interaction between acute rejection and recipient age on long-term renal allograft survival. Transplant Proc 33: 3425–3426.
14. Moreso F, Alonso A, Gentil MA, Gonzalez-Molina M, Capdevila L, et al. (2010) Improvement in late renal allograft survival between 1990 and 2002 in Spain: results from a multicentre case-control study. Transpl Int 23: 907–913.

15. Morales JM, Marcen R, Del CD, Andres A, Gonzalez-Molina M, et al. (2012) Risk factors for graft loss and mortality after renal transplantation according to recipient age: a prospective multicentre study. Nephrol Dial Transplant 27 Suppl 4: v39–v46.

16. Meier-Kriesche HU, Port FK, Ojo AO, Rudich SM, Hanson JA, et al. (2000) Effect of waiting time on renal transplant outcome. Kidney Int 58: 1311–1317.

17. Goldfarb-Rumyantzev A, Hurdle JF, Scandling J, Wang Z, Baird B, et al. (2005) Duration of end-stage renal disease and kidney transplant outcome. Nephrol Dial Transplant 20: 167–175.

18. Remport A, Keszei A, Vamos EP, Novak M, Jaray J, et al. (2011) Association of pre-transplant dialysis duration with outcome in kidney transplant recipients: a prevalent cohort study. Int Urol Nephrol 43: 215–224.

19. Helantera I, Salmela K, Kyllonen L, Koskinen P, Gronhagen-Riska C, et al. (2014) Pretransplant dialysis duration and risk of death after kidney transplantation in the current era. Transplantation 98: 458–464.

20. Himmelfarb J, Ikizler TA (2010) Hemodialysis. N Engl J Med 363: 1833–1845.

21. Brennan DC (2001) Cytomegalovirus in renal transplantation. J Am Soc Nephrol 12: 848–855.

22. Cainelli F, Vento S (2002) Infections and solid organ transplant rejection: a cause-and-effect relationship? Lancet Infect Dis 2: 539–549.

23. George MJ, Snydman DR, Werner BG, Griffith J, Falagas ME, et al. (1997) The independent role of cytomegalovirus as a risk factor for invasive fungal disease in orthotopic liver transplant recipients. Boston Center for Liver Transplantation CMVIG-Study Group. Cytogam, MedImmune, Inc. Gaithersburg, Maryland. Am J Med 103: 106–113.

24. De Keyzer K, Van Laecke S, Peeters P, Vanholder R (2011) Human cytomegalovirus and kidney transplantation: a clinician's update. Am J Kidney Dis 58: 118–126.

25. Ahmed J, Velarde C, Ramos M, Ismail K, Serpa J, et al. (2004) Outcome of low-dose ganciclovir for cytomegalovirus disease prophylaxis in renal-transplant recipients. Transplantation 78: 1689–1692.

26. Martins PN, Pratschke J, Pascher A, Fritsche L, Frei U, et al. (2005) Age and immune response in organ transplantation. Transplantation 79: 127–132.

27. Meier-Kriesche HU, Ojo AO, Hanson JA, Kaplan B (2001) Exponentially increased risk of infectious death in older renal transplant recipients. Kidney Int 59: 1539–1543.

28. Kauffman HM, McBride MA, Cors CS, Roza AM, Wynn JJ (2007) Early mortality rates in older kidney recipients with comorbid risk factors. Transplantation 83: 404–410.

29. Doyle SE, Matas AJ, Gillingham K, Rosenberg ME (2000) Predicting clinical outcome in the elderly renal transplant recipient. Kidney Int 57: 2144–2150.

30. Tao SC, Huang ZD, Wu XG, Zhou BF, Xiao ZK, et al. (1989) CHD and its risk factors in the People's Republic of China. Int J Epidemiol 18: S159–S163.

31. Campbell TC, Parpia B, Chen J (1998) Diet, lifestyle, and the etiology of coronary artery disease: the Cornell China study. Am J Cardiol 82: 18T–21T.

32. Ueshima H, Sekikawa A, Miura K, Turin TC, Takashima N, et al. (2008) Cardiovascular disease and risk factors in Asia: a selected review. Circulation 118: 2702–2709.

33. Fabrizii V, Winkelmayer WC, Klauser R, Kletzmayr J, Saemann MD, et al. (2004) Patient and graft survival in older kidney transplant recipients: does age matter? J Am Soc Nephrol 15: 1052–1060.

20

Rhegmatogenous Retinal Detachment Surgery in Elderly People over 70 Years Old: Visual Acuity, Quality of Life, and Cost-Utility Values

Yingyan Ma[1⋑], Xiaohua Ying[2⋑], Haidong Zou[1,3]*, Xiaocheng Xu[2], Haiyun Liu[1], Lin Bai[1], Xun Xu[1], Xi Zhang[1]

1 Department of Ophthalmology, Shanghai First People's Hospital, Shanghai Jiao Tong University, Shanghai, China, 2 School of Public Health, Fudan University, Shanghai, China, 3 Shanghai Eye Disease Prevention & Treatment Center, Shanghai, China

Abstract

Background and Purpose: To evaluate the influence of rhegmatogenous retinal detachment (RRD) surgery on elderly patients in terms of visual acuity, vision-related quality of life and its cost-effectiveness.

Methods: Elderly patients over 70 years old, who were diagnosed and underwent RRD surgery at Shanghai First People's Hospital, Shanghai Jiao Tong University, China, from January 1, 2009, through January 1, 2013. The participants received scleral buckling surgery and vitreous surgery with or without scleral buckling under retrobulbar anesthesia. We followed the patients for 1 year and collected best-corrected visual acuity (BCVA), vision-related quality of life, and direct medical costs data. Utility values elicited by time-trade-off were analyzed to determine the quality of life. Quality-adjusted life years (QALYs) gained in life expectancy were calculated and discounted at 3% annually. Costs per QALY gained were reported using the bootstrap method. Further analyses were made for two age groups, age 70–79 and age over 80 years. Sensitivity analyses were performed to test stability of the results.

Results: 98 patients were included in the study. The BCVA significantly improved by 0.53 ± 0.44 (Logarithm of the Minimum Angle of Resolution (logMAR)) at the 1-year postoperative time point ($p < 0.001$). Utility values increased from 0.77 to 0.84 ($p < 0.001$), and an average of 0.4 QALYs were gained in the life expectancy. Costs per QALY gained from the RRD surgery were 33,186 Chinese Yuan (CNY) (5,276 US dollars (USD))/QALY; 24,535 CNY (3,901 USD)/QALY for the age group of 70–79 years and 71,240 CNY (11,326 USD)/QALY for the age group over 80 years.

Conclusions: RRD surgery improved the visual acuity and quality of life in the elderly patients over 70 years old. According to the World Health Organization's recommendation, at a threshold of willingness to pay of 115,062 CNY (18,293 USD)/QALY, RRD surgery is cost effective in the elderly patients.

Editor: Haotian Lin, Sun Yat-sen University, China

Funding: This study was funded by a key grant from the Shanghai Health Bureau (20114007), a grant from the Shanghai Leading Talent Reserve Programme (40311), and a grand from National Population and Family Planning Commission: Researches on modern hospital management system-costs calculation in hospital (SJYF2014XD010B). ZHD received the funding. The funders had no role in study design, data collection and analysis, decision to publish, or preparation of the manuscript.

Competing Interests: The authors have declared that no competing interests exist.

* Email: zouhaidong@hotmail.com

⋑ These authors contributed equally to this work.

Introduction

Rhegmatogenous retinal detachment (RRD) is the most common type of retinal detachment, and it severely threatens visual acuity and vision-related quality of life [1–3]. Proper and timely treatments, such as scleral buckling surgery and vitreous surgery, can largely restore visual acuity and permit a certain degree of improvement in vision-related quality of life [4], [5]. However, in most developing countries with limited medical resources, the treatment for retinal detachment has been a low priority [6]. Despite the effectiveness of RRD surgery, the costs are

not small. Brown and associates reported the costs for vitreoretinal surgery to be between 7,109 US dollars (USD) and 9,607 USD in patients with severe proliferative vitreoretinopathy [7]. Two recent studies performed in America calculated the costs for the two types of surgery varying from 4,048 USD to 7,940 USD [8], [9]. In our previous study, an average cost of 11,384 Chinese Yuan (CNY) (1,810 USD, 1 USD = 6.29 CNY, 2012.12.31) was determined for RRD surgery in Shanghai [10]. Although comparatively lower than the cost reported in America, it is still a large burden for most families in China.

The annual incidence of RRD ranged from 6.3 to 17.9 per 100,000 population globally [11]. Age is one risk factor for RRD [11–13]. In elderly people who are 70 to 79 years old, the incidences vary from 15.21 to 50 per 100,000 worldwide [11]. In a recent study conducted in the Netherlands, the annual incidence of RRD was reported to be 21.43 per 100,000 for people aged 85–89 years old [14]. However, age was also a negative predictor for optimal visual outcomes after RRD surgery. As demonstrated in many previous studies, patients of older age have inferior functional results, namely best-corrected visual acuity, than younger patients [15–19]. Therefore, in clinical practice, it is not unusual that many elderly people give up on the surgery considering the expensive medical costs, the uncertain visual outcomes, and the relatively short remaining life years. These elderly people will definitely experience severe visual impairment, and as a result, losses of quality of life. As shown in a survey of a community population aged over 60 years in Shanghai, retinal detachment was the fifth leading cause of blindness [20].

Cost-utility analysis is one method of economic evaluation that incorporates the utility value in the form of quality-adjusted life years (QALYs) with costs to calculate how much money should be spent on each QALY gained for certain medical interventions [21], [22]. One advantage of cost-utility analysis is that it allows comparison among different disciplines by a common unit of measure (costs/QALY). Therefore, policymakers can identify relative priorities when determining resource allocation among medical interventions [21], [22]. In Brown's study, the costs/QALY were between 40,252 USD/QALY and 62,383 USD/QALY for vitreous surgery in patients complicated with severe proliferative vitreoretinopathy [7]. In the recent American study, the costs/QALY varied from 1,377 USD/QALY to 2,243 USD/QALY for scleral buckling and vitreous surgery [9]. In Shanghai, the costs/QALY were 13,794 CNY (2,193 USD)/QALY for normal RRD patients throughout their life expectancies [10]. However, the cost-effectiveness of RRD surgery for elderly patients has not been evaluated in the existing literatures.

As we enter an aging society, along with the popularity of cataract surgery and high rates of myopia, we anticipate a greater number of elderly patients suffering from RRD [11]. Therefore, it is worthwhile to explore how much the elderly people could benefit from RRD surgery and whether performing RRD surgery is cost-effective in this population. This study presented the outcomes of RRD surgery in terms of visual acuity and vision-related quality of life and calculated its cost-effectiveness in an elderly population.

Methods

Ethics

All participants gave their written informed consent. The study was conducted according to the tenets of the Declaration of Helsinki and was approved by the Institutional Review Board at Shanghai First People's Hospital, Shanghai Jiao Tong University.

Participants and investigations

Between January 1, 2009, and January 1, 2013, study participants included elderly patients over the age of 70 years who were newly diagnosed with RRD (in at least one eye) and subsequently underwent surgery in the Shanghai First People's Hospital, Shanghai Jiao Tong University. Patients were excluded if they had other severe eye diseases, physical disability or mental disorders.

Participants were interviewed before and one year after surgery. Data were collected for age, gender, educational level, systemic

diseases, duration of time from RRD symptoms to RRD surgery (or, if no symptoms, time since diagnosis), range of detachment in quadrants, macular-on or macular-off, RRD surgery type, surgical procedures, best-corrected visual acuity (BCVA), costs, utility value, and complications of surgery. BCVA was also collected at the 3-month postoperative time point. Surgical procedures were classified as scleral buckling surgery and vitreous surgery with or without scleral buckling. A skilled interviewer (HDZ), who did not take part in any of the examinations or follow-up with the participants, administered the questionnaire and provided assistance when required.

Utility values and costs

Utility values were obtained by using the time trade-off (TTO) method at pre-operative and 1-year post-operative time points. Participants were asked how many additional years they expected to live and how many of these theoretical remaining years they would be willing to give up in return for guaranteed, permanently perfect vision. The utility value was then calculated by subtracting the quotient of these numbers (years given up/years to live) from 1.0 [23]. For example, if a 70-year-old RRD patient with a self-perceived life expectancy of 10 additional years would like to trade 2 years to get rid of his or her visual impairment caused by RRD, the utility value related to his or her RRD would be $(1.0 - 2/10) = 0.8$.

Costs were calculated from the patient perspective, and all of these costs were inflated to 2012 values by utilizing the consumer price index for health care [24]. Self-designed investigation forms were distributed to record the medical costs associated with RRD surgery for the first diagnosed eye, including costs of pharmaceuticals, examinations, treatment, anesthesia, surgery, hospitalization, and transportation fees. Downstream costs induced by surgery were also collected during the 1-year follow up, such as the costs for the removal of silicone oil and treatment for complications including cataract surgery, treatment of corneal edema, and intraocular hypertension. If the second eye also received RRD surgery during the 1-year study period, costs incurred by this surgery were also recorded. The costs collected in this research were associated with the Chinese medical insurance unified prices; hence, they were representative of the medical costs charged by other hospitals in Shanghai and in other cities in China. Only direct costs were included. Indirect costs, such as loss of productivity and leisure time, were not incorporated into this investigation.

Model design

According to our previous research [25], we assumed that the utility value in RRD patients increased steadily in the first year and then remained stable. Hypothetical patients designed as no-treatment controls were expected to obtain the same pre-operative utility values as the participants. Additionally, it was assumed that their utility values remained constant and that no medical costs related to RRD treatment had ever been incurred in our hypothetical patients.

Because the benefits of RRD surgery are life-long, we carried out a cost-utility analysis over the remaining life expectancy for RRD surgery. Lacking evidence of utility change over the remaining lifetime of RRD patients, and in accord with other economic evaluations within ophthalmology [7], [26], [27], we assumed that the vision-related quality of life would remain constant over the life expectancy. The age and gender-specific life expectancy table from the Health Profile China was used to calculate life expectancy QALYs gained [28]. In the control group, hypothetical patients who did not receive surgery would also

Table 1. Characteristics and surgical data for 98 elderly RRD patients.

	Total	70s	80s	P value*
No. of patients	98	57	41	
Average age [Mean (SD)]	78.49(4.36)	75.33(2.48)	82.88(1.90)	<0.001
Male [No. (%)]	54(55.1)	35(61.40)	19(46.34)	0.139
Education time >10 years [No. (%)]	50(51.02)	32(56.14)	18(43.90)	0.232
Duration of symptoms [Weeks, Median (Range)]	5[1–27]	6[1–23]	4[1–27]	0.550
More than 2 quadrants detached [No. (%)]	78(79.60)	46(80.70)	32(78.05)	0.748
Macular-off [No. (%)]	68(69.39)	40(70.18)	28(68.29)	0.842
Types of surgery				0.191
Scleral buckling surgery [No. (%)]	31(31.63)	21(36.84)	10(24.39)	
Vitreous surgery [No. (%)]	67(68.37)	36(63.16)	31(75.61)	
Bilateral surgery rate [No. (%)]	13(13.27)	9(15.79)	4(9.76)	0.385
Complication rate [No. (%)]	66(67.35)	35(61.40)	31(75.61)	0.139

*A comparison was made between age groups of patients in their 70s and 80s. An independent sample t-test was used for continual data of normal distribution, a Mann Whitney U test for non-normal distribution data, and the Pearson chi-square test for the categorical data. A value of P<0.05 was regarded as statistically significant. RRD, rhegmatogenous retinal detachment; SD, standard deviation.

remain at their preoperative health status throughout their life expectancies with no medical expenditures related to RRD. The QALYs were discounted at 3% annually in the baseline analysis. Because all medical costs were paid over a 1-year period, they were not discounted. The incremental cost-effectiveness ratio (ICER) was then calculated to evaluate the life-span cost-utility result of RRD surgery, compared with the no-treatment option.

Moreover, we performed subgroup analyses by dividing the participants into two age groups: 70–79-year-olds and over 80-year-olds. Costs, QALYs gained, and the ICER were calculated for each age group to explore the cost-effectiveness of RRD surgery in different age intervals. Additional analyses for scleral buckling surgery and vitreous surgery were also calculated.

Threshold ratio of willingness to pay

In China, there is no official guiding document or consensus on the threshold ratio of willingness to pay (WTP); hence, we adopted the standard posed by the World Health Organization (WHO). As recommended by the WHO, if the ICER is less than three times the gross domestic product (GDP) per capita, it can be regarded as cost-effective, and if the ICER is less than the GDP per capita, the intervention can be regarded as highly cost-effective [29]. This approach has already been utilized in several economic evaluations in China [30], [31]. With a 2012 GDP per capita in China of

38,354 CNY, we used 115,062 CNY (18,293 USD)/QALY as the threshold ratio of willingness to pay to determine whether the RRD surgery was cost-effective in the elderly population.

Statistical analysis

Costs and QALYs are usually highly skewed, and the uncertainty of the ICER is difficult to present using traditional statistical methods; therefore, we performed a bootstrapping with 1,000 replications to calculate mean costs, mean QALYs, the ICERs and the uncertainty of those results [32–34]. The percentile method (2.5 and 97.5 percentiles from the bootstrapped sample) was used to estimate 95% confidence intervals (CIs) for the incremental costs and QALYs [21], [33]. Furthermore, cost-effectiveness acceptability curves (CEACs) were drawn, representing the probability of RRD surgery being more cost-effective than no treatment for different thresholds of willingness to pay per QALY [35], [36]. The Mann-Whitney U test was used to compare the differences of costs, utility values, QALYs, and duration time of RRD between the two age groups for the non-normal distribution of the variables. An independent sample t-test was used for continual data of normal distribution, and the Pearson chi-square test was used for the categorical data. The paired sample t-test was used for testing differences between BCVA

Table 2. Outcomes of visual acuity for RRD surgery in an elderly population (n = 98).

	Total	70s	80s	P value*
BCVA before surgery [LogMAR, Mean (SD)]	1.06(0.50)	1.05(0.50)	1.09(0.52)	0.682
BCVA 3 months after surgery [LogMAR, Mean (SD)]	0.74(0.35)	0.71(0.34)	0.78(0.36)	0.334
Difference of BCVA during the 3 months [LogMAR, Mean (SD)]	0.32(0.35)	0.34(0.36)	0.31(0.34)	0.709
BCVA 1 year after surgery [LogMAR, Mean (SD)]	0.54(0.26)	0.53(0.25)	0.55(0.29)	0.650
Difference of BCVA during the 1 year [LogMAR, Mean (SD)]	0.53(0.44)	0.52(0.40)	0.54(0.49)	0.845

*A comparison was made between age groups of patients who were in their 70s and 80s using independent samples t-tests. A value of P<0.05 was regarded as statistically significant.
RRD, rhegmatogenous retinal detachment; BCVA, best-corrected visual acuity; LogMAR, Logarithm of the Minimum Angle of Resolution; SD, standard deviation.

Table 3. Results of the baseline cost-utility analysis for RRD surgery in an elderly population (bootstrap, n = 1000).

	Total	70s	80s	P value*
Utility value before surgery [Mean (SD)]	0.77(0.12)	0.76(0.13)	0.79(0.11)	0.131
Utility value 1-year after surgery [Mean (SD)]	0.84(0.08)	0.84(0.07)	0.84(0.09)	0.352
Difference of utility values during the 1 year [Mean (SD)]	0.07(0.07)	0.08(0.08)	0.05(0.06)	0.096
QALYs gained in life-expectancy [Mean (95% CI)]	0.40(0.31–0.50)	0.55(0.41–0.72)	0.18(0.12–0.24)	
Mean Costs [CNY(USD)]	12,992(2,066)	13,319(2,117)	12,484(1,985)	
Costs 95% CI [CNY(USD)]	11,984(1,905) −14,088(2,239)	11,818(1,879)− 14,800(2,353)	11,131(1,769)− 13,910(2,211)	
Mean ICER [CNY(USD)/QALY]	33,186(5,276)	24,536(3,901)	71,240(11,326)	

*Comparisons were made between age groups of patients in their 70s and 80s using a Mann Whitney U test. A value of P<0.05 was regarded as statistically significant. RRD, rhegmatogenous retinal detachment; CNY, Chinese Yuan; USD, US dollar; SD, standard deviation; QALY, quality-adjusted life year; CI, confidence interval; ICER, incremental cost-effectiveness ratio.

before and after surgery, and the Wilcoxon signed rank test was used for differences between utility values.

A value of P<0.05 was regarded as statistically significant. All bootstrap analyses were performed using Microsoft Excel 2007 software, and other analyses were calculated by SPSS 16.0.

Sensitivity analyses

We conducted sensitivity analyses to test the robustness of the results. First, we tested the impact of varying the discount rate from the 3% assumed in the baseline scenario to between 0% and 5% for lifespan analyses, as recommended [21]. Second, we floated the costs and QALYs to 10% individually and simultaneously. Subsequently, we calculated the upper limits for the extent of the increasing costs, or the decreasing QALYs, to overturn the final determination. Finally, we performed an

additional analysis by excluding patients who had undergone bilateral RRD surgery, which might have had a potential influence on the results [7].

Results

A total of 98 patients fulfilled study inclusion criteria, with 57 patients aged 71 to 79 years old and 41 patients aged 81 to 87 years old. Basic socio-demographic and clinical data for the patients appear in Table 1. There was no significant difference between the two age groups in terms of basic characteristics, including type of surgery. During the 1-year follow up, no severe systemic diseases occurred in any participant.

The best-corrected visual acuity significantly improved at the 3-month post-operative time point compared with the preoperative time (paired sample t-test, p<0.001 for overall participants,

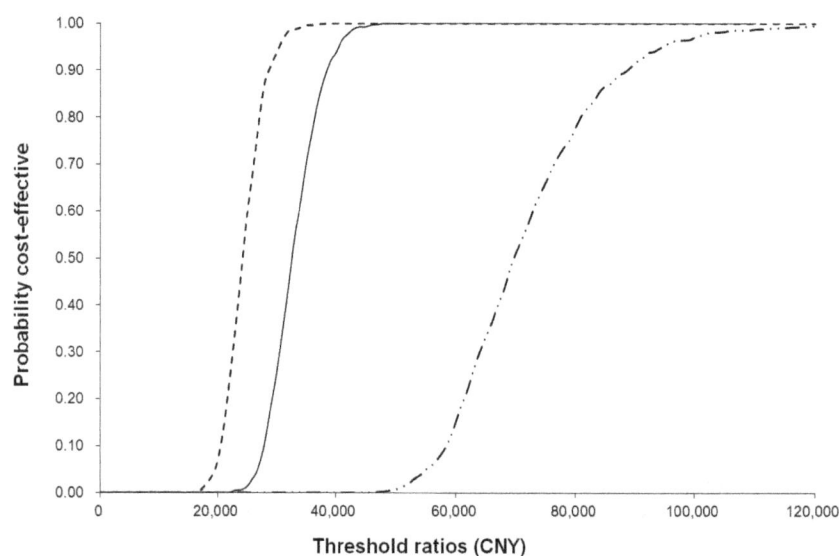

Figure 1. CEACs of life expectancy analysis for RRD surgery in the 70–79-year-olds, the above-80-year-olds, and all the elderly patients. The upper most dashed line represents the CEAC for RRD surgery in the 70–79-year-olds. The solid line represents the CEAC for RRD surgery in all of the elderly people. The dot-dashed line represents the CEAC for RRD surgery in the above-80-year-olds. RRD, Rhegmatogenous retinal detachment; CNY, Chinese yuan; QALY, quality-adjusted life year; CEAC, Cost-effectiveness acceptability curve.

Table 4. Threshold ratios of WTP (CNY (USD)/QALY) for RRD surgery to be cost-effective at probabilities of 50%, 70% and 90% compared with no treatment option.

Probability of being cost-effective	WTP [CNY(USD)/QALY]		
	All (n = 98)	70s (n = 57)	80s (n = 41)
50%	33,000(5,246)	24,000(3,816)	70,000(11,129)
70%	35,000(5,564)	26,000(4,134)	76,000(12,083)
90%	39,000(6,200)	29,000(4,610)	88,000(13,991)

WTP, willingness to pay; CNY, Chinese Yuan; USD, US dollar; QALY, quality-adjusted life year.

patients in their 70s, and patients in their 80s). At the 1-year post-operative time point, BCVA also improved significantly (paired sample t-test, p<0.001 for overall participants, patients in their 70s, and patients in their 80s) (Table 2). The utility values significantly increased 1 year after the surgery (Wilcoxon signed rank test, p<0.001 for the whole group, patients in their 70s, and patients in their 80s). The results of the baseline cost-utility analysis for the two age groups are shown in Table 3.

Over their remaining life expectancies, participants could achieve an average of 0.4 QALYs by having the retinal detachment surgery. For patients in their 70s, the QALYs gained were more than three times greater than for those of the patients in their 80s. According to the threshold willingness to pay, which was 115,062 CNY (18,293 USD)/QALY in 2012, the retinal detachment surgery is cost-effective for all elderly patients. The ICER for patients in their 80s is approximately three times higher than that of those in their 70s, though it is still a cost-effective intervention.

With a WTP of 115,062 CNY (18,293 USD) per QALY, there is a 100%, 100%, and 99.2% chance of RRD surgery being cost-effective for all of the elderly, patients in their 70s, and patients in their 80s, respectively. The CEAC (Figure 1) of the over-age-80 group is lower than that of the 70–79-year-old group, which indicates that RRD surgery is more cost-effective for those in their 70s than in their 80s. In the absence of an officially recognized threshold WTP, we further listed the threshold ratios of WTP for the surgery with cost-effective chances of 50%, 70%, and 90% (Table 4).

The results of additional analyses for the two major types of surgery were presented in table 5. The vitreous surgery was a little more expensive than the scleral buckling surgery, however obtained more QALYs for the elderly patients as well; hence, the costs per QALYs for vitreous surgery were less expensive than for scleral buckling surgery in the elderly population.

Table 6 presents the results of the sensitivity analyses. In general, the sensitivity analyses do not influence the decisions based on the results of the baseline analysis. Altering the discount rate from 3% in the baseline scenario to 0% decreases the ICERs; however, using a 5% discount rate increases the ICERs. Raising the costs by 10% and reducing the QALYs gained by 10% mildly increases the ICERs. With changes in both the costs and the QALYs, the ICERs still did not exceed the threshold of 115,062 CNY (18,293 USD)/QALY. To overturn the cost-effectiveness of the RRD surgery, the costs have to be 2.5 times more than the existing costs and the QALYs gained should be decreased by 75% from the baseline. Excluding bilateral RRD patients enhances the ICERs and makes RRD surgery less cost-effective for all of the elderly patients and in each age group.

Discussion

This article is the first to evaluate the visual outcomes and health economic value of RRD surgery in the elderly population. RRD surgery improved the visual acuity and quality of life for the elderly patients and was cost-effective in consideration of their life expectancies, with ICERs ranging from 30,142 CNY (4,792 USD)/QALY to 40,607 CNY (6,456 USD)/QALY. For patients above 80 years of age, although the ICER was about three times higher than that for patients aged 70–79 years, the RRD surgery remained a cost-effective intervention.

Compared with other studies, the patients in this study are relatively older, as most studies included patients with an average age of approximately 60 years old [37–39]. Additionally, the duration of symptoms until surgery is longer, although it is similar to those reported in developing countries [40], [41]. In China, 60–70% of RRD patients reside in remote areas or small villages and lack knowledge about RRD [42]; thus, the elderly patients received treatment after a longer time period from their diagnoses, which resulted in relatively poorer preoperative visual acuity and higher rates of macular-off compared with participants in other studies.

Table 5. Results of cost-utility analysis for the two surgery types in an elderly RRD population (bootstrap, n = 1000).

	Scleral buckling surgery (n = 31)	Vitreous surgery (n = 67)
Mean Costs [CNY(USD)]	12,804(2,036)	13,027(2,071)
Costs 95% CI [CNY(USD)]	10,813(1,719) – 14,737(2,343)	11,698(1,859) – 14,343(2,281)
QALYs gained in life-expectancy [Mean (95% CI)]	0.36(0.24–0.50)	0.41(0.29–0.56)
Mean ICER [CNY(USD)/QALY]	36,513(5,805)	32,287(5,133)

RRD, rhegmatogenous retinal detachment; CNY, Chinese Yuan; USD, US dollar; QALY, quality-adjusted life year; ICER, incremental cost-effectiveness ratio.

Table 6. A summary of ICERs (CNY (USD)/QALY) in sensitivity analyses for RRD surgery in an elderly population (n = 98).

	All	70s	80s
0% discount	30,142(4,792)	22,072(3,509)	69,756(10,091)
5% discount	35,092(5,579)	25,933(4,123)	73,961(11,758)
Cost+10%	36,111(5,740)	26,849(4,269)	78,790(12,526)
QALYs−10%	37,049(5,891)	27,160(4,318)	80,863(12,856)
Costs+10% and QALYs−10%	40,607(6,456)	29,743(4,729)	89,210(14,183)
Costs limit	+250%	+365%	+68%
QALYS limit	−75%	−81%	−42%
Excluding bilateral RRD patients	38,243(6,080)	25,825(4,106)	72,250(11,486)

ICER, incremental cost-effectiveness ratio; CNY, Chinese Yuan; USD, US dollar; RRD, rhegmatogenous retinal detachment; QALY, quality-adjusted life year.

However, the surgery brought significant improvement to the visual acuity of these patients. The BCVA of the elderly patients increased continuously from 3 months to 1 year postoperatively in the study. The average improvement in BCVA was 0.53 ± 0.44 at the 1-year postoperative time point for all of the participants. Although age was reported to be a negative predictor of visual acuity outcomes after RRD surgery in many publications [15–19], the increase in BCVA in our study was no less than that reported in other studies that also included younger patients whose average age was approximately 60 years old [25], [37], [38], [43]. Similarly, in the SPR study, no relationship was observed between age and inferior visual outcomes [44]. Due to the inconsistency of the baseline status of RRD between the different study groups, the results in our study cannot be directly compared with other studies

and we are therefore not be able to conclude whether age is a negative predictor for visual outcome. In any case, the significant improvement in BCVA indicates that RRD surgery is beneficial for patients over 80 years old as well as patients 70–79 years old.

In recent years, increasing emphasis has been put on evaluating the vision-related quality of life in ocular diseases. To reflect how the retinal detachment surgery influences the patients' quality of life, we investigated preference-based utility values before and 1 year after the surgery among the elderly patients. Utility analysis, unlike some other quality of life measurements, enables comparisons of quality of life across different health statuses in medicine and further analyses of cost-utility results for resource allocations [45]. The patients reported statistically significant increases in utility values postoperatively, rising from an average of 0.77 to

Table 7. Comparisons of surgical outcomes between the normal RRD patients and the elderly patients [4], [10].

	Normal population	Elderly population	P value*
No. of Patients	117	98	
Age [Mean (SD)]	54.28(10.30)	78.49(4.36)	<0.001
Type of surgery			<0.001
Scleral buckling surgery [No. (%)]	68(58.12)	31(31.63)	
Vitreous surgery [No. (%)]	49(41.89)	67(68.37)	
Preoperative BCVA	1.06(0.63)	1.06(0.50)	0.832
BCVA after 3 months	0.68(0.40)	0.74(0.35)	0.227
BCVA after 1 year	0.51(0.32)	0.54(0.26)	0.456
Difference of BCVA in 3 months	0.38(0.40)	0.32(0.35)	0.314
Difference of BCVA in 1 year	0.55(0.48)	0.53(0.44)	0.773
Utility value before surgery	0.77(0.12)	0.77(0.12)	0.806
Utility value after 1 year	0.83(0.10)	0.84(0.08)	0.610
Difference of utility value in 1 year	0.06(0.09)	0.07(0.07)	0.427
Costs [Bootstrap 1000 times; Mean (95% CI); CNY]	11,384(10,338–12,563)	12,992(11,984–14,088)	
QALYs gained in life time [Bootstrap 1000 times; Mean (95% CI)]	0.88(0.64–1.13)	0.40(0.31–0.50)	
ICERs [Bootstrap 1000 times; Mean; CNY/QALY]	13,794	33,186	

*An independent sample t-test was used for continual data of normal distribution, a Mann Whitney U test for non-normal distribution data, and the Pearson chi-square test for the categorical data. A value of P<0.05 was regarded as statistically significant.
RRD, rhegmatogenous retinal detachment; SD, standard deviation; BCVA, best -corrected visual acuity; CI, confidence interval; CNY, Chinese Yuan; QALY, quality-adjusted life year.

0.84. The patients above 80 years old seem to benefit less than those in the 70 to 79 years old group do, as demonstrated by the 1-year postoperative utility value; however, the ambiguous p value (0.096) makes it difficult to determine whether this difference is meaningful. Moreover, the change in utility values in the elderly population is similar to what we investigated in a younger population with an average age of 54 years old (P = 0.427) [4]. A summary of comparisons with our previous study is presented in Table 7.

When the benefit of lifetime was considered, the QALYs gained in patients aged 70–79 years old were approximately three times greater than in patients over 80 years old. Compared with our previous study [10], the QALYs gained in the elderly population were relatively small: 0.40 QALYs for the elderly compared to 0.88 QALYs for an average group of patients (Table 7). This is likely because older people have theoretically fewer remaining life years than younger people do. Consequently, the ICER, which combined the costs and QALYs gained, was higher in the elderly population compared to an average group of patients. The ICER in patients over 80 years old was three times higher than that in patients in their 70s. Despite the lower cost-effectiveness of RRD surgery in the elderly patients, the treatment was still below the threshold of willingness to pay of China, even for patients over 80 years old.

In the subgroup analyses for the two types of surgery, the vitreous surgery was less expensive for each QALYs gained than scleral buckling surgery in the elderly population, however, the discrepancy was not large. Unlike what we observed in the normal patients [10], the elderly people seemed to benefit less from scleral buckling surgery, probably because that the elderly patients usually have more complicated and diverse conditions than the normal patients do, which enables the comparable costs for the two types surgery. This might also be the reason that the proportion of vitreous surgery was higher in the elderly population than in the normal patients (Table 7), since surgeons' preference of choosing the vitreous surgery for complicated situation.

Elderly patients do not always accept surgery for RRD. On the one hand, the costs of RRD surgery are still relatively high for most people in our country, despite the fact that the National Health Insurance policy might cover some of the expenses [46]. On the other hand, elderly people might have fewer demands for vision-related quality of life because daily life activities are reduced and their life expectancy is relatively short. Additionally, lacking knowledge about health, they might be anxious about the disadvantages of the surgery, such as discomfort, complications, or risk of death. As a result, quite a few elderly people ultimately choose not to undertake the surgical option, which is the reason for the relatively small sample size in this population. It is difficult to persuade such patients to have surgery, yet it is considered unethical for an ophthalmologist to allow these patients to return home without treatment. Our study provides evidence that RRD surgery can improve visual acuity and the quality of life, and it is a cost-effective intervention in people over 70 years old. Therefore, ophthalmologists should persuade such elderly RRD patients to have surgery. In the interim, this health economic evaluation of RRD surgery may also provide a valuable tool for governmental agencies in formulating the National Health Insurance policy.

There are some limitations of this study. First, the study lacks real patient controls; however, not offering treatment for RRD patients violates the tenets of the Declaration of Helsinki, preventing approval by an ethical committee. Secondly, the study period was not long enough to truly reflect the long-term cost-utility of RRD surgery. The results of the long-term analysis were based on the assumption that no more costs associated with RRD surgery would be incurred and that patients would retain their utility value of the 1-year postoperative time point throughout their remaining life years. In the real world, outpatient service fees and transportation fees should be included as well, even if the costs are trivial compared with the surgery expenditures during the first year. Additionally, the utility value would deteriorate both in the treatment group and in the control group over the course of the life expectancy; however, some of the declining factors might counteract each other, making their influence unclear. Third, the study population was relatively small, and all the participants were from one teaching hospital. The results might be more presentative for large cities with similar economic conditions as Shanghai than for small towns in China. In future work, studies with more participants from different regions and longer follow-up times are desirable to facilitate cost-utility analyses that are more comprehensive. Finally, we did not include indirect costs, and this exclusion would probably underestimate the economic value of the surgery, as people in the control group had severe visual impairment, which might influence their living independency and incur expenses for nursing.

To conclude, the RRD surgery greatly improves visual acuity and the quality of life in elderly people in China. Compared to other studies that include younger populations, the visual acuity and vision-related quality of life outcomes were similar. Considering the shorter life expectancy, the elderly patients obtain fewer QALYs from RRD surgery, and thus, a higher cost per QALY was found. However, it is still cost-effective for elderly people to have RRD surgery, even for patients over 80 years old.

Author Contributions

Conceived and designed the experiments: HDZ XZ XX. Performed the experiments: HYL LB. Analyzed the data: YYM XHY XCX. Contributed reagents/materials/analysis tools: XHY XCX. Contributed to the writing of the manuscript: YYM. Final approval of the version to be published: HDZ. Help to interpret data: HYL LB. Modified the manuscript: XX XZ HDZ.

References

1. Ross WH, Stockl FA (2000) Visual recovery after retinal detachment. Curr Opin Ophthalmol 11: 191–194.
2. Zou H, Zhang X, Xu X, Liu H (2008) Quality of life in subjects with rhegmatogenous retinal detachment. Ophthal Epidemiol 15: 215–217.
3. Okamoto F, Okamoto Y, Hiraoka T, Oshika T (2008) Vision-related quality of life and visual function after retinal detachment surgery. Am J Ophthalmol 1461: 85–90.
4. Zou H, Zhang X, Xu X, Liu H, Bai L, et al. (2011) Utility value and retinal detachment surgery. Ophthalmology 118: 601.
5. Sodhi A, Leung LS, Do DV, Gower EW, Schein OD, et al. (2008) Recent trends in the management of rhegmatogenous retinal detachment. Surv Ophthalmol 53: 50–67.
6. Yorston D, Jalali S (2002) Retinal detachment in developing countries. Eye 16: 353–358.
7. Brown GC, Brown MM, Sharma S, Busbee B, Landy J (2002) A cost-utility analysis of interventions for severe proliferative vitreoretinopathy. Am - J Ophthalmol 133: 365–372.
8. Seider MI, Naseri A, Stewart JM (2013) Cost comparison of scleral buckle versus vitrectomy for rhegmatogenous retinal detachment repair. Am J Ophthalmol 156: 661–666.
9. Chang JS, Smiddy WE (2014) Cost-effectiveness of retinal detachment repair. Ophthalmology 121: 946–951.
10. Ma Y, Ying X, Zou H, Xu X, Liu H, et al. (2014) Cost-utility Analysis of Rhegmatogenous Retinal Detachment Surgery in Shanghai, China. Ophthalmic Epidemiol, doi:10.3109/09286586.2014.884601.
11. Mitry D, Charteris DG, Fleck BW, Campbell H, Singh J (2010) The epidemiology of rhegmatogenous retinal detachment: geographical variation and clinical associations. Br J Ophthalmol 94: 678–684.

12. Park SJ, Choi NK, Park KH, Woo SJ (2013) Five year nationwide incidence of rhegmatogenous retinal detachment requiring surgery in Korea. PloS one. Available at http://www.plosone.org/article/info%3Adoi%2F10.1371%2Fjournal.pone.0080174#pone-0080174-g001. Accessed May 1,2014.

13. Mitry D, Charteris DG, Yorston D, Siddiqui MA, Campbell H, et al. (2010) The epidemiology and socioeconomic associations of retinal detachment in Scotland: a two-year prospective population-based study. Invest Ophthalmol Vis Sci 51: 4963–4968.

14. Van de Put MA, Hooymans JM, Los LI, Dutch Rhegmatogenous Retinal Detachment Study Group (2013) The incidence of rhegmatogenous retinal detachment in The Netherlands. Ophthalmology 120: 616–622.

15. Ross WH (2002) Visual recovery after macula-off retinal detachment. Eye (Lond) 16: 440–446.

16. Ahmadieh H, Entezari M, Soheilian M, Azarmina M, Dehghan MH, et al. (2000) Factors influencing anatomic and visual results in primary scleral buckling. Eur J Ophthalmol 10: 153–159.

17. Mowatt L, Shun Shin GA, Arora S, Price N (2005) Macula off retinal detachments. How long can they wait before it is too late? Eur J Ophthalmol 15: 109–117.

18. Pastor JC, Fernández I, Rodríguez de la Rúa E, Coco R, Sanabria Ruiz Colmenares MR, et al. (2008) Surgical outcomes for primary rhegmatogenous retinal detachments in phakic and pseudophakic patients: the Retina 1 Project–report 2. Br J Ophthalmol 92: 378–382.

19. Liu F, Meyer CH, Mennel S, Hoerle S, Kroll P (2006) Visual recovery after scleral buckling surgery in macula-off rhegmatogenous retinal detachment. Ophthalmologica 220: 174–180.

20. Huang XB, Zou HD, Wang N, Wang WW, Fu J, et al. (2009) A prevalence survey of blindness and visual impairment in adults aged equal or more than 60 years in Beixinjing blocks of Shanghai, China. Zhonghua Yan Ke Za Zhi 45: 786–792.

21. Drummond MF (2005) Methods for the economic evaluation of Health Care Programmes. United States: Oxford university press. 7–269p.

22. Muennig P (2008) Cost-effectiveness analyses in health: a practical approach. United States: John Wiley & Sons. 1–18p.

23. Sharma S, Brown GC, Brown MM, Hollands H, Robins R, et al. (2002) Validity of the time trade-off and standard gamble methods of utility assessment in retinal patients. Br J Ophthalmol 86: 493–496.

24. National Bureau of Statistics of China (2014) Statistical Communique of the People's Republic of China. Available at: http://www.stats.gov.cn/tjsj/tjgb/ndtjgb/. Accessed May 1, 2014.

25. Zou H, Zhang X, Xu X, Liu H, Bai L, et al. (2011) Vision-Related Quality of Life and Self-Rated Satisfaction Outcomes of Rhegmatogenous Retinal Detachment Surgery: 3-Year Prospective Study. PLoS one. Available at: http://www.plosone.org/article/info%3Adoi%2F10.1371%2Fjournal.pone.0028597. Accessed December 5, 2013.

26. Sach TH, Foss AJ, Gregson RM, Zaman A, Osborn F, et al. (2010) Second-eye cataract surgery in elderly women: a cost-utility analysis conducted alongside a randomized controlled trial. Eye (Lond) 24: 276–283.

27. Sharma S, Hollands H, Brown GC, Brown MM, Shah GK, et al. (2001) The cost-effectiveness of early vitrectomy for the treatment of vitreous hemorrhage in diabetic retinopathy. Curr Opin Ophthalmol 12: 230–234.

28. World Health Rankings. Health profile China. Available at http://www.worldlifeexpectancy.com/country-health-profile/china. Accessed Dec 3, 2013.

29. Commission on Macroeconomics, HealthWorld Health Organization (2001) Macroeconomics and Health: Investing in Health for Economic Development-Report of the Commission on Macroeconomics and HealthWorld Health Organization, Geneva, Switzerland.

30. Yuan Y, lloeje U, Li H, Hay J, Yao GB (2008) Economic implications of entecavir treatment in suppressing viral replication in chronic hepatitis B (CHB) patients in China from a perspective of the Chinese Social Security program. Value Health 11(Suppl): 11–22.

31. Yang L, Christensen T, Sun F, Chang J (2012) Cost-effectiveness of switching patients with type 2 diabetes from insulin glargine to insulin detemir in Chinese setting: a health economic model based on the PREDICTIVE study. Value Health 15(Suppl): 56–59.

32. Briggs AH, Gray AM (1999) Handling uncertainty when performing economic evaluation of healthcare interventions. Health Technol Assess 3: 1–134.

33. Polsky D, Glick HA, Willke R (1997) Confidence intervals for cost-effectiveness ratios: a comparison of four methods. Health Econ 6: 243–252.

34. Barber JA, Thompson SG (2000) Analysis of cost data in randomized trials: an application of the nonparametric bootstrap. Stat Med 19: 3219–3236.

35. van Hout BA, Al MJ, Gordon GS, Rutten FF (1994) Costs, effects and C/E-ratios alongside a clinical trial. Health Econ 3: 309–319.

36. Fenwick E, Claxton K, Sculpher M (2001) Representing uncertainty: the role of cost-effectiveness acceptability curves. Health Econ 10: 779–787.

37. Heimann H, Zou X, Jandeck C, Kellner U, Bechrakis NE, et al. (2006) Primary vitrectomy for rhegmatogenous retinal detachment: an analysis of 512 cases. Graefes Arch Clin Exp Ophthalmol 244: 69–78.

38. Salicone A, Smiddy WE, Venkatraman A, Feuer W (2006) Visual recovery after scleral buckling procedure for retinal detachment. Ophthalmology 113: 1734–1742.

39. Schneider EW, Geraets RL, Johnson MW (2012) Pars plana vitrectomy without adjuvant procedures for repair of primary rhegmatogenous retinal detachment. Retina 32: 213–219.

40. Ahmadieh H, Moradian S, Faghihi H, Parvaresh MM, Ghanbari H, et al (2005) Anatomic and visual outcomes of scleral buckling versus primary vitrectomy in pseudophakic and aphakic retinal detachment: six-month follow-up results of a single operation–report no. 1. Ophthalmology 112: 1421–1429.

41. Azad RV, Chanana B, Sharma YR, Vohra R (2007) Primary vitrectomy versus conventional retinal detachment surgery in phakic rhegmatogenous retinal detachment. Acta Ophthalmol Scand 85: 540–545.

42. Li X, Beijing Rhegmatogenous Retinal Detachment Study Group (2003) Incidence and epidemiological characteristics of rhegmatogenous retinal detachment in Beijing, China. Ophthalmology 110: 2413–2417.

43. Heimann H, Bartz Schmidt KU, Bornfeld N, Weiss C, Hilgers RD, et al. (2007) Scleral Buckling versus Primary Vitrectomy in Rhegmatogenous Retinal Detachment Study Group. Scleral buckling versus primary vitrectomy in rhegmatogenous retinal detachment: a prospective randomized multicenter clinical study. Ophthalmology 114: 2142–2154.

44. Heussen N, Feltgen N, Walter P, Hoerauf H, Hilgers RD, et al. (2011) Scleral buckling versus primary vitrectomy in rhegmatogenous retinal detachment study (SPR Study): predictive factors for functional outcome. Study report no. 6. Graefes Arch Clin Exp Ophthalmol 249: 1129–1136.

45. Brown MM, Brown GC, Sharma S, Busbee B (2003) Quality of life associated with visual loss: a time tradeoff utility analysis comparison with medical health states. Ophthalmology 110: 1076–1081.

46. Shanghai Health Insurance. Information of urban basic health insurance programs in Shanghai. Available at http://www.shyb.gov.cn/ybzc/zcfg/03/201111/t20111101_1134638.shtml. Accessed Dec 3, 2013.

21

Zinc Supplementation Inhibits Complement Activation in Age-Related Macular Degeneration

Dzenita Smailhodzic[1,9,¶], **Freekje van Asten**[1,9,¶], **Anna M. Blom**[2], **Frida C. Mohlin**[2], **Anneke I. den Hollander**[1,3], **Johannes P. H. van de Ven**[1], **Ramon A. C. van Huet**[1], **Joannes M. M. Groenewoud**[4], **Yuan Tian**[5], **Tos T. J. M. Berendschot**[5], **Yara T. E. Lechanteur**[1], **Sascha Fauser**[6], **Chris de Bruijn**[7], **Mohamed R. Daha**[8], **Gert Jan van der Wilt**[4], **Carel B. Hoyng**[1], **B. Jeroen Klevering**[1]*

1 Department of Ophthalmology, Radboud university medical center, Nijmegen, the Netherlands, 2 Section of Medical Protein Chemistry, Department of Laboratory Medicine Malmo, Lund University, Malmo, Sweden, 3 Department of Human Genetics, Radboud university medical center, Nijmegen, the Netherlands, 4 Department for Health Evidence, Radboud university medical center, Nijmegen, the Netherlands, 5 University Eye Clinic Maastricht, Maastricht, the Netherlands, 6 Department of Ophthalmology, University of Cologne, Cologne, Germany, 7 Innomedics, Düsseldorf, Germany, 8 Department of Nephrology, Leiden University Medical Center, Leiden, the Netherlands

Abstract

Age-related macular degeneration (AMD) is the leading cause of blindness in the Western world. AMD is a multifactorial disorder but complement-mediated inflammation at the level of the retina plays a pivotal role. Oral zinc supplementation can reduce the progression of AMD but the precise mechanism of this protective effect is as yet unclear. We investigated whether zinc supplementation directly affects the degree of complement activation in AMD and whether there is a relation between serum complement catabolism during zinc administration and the *complement factor H (CFH)* gene or the *Age-Related Maculopathy susceptibility 2 (ARMS2)* genotype. In this open-label clinical study, 72 randomly selected AMD patients in various stages of AMD received a daily supplement of 50 mg zinc sulphate and 1 mg cupric sulphate for three months. Serum complement catabolism–defined as the C3d/C3 ratio–was measured at baseline, throughout the three months of supplementation and after discontinuation of zinc administration. Additionally, downstream inhibition of complement catabolism was evaluated by measurement of anaphylatoxin C5a. Furthermore, we investigated the effect of zinc on complement activation *in vitro*. AMD patients with high levels of complement catabolism at baseline exhibited a steeper decline in serum complement activation (p<0.001) during the three month zinc supplementation period compared to patients with low complement levels. There was no significant association of change in complement catabolism and *CFH* and *ARMS2* genotype. *In vitro* zinc sulphate directly inhibits complement catabolism in hemolytic assays and membrane attack complex (MAC) deposition on RPE cells. This study provides evidence that daily administration of 50 mg zinc sulphate can inhibit complement catabolism in AMD patients with increased complement activation. This could explain part of the mechanism by which zinc slows AMD progression.

Trial Registration: The Netherlands National Trial Register NTR2605

Editor: Margaret M. DeAngelis, University of Utah, United States of America

Funding: This work was supported by the Netherlands Organisation for Scientific Research (grant 016.096.309), the MD Fonds, the Oogfonds, the Landelijke Stichting voor Blinden en Slechtzienden, the Algemene Nederlandse Vereniging ter Voorkoming van Blindheid, the Stichting Researchfonds Oogheelkunde, the Stichting Nederlands Oogheelkundig Onderzoek, the Stichting Blindenhulp, the Gelderse Blindenstichting, the Swedish Research Council (K2012-66X-14928-09-5) and the grant for clinical research (ALF). Zinc sulphate and cupric sulphate capsules were a generous gift from Sanmed, Almere, the Netherlands. The funders had no role in study design, data collection and analysis, decision to publish, or preparation of the manuscript.

Competing Interests: Prof. C. De Bruijn was affiliated with the company Innomedics and had a consulting role in this study which was unrelated to his employment at Innomedics. Zinc sulphate and cupric sulphate capsules were a gift from Sanmed, Almere, the Netherlands. None of these commercial companies had a role in the study design, data collection and analysis, decision to publish, or preparation of the manuscript.

* Email: Jeroen.Klevering@radboudumc.nl

⑨ These authors contributed equally to this work.

¶ DS and FA are equivalent and joint first authors on this work.

Introduction

Worldwide, age-related macular degeneration (AMD) affects 30–50 million people and is the leading cause of blindness in the Western world [1–4]. AMD is a complex, multifactorial disease that manifests clinically as a loss of central vision resulting in an inability to read, recognize faces or discriminate colors. The hallmark lesions of early stage AMD are drusen, which are pathological deposits of extracellular material that form between the retinal pigment epithelium and Bruch membrane [5]. The late stages of AMD can be separated into geographic atrophy and neovascular AMD [5]. In patients with neovascular AMD, choroidal blood vessels invade the central retina and subretinal space causing a rapidly progressive loss of vision [5]. Although the neovascular AMD accounts for 10% of all AMD patients, it is responsible for the majority of AMD-related severe visual impairment [6–9]. Despite the beneficial effects of intraocular injections of vascular endothelial growth factor A (VEGF-A) inhibitors [10–11], a large percentage of neovascular AMD patients continue to lose vision [12–13]. In patients with geographic atrophy, loss of the RPE and photoreceptor cells in the central retina result in a progressive decline of vision at a much slower rate than neovascular AMD [5]. Unfortunately, an effective therapy for treating geographic atrophy has yet to be developed.

Pivotal studies performed during the past decade have changed our understanding of the molecular mechanisms underlying AMD. These findings have led to the exploration of a new therapeutic paradigm for managing AMD, namely the targeting of specific molecular components in the complement pathway [14–15]. The complement system is a major component of innate immunity with crucial roles in the first line defense against invading microorganisms, clearance of the apoptotic cells and modulation of the adaptive immune response [16]. There are three pathways of complement activation: the classical, the lectin and the alternative pathway [16]. The most important step of the alternative complement pathway activation is the formation of unstable C3 convertase C3bBb, which cleaves C3 to generate the active fragment C3b. Deposition of C3b on the target surface triggers the effector molecules C3a, C5a and the membrane attack complex (MAC), resulting in inflammation and cell lysis. The discovery that drusen contain proteins of the alternative complement pathway led to the hypothesis that drusen could be involved in local complement-mediated inflammation [17–18]. Moreover, the discovery of a strong association between AMD and genetic variants in *CFH* gene, a major inhibitor of the alternative pathway, provided a second line of evidence in support of the inflammation model [19–22]. In addition to *CFH*, several other AMD risk variants have been found in genes underlying the alternative pathway [23–26]. A third line of evidence supporting complement involvement in AMD came from studies that showed that AMD patients have higher levels of complement activation products in their blood [27–30]. However, it is likely to be several years before any of the complement inhibiting drugs will be approved for routine use in clinical practice, assuming they are eventually found to be safe and effective.

In 2001, the data collected from the Age-Related Eye Disease Study (AREDS) revealed that patients who were treated with zinc–either alone or in combination with vitamins–had reduced progression to advanced AMD [31]. Based on these results, AREDS recommends that persons who are older than 55 years of age and who are at risk for developing advanced AMD should consider taking vitamin supplements plus zinc [31]. A report published by the Blue Mountains Eye Study, a population-based study, confirmed the beneficial effect of zinc in AMD patients [32]. The large population-based Rotterdam Study supported the hypothesis of biological interactions between the *CFH* gene Y402H variant and zinc, β-carotene, lutein/zeaxanthin and omega-3 fatty acids and between the *ARMS2* gene A69S variant and zinc and omega-3 fatty acids [33]. As a result of these findings, the Rotterdam Study recommended that clinicians give dietary advice to young individuals who are at risk for AMD [33]. More recently, AREDS2 demonstrated that addition of lutein, zeaxanthin and omega-3 long-chain polyunsaturated fatty acids to the AREDS formulation, did not further reduce risk of progression to

advanced AMD [34]. However, exploratory subgroup analyses demonstrated that addition of lutein and zeaxanthin to the AREDS formulation, resulted in a significant reduction of progression to advanced AMD for persons in the lowest quintile of dietary intake, suggesting different treatment effects within subgroups of AMD patients [34]. Despite the widespread use of zinc and antioxidants among AMD patients, the mechanism by which zinc exerts its beneficial effects in AMD patients has not yet been identified. The design of optimal and appropriate therapies require a comprehensive understanding of the factors that drive and delay pathogenesis of AMD. To add to current knowledge we designed the present study to investigate whether zinc affects the activity of the alternative complement pathway in patients with AMD, which might explain how zinc slows AMD progression in subgroups of patients with AMD. Secondly, we correlate the response to zinc supplements to the *CFH* and *ARMS2* genotype status. Lastly, we conducted an in vitro experiment to evaluate whether there is a direct effect of zinc on complement activation.

Methods

Study population of the clinical study

This study was performed in accordance with the Declaration of Helsinki and the Dutch Medical Research Involving Human Subjects Act. Prior to the study, we obtained approval from the local ethics committee (Commissie Mensgebonden Onderzoek regio Arnhem-Nijmegen, April 20th 2010) as well as written informed consent from all participants. This clinical study was registered with The Netherlands National Trial Register (number NTR2605) shortly after recruitment began due to an administrative error. The authors confirm that all ongoing and related trials for this drug/intervention are registered. The protocol for this trial and supporting TREND checklist are available as supporting infromation (Protocol S1 and Checklist S1). The study participants were enrolled in EUGENDA (www.eugenda.org), a multicenter database for the clinical and molecular analysis of AMD, between March 2006 and August 2009. Patients with various stages of AMD were selected at random from the EUGENDA database and were included between June 2010 and February 2011. Follow-up ranged between 14 and 22 months. All data were collected at the department of Ophthalmology of the Radboud university medical center. We excluded individuals who had a core body temperature above 38°C and/or received antibiotics at baseline. In addition, we excluded patients who were receiving intraocular anti-angiogenic treatment, individuals with atypical hemolytic uremic syndrome or membranoproliferative glomerulonephritis type 2 and patients who received local or systemic steroid therapy within the three months prior to the trial. A total of 72 AMD patients were included in this study (Figure 1).

Study design

To study the effect of zinc on complement activation in patients with AMD, 72 AMD patients received a daily oral supplement containing 50 mg zinc sulphate and 1 mg cupric sulphate in capsule form. The capsules were to be taken at home for a period of three months. These components were donated by Sanmed, Almere, the Netherlands. The 50 mg dose of zinc was lower than in the original AREDS formulation and was chosen to minimize the chance of side-effects. Also, we chose zinc sulphate instead of zinc oxide (as used in the AREDS study), because most over-the-counter supplements contain zinc sulphate and in addition there is evidence that the bioavailability may be higher [35,36]. The primary endpoint of the study was a change in serum complement catabolism during the three months of zinc supplementation.

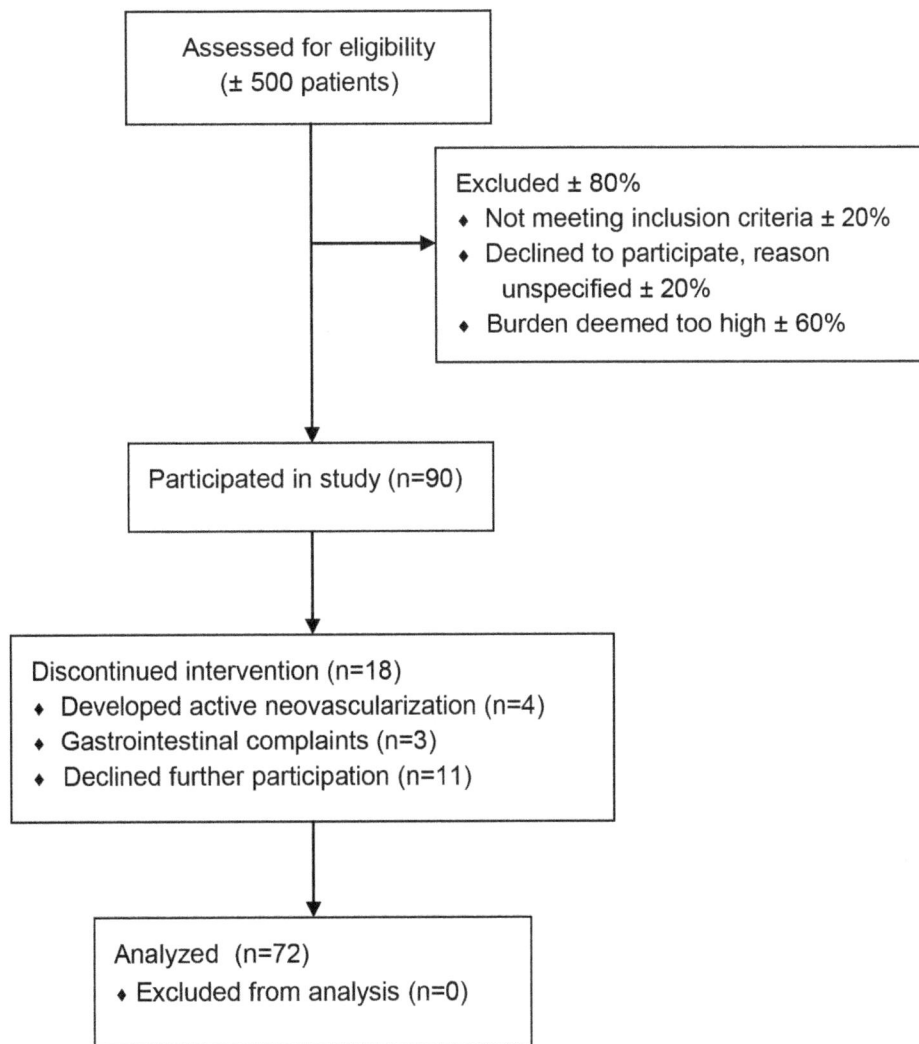

Figure 1. Flow diagram of patient inclusion.

AMD patients have increased serum levels of C3 and the metabolic byproduct C3d, the most prominent marker of chronic activation of the alternative complement pathway [30]. To correct for individual variations in the level of C3, complement activation was defined as the C3d/C3 ratio as described previously [30]. Anaphylatoxin C5a levels are also elevated in AMD patients and promote choroidal neovascularization [28,29,37]. In order to explore downstream inhibitory effects of zinc on complement catabolism, we additionally measured serum C5a levels during the study period. The second objective was to study the association of serum complement catabolism during zinc administration and genotypes of AMD risk variants in *CFH* or *ARMS2*.

During the course of the study, six venous blood samples were collected. One sample was collected prior to zinc supplementation and served as the baseline sample. Three samples were collected at the end of months 1, 2 and 3 of the three-month period of zinc supplementation. We collected a fifth blood sample two months after ending the zinc administration (i.e., at the end of month 5) to check for any reversible effects on complement activation. A final blood sample was collected in months 14–22. From one month prior to zinc supplementation through the end of month 5, the patients were prohibited to take any type of nutritional supple-

ment; from month 5 onwards, the patients were free to take supplements at their own discretion.

To identify clinical manifestations associated with intermittent infections, at every visit, we performed a general physical examination, measured the serum C-reactive protein (CRP) levels and administered a questionnaire that was aimed at identifying clinical manifestations associated with intermittent infections. At every visit, patients were asked whether they had been taking the zinc supplements daily to promote compliance. We also assessed the best-corrected visual acuity using Early-Treatment Diabetic Retinopathy Study (ETDRS) charts at every visit. In addition, we imaged the retinas using high-resolution spectral-domain optical coherence tomography (SD-OCT) to detect active neovascular manifestation of AMD. We performed color fundus photography at baseline to assist in AMD grading based on the 5-grade Clinical Age-Related Maculopathy Staging (CARMS) classification scale [38].

Complement measurements and genotyping in AMD patients

Serum was prepared by coagulation at room temperature and after centrifugation the samples were stored at $-80°C$ within one hour after collection. C3 and C3d were measured in serum samples as described [39,40]. All C3 and C3d measurements in this study were performed in a single experiment, except for the final sample in months 14–22. C5a was measured by ELISA at a 1/10 dilution using a commercially available development kit (DuoSet) for human complement component C5a (R&D Systems, Minneapolis, USA). All the samples collected at baseline to month 5 were measured in a single run.

The *CFH* (Y402H; rs1061170) and *ARMS2* (A69S; rs10490924) SNPs were genotyped as described [41]. Serum zinc concentration was measured by atomic absorption spectroscopy with the spectrophotometer 1100 B from Perkin Elmer. CRP levels were measured by Abbott Architect C16000 system. The immunoturbidimetric test for CRP was provided by Abbott Diagnostics (Abbott Diagnostics).

In vitro hemolytic assays and membrane attack complex (MAC) deposition on RPE cells

We designed in vitro experiments to provide evidence of a direct effect of zinc on the complement pathway. Human serum was prepared from blood of several healthy volunteers after written informed consent had been obtained with the specific permit (418/2008) from the ethics committee of Lund University. Commercially available rabbit erythrocytes (Håtunalab, Bro, Sweden) were washed in 2.5 mM veronal buffer pH 7.3, supplemented with 70 mM NaCl, 140 mM glucose, 0.1% porcine gelatin and 7 mM $MgCl_2$. Different concentrations (0–64 μM) of zinc sulphate (Merck) were pre-incubated with 2% serum in the same buffer for 1.5 h at 37°C, followed by 1 h incubation at 37°C together with the erythrocytes. The amount of lysed erythrocytes was determined from the amount of released hemoglobin at 405 nm using Cary 50 MPR microplate reader (Varian).

To study the effect of zinc on membrane MAC deposition on human RPE cells, RPE cells (ARPE-19, ATCC) were cultured in DMEM/F12 media (HyClone), supplemented with 10% FCS (Gibco) and antibiotics (HyClone). After detachment using trypsin, the cells were incubated in medium containing 10 mM H_2O_2 for 2 h at 37°C, to mimic oxidative damage and make them amenable to attack from complement [42,43]. After washing with PBS, the cells were incubated with 5% human serum, together with 0–250 μM zinc sulphate, in the veronal buffer defined above, for 1 h at 37°C. The amount of MAC deposited on the RPE cells was detected using a monoclonal C9 neoepitope antibody (aE11, Hycult), which only recognizes C9 in the C5b-9 complex, followed by a FITC-conjugated secondary antibody and flow cytometric analysis (Partec).

Statistical analysis

A sample size of 70 was calculated to detect a decrease in serum C3d/C3 of 10% after 3 months, using the complement levels from a previous study to estimate variation [30], with $\alpha = 0.05$ and a power of 80%.

Change in serum zinc, change in C3d/C3 ratio and change in C5a over the entire study period (0 to 14–22 months) were all modeled separately. Changes in serum zinc concentration were analyzed using a linear mixed-effects model with zinc concentration as the dependent variable. To make optimal use of repeated measures and to allow for correction of baseline differences, changes in C3d/C3 and C5a levels level were analyzed using linear mixed-effects models with C3d/C3 ratio or C5a as the dependent variable. The interaction between time and baseline complement levels was included in a linear mixed-effects model to study any baseline effects. To illustrate the effect of the baseline

C3d/C3 ratio we plotted the course of the C3d/C3 ratio for 3 groups with different baseline ratios using the raw data. In a recent study we measured C3d/C3 levels in 150 unaffected control subjects of 65 years and older [30], and we used the mean value (1.5) and standard deviation (0.6) to determine the cut-off points. The cut-off values for the different groups were selected by taking the mean C3d/C3 ratio and one standard deviation above and below the mean of the healthy control group. Our population was not large enough to create groups of individuals with two standard deviations above and below the mean. This resulted in the following three groups: 1. patients with baseline ratio ≥2.1 (n = 16); 2. patients with ratios between 1.5–2.1 (n = 29); and 3. patients with ratio <1.5 (n = 31). Only very few subjects (n = 3) had a baseline ratio more than one standard deviation below the mean, so these individuals were included in group 3. The associations between the complement levels throughout the study and *CFH* and *ARMS2* genotype, age, gender, CRP level and zinc level were also studied using a linear mixed-effects model. In the final models for the change in zinc, C3d/C3 and C5a, only significant predictors were used (p<0.05). For the final serum zinc and C5a models this meant the inclusion of time and baseline values as the independent variables. In the final C3d/C3 model the independent variables were time, baseline C3d/C3 and the interaction between time and baseline C3d/C3.

To further explore the relationship between baseline complement catabolism and other patient characteristics at baseline, we assessed the associations of age and baseline visual acuity with baseline C3d/C3 ratio and C5a using the Pearson correlation and the Spearman's rank correlation coefficient. The difference in baseline complement catabolism between different genotypes was assessed using one-way ANOVA.

Because patients often display different stages of AMD in each eye, we created five groups for both eyes. These groups were based on the CARMS classification as follows: (CARMS grade 2:2), small drusen and/or RPE changes in both eyes; (CARMS grade 3:3), large drusen and/or drusenoid RPE detachment in both eyes; (CARMS grade 2:4–5), small drusen and/or RPE changes in one eye and geographic atrophy or choroidal neovascularisation in the other eye; (CARMS grade 3:4–5), large drusen and/or drusenoid RPE detachment in one eye and geographic atrophy or choroidal neovascularisation in the other eye; and (CARMS grade 4–5:4–5), geographic atrophy or choroidal neovascularisation in both eyes. The association between baseline systemic complement catabolism and CARMS classification was tested using one-way ANOVA with a post-hoc Bonferroni correction. The correlation between baseline visual acuity and CARMS was tested using the Spearman's rank correlation coefficient.

Visual acuity changes during the course of the study were assessed by generalized estimated equations (GEE). The GEE model estimated the probability of low vision (LogMAR <0.5) versus high vision (LogMAR >0.5), with time and baseline C3d/C3 ratio as predictors. Data for the hemolytic assay and the RPE cell assay were analyzed using one-way ANOVA with Dunnett's multiple comparison test.

Reported p-values are two-sided, and differences were considered to be statistically significant if lower than 0.05. All statistical analyses were performed using SPSS, version 18.0.

Results

To evaluate the effect of receiving zinc supplements on systemic complement catabolism, AMD patients received oral zinc sulphate. The baseline characteristics of the study population are presented in Table 1. Serum zinc concentration increased significantly during the supplementation period (p<0.001) and returned to baseline levels two months after the zinc supplements were discontinued (Figure 2). The mean complement activation level, defined as the C3d/C3 ratio, in the 72 patients showed tendency to decline (albeit not significantly; p = 0.149) during the three months of zinc supplementation (Figure 2). From month five onwards, 36 patients indicated they had been using over-the-counter zinc supplements, but generally in lower dosages than used in this study.

Exploration of effect of zinc supplementation on complement catabolism

We conducted further exploratory analyses whether zinc supplementation may have different effects within patients with different levels of baseline complement catabolism defined as C3d/C3 ratio. In this analysis, we observed a strong interaction between baseline C3d/C3 ratio and change in C3d/C3 ratio during zinc supplementation (p<0.001). The AMD patients with relatively high baseline levels of serum complement catabolism exhibited a more pronounced decline in their C3d/C3 ratio during the administration of zinc sulphate, compared to those AMD patients with lower baseline levels. After the zinc supplementation period, the decline in C3d/C3 ratio remained at this lower level for the following two months. Measurements performed at least nine months later (in months 14–22) showed that complement activation had returned to baseline levels. The AMD patients who already had a relatively low C3d/C3 ratio at baseline showed no decline in C3d/C3 ratio throughout the treatment period. Figure 3 illustrates the course of serum C3d/C3 ratio over time in three groups with different baseline C3d/C3 ratios. The statistical model was not based on these cut-off points. There was no significant association between C3d/C3 ratio and age or gender throughout the course of the study. C5a levels decreased significantly over the three-month supplementation

period (p = 0.019) (Figure 4). We observed a similar baseline effect for the course of C5a levels, however, the interaction between baseline and time was not significant and therefore not included in the final model (p = 0.065).

Association between the stage of AMD and serum complement catabolism

We further analyzed the clinical characteristics of AMD patients with a relatively high baseline complement catabolism. Higher baseline C3d/C3 ratio was significantly associated with younger age (r = −0.33, p = 0.005) and better visual acuity (OD: r = 0.25, p = 0.031 and OS: r = 0.36, p = 0.002). Also, baseline C3d/C3 ratio was associated with the CARMS classification based on both eyes (p = 0.010). Post hoc analysis revealed that patients with large drusen and/or drusenoid RPE detachment in one eye and geographic atrophy or choroidal neovascularization in the other eye (3:4–5) had higher baseline complement catabolism compared to geographic atrophy or choroidal neovascularization in both eyes (4–5:4–5) (Table 2). There was no association with baseline C5a and age (r = 0.068, p = 0.583), visual acuity (OD: r = −0.110, p = 0.381 and OS: r = −0.023, p = 0.855) or the CARMS classification based on both eyes (p = 0.947). C3d/C3 ratio and C5a levels were measured in separate experiments and were not correlated (r = 0.086, p = 0.490). As expected, baseline visual acuity for each eye was strongly associated with the CARMS classification per eye (OD: r = −0.69, p<0.001 and OS: r = −0.65, p<0.001) (Table S1).

Correlation between the serum complement catabolism and the genotype

The baseline C3d/C3 ratios did not differ significantly between wildtype/heterozygous Y402H *CFH* genotype and the homozygous Y402H genotype (p = 0.934) nor between *ARMS2* genotypes (p = 0.729). There was also no difference in baseline C5a between *CFH* (p = 0.597) and *ARMS2* genotypes (p = 0.412). Change in

Table 1. The baseline characteristics of the study population.

Baseline characteristics	AMD, n = 72
Mean age – years ± SD	73.9±8.3
Sex, male – No. (%)	29 (40.3)
Visual acuity OD – median (1st–3rd quartile)	20/83 (20/400–20/25)
Visual acuity OS – median (1st–3rd quartile)	20/55 (20/333–20/26)
Mean C3d/C3 ratio ± SD	1.65±0.69
Mean zinc level – µmol/l ± SD	13.33±2.83
CFH (Y402H; rs1061170) genotypes, No. (%)	
CFH TT genotype (wildtype)	1 (1.4)
CFH CT genotype	36 (50.0)
CFH CC genotype	34 (47.2)
ARMS2 (A69S; rs10490924) genotypes, No. (%)	
ARMS2 GG genotype (wildtype)	19 (26.4)
ARMS2 TG genotype	30 (41.7)
ARMS2 TT genotype	22 (30.6)
Serum C-reactive protein (CRP), No. (%)	
<5 – mg/l	52 (72.2)
5–15 – mg/l	18 (25.0)
16–45 – mg/l	2 (2.8)

SD = Standard deviation, visual acuity in Snellen.

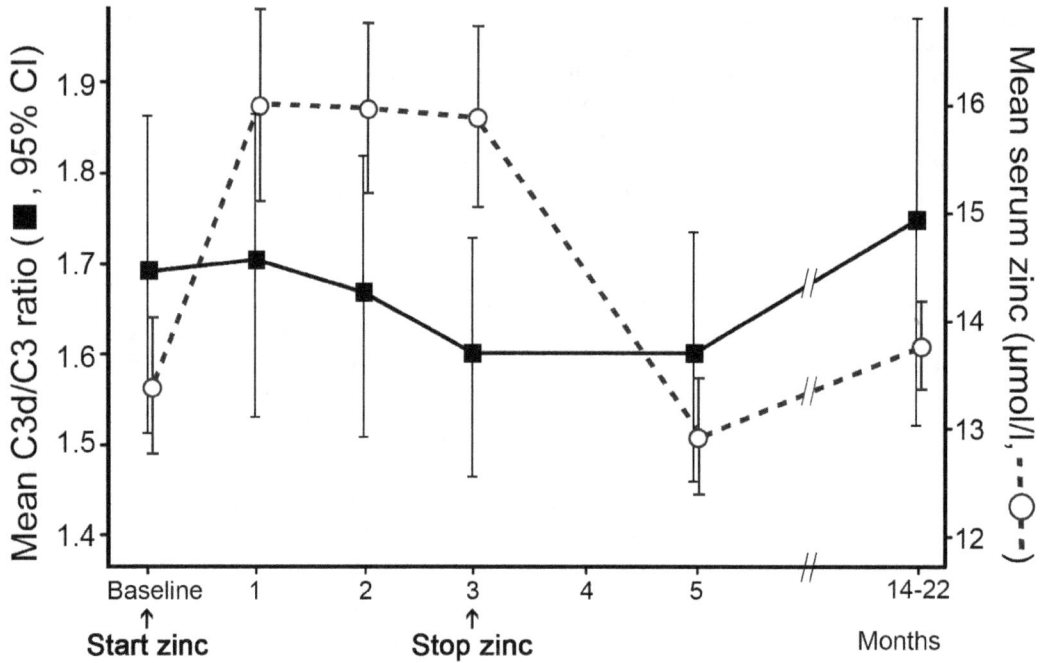

Figure 2. Serum zinc concentration and C3d/C3 ratio throughout the study period. During the three months daily zinc supplementation, serum zinc concentration increased significantly (p<0.001). After zinc supplementation was discontinued, the serum zinc levels returned to baseline levels within 2 months. The C3d/C3 ratio showed non-significant decline during zinc supplementation (p=0.149).

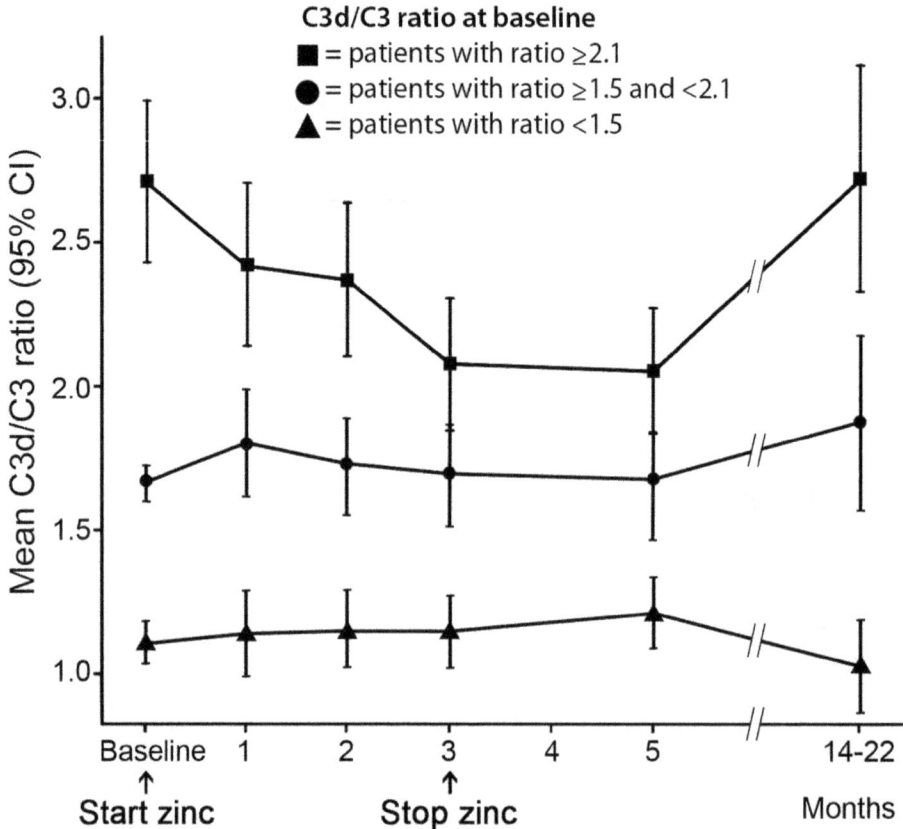

Figure 3. The effect of zinc supplementation on patients with different level of complement catabolism at baseline. The patients with high serum complement catabolism had a steeper decline in C3d/C3 ratio during the administration of zinc sulphate (p<0.001).

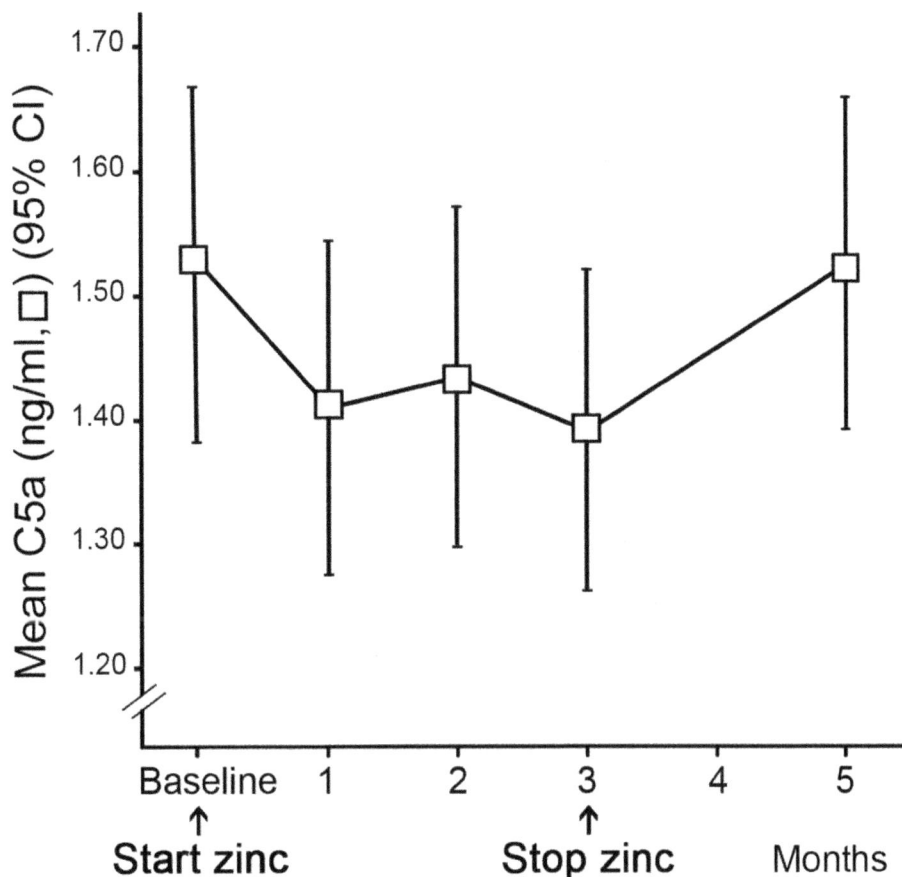

Figure 4. C5a concentration throughout the study period. The C5a levels decreased significantly during the three months of zinc supplementation and returned to baseline level within 2 months after the cessation of zinc supplementation.

C3d/C3 ratio or C5a levels were not related to *CFH* or *ARMS2* genotypes.

Intermittent infections and the C3d/C3 ratio

Serum CRP levels were measured at every visit and were not significantly associated with the C3d/C3 ratio (p = 0.168) nor the C5a levels (p = 0.942). Questionnaires demonstrated that antibiotics were prescribed in 10 patients during the study period. Use of antibiotics was not related to increased CRP levels, increased body

temperature or elevated C3d/C3 ratio (data not shown) in these individuals.

Effect of zinc on complement catabolism *in vitro*

To demonstrate the *in vitro* effect of zinc on the complement activity of human serum and to better understand the effect observed in vivo in the patients, we performed an alternative pathway hemolytic assay. Results showed that zinc sulphate inhibits the lysis of rabbit erythrocytes in a dose-dependent

Table 2. Association between the stage of AMD and serum complement catabolism.

Clinical Age-Related Maculopathy Staging (CARMS) for both eyes	Mean C3d/C3 ratio (SE)	No. (%)	p*
Grade 2 in both eyes (2:2)	1.64 (0.30)	4 (5.6)	1.000
Grade 2 in the first eye and grade 4 or 5 in the second eye (2:4–5)	1.69 (0.31)	9 (12.7)	1.000
Grade 3 in both eyes (3:3)	1.86 (0.17)	10 (14.1)	0.263
Grade 3 in the first and stages 4 or 5 in the second eye (3:4–5)	2.01 (0.20)	19 (26.8)	0.006
Grades 4 or 5 in both eyes (4–5:4–5)	1.32 (0.06)	29 (40.8)	Ref.

Compared to the patients with intermediate AMD in one eye and late AMD in the other eye (CARMS stage 3:4–5), the patients who had late AMD in both eyes (CARMS 4–5:4–5) had significantly lower C3d/C3 levels (p = 0.006).
*p-value from one-way ANOVA with post hoc Bonferroni correction.

manner (Figure 5A). Retina is exposed to high levels of oxidative stress from light exposure and metabolic processes [44]. We tested *in vitro* whether zinc could also protect the RPE from a oxidative stress related damage from the complement system. The test results show that the amount of MAC deposited on RPE cells exposed to oxidative stress can be reduced in a dose dependent manner by zinc sulphate (Figure 5B–C). In the negative controls, zinc and serum were omitted.

Discussion

In the past decade, it has become increasingly clear that complement-mediated inflammation plays a fundamental role in the etiology of AMD [18,45]. All current therapies for treating neovascular AMD are designed to reduce the ongoing VEGF stimulus–and hence inhibit the growth of new vessels–but do not address the underlying pathology. Moreover, no effective therapy has been developed for treating early AMD or geographic atrophy. The discovery of complement as a major contributing factor to AMD pathogenesis has sparked considerable interest in this system as a potential therapeutic target, and various complement inhibitors are currently being tested in clinical trials [14,15].

Our findings suggest that increased complement catabolism, defined as the C3d/C3 ratio, in AMD patients can be reduced by the daily oral administration of 50 mg zinc sulphate. However, the effect of complement inhibition seemed to be limited to patients with a high baseline level of complement catabolism. The C3d/C3 ratio returned to its baseline value after the supplementation period, indicating a reversible effect of zinc supplementation on complement activation. Continuous zinc supplementation may therefore be necessary to inhibit complement activity over longer periods of time. Approximately 50% of patients indicated they had been using zinc supplements during the period before the last measurement. However, the zinc dosage and possibly compliance in these patients was apparently too low to exert a clear effect on complement levels.

We then linked the degree of serum complement activation to the clinical stages of AMD and found that the level of serum complement activation is correlated with patients having large drusen and/or drusenoid RPE detachment. It has been demonstrated that 42% of patients with drusenoid RPE detachment progress to end-stage AMD and develop profound and irreversible visual loss within five years [46]. The AREDS1 study showed that this group in particular benefits from zinc plus antioxidant supplementation. Our results suggest that this may be related to increased activation of the alternative complement pathway in this group, which would support the notion that patients with large drusen and/or drusenoid RPE detachment should receive supplements. Although correlation coefficients were modest, higher complement levels at baseline were mostly observed in younger patients with better visual acuity, corresponding with less advanced disease. This could indicate that the use of supplements should not be postponed until more advanced stages of the disease.

C5a showed a significant decrease during zinc supplementation, indicating that zinc inhibition of the complement pathway can also be detected further downstream. We observed a similar pattern of increased inhibitory effect in patients with higher baseline C5a levels, but this was not as profound as for the C3d/C3 ratio. This could be explained by the more unstable nature of C5a as compared to the C3d/C3 ratio which corrects for intrapersonal fluctuations. C5a returned to its baseline value within 2 months after the supplementation period also suggesting a reversible effect of zinc on C5a.

The exact role of genotype in the response to zinc and antioxidant supplements remains unclear. The Rotterdam study showed that high dietary zinc intake reduces the risk of AMD associated with the *CFH* Y402H variant, suggesting a relationship between zinc and this genotype [33]. A recent subgroup analysis, utilizing data from the AREDS study, showed that the response to zinc and antioxidants may be influenced by *CFH* and *ARMS2* genotype. Their results suggested that patients carrying the *CFH* Y402H risk allele have no benefit from zinc supplementation on the 10-year disease progression [47]. In previous studies by AREDS study researchers on the interaction between genotype and treatment response, they found that the AREDS supplements may be less effective in reducing progression in carriers of the *CFH* risk allele [48]. But in a later publication they could not corroborate the interaction and could not find any relation with response to zinc or antioxidants and genotype [49]. Notably, a biochemical study of zinc and factor H showed that the interaction between zinc and the factor H protein was not influenced by the *CFH* Y402H variant [50]. In our study, genotype did not have an effect on baseline or change of complement activation levels. Given the small number of study participants our study probably lacks the power to detect a possible interaction between *CFH* or *ARMS2* genotype and zinc supplementation.

Changes in C3 activation over time can also be caused by various factors related to immune defense in case of infection [51]. Since serum CRP levels were not significantly associated with C3d/C3 ratio, it is unlikely that the observed change in complement catabolism can be ascribed to an intermittent

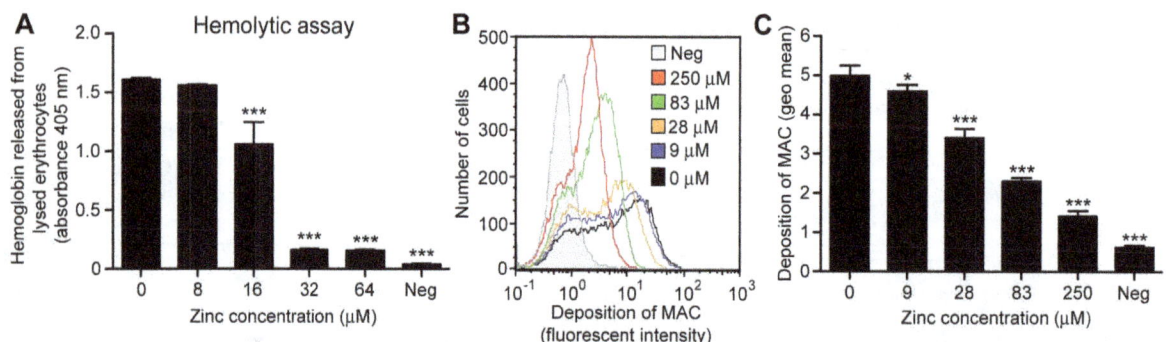

Figure 5. The effect of zinc on the hemolytic activity of human serum and on the membrane attack complex (MAC) deposition on retinal pigment epithelial (RPE) cells. (A) Zinc sulphate inhibits the lysis of rabbit erythrocytes in a dose-dependent manner. (B–C) the amount of MAC deposited on RPE cells exposed to oxidative stress can be reduced in a dose dependent manner by zinc. *p<0.05 and ***p<0.001.

infection. Data obtained from a general physical examination and a questionnaire aimed at identifying clinical manifestations of intermittent infections also did not point to an infectious cause for the change in complement levels in these AMD patients. Finally, it is unlikely that the study results were influenced by the statistical phenomenon of 'regression to the mean' because the C3d/C3 ratio returned to baseline levels for after discontinuation of zinc administration.

In further support of our hypothesis that zinc administration affects complement catabolism, we demonstrated *in vitro* that zinc sulphate directly inhibits complement activation in human serum in a dose-dependent manner. In addition, we demonstrated that during oxidative challenge the presence of zinc sulphate diminishes MAC deposition on RPE cells, thereby preventing complement-mediated cytolysis and apoptosis. This implies that zinc not only has the ability to reduce systemic activation of the alternative complement pathway, but may also diminish complement activation locally on RPE cells. Important to note is that zinc concentrations were in physiological levels [44,52], and therefore have biomedical significance. A previous biochemical study showed that oligomerization of the CFH protein occurs in the presence of zinc, theoretically leading to increased complement activation [53]. A more recent biochemical study from researchers of the same study group demonstrated that factor H-C3b complexes are precipitated by zinc which would inhibit complement activation [54]. Thus we cannot pinpoint the exact molecular mechanism behind our observations, however, we can conclude that zinc inhibits systemic complement activation and local MAC deposition preventing RPE cell damage.

This study has some limitations that should be addressed. A relatively small number of subjects were included, and zinc was administered for a relatively brief period of time. Patient compliance was monitored through questionnaires, which could potentially underestimate zinc intake. However, a steep increase in serum zinc following the initiation of treatment indicated that supplementation had been successful. Because of the slow natural progression of AMD, this study was never designed to measure a direct protective effect of zinc on visual acuity. Larger patient cohorts and a longer period of zinc supplementation should also be studied to corroborate and extend our findings.

In summary, in our study increased levels of serum complement catabolism correlates with the stage of AMD. Our study demonstrate that increased levels of complement catabolism can be normalized by the daily oral administration of 50 mg zinc sulphate. Findings from the present study might explain how zinc slows AMD progression in subgroups of patients with AMD.

Supporting Information

Table S1   Visual acuity per CARMS classification grade. Baseline median visual acuity in Snellen per Clinical Age-Related Maculopathy Staging (CARMS) classification grade for the separate eyes. Visual acuity decreases as CARMS classification increases.

Acknowledgments

During the trial phase of this study our colleague Professor Chris de Bruijn has unfortunately passed away. We would like to acknowledge his important contributions to this work.

Author Contributions

Contributed to the writing of the manuscript: DS FA BJK CBH AMB AIH. Conceived and designed the experiments: CBH DS BJK AMB GJW CB MRD. Performed the experiments: DS FCM JPHV RACH YTEL FA TTJMB YT FCM AMB. Analyzed the data: FA DS JMMG FCM BJK AIH AMB GJW MRD CBH. Contributed reagents/materials/analysis tools: DS FA YT TTJMB MRD SF CB RACH AMB FCM AIH.

References

1. Kawasaki R, Yasuda M, Song SJ, Chen SJ, Jonas JB, et al. (2010) The prevalence of age-related macular degeneration in Asians: a systematic review and meta-analysis. Ophthalmology 117: 921–927.
2. Krishnan T, Ravindran RD, Murthy GV, Vashist P, Fitzpatrick KE, et al. (2010) Prevalence of early and late age-related macular degeneration in India: the INDEYE study. Invest Ophthalmol Vis Sci 51: 701–707.
3. Rein DB, Wittenborn JS, Zhang X, Honeycutt AA, Lesesne SB, et al. (2009) Forecasting age-related macular degeneration through the year 2050: the potential impact of new treatments. Arch Ophthalmol 127: 533–540.
4. Smith W, Assink J, Klein R, Mitchell P, Klaver CC, et al. (2001) Risk factors for age-related macular degeneration: Pooled findings from three continents. Ophthalmology 108: 697–704.
5. de Jong PT (2006) Age-related macular degeneration. N Engl J Med 355: 1474–1485.
6. Friedman DS, O'Colmain BJ, Munoz B, Tomany SC, McCarty C, et al. (2004) Prevalence of age-related macular degeneration in the United States. Arch Ophthalmol 122: 564–572.
7. Klaver CC, Wolfs RC, Vingerling JR, Hofman A, de Jong PT (1998) Age-specific prevalence and causes of blindness and visual impairment in an older population: the Rotterdam Study. Arch Ophthalmol 116: 653–658.
8. Klein R, Klein BE, Tomany SC, Meuer SM, Huang GH (2002) Ten-year incidence and progression of age-related maculopathy: The Beaver Dam eye study. Ophthalmology 109: 1767–1779.
9. Mitchell P, Smith W, Attebo K, Wang JJ (1995) Prevalence of age-related maculopathy in Australia. The Blue Mountains Eye Study. Ophthalmology 102: 1450–1460.
10. Martin DF, Maguire MG, Ying GS, Grunwald JE, Fine SL, et al. (2011) Ranibizumab and bevacizumab for neovascular age-related macular degeneration. N Engl J Med 364: 1897–1908.
11. Rosenfeld PJ, Brown DM, Heier JS, Boyer DS, Kaiser PK, et al. (2006) Ranibizumab for neovascular age-related macular degeneration. N Engl J Med 355: 1419–1431.
12. Ip MS, Scott IU, Brown GC, Brown MM, Ho AC, et al. (2008) Anti-vascular endothelial growth factor pharmacotherapy for age-related macular degeneration: a report by the American Academy of Ophthalmology. Ophthalmology 115: 1837–1846.
13. Smailhodzic D, Muether PS, Chen J, Kwestro A, Zhang AY, et al. (2012) Cumulative effect of risk alleles in CFH, ARMS2, and VEGFA on the response to ranibizumab treatment in age-related macular degeneration. Ophthalmology 119: 2304–2311.
14. Troutbeck R, Al-Qureshi S, Guymer RH (2012) Therapeutic targeting of the complement system in age-related macular degeneration: a review. Clin Experiment Ophthalmol 40: 18–26.
15. Yehoshua Z, de Amorim Garcia Filho CA, Nunes RP, Gregori G, Penha FM, et al. (2014) Systemic complement inhibition with eculizumab for geographic atrophy in age-related macular degeneration: the COMPLETE study. Ophthalmology 121: 693–701.
16. Walport MJ (2001) Complement. First of two parts. N Engl J Med 344: 1058–1066.
17. Anderson DH, Mullins RF, Hageman GS, Johnson LV (2002) A role for local inflammation in the formation of drusen in the aging eye. Am J Ophthalmol 134: 411–431.
18. Anderson DH, Radeke MJ, Gallo NB, Chapin EA, Johnson PT, et al. (2010) The pivotal role of the complement system in aging and age-related macular degeneration: hypothesis re-visited. Prog Retin Eye Res 29: 95–112.
19. Edwards AO, Ritter R 3rd, Abel KJ, Manning A, Panhuysen C, et al. (2005) Complement factor H polymorphism and age-related macular degeneration. Science 308: 421–424.
20. Hageman GS, Anderson DH, Johnson LV, Hancox LS, Taiber AJ, et al. (2005) A common haplotype in the complement regulatory gene factor H (HF1/CFH) predisposes individuals to age-related macular degeneration. Proc Natl Acad Sci U S A 102: 7227–7232.

21. Haines JL, Hauser MA, Schmidt S, Scott WK, Olson LM, et al. (2005) Complement factor H variant increases the risk of age-related macular degeneration. Science 308: 419–421.

22. Klein RJ, Zeiss C, Chew EY, Tsai JY, Sackler RS, et al. (2005) Complement factor H polymorphism in age-related macular degeneration. Science 308: 385–389.

23. Fagerness JA, Maller JB, Neale BM, Reynolds RC, Daly MJ, et al. (2009) Variation near complement factor I is associated with risk of advanced AMD. Eur J Hum Genet 17: 100–104.

24. Gold B, Merriam JE, Zernant J, Hancox LS, Taiber AJ, et al. (2006) Variation in factor B (BF) and complement component 2 (C2) genes is associated with age-related macular degeneration. Nat Genet 38: 458–462.

25. Maller JB, Fagerness JA, Reynolds RC, Neale BM, Daly MJ, et al. (2007) Variation in complement factor 3 is associated with risk of age-related macular degeneration. Nat Genet 39: 1200–1201.

26. Yates JR, Sepp T, Matharu BK, Khan JC, Thurlby DA, et al. (2007) Complement C3 variant and the risk of age-related macular degeneration. N Engl J Med 357: 553–561.

27. Hecker LA, Edwards AO, Ryu E, Tosakulwong N, Baratz KH, et al. (2010) Genetic control of the alternative pathway of complement in humans and age-related macular degeneration. Hum Mol Genet 19: 209–215.

28. Reynolds R, Hartnett ME, Atkinson JP, Giclas PC, Rosner B, et al. (2009) Plasma complement components and activation fragments: associations with age-related macular degeneration genotypes and phenotypes. Invest Ophthalmol Vis Sci 50: 5818–5827.

29. Scholl HP, Charbel Issa P, Walier M, Janzer S, Pollok-Kopp B, et al. (2008) Systemic complement activation in age-related macular degeneration. PLoS One 3: e2593.

30. Smailhodzic D, Klaver CC, Klevering BJ, Boon CJ, Groenewoud JM, et al. (2012) Risk alleles in CFH and ARMS2 are independently associated with systemic complement activation in age-related macular degeneration. Ophthalmology 119: 339–346.

31. Age-Related Eye Disease Study Research Group (2001) A randomized, placebo-controlled, clinical trial of high-dose supplementation with vitamins C and E, beta carotene, and zinc for age-related macular degeneration and vision loss: AREDS report no. 8. Arch Ophthalmol 119: 1417–1436.

32. Tan JS, Wang JJ, Flood V, Rochtchina E, Smith W, et al. (2008) Dietary antioxidants and the long-term incidence of age-related macular degeneration: the Blue Mountains Eye Study. Ophthalmology 115: 334–341.

33. Ho L, van Leeuwen R, Witteman JC, van Duijn CM, Uitterlinden AG, et al. (2011) Reducing the genetic risk of age-related macular degeneration with dietary antioxidants, zinc, and omega-3 fatty acids: the Rotterdam study. Arch Ophthalmol 129: 758–766.

34. Age-Related Eye Disease Study 2 Research Group (2013) Lutein + zeaxanthin and omega-3 fatty acids for age-related macular degeneration: the Age-Related Eye Disease Study 2 (AREDS2) randomized clinical trial. JAMA 309: 2005–2015.

35. Wedekind KJ, Baker DH (1990) Zinc bioavailability in feed-grade sources of zinc. J Anim Sci 68: 684–689.

36. Schell TC, Kornegay ET (1996) Zinc concentration in tissues and performance of weanling pigs fed pharmacological levels of zinc from ZnO, Zn-methionine, Zn-lysine, or ZnSO4. J Anim Sci 74: 1584–1593.

37. Nozaki M, Raisler BJ, Sakurai E, Sarma JV, Barnum SR, et al. (2006) Drusen complement components C3a and C5a promote choroidal neovascularization. Proc Natl Acad Sci U S A 103: 2328–2333.

38. Seddon JM, Sharma S, Adelman RA (2006) Evaluation of the clinical age-related maculopathy staging system. Ophthalmology 113: 260–266.

39. Reddingius RE, Schroder CH, Daha MR, Monnens LA (1993) The serum complement system in children on continuous ambulatory peritoneal dialysis. Perit Dial Int 13: 214–218.

40. Siezenga MA, Chandie Shaw PK, van der Geest RN, Mollnes TE, Daha MR, et al. (2009) Enhanced complement activation is part of the unfavourable cardiovascular risk profile in South Asians. Clin Exp Immunol 157: 98–103.

41. Hawkins JR, Khripin Y, Valdes AM, Weaver TA (2002) Miniaturized sealed-tube allele-specific PCR. Hum Mutat 19: 543–553.

42. Kim MH, Chung J, Yang JW, Chung SM, Kwag NH, et al. (2003) Hydrogen peroxide-induced cell death in a human retinal pigment epithelial cell line, ARPE-19. Korean J Ophthalmol 17: 19–28.

43. Bandyopadhyay M, Rohrer B (2012) Matrix metalloproteinase activity creates pro-angiogenic environment in primary human retinal pigment epithelial cells exposed to complement. Invest Ophthalmol Vis Sci 53: 1953–1961.

44. Wills NK, Ramanujam VM, Kalariya N, Lewis JR, van Kuijk FJ (2008) Copper and zinc distribution in the human retina: relationship to cadmium accumulation, age, and gender. Exp Eye Res 87: 80–88.

45. Charbel Issa P, Chong NV, Scholl HP (2011) The significance of the complement system for the pathogenesis of age-related macular degeneration - current evidence and translation into clinical application. Graefes Arch Clin Exp Ophthalmol 249: 163–174.

46. Cukras C, Agron E, Klein ML, Ferris FL, 3rd, Chew EY, et al. (2010) Natural history of drusenoid pigment epithelial detachment in age-related macular degeneration: Age-Related Eye Disease Study Report No. 28. Ophthalmology 117: 489–499.

47. Awh CC, Lane AM, Hawken S, Zanke B, Kim IK (2013) CFH and ARMS2 genetic polymorphisms predict response to antioxidants and zinc in patients with age-related macular degeneration. Ophthalmology 120: 2317–2323.

48. Klein ML, Francis PJ, Rosner B, Reynolds R, Hamon SC, et al. (2008) CFH and LOC387715/ARMS2 genotypes and treatment with antioxidants and zinc for age-related macular degeneration. Ophthalmology 115: 1019–1025.

49. Chew EY, Klein ML, Clemons TE, Agron E, Ratnapriya R, et al. (2014) No Clinically Significant Association between CFH and ARMS2 Genotypes and Response to Nutritional Supplements: AREDS Report Number 38. Ophthalmology.

50. Nan R, Farabella I, Schumacher FF, Miller A, Gor J, et al. (2011) Zinc binding to the Tyr402 and His402 allotypes of complement factor H: possible implications for age-related macular degeneration. J Mol Biol 408: 714–735.

51. Zipfel PF, Skerka C (2009) Complement regulators and inhibitory proteins. Nat Rev Immunol 9: 729–740.

52. Lowe NM, Medina MW, Stammers AL, Patel S, Souverein OW, et al. (2012) The relationship between zinc intake and serum/plasma zinc concentration in adults: a systematic review and dose-response meta-analysis by the EURRECA Network. Br J Nutr 108: 1962–1971.

53. Nan R, Gor J, Lengyel I, Perkins SJ (2008) Uncontrolled zinc- and copper-induced oligomerisation of the human complement regulator factor H and its possible implications for function and disease. J Mol Biol 384: 1341–1352.

54. Nan R, Tetchner S, Rodriguez E, Pao PJ, Gor J, et al. (2013) Zinc-induced self-association of complement C3b and Factor H: implications for inflammation and age-related macular degeneration. J Biol Chem 288: 19197–19210.

22

Gender Disparities in Latent Tuberculosis Infection in High-Risk Individuals: A Cross-Sectional Study

Wen-Ying Ting[1], Shiang-Fen Huang[2,3], Ming-Che Lee[1], Yung-Yang Lin[4,5], Yu-Chin Lee[1,3], Jia-Yih Feng[1,6]*◊, Wei-Juin Su[1,3]*◊

1 Department of Chest Medicine, Taipei Veterans General Hospital, Taipei, Taiwan, R.O.C., 2 Division of Infectious Disease, Department of Internal Medicine, Taipei Veterans General Hospital, Taipei, Taiwan, R.O.C., 3 School of Medicine, National Yang-Ming University, Taipei, Taiwan, R.O.C., 4 Institute of Clinical Medicine and Institute of Brain Science, National Yang-Ming University, Taipei, Taiwan, R.O.C., 5 Laboratory of Neurophysiology and Department of Neurology, Taipei Veterans General Hospital, Taipei, Taiwan, R.O.C., 6 Institute of Clinical Medicine, School of Medicine, National Yang-Ming University, Taipei, Taiwan, R.O.C.

Abstract

Male predominance in active tuberculosis (TB) is widely-reported globally. Gender inequalities in socio-cultural status are frequently regarded as contributing factors for disparities in sex in active TB. The disparities of sex in the prevalence of latent TB infection (LTBI) are less frequently investigated and deserve clarification. In this cross-sectional study conducted in a TB endemic area, we enrolled patients at high-risk for LTBI and progression from LTBI to active TB from 2011 to 2012. Diagnosis of LTBI was made by QuantiFERON-TB Gold In-Tube (QFT-GIT). Differences in sex in terms of prevalence of LTBI and clinical predictors for LTBI were investigated. Associations among age, smoking status, and sex disparities in LTBI were also analyzed. A total of 1018 high-risk individuals with definite QFT-GIT results were included for analysis, including 534 males and 484 females. The proportion of LTBI was significantly higher in males than in females (32.6% vs. 25.2%, $p = 0.010$). Differences in the proportion of LTBI between sexes were most prominent in older patients (age ≥55 years). In multivariate analysis, independent clinical factors associated with LTBI were age ($p = 0.014$), smoking ($p = 0.048$), and fibro-calcified lesions on chest radiogram ($p = 0.009$). Male sex was not an independent factor for LTBI ($p = 0.88$). When stratifying patients according to the smoking status, the proportion of LTBI remained comparable between sexes among smokers and non-smokers. In conclusion, although the proportion of LTBI is higher in men, there is no significant disparity in terms of sex in LTBI among high-risk individuals after adjusting for age, smoking status, and other clinical factors.

Editor: Scarlett L. Bellamy, University of Pennsylvania School of Medicine, United States of America

Funding: This study was funded by the Institute for Biotechnology and Medicine Industry of Taiwan and by Taipei Veterans General Hospital (V99C1-181, V99A-023, V100A-002, V101B-027, and V102B-030). The funders had no role in study design, data collection and analysis, decision to publish, or preparation of the manuscript.

Competing Interests: The authors have declared that no competing interests exist.

* Email: jyfeng@vghtpe.gov.tw (JYF); wjsu@vghtpe.gov.tw (WJS)

◊ These authors contributed equally to this work.

Introduction

Tuberculosis (TB) is caused by *Mycobacterium tuberculosis* (MTB) and is one of the deadliest infectious diseases worldwide. Despite recent progress in molecular diagnosis and effective medications, its morbidity and mortality remain high. The World Health Organization (WHO) reported that 8.7 million people developed active TB in 2011 and 1.4 million people died from it [1]. Meanwhile, one-third of the world's population is estimated to be infected by MTB. Latent TB infection (LTBI) is defined by evidence of immunological responses by *Mycobacterium tuberculosis* (MTB) proteins in the absence of clinical symptoms/signs of active diseases [2]. An estimated 30% of the people exposed to MTB will have evidence of LTBI by tuberculin skin test [3]. By definition, LTBI cases do not have clinical or radiographic evidence of the disease and will not cause transmission. However, a significant proportion of patients with LTBI will progress to active disease and it is preventable by effective treatment. Therefore, identifying and sterilizing latently infected individuals, especially those at high risk, are of paramount importance for eliminating TB [4].

Sex differences in the epidemiology and treatment outcomes of active TB are remarkable and have been well-described in previous reports [5–8]. In general, men are more likely to be diagnosed with active TB than women, with a male-to-female ratio of 2:1 to 3:1 globally [1]. Males with active TB also have worse outcomes, including delayed sputum conversion, higher reactivation rate, and higher mortality rate, compared to females [9–11]. The impact of smoking, inequalities in socio-economic status, differences in medical accessibility, and sex hormone-related differences in immunity are reported as possible causes for the disparities in sexes in active TB [12–15]. However, the exact mechanisms remain unclear.

Compared to numerous reports on active TB, disparities between sexes in LTBI are less frequently analyzed and have inconsistent findings. Male sex has been identified as an independent risk factor associated with LTBI in some studies [16–18], but several studies also report insignificant correlation between sex and LTBI [19,20]. Most studies have focused on specific populations with relatively few case numbers. Important clinical characteristic profiles, especially smoking status, are also lacking. Given the uncertainty of the mechanisms related to sex disparities in active TB, analyzing sex differences in LTBI from an active case-finding setting will be helpful in elucidating the issue. The present study aimed to investigate differences between sexes in LTBI among high-risk individuals. The associated clinical factors, especially age and smoking habits, and their impact on sex disparities, were also evaluated.

Materials and Methods

Study Design and Settings

This cross-sectional study was conducted at Taipei Veterans General Hospital, a 3000-bed tertiary medical center in Taiwan where more than 450 active TB cases are diagnosed each year. As a TB endemic area with moderate TB burden, Taiwan had 12,634 newly diagnosed TB cases in 2011, with an annual incidence of 54.5 cases/100,000 population [21]. From 2005 to 2010, there was a 23.3% decrease in number of TB cases and 24.8% decrease in incidence rate.

Patients and Data Collection

From January 2011 to December 2012, in-patients and out-patients who were considered at risk for LTBI and progression to active TB disease were eligible for enrollment. These high-risk individuals included people with active TB contact, health care workers, and patients with malignancy, end-stage renal disease, liver cirrhosis, post-organ transplantation, autoimmune diseases, and fibro-calcified lesions suggestive of prior TB on chest radiogram [22].

Patients who were under anti-TB treatment were excluded, as well as those who were diagnosed with active TB (based on the TB registration database of the Centers for Disease Control, Taiwan) within two months of enrollment. The other exclusion criteria included patients younger than 20 years of age, pregnant women, and those with a history of previous anti-TB treatment.

Demographic profiles (age, sex, and co-morbidities) and clinical characteristics (TB contact history, BCG scars, and smoking habit) were obtained by enrollment interviews and medical records. Smoking habit was defined as smoked at least one cigarette a day for at least one year. Body mass index (BMI) was calculated on the day of enrollment. Chest radiographs were taken on enrollment and read by a chest physician who was blinded to the LTBI testing results. Fibro-calcified lesions suggestive of previous TB infection were recorded. The hospital's Institutional Review Board approved this study and all of the patients or their authorized representative(s) provided written informed consent before enrollment.

Diagnosis of LTBI

The diagnosis of LTBI was determined by interferon-γ release assays, which was performed by the QuantiFERON-TB Gold In-Tube (QFT-GIT; QFT-GIT; Qiagen, Germany) according to the manufacturer's instructions. Peripheral blood (3–5 ml) was obtained from the patients on the day of enrollment. Blood was collected in three special tubes: one coated with MTB-specific peptides (TB antigen), one coated with phytohemaglutinin (mitogen) as a positive control, and one without antigen coating as a negative control (Nil).

Within 8 hours of blood sampling, the tubes were incubated for 16–24 hours at 37°C, centrifuged, and stored at 4°C until assay. The plasma interferon-γ concentration was measured by QFT-GIT enzyme-linked immuno-sorbent assay (ELISA). The test results were determined as negative, intermediate, or positive (cut-off at 0.35 IU/ml) according to the manufacturer's software.

Statistical Analysis

Statistical analysis was performed using the SPSS version 17.0 software (SPSS, Inc., Chicago, IL, USA). Continuous variables such as age and BMI between sub-groups were compared by Mann-Whitney U tests, while categorical variables were compared using Pearson's chi-square or Fisher's exact tests, as appropriate. Binary logistic regression analysis with stepwise selection was performed to determine the independent variables associated with LTBI in the overall study population and by male and female populations. Crude and adjusted odds ratios (ORs) with their 95% confidence intervals (CI) were presented. A $p < 0.1$ in the univariate analysis was required for a variable to be entered into the multivariate model. Patients with indeterminate QFT-GIT results were excluded from the analysis. All tests were two-tailed and $p < 0.05$ was considered statistically significant.

Results

Study Population

From January 2011 to December 2012, 1230 high-risk in-patients and out-patients were eligible for recruitment. After a process of exclusion (Figure 1), 1113 patients were enrolled, including 296 (26.6%) who were QFT-GIT positive, 722 (64.9%) who were QFT-GIT negative, and 95 (8.5%) with indeterminate QFT-GIT results. Ultimately, 1018 high-risk individuals composed of 534 (52.5%) males and 484 (47.5%) females with determinate QFT-GIT results were included for analysis. Among them, 152 (14.9%) had recent contact history with active TB cases, 42 (4.1%) were health care workers, 147 (14.4%) had diabetes mellitus, 351 (34.5%) had malignancies, 22 (2.2%) had end-stage renal disease, 44 (4.3%) had liver cirrhosis, 12 (1.2%) had history of organ transplantations, 140 (13.8%) had some autoimmune diseases, and 216 (21.2%) had fibro-calcified lesions on chest radiograms.

Compared to female patients, males were older ($p = 0.001$), more likely to have a smoking habit ($p < 0.001$), had COPD ($p < 0.001$), had some malignancies ($p < 0.001$), and had fibro-calcified lesions on chest radiograms ($p = 0.012$) (Table 1). Males were less likely to have TB contact history ($p < 0.001$), be health care workers ($p < 0.001$), and have autoimmune disorders ($p < 0.001$). The proportion of LTBI in male and females were 32.6% and 25.2% respectively, with statistically significant difference ($p = 0.010$).

LTBI between Sexes

The demographic characteristics of individuals with and without LTBI between sexes (Table 1) revealed that in males, patients with LTBI were older ($p < 0.001$), more likely to have a smoking habit ($p < 0.001$), had COPD ($p = 0.005$), had fibro-calcified lesions on chest radiogram ($p < 0.001$), and less likely to have BCG vaccination history ($p = 0.001$) compared with those without LTBI. In females, patients with LTBI were more likely to have a history of gastrectomy ($p = 0.016$).

Because older age was associated with LTBI in both males and females, the proportion of LTBI between sexes in various age groups was analyzed. The proportion of LTBI in males dramatically increased with increasing age, especially in those older than 55 years old (Figure 2). The proportion of LTBI in females also increased with increasing age but the differences were less remarkable. Sex disparities in LTBI were most prominent in patients with age ranged of 55–84 years. The proportion of LTBI declined in the extremely old population, i.e. >85 years old, in both sexes.

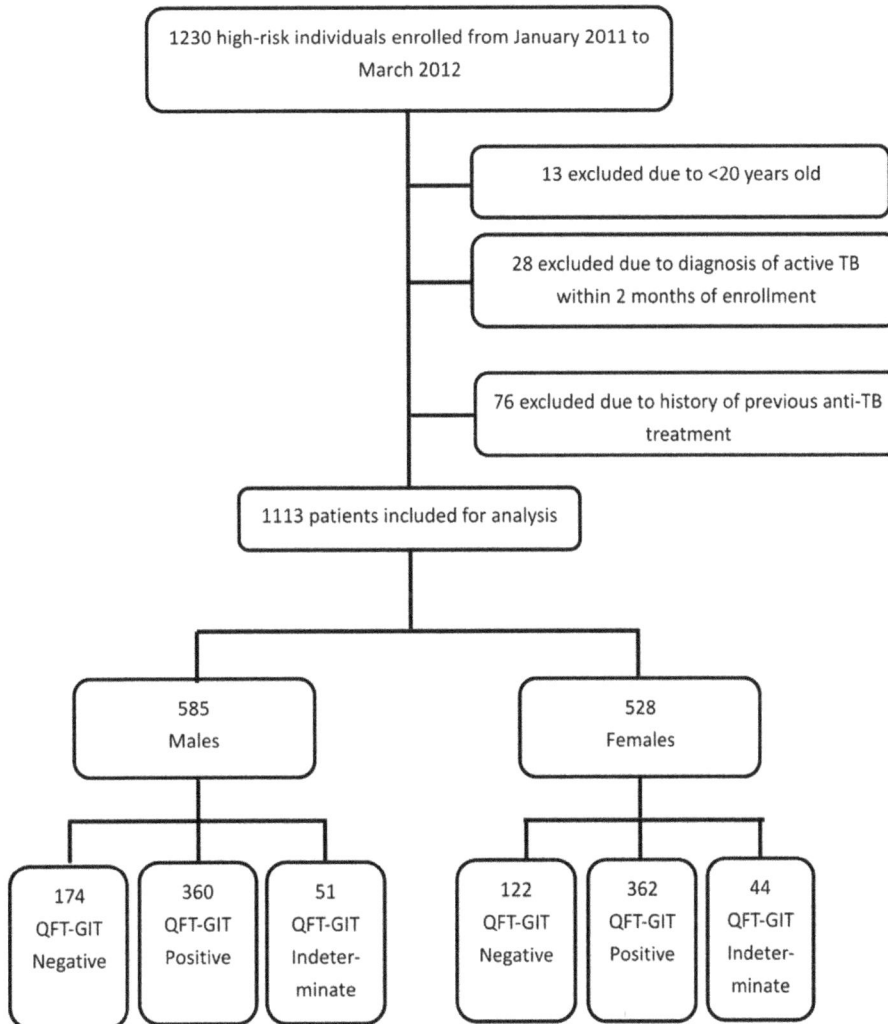

Figure 1. Study profile demonstrating the number of cases and reasons for exclusion.

Clinical Factors Associated with LTBI

In multivariate analysis (Table 2), the independent clinical factors associated with LTBI in the overall population included older age (OR 1.013, 95% CI 1.003–1.023; $p = 0.014$), smoking habit (OR 1.46, 95% CI 1.003–2.115; p = 0.048), and fibro-calcified lesions on chest radiogram(OR 1.56, 95% CI 1.12–2.17; $p = 0.009$). Male sex was not a significant factor (OR 1.03, 95% CI 0.72–1.46; $p = 0.88$).

The patients were further stratified by sex and the predictors for LTBI analyzed accordingly (Table 3). In males, the independent factors associated with LTBI included smoking habit (OR 1.59, 94% CI 1.05–2.40; p = 0.027) and fibro-calcified lesions on chest radiogram (OR 1.80, 95% CI 1.17–2.78, p = 0.008). In females, the independent factors associated with LTBI included older age (OR 1.02, 95% CI 1.004–1.032; $p = 0.009$), absence of malignancy (OR 0.50, 95% CI 0.28–0.87; $p = 0.016$), and history of gastrectomy (OR 11.15, 95% CI 1.22–101.84; $p = 0.033$).

In order to clarify the effects of smoking on LTBI between sexes, the proportion of LTBI between sexes among smokers and non-smokers were compared. Among smokers, the proportions of LTBI were 39.3% in males and 18.8% in females. Among non-smokers, the proportions were 23.9% in males and 25.4% in females. There were no statistically significant differences in the proportions of LTBI between sexes in both smokers (p = 0.10) and non-smokers (p = 0.67) (Figure 3).

Discussion

This cross-sectional study enrolled high-risk individuals from a TB-endemic area and analyzed the disparities in terms of sex in LTBI. More than 25% of patients had LTBI. By univariate analysis, the proportion of LTBI was significantly higher in men than in women. The proportion of LTBI significantly increased with increasing age in both men and women, and the sex disparity was most prominent in the elderly populations. When stratifying the patients according to their smoking habit, the proportions of LTBI were comparable between sexes in both smokers and non-smokers. By multivariate analysis, male sex was not an independent factor associated with LTBI. Other independent factors associated with LTBI included age, smoking habit, and fibro-calcified lesions on chest radiograms.

As sex disparities in active TB are widely reported globally, several possible causes are proposed to explain the observations. The gender inequalities in cultural and social aspects are enormous in some developing countries that are also TB-endemic

Table 1. Demographic characteristic between sexes with and without latent TB infection in high-risk individuals[a, b].

	Males n=534	Females n=484	p value	Males, n=534			Females, n=484		
				With LTBI n=174	Without LTBI n=360	p value	With LTBI n=122	Without LTBI n=362	p value
Mean Age (SD)[c]	60.7 (18.9)	57.1 (16.9)	<0.001	65.7 (15.5)	58.3 (19.9)	<0.001	59.8 (15.0)	56.1 (17.4)	0.05
BMI[c]	23.0 (4.3)	22.7 (4.0)	0.015	22.9 (4.0)	23.1 (4.5)	0.84	23.0 (4.0)	22.5 (4.0)	0.36
TB contact history	57 (10.7%)	95 (19.6%)	<0.001	13 (7.5%)	44 (12.2%)	0.10	30 (24.6)	65 (18%)	0.11
Smoking habit	300 (56.2%)	16 (3.3%)	<0.001	118 (67.8%)	182 (50.6%)	<0.001[d]	3 (2.5%)	13 (3.6%)	0.77[d]
BCG vaccination	337 (63.1%)	333 (68.8%)	0.06	93 (53.4%)	244 (67.8%)	0.001	79 (64.8%)	254 (70.2%)	0.27
Health care worker	10 (1.9%)	32 (6.6%)	<0.001	4 (2.3%)	6 (1.7%)	0.61[d]	11 (9%)	21 (5.8%)	0.22
Co-morbidity									
Diabetes	80 (15%)	67 (13.8%)	0.61	32 (18.4%)	48 (13.3%)	0.13	16 (13.1%)	51 (14.1%)	0.79
COPD	33 (6.2%)	0	<0.001	18 (10.3%)	15 (4.2%)	0.005	0	0	
Malignancy	243 (45.5%)	108 (22.3%)	<0.001	86 (49.4%)	157 (43.6%)	0.21	20 (16.4%)	88 (24.3%)	0.07
Renal insufficiency	14 (2.6%)	8 (1.7%)	0.29	4 (2.3%)	10 (2.8%)	0.75[d]	3 (2.5%)	5 (1.4%)	0.42[d]
HIV positive	0	0		0	0		0	0	
Post gastrectomy	14 (2.6%)	5 (1%)	0.06	6 (3.4%)	8 (2.2%)	0.40[d]	4 (3.3%)	1 (0.3%)	0.016[d]
Liver cirrhosis	28 (5.2%)	16 (3.3%)	0.13	10 (5.7%)	18 (5%)	0.72	1 (1.1%)	15 (4.1%)	0.08[d]
Autoimmune disorders	41 (7.7%)	99 (20.4%)	<0.001	12 (6.9%)	29 (8.1%)	0.64	22 (18%)	77 (21.3%)	0.65
Organ transplantation	7 (1.3%)	5 (1%)	0.68	0	7 (1.9%)	0.10[d]	0	5 (1.4%)	0.34[d]
Fibro-calcified lesions on chest radiogram	128 (24%)	85 (17.6%)	0.012	59 (33.9%)	69 (19.2%)	<0.001	27 (22.1%)	59 (16.3%)	0.15
Latent TB infection	174 (32.6%)	122 (25.2%)	0.010						

[a]Data are presented as mean ± SD or n (%), unless otherwise stated.
[b]Only patients with determinate QFT-GIT test results were included for analysis.
[c]Analyses were performed by Mann-Whitney U test.
[d]Analyses were performed by Fisher's exact test.
BCG, bacille Calmette-Guerin; BMI, body mass index; COPD, chronic obstructive pulmonary disorder; HIV, human immunodeficiency virus; TB, tuberculosis.

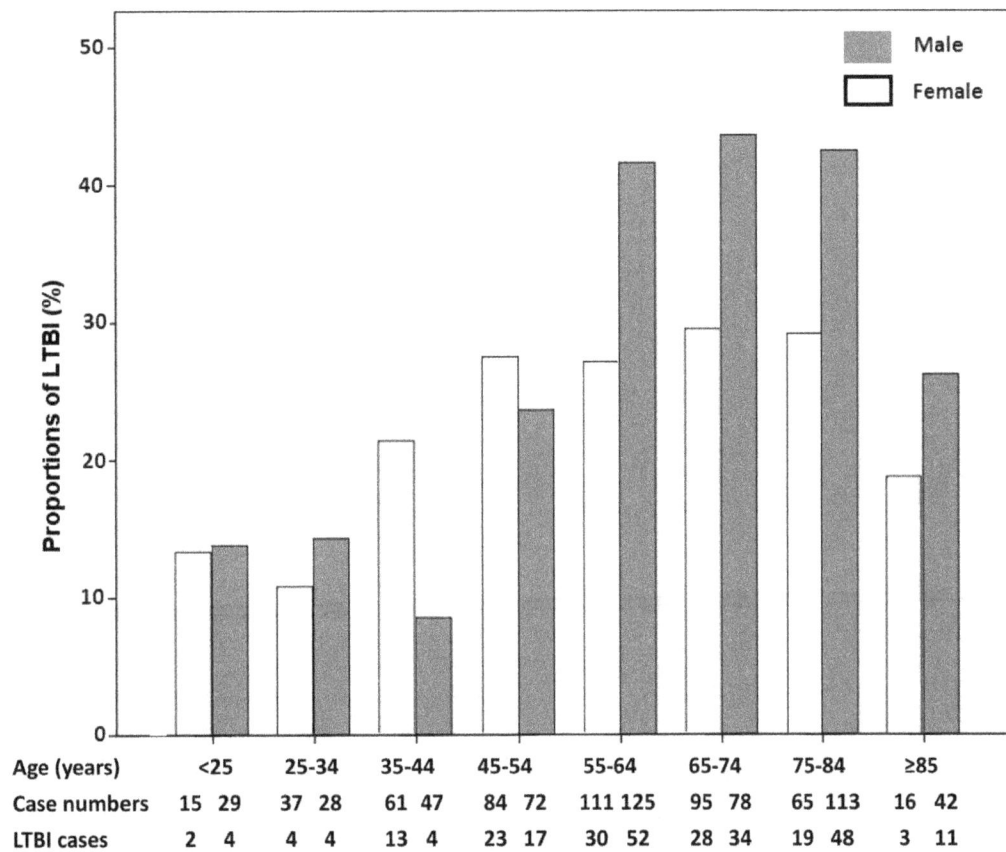

Figure 2. Proportions of latent TB infection between sexes in various age groups.

areas. These inequalities affect the help-seeking behaviors and reduce the access of women to health care services. The under-notification of active TB cases in females may be due to the gender bias in these areas, especially in a passive case-finding setting [12,13,23]. Moreover, men may have more social contact than women and thus lead to an increased risk of exposure to contagious case [24]. However, in a large population prevalence survey carried out in Bangladesh that used an active-case finding strategy, excess TB cases in males with male-to-female ratio of 3:1 was still reported [25]. Although the authors concluded that disparities between sexes in active TB are real, several potential confounding factors like smoking, drug use, and air pollution exposure were not adjusted in their study [26,27].

The present study analyzed the prevalence of LTBI between sexes in a TB endemic area. Since cases with LTBI were asymptomatic, this cross-sectional study was in an active case-finding setting. Socio-cultural disparities between sexes are less remarkable in Taiwan. In addition, there is high medical accessibility since 99% of the population has universal medical coverage by the National Health Insurance Program. In our study, although men have higher proportion of LTBI than women, with odds ratio of 1.43 in univariate analysis, male sex is not an independent factor associated with LTBI after adjusting for age,

Table 2. Univariate and multivariate analysis of clinical factors associated with latent TB infection in high-risk individuals[a].

	Univariate analysis		Multivariate analysis	
	OR (95% CI)	p value	OR (95% CI)	p value
Age	1.02 (1.01–1.03)	<0.001	1.013 (1.00–1.02)	0.014
Male sex	1.43 (1.09–1.89)	0.010	1.03 (0.72–1.46)	0.88
BCG vaccination	0.62 (0.47–0.83)	0.001	0.99 (0.69–1.41)	0.96
Smoking habit	1.87 (1.41–2.48)	<0.001	1.46 (1.00–2.12)	0.048
COPD	2.05 (1.52–6.14)	0.002	1.96 (0.94–4.10)	0.07
Fibro-calcified lesions on chest radiograms	1.87 (1.36–2.56)	<0.001	1.56 (1.12–2.17)	0.009

[a]Odds ratios and 95% confidence intervals were derived from the logistic regression analysis.
OR, odds ratio; CI, confidence interval; COPD, chronic obstructive pulmonary disorder; TB, pulmonary tuberculosis; BCG, bacille Calmette-Guerin.

Table 3. Univariate and multivariate analysis of clinical factors associated with latent TB infection between sexes[a].

	Male				Female			
	Univariate analysis		Multivariate analysis		Univariate analysis		Multivariate analysis	
	OR (95% CI)	p value	OR (95% CI)	p value	OR (95% CI)	p value	OR (95% CI)	p value
Age	1.02 (1.01–1.03)	<0.001	1.01 (1.00–1.03)	0.09	1.01 (1.00–1.03)	0.040	1.02 (1.00–1.03)	0.009
BCG vaccination	0.55 (0.38–0.79)	0.001	0.97 (0.61–1.64)	0.91	0.78 (0.51–1.21)	0.27		
Smoking habit	2.06 (1.41–3.01)	<0.001	1.59 (1.05–2.40)	0.027	0.68 (1.90–2.42)	0.55		
COPD	2.65 (1.30–5.40)	0.007	1.93 (0.91–4.09)	0.09				
Malignancy	1.26 (0.88–1.82)	0.21			0.61 (0.36–1.04)	0.07	0.50 (0.28–0.87)	0.016
Post gastrectomy	1.57 (0.54–4.60)	0.41			12.20 (1.35–110.26)	0.026	11.15 (1.22–101.84)	0.033
Autoimmune diseases	0.85 (0.42–1.70)	0.64			0.81 (0.48–1.35)	0.41		
Liver cirrhosis	1.16 (0.52–2.57)	0.72			0.19 (0.03–1.46)	0.11		
Fibro-calcified lesions on chest radiograms	2.16 (1.44–3.26)	<0.001	1.80 (1.17–2.78)	0.008	1.46 (0.88–2.43)	0.15		

[a]Odds ratios and 95% confidence intervals were derived from the logistic regression analysis.
OR, odds ratio; CI, confidence interval; COPD, chronic obstructive pulmonary disorder; TB, pulmonary tuberculosis; BCG, bacille Calmette-Guerin.

smoking habit, and other clinical factors. These results support previous observations that males have higher a probability of having TB infection with active disease progression. However, the results also indicate that age and smoking may play important roles in sex disparities in TB.

Because males in the enrolled population are older and more likely to have a smoking habits, the patients were further stratified by age and smoking status to evaluate their roles in sex disparities. Disparities between sexes were most prominent in the elderly population and the proportion of LTBI is comparable between sexes in patients younger than 45 years old. Such findings are comparable with those reported in Bangladesh as their female-to-male ratio also declined rapidly in patients older than 45 years old [25]. Elderly males may have more co-morbidities that lead to a higher proportion of LTBI. Prolonged smoke exposure in elderly male is also a possible factor.

Smoking is a well-established risk factor for lung disorders, including TB [28]. Some animal studies demonstrate that smoke exposure impairs pulmonary immunity and increased susceptibilities to mycobacterial infection [29,30]. Thus, the higher smoking rate in males and longer duration of smoking in elderly males may be other important factors for sex disparities. Interestingly, the proportion of LTBI is comparable between men and women without smoking. Among smokers, the proportion of LTBI is higher in men but without statistical significance. Due to the small case number of females with a smoking habit, the impact of smoking on LTBI in females cannot be readily evaluated in the present study. Nonetheless, the findings here strongly suggest that smoke exposure plays at least a partial role in sex disparities in LTBI in Taiwan. The anti-smoking campaign and smoke cessation program are important for TB control and should be incorporated in any TB control program.

The present study has several limitations. The participants were from a referral medical center. Patients with older age and more co-morbidities were more likely to be enrolled. The study included high-risk individuals with different disease entities so the patient population was heterogeneous, which made the findings applicable to various high-risk individuals. However, it also limited our findings to be applied in general populations. Although patients with previous and current anti-TB treatment were excluded, a significant portion of the patients had fibro-calcified lesions on chest radiograms, which is suggestive of previous TB disease. The remote immune memory may confound the QFT-GIT results. Nevertheless, their impact has been adjusted in the multivariate analysis. Few cases of female smokers have been enrolled in the present study. Further studies with larger sample sizes are needed to elucidate the impact of smoking on LTBI in females. Lastly, Taiwan is a TB-endemic area with a low prevalence for HIV. Testing for HIV was not routinely conducted among the enrolled patients. This limits the applicability of the findings to countries with a low prevalence of TB- or HIV-endemic areas.

In conclusion, male high-risk individuals in Taiwan have a higher proportion of LTBI compared to females. The proportion of LTBI increases with increasing age in both men and women, and disparities in sex are most prominent in the elderly populations. Male sex is not an independent predictor for LTBI by multivariate analysis. There is also no statistically significant difference in the proportion of LTBI between sexes in both smokers and non-smokers. Other independent factors associated with LTBI include age, smoking, and fibro-calcified lesions on chest radiograms. The role of smoking in disparities in sexes in LTBI deserves further studies and highlights the importance of the anti-smoking campaign in TB control.

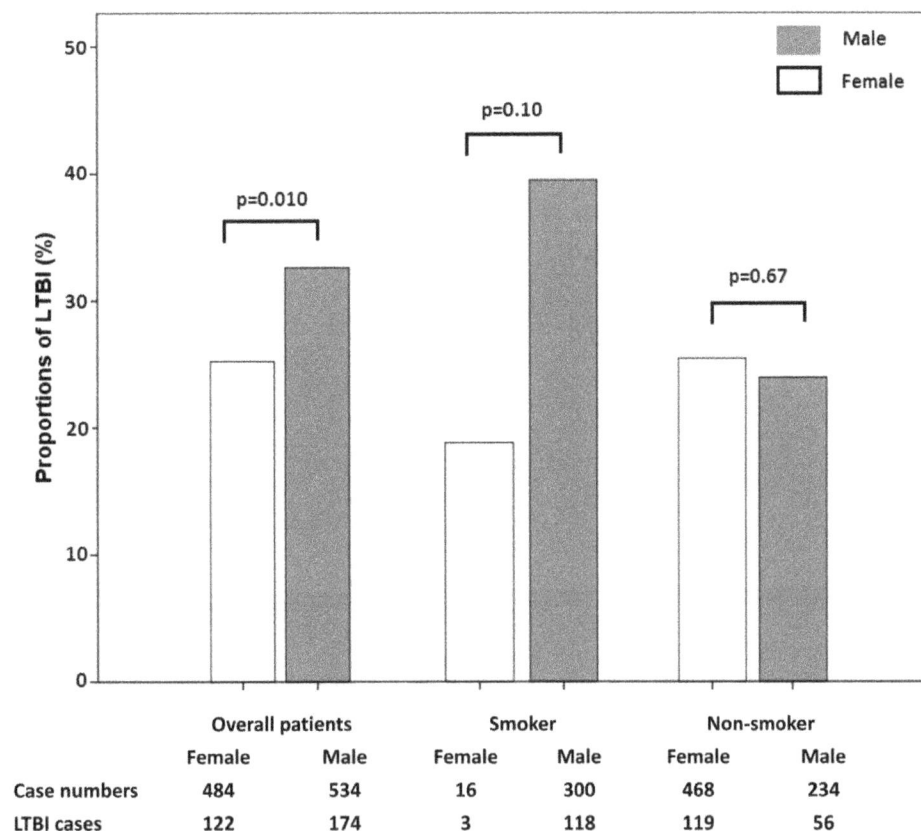

	Overall patients		Smoker		Non-smoker	
	Female	Male	Female	Male	Female	Male
Case numbers	484	534	16	300	468	234
LTBI cases	122	174	3	118	119	56

Figure 3. Proportions of LTBI between sexes in smokers and non-smokers.

Acknowledgments

We thank for the Medical Science & Technology Building of Taipei Veterans General Hospital for providing experimental space and facilities.

Author Contributions

Conceived and designed the experiments: JYF YCL WJS YYL. Performed the experiments: WYT SFH MCL. Analyzed the data: JYF WJS SFH. Contributed reagents/materials/analysis tools: WYT SFH MCL. Wrote the paper: WYT JYF.

References

1. WHO Global tuberculosis report (2013) Geneva, Switzerland: WHO, 2013. Available at http://apps.who.int/iris/bitstream/10665/91355/1/9789241564656_eng.pdf. Accessed 2014 September 24.

2. Barry CE 3rd, Boshoff HI, Dartois V, Dick T, Ehrt S, et al. (2009) The spectrum of latent tuberculosis: rethinking the biology and intervention strategies. Nat Rev Microbiol 7: 845–855.

3. Jereb J, Etkind SC, Joglar OT, Moore M, Taylor Z (2003) Tuberculosis contact investigations: outcomes in selected areas of the United States, 1999. Int J Tuberc Lung Dis 7: S384–390.

4. Diel R, Loddenkemper R, Zellweger JP, Sotgiu G, D'Ambrosio L, et al. (2013) Old ideas to innovate tuberculosis control: preventive treatment to achieve elimination. Eur Respir J 42: 785–801.

5. Feng JY, Huang SF, Ting WY, Chen YC, Lin YY, et al. (2012) Gender differences in treatment outcomes of tuberculosis patients in Taiwan: a prospective observational study. Clin Microbiol Infect 18: E331–337.

6. Onifade DA, Bayer AM, Montoya R, Haro M, Alva J, et al. (2010) Gender-related factors influencing tuberculosis control in shantytowns: a qualitative study. BMC Public Health 10: 381.

7. Jimenez-Corona ME, Garcia-Garcia L, DeRiemer K, Ferreyra-Reyes L, Bobadilla-del-Valle M, et al. (2006) Gender differentials of pulmonary tuberculosis transmission and reactivation in an endemic area. Thorax 61: 348–353.

8. Lin CY, Chen TC, Lu PL, Lai CC, Yang YH, et al. (2013) Effects of gender and age on development of concurrent extrapulmonary tuberculosis in patients with pulmonary tuberculosis: a population based study. PLoS One 8: e63936.

9. Feng JY, Su WJ, Chiu YC, Huang SF, Lin YY, et al. (2011) Initial presentations predict mortality in pulmonary tuberculosis patients—a prospective observational study. PLoS One 6: e23715.

10. Visser ME, Stead MC, Walzl G, Warren R, Schomaker M, et al. (2012) Baseline predictors of sputum culture conversion in pulmonary tuberculosis: importance of cavities, smoking, time to detection and W-Beijing genotype. PLoS One 7: e29588.

11. Fortun J, Martin-Davila P, Molina A, Navas E, Hermida JM, et al. (2007) Sputum conversion among patients with pulmonary tuberculosis: are there implications for removal of respiratory isolation? J Antimicrob Chemother 59: 794–798.

12. Yamasaki-Nakagawa M, Ozasa K, Yamada N, Osuga K, Shimouchi A, et al. (2001) Gender difference in delays to diagnosis and health care seeking behaviour in a rural area of Nepal. Int J Tuberc Lung Dis 5: 24–31.

13. Vlassoff C, Garcia Moreno C (2002) Placing gender at the centre of health programming: challenges and limitations. Soc Sci Med 54: 1713–1723.

14. Neyrolles O, Quintana-Murci L (2009) Sexual inequality in tuberculosis. PLoS Med 6: e1000199.

15. Yamamoto Y, Tomioka H, Sato K, Saito H, Yamada Y, et al. (1990) Sex differences in the susceptibility of mice to infection induced by Mycobacterium intracellulare. Am Rev Respir Dis 142: 430–433.

16. Kim SY, Jung GS, Kim SK, Chang J, Kim MS, et al. (2013) Comparison of the tuberculin skin test and interferon-gamma release assay for the diagnosis of latent tuberculosis infection before kidney transplantation. Infection 41: 103–110.

17. Soysal A, Toprak D, Koc M, Arikan H, Akoglu E, et al. (2012) Diagnosing latent tuberculosis infection in haemodialysis patients: T-cell based assay (T-SPOT.TB) or tuberculin skin test? Nephrol Dial Transplant 27: 1645–1650.

18. Pareek M, Watson JP, Ormerod LP, Kon OM, Woltmann G, et al. (2011) Screening of immigrants in the UK for imported latent tuberculosis: a multicentre cohort study and cost-effectiveness analysis. Lancet Infect Dis 11: 435–444.

19. Zhang X, Jia H, Liu F, Pan L, Xing A, et al. (2013) Prevalence and Risk Factors for Latent Tuberculosis Infection among Health Care Workers in China: A Cross-Sectional Study. PLoS One 8: e66412.
20. Yen YF, Hu BS, Lin YS, Li LH, Su LW, et al. (2013) Latent tuberculosis among injection drug users in a methadone maintenance treatment program, Taipei, Taiwan: TSPOT.TB versus tuberculin skin test. Scand J Infect Dis 45: 504–511.
21. Kim HR, Hwang SS, Ro YK, Jeon CH, Ha DY, et al. (2008) Solid-organ malignancy as a risk factor for tuberculosis. Respirology 13: 413–419.
22. (2000) Targeted tuberculin testing and treatment of latent tuberculosis infection. American Thoracic Society. MMWR Recomm Rep 49: 1–51.
23. Weiss MG, Sommerfeld J, Uplekar MW (2008) Social and cultural dimensions of gender and tuberculosis. Int J Tuberc Lung Dis 12: 829–830.
24. Diwan VK, Thorson A (1999) Sex, gender, and tuberculosis. Lancet 353: 1000–1001.
25. Hamid Salim MA, Declercq E, Van Deun A, Saki KA (2004) Gender differences in tuberculosis: a prevalence survey done in Bangladesh. Int J Tuberc Lung Dis 8: 952–957.
26. Slama K, Chiang CY, Enarson DA, Hassmiller K, Fanning A, et al. (2007) Tobacco and tuberculosis: a qualitative systematic review and meta-analysis. Int J Tuberc Lung Dis 11: 1049–1061.
27. Lin HH, Ezzati M, Murray M (2007) Tobacco smoke, indoor air pollution and tuberculosis: a systematic review and meta-analysis. PLoS Med 4: e20.
28. Lin HH, Ezzati M, Chang HY, Murray M (2009) Association between tobacco smoking and active tuberculosis in Taiwan: prospective cohort study. Am J Respir Crit Care Med 180: 475–480.
29. Shaler CR, Horvath CN, McCormick S, Jeyanathan M, Khera A, et al. (2013) Continuous and discontinuous cigarette smoke exposure differentially affects protective Th1 immunity against pulmonary tuberculosis. PLoS One 8: e59185.
30. Shang S, Ordway D, Henao-Tamayo M, Bai X, Oberley-Deegan R, et al. (2011) Cigarette smoke increases susceptibility to tuberculosis—evidence from in vivo and in vitro models. J Infect Dis 203: 1240–1248.

23

A Prospective Cohort Study to Examine the Association between Dietary Patterns and Depressive Symptoms in Older Chinese People in Hong Kong

Ruth Chan[1]*, Dicken Chan[2], Jean Woo[1]

1 Department of Medicine and Therapeutics, The Chinese University of Hong Kong, Shatin, Hong Kong, 2 The Jockey Club School of Public Health and Primary Care, The Chinese University of Hong Kong, Shatin, Hong Kong

Abstract

Introduction: Dietary patterns are culturally specific and there is limited data on the association of dietary patterns with late-life depression in Chinese. This study examined the associations between dietary patterns and baseline and subsequent depressive symptoms in community-dwelling Chinese older people in Hong Kong.

Methods: Participants aged ≥65 year participating in a cohort study examining the risk factors for osteoporosis completed a validated food frequency questionnaire at baseline between 2001 and 2003. Factor analysis was used to identify three dietary patterns: "vegetables-fruits" pattern, "snacks-drinks-milk products" pattern, and "meat-fish" pattern. Depressive symptoms were measured at baseline and 4-year using the validated Geriatric Depression Scale. Multiple logistic regression was used for cross-sectional analysis (n = 2,902) to assess the associations between dietary patterns and the presence of depressive symptoms, and for longitudinal analysis (n = 2,211) on their associations with 4-year depressive symptoms, with adjustment for socio-demographic and lifestyle factors.

Results: The highest quartile of "vegetables-fruits" pattern score was associated with reduced likelihood of depressive symptoms [Adjusted OR = 0.55 (95% CI: 0.36–0.83), p_{trend} = 0.017] compared to the lowest quartile at baseline. Similar inverse trend was observed for the highest quartile of "snacks-drinks-milk products" pattern score [Adjusted OR = 0.41 (95% CI: 0.26–0.65), p_{trend}<0.001] compared to the lowest quartile. There was no association of "meat-fish" pattern with the presence of depressive symptoms at baseline. None of the dietary patterns were associated with subsequent depressive symptoms at 4-year.

Conclusion: Higher "vegetables-fruits" and "snacks-drinks-milk products" pattern scores were associated with reduced likelihood of baseline depressive symptoms in Chinese older people in Hong Kong. The longitudinal analyses failed to show any causal relationship between dietary patterns and depressive symptoms in this population.

Editor: Robert Stewart, Institute of Psychiatry, United Kingdom

Funding: This study was supported by grants from the Research Grants Council of Hong Kong, CUHK 4101/02M; the Hong Kong Jockey Club Charities Trust; the SH Ho Centre for Gerontology and Geriatric and the Centre for Nutritional Studies, The Chinese University of Hong Kong. The funders had no role in study design, data collection and analysis, decision to publish, or preparation of the manuscript.

Competing Interests: The authors have declared that no competing interests exist.

* Email: ruthchansm@cuhk.edu.hk

Introduction

Depression is a common mental health disorder. It affects over 350 million people worldwide and it is expected that depression will become the world's leading cause of disease burden by the year 2030 [1]. Depression is less prevalent among older adults than among younger counterparts [2]. However, late-life depression is considered as an important public health problem due to its devastating consequences, including increased risk of morbidity and reduced physical, cognitive, and social functioning [3,4]. As a result, to identify modifiable risk factors for depression is inevitably important [5].

Recent evidence suggests that diet modifies key biological factors associated with the development of depression, and diet rich in fruits, vegetables, whole grains and fish is in general associated with lower risk of depression [6,7]. Studies have shown that the antioxidant compounds in fruit and vegetables could reduce neuronal damage induced by oxidative-stress whereas long-chain omega-3 polyunsaturated fatty acids could possibly affect mood by an alteration of the brain serotonergic function and its immune-neuroendocrine effects [6,7]. However, the examination of diet as a risk factor for depression has traditionally focused on the effect of single foods and nutrients, and the findings thus far are inconsistent [8]. Since diet is a combination of food and nutrients, there has been an increasing interest in using dietary pattern analysis in epidemiological studies [9]. There are two main approaches to define dietary patterns [9,10]. One approach is the *a priori* approach in which dietary indices are constructed based on prevailing dietary recommendations. Another approach is the *a posteriori* approach in which dietary patterns are derived from statistical modeling, such as factor analysis, using data from dietary records or food frequency questionnaires (FFQ).

Data on the association between dietary patterns and depression are limited. Some cross-sectional studies have been carried out in Caucasians and Japanese to evaluate the association between dietary patterns and depression or depressive symptoms in adulthood [11–16]. To our knowledge, nine prospective studies have examined the role of dietary patterns and depression or depressive symptoms in adulthood [17–25] and two prospective studies have evaluated this association in adolescents [26,27]. Few studies have investigated the association between depression and diet in Chinese older people, and these studies mainly focused on the effect of single foods and nutrients [28,29]. Only one cross-sectional study has examined the association of dietary patterns with depressive symptoms in Chinese but it was done in adolescents [27].

Since dietary patterns are culturally specific and there is limited data on the association of dietary patterns with late-life depression in Chinese, we evaluated the association between dietary patterns and baseline and subsequent depressive symptoms in older Chinese people, using data from a sample of community-dwelling men and women aged 65 and over participating in a prospective study in Hong Kong. We hypothesized that dietary patterns are associated with baseline and subsequent depressive symptoms in this population.

Methods

Study population

Subjects were participants of a cohort study examining the risk factors for osteoporosis in Hong Kong [30]. 2,000 men and 2,000 women aged 65 years and over living in the community were recruited in a health survey between August 2001 and December 2003 by recruitment notices and talks in community centers and housing estates. Participants were volunteers and were able to walk or take public transport to the study site. They were recruited using a stratified sample so that approximately 33% would be in each of these age groups: 65–69, 70–74, 75+. Compared with the official population statistics, participants had higher educational level than the overall older population in Hong Kong (12–18% vs. 3–9% with tertiary education in the age groups 80+, 75–79, 70–74, and 65–69 years) [31]. The 4-year follow-up was held between August 2005 and November 2007. Follow-up was done by a mailed reminder for a follow-up body check appointment. Phone reminders were given again close to the appointment dates, and defaulters were given a second appointment to enhance attendance rates. Mean (SD) follow-up year was 3.9 (0.1) years.

We excluded participants who did not have dietary data (n = 5), those with extreme daily energy intake at the first- and last-half percentiles of the sex-specific range (n = 37), those who had missing data for the variables included for the analyses (n = 6), and those who were probable dementia defined using the cognitive part of the Community Screening Instrument for Dementia (CSI-D) with the cutoff point of ≤28.4 [32] (n = 1,050). The baseline analysis was performed on 2,902 participants. For the longitudinal analysis, we further excluded 218 participants who had depressive symptoms at baseline and 473 participants who did not attend the 4-year follow-up. 2,211 participants were therefore included for the 4-year incidence analysis (Figure 1). This study was conducted in accordance with the Declaration of Helsinki. This study was approved by the Clinical Research Ethics Committee of the Chinese University of Hong Kong. Written informed consent was obtained from all participants.

Demographic and overall health characteristics

A standardized interview was performed to collect information on age, gender, education level, marital status, smoking habit, alcohol use and medical history. Information on the duration and

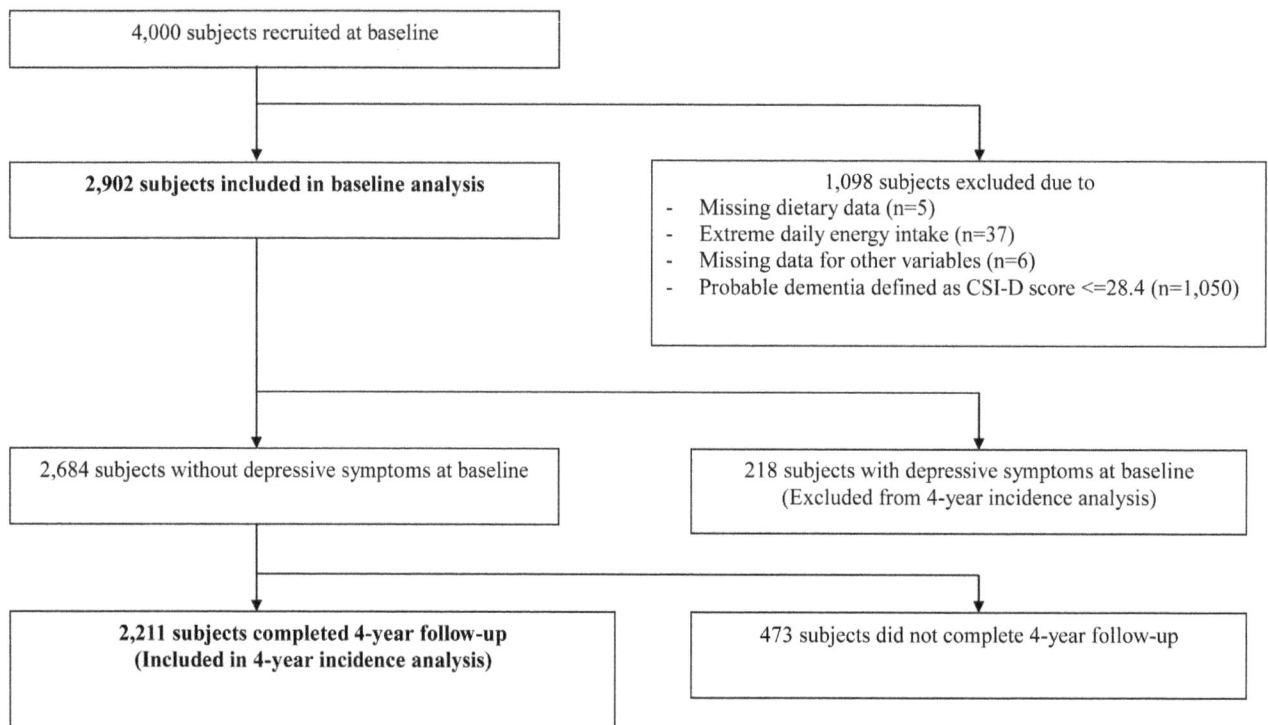

Figure 1.Number of subjects included and excluded for baseline and 4-year follow-up analyses.

level of past and current use of cigarettes, cigars and pipes was obtained. Smoking history was classified in terms of former smoking (at least 100 cigarettes smoked in a lifetime), current smoking and never smoking. Drinking status was defined as never, former (ever drank at least 5 drinks daily in a lifetime) or current drinker. Baseline disease status was obtained by self-report of their doctors' diagnoses, supplemented by the identification of drugs brought to the interviewers.

Anthropometric data

Body weight was measured to the nearest 0.1 kg with participants wearing a light gown, using the Physician Balance Beam Scale (Healthometer, Illinois, USA). Height was measured to the nearest 0.1 cm using the Holtain Harpenden stadiometer (Holtain Ltd, Crosswell, UK). Body mass index (BMI) was calculated as body weight in kg / (height in m)^2.

Physical activity assessment

Physical activity was assessed by the Physical Activity Scale for the Elderly (PASE) [33], which was adapted for use in elderly Hong Kong Chinese [34]. This is a 12-item scale measuring the average number of hours per day spent in leisure, household, and occupational physical activities over the previous 7-day period. Activity weights for each item were determined based on the amount of energy spent, and each item score was calculated by multiplying the activity weight with daily activity frequency. A composite PASE score of all the items was yielded. A higher PASE score reflects higher physical activity level.

Number of instrumental activities of daily living (IADLs) were assessed using specific questions and participants were asked to self-report of any impairment in walking two to three blocks outdoors on level ground, climbing 10 steps without resting, preparing own meals, doing heavy housework like scrubbing floors or washing windows, and shopping for groceries or clothes. A summed score from 0 to 5 was calculated from these activities as the degree of impairment in IADLs, with higher score indicating greater impairment.

Assessment of cognitive function

Since depression may be associated with cognitive impairment, in the analysis of factors associated with depression, the presence of cognitive impairment was adjusted for as a confounding factor. Cognitive function was assessed by trained research staff using the cognitive part of the Community Screening Instrument for Dementia (CSI-D) [32], validated in different cultural and educational settings [32]. The cognitive part of the CSI-D consists of 32 items in six cognitive domains: orientation to time, orientation to place, praxis, abstract thinking, language and memory. A summary score ranged from 0 to 33 was generated, with higher score meaning better cognitive function. The cutoff point for probable dementia is ≤28.4.

Assessment of depressive symptoms

Depressive symptoms was assessed by face-to-face interviews using a validated Chinese version of the Geriatric Depression Scale (GDS) [35,36]. The GDS short form was found to be a highly reliable (reliability coefficient of 0.90) and valid screening device (sensitivity of 96.3% and specificity of 87.5%) for assessing geriatric depression in Hong Kong Chinese [36]. The GDS short form consists of 15 questions relevant to depression, such as motivation, self-image, losses, agitation and mood. A yes/no format was designed for each question. A summary score ranged from 0 to 15 was generated, and a cut-off of 8 or more was used to define the presence of depressive symptoms.

Dietary assessment

Baseline dietary intake was assessed using a validated FFQ developed in a population survey [37]. Daily nutrient intake was calculated using food tables derived from McCance and Widdowson [38] and the Chinese Medical Sciences Institute [39]. The FFQ consisted of 280 food items. Each participant reported the frequency and the usual amount of consumption of each food item over the past year. For each food 9 different categories were given from never or seldom to more than once a day. Portion size was explained to participants using a catalogue of pictures of individual food portions. For seasonally consumed vegetables and fruits, participants were asked about the months of food consumption over the past year. The amount of cooking oil was estimated according to the usual cooking methods of preparing standardized portion of different foods and the usual portion of different foods consumed by the participants.

Dietary patterns derived by factor analysis

Details of dietary pattern scores derived by the factor analysis have been described elsewhere [40]. In brief, individual food items from the FFQ were aggregated into 32 food groups based on similarity of type of food and nutrient composition. The food groups were energy adjusted by dividing the energy intake from each food group by total energy intake and multiplying by 100, and were expressed as percentage contribution to total energy [41]. Factor analysis was conducted with varimax rotation using the 32 food groups [9]. Factors were retained based on an eigenvalues greater than 1.0, a scree plot, and the interpretability [42]. The factor scores for each pattern were calculated for each participant by summing intakes of food items weighted by their factor loadings. A higher score indicated greater conformity with the pattern being calculated.

Statistical analysis

Statistical analyses were performed using the statistical package SPSS version 21.0 (SPSS Inc., Illinois, US). Data were checked for normality using histograms and logarithmic transformation was applied whenever appropriate. Dietary pattern scores derived by factor analysis were stratified into quartiles based on the distribution of each sex. Pearson's correlation was used to examine the correlation between each dietary pattern score and intakes of various nutrients. Independent t test and chi square test were used to examine baseline differences in mean age, BMI, PASE, CSI-D score, energy intake, and also differences in the distribution of sex, education level, smoking status, alcohol use, number of IADLs, self-reported disease status, quartiles of each dietary pattern score between participants with depressive symptoms and participants without depressive symptoms at baseline. These tests were also used to examine differences in baseline characteristics between participants who included and excluded in the baseline analysis, and between participants who completed and participants who did not complete the 4-year follow-up.

Multivariate logistic regression was used to estimate the odds ratio (OR) and 95% confidence intervals (CIs) for both the baseline and the subsequent depressive symptoms according to quartiles of each dietary pattern score. Model 1 was adjusted for baseline age (years), sex, and daily energy intake (kcal). Model 2 was further adjusted for baseline BMI, PASE, number of IADLs (no difficulty/some difficulties), smoking habit (never/past/current), alcohol use (never/past/current), education level (no education/primary or below/secondary or matriculation/University or above), and marital status (married or living with a partner/ widowed, separated or divorced/single). Model 3 was further adjusted for baseline self-reported history of diabetes (yes/no), hypertension (yes/no), and CVD or stroke (yes/no), and CSI-D score. Test for trend was examined by entering quartiles of each dietary pattern score in all models. An α level of 5% was used as the level of significance. Interaction between sex and quartiles of each dietary pattern score was tested by addition of cross-product terms to the multivariate models. Interactions were not significant, thus all analyses are presented in the total population.

To check the possibility of reverse causation, a sensitivity analysis excluding participants with extreme GDS at the top two percentiles (GDS$\geq$11) was performed for the cross-sectional data. Considering that GDS is a screening scale and may be limited as a case-defining instrument compared to other diagnostic instruments [43], multivariate logistic regression models were repeated using a group whose depressive symptom levels had clearly increased over 4-year (i.e. with an increase in GDS score at 4 and over from baseline to four years) as an outcome variable. This cut-off value was chosen because 142 participants (6.4%) could be classified as the worsening cases and this number of cases may be more sufficient and powerful for statistical analysis than using an increase in GDS score at 5 and over as a cut-off value (i.e. n = 85). All models were adjusted for the same variables mentioned above.

Results

Dietary patterns of the participants

Factor analysis identified three dietary patterns (Table 1). The first factor (vegetables-fruits pattern) was dominated by frequent intake of vegetables, fruits, soy and soy products, and legumes. The second factor (snacks-drinks-milk products pattern) was composed of a mixture of healthy and unhealthy food groups. It was characterized by frequent intake of condiments, drinks, fast food, French fries, potato chips, sweets and desserts, nuts, milk products, and whole grains. The third factor (meat-fish pattern) included frequent intake of dim sum, red and processed meats, poultry, fish and seafood, and wine.

'Vegetables-fruits' dietary pattern scores were inversely associated with total fat, saturated fat, monounsaturated fat and polyunsaturated fat intakes, and positively associated with intakes of protein, fiber, isoflavones, most vitamins and minerals. 'Snacks-drinks-milk products' dietary pattern scores were inversely associated with intakes of polyunsaturated fat and vitamin K, and positively associated with intakes of carbohydrates, protein, total fat, saturated fat, monounsaturated fat, cholesterol, fiber, most minerals and vitamins. Whilst 'snacks-drinks-milk products' dietary pattern scores were also positively associated with intakes of fiber and most minerals and vitamins, the associations were less strong than those with 'vegetables-fruits' dietary pattern scores. 'Meat-fish' dietary pattern scores were weakly positively associated with intakes of polyunsaturated fat and most micronutrients, moderately positively associated with intakes of protein, total fat and monounsaturated fat, and strongly positively associated with saturated fat and cholesterol intakes. The positive associations of protein, total fat, different kinds of fat and cholesterol with 'meat-fish' dietary pattern scores were stronger than those with 'snacks-drinks-milk products' dietary pattern scores (Table 2).

Participants' characteristics by baseline depressive status

Participants who were excluded in the cross-sectional analysis were older and less physically active, had lower education level, and were more likely to be female, widowed, separated, divorced or single, and to have self-reported history of diabetes than those who were included in the cross-sectional analysis ($p<0.05$). Those who discontinued the 4-year follow-up were older, less physically active, and were more likely to be divorced or single as compared to those who completed the 4-year follow-up ($p<0.05$) (details not shown).

Among 2,902 participants included in the cross-sectional analysis, there were 218 (7.5%) participants who were classified as having depressive symptoms at baseline. For the longitudinal analysis, 81 (3.7%) cases were newly identified as having depressive symptoms out of 2,211 participants at the 4-year follow-up. The characteristics of participants with depressive symptoms and participants without depressive symptoms at baseline are shown in Table 3. Those who had depressive symptoms had lower CSI-D score, lower education level, more impairments in IADLs, and were more likely to be widowed, separated, divorced or single, and current smokers, and were more likely to have self-reported history of heart diseases or stroke. Those who had depressive symptoms also showed lower 'vegetables-fruits' dietary pattern scores and lower 'snacks-drinks-milk products' dietary pattern scores.

Dietary patterns and the presence of depressive symptoms at baseline and 4-year

In the cross-sectional analysis, participants in the highest quartile of "vegetables-fruits" pattern score had reduced likelihood of depressive symptoms [Adjusted OR = 0.55 (95% CI: 0.36–0.83), $p_{trend} = 0.017$] compared to participants in the lowest quartile. Participants in the highest quartile of "snacks-drinks-milk products" pattern score also showed reduced likelihood of depressive symptoms [Adjusted OR = 0.41 (95% CI: 0.26–0.65), $p_{trend} < 0.001$] compared to those in the lowest quartile. There was no association of "meat-fish" pattern with depressive status at baseline (Table 4). Longitudinal analysis showed that none of the dietary patterns were associated with the presence of depressive symptoms at 4-year (Table 5).

Sensitivity analysis excluding participants with extreme GDS (i.e. GDS$\geq$11 (n = 56)) showed similar results for the cross-sectional data (details not shown). Multivariate logistic regression models that were repeated using a group with an increase in GDS score $> = 4$ over four years as an outcome also showed no association between each dietary pattern and the presence of depressive symptoms at 4-year (details not shown).

Discussion

This study found an inverse association between "vegetables-fruits' and 'snacks-drinks-milk products' dietary pattern scores and baseline depressive symptoms. However, no significant associations between 'meat-fish' dietary pattern scores and baseline depressive symptoms were observed. Moreover, we did not observe significant associations between baseline dietary pattern scores and subsequent depressive symptoms at 4-year.

Previous cross-sectional studies have evaluated the association between dietary patterns and depression or depressive symptoms. However, the results are inconclusive [13–16,22]. Similar to our findings, two recent studies from Japan showed that a healthy Japanese dietary pattern characterized by high intakes of plant foods including vegetables, fruit, mushrooms and soy products was associated with fewer depressive symptoms [14,16]. Our results were also consistent with the findings from an Australian study which showed that a diet characterized by high intakes of fruits, vegetables, and plant based foods was associated with fewer depressive symptoms[13]. Compared to the "snacks-drinks-milk products" pattern and the "meat-fish" pattern, the "vegetables-fruits" pattern showed the highest correlations with fiber and other

Table 1. Food group factor loading[a] for three dietary patterns.

Food groups	Dietary patterns		
	Factor 1: Vegetables-fruits	Factor 2: Snacks-drinks-milk products	Factor 3: Meat-fish
Other vegetables	**0.60**	-0.08	0.03
Cruciferous vegetables	**0.48**	−0.08	−0.06
Tomatoes	**0.47**	0.05	−0.04
Soy	**0.43**	0.03	0.10
Dark green & leafy vegetables	**0.42**	−0.27	−0.04
Starchy vegetables	**0.42**	0.07	−0.03
Fruits	**0.39**	0.06	0.03
Legumes	**0.35**	−0.06	0.02
Mushroom & fungi	**0.25**	0.07	−0.06
Fats and oils	**−0.39**	−0.20	0.11
Condiments	−0.06	**0.48**	−0.06
Coffee	−0.15	**0.41**	−0.15
Nuts	0.12	**0.39**	−0.03
Fast food	−0.02	**0.35**	0.14
French fries and potato chips	−0.02	**0.34**	0.14
Milk and milk products	0.11	**0.33**	−0.10
Whole grains	0.16	**0.32**	−0.16
Sweets and desserts	0.01	**0.27**	0.19
Beverages	−0.02	**0.22**	0.10
Eggs	0.08	**0.22**	0.05
Dim sum	−0.17	−0.17	**0.51**
Red and processed meats	−0.07	−0.03	**0.47**
Poultry	0.06	0.03	**0.47**
Fish and seafood	0.20	−0.26	**0.33**
Cakes, cookies, pies and biscuits	0.07	0.12	**0.24**
Wine	−0.15	0.07	**0.22**
Refined grains	−0.24	−0.42	**−0.74**
Organ meats	−0.08	0.13	0.12
Others	0.01	0.07	0.05
Preserved vegetables	0	0.10	0.01
Soups	0	0	−0.01
Tea	−0.03	0.17	0.05
% variance explained	**6.5**	**5.2**	**5.2**

[a]Factor loadings with absolute value ≥0.2 are shown in bold (Field 2005). For food group loads more than one dietary pattern, only the highest absolute value of loading is bolded.

nutrients, such as vitamin C that are considered as beneficial for brain health [6]. It is possible that the "vegetables-fruits" pattern is associated with reduced oxidative stress, higher anti-inflammatory property, and higher antioxidant capacity, the potential biological mechanisms that are linked with better mood and brain health [44]. The potential protective effect of the 'vegetables-fruits' pattern could also come from folate that is rich in some cruciferous vegetables, leafy vegetables, and other green vegetables. There has been evidence to suggest that folate deficiency impairs the synthesis of homocysteine to methionine and S-adenosyl-methionine. The latter is a methyl donor and is involved in the synthesis and metabolism of neurotransmitters [45]. There is also substantial evidence from observational studies and randomized con-

trolled trials to suggest that folate deficiency is associated with increased risk of depression [7,46].

Our study showed that 'snacks-drinks-milk products' dietary pattern was linked to a fewer depressive symptoms. Such an inverse association was less easy to interpret. In comparison to the 'vegetable-fruit' dietary pattern, the positive association of this pattern with intakes of fiber and most minerals and vitamins was less strong. However, this pattern was composed of healthy and unhealthy food groups. This pattern was dominated by the intake of condiments, drinks, sweets and desserts, fast food, French fries, potato chips, nuts, milk and milk products, and whole grains. Past studies have examined the role of these food groups in depression [47–49]. Greater intake of high-calorie sweet foods and fast foods appeared to be associated with more depressive symptoms [47,48].

Table 2. Pearson's correlations between each dietary pattern score and nutrient intakes at baseline (n = 2,902).

Nutrients	Vegetables-fruits		Snacks-drinks-milk products		Meat-fish	
	r	p	r	p	r	P
Energy (kcal)	−0.05	0.006	0.21	<0.001	0.22	<0.001
Carbohydrates (g)	−0.01	0.456	0.17	<0.001	−0.11	<0.001
Protein (g)	0.13	<0.001	0.21	<0.001	0.39	<0.001
Fat (g)	−0.12	<0.001	0.18	<0.001	0.48	<0.001
SFA (% energy)	−0.17	<0.001	0.14	<0.001	0.57	<0.001
MUFA (% energy)	−0.06	0.001	0.06	0.001	0.36	<0.001
PUFA (% energy)	−0.13	<0.001	−0.11	<0.001	0.15	<0.001
Cholesterol (mg) [†]	0.03	0.168	0.15	<0.001	0.55	<0.001
Fiber (g) [†]	0.60	<0.001	0.17	<0.001	0.04	0.019
Vitamin A (IU) [†]	0.57	<0.001	0.05	0.006	0.11	<0.001
Vitamin C (mg) [†]	0.52	<0.001	0.03	0.103	0.12	<0.001
Calcium (mg)	0.36	<0.001	0.31	<0.001	0.02	0.258
Phosphorus (mg)	0.19	<0.001	0.33	<0.001	0.07	<0.001
Iron (mg) [†]	0.28	<0.001	0.26	<0.001	0.18	<0.001
Potassium (mg) [†]	0.24	<0.001	0.08	<0.001	0.33	<0.001
Magnesium (mg) [†]	0.38	<0.001	0.07	<0.001	−0.01	0.645
Sodium (mg) [†]	0.12	<0.001	0.23	<0.001	0.31	<0.001
Zinc (mg)	0.20	<0.001	0.15	<0.001	0.28	<0.001
Isoflavones (mg) [†]	0.35	<0.001	0.09	<0.001	0.13	<0.001
Vitamin K (µg) [†]	0.52	<0.001	−0.13	<0.001	0.07	<0.001
Vitamin D (IU) [†]	0.10	<0.001	0.30	<0.001	0.06	0.001

SFA, Saturated fatty acids; MUFA, Monounsaturated fatty acids; PUFA, Polyunsaturated fatty acids.
[†]log transformed nutrient intake.

In contrast, there is evidence to suggest that increased intake of milk and dairy products, in particular the low-fat milk and dairy products is associated with better brain function and mood [49].

Our longitudinal analysis did not show significant associations between baseline dietary pattern scores and subsequent depressive symptoms at 4-year. Sensitivity analysis by repeating the multivariate logistic regression models with an outcome of a group with an increase in GDS score $> = 4$ over four years also confirmed these negative findings. Furthermore, in order to investigate the relationship between diet and depression persistence at 4-year, we tried to repeat the multivariate logistic regression models for participants with depressive symptoms at baseline. No association between dietary patterns and the presence of depressive symptoms was observed at 4-year among this group of baseline depressive participants and these findings further confirmed our negative longitudinal findings. Several prospective studies have examined the role of dietary patterns and incident depression or depressive symptoms in adulthood [17–25], and the findings generally support the role of dietary patterns in the development of depression. Most studies reported significant associations between dietary patterns and incident depression or depressive symptoms [17–19,21–25], but one recent study showed no clear associations between dietary patterns and depression incidence [20]. Using data of 3,486 men and women of the Whitehall II prospective cohort, Akbaraly and colleagues showed a higher odds of depressive symptoms with a "processed food pattern" which was heavily loaded by high intake of sweetened desserts, chocolates, fried food, processed meat, pies, refined grains, high-fat dairy products and condiments [18]. In the

GAZEL cohort, Le Port et al. [19] reported that healthy pattern (characterized by vegetables consumption) were associated with fewer depressive symptoms in men and women, and traditional pattern (characterized by fish and fruit consumption) were associated with lower risk of incident depression in women. Furthermore, the highest quartile of low-fat, western, high snack and high fat-sweet diets in men and low-fat and high snack diets in women were associated with higher likelihood of depressive symptoms compared to the lowest quartile. However, recent findings among women in the Nurses' Health Study did not suggest clear associations between dietary Prudent and Western pattern scores and incident depression risk [20]. Differences in the study design, such as tools for assessing depression (i.e. self-reported scale vs. clinical diagnosis), inclusion and exclusion criteria for the subjects, and covariates that were included in the statistical models may account for the variations in the study findings [50]. Recent findings from a multicenter, randomized, primary prevention filed trial suggest that a Mediterranean diet supplemented with nuts could possibly reduce the risk of depression in patients with type 2 diabetes [51]. Therefore, the role of diet in depression warrants further investigation.

Strengths of our study are inclusion of both cross-sectional and longitudinal study design, and adjustment for several potential confounders. However, our study had several limitations. First, the use of the self-reported measure of depression (GDS) and cognitive impairment (CSI-D) may be one of the limitations. However, the sensitivity of these measures is high and has been validated in Chinese populations [32,36]. Second, the low number of participants with depressive symptoms at the 4-year follow-up

Table 3. Subject characteristics by baseline depressive status (n = 2,902).

	Subjects without depressive symptoms (GDS<8) (n = 2,684)		Subjects with depressive symptoms (GDS> = 8) (n = 218)		P value[1]
	Mean/n	(SD/%)	Mean/n	SD/%	
Age (years)	71.8	(4.8)	72.2	(5.0)	0.310
BMI (kg/m^2)	23.6	(3.2)	23.4	(3.3)	0.203
PASE score	94.1	(44.7)	91.5	(40.2)	0.399
CSI-D score	31.2	(0.9)	31.0	(0.8)	**0.001**
Daily energy intake (kcal)	1913.8	(571.4)	1876.3	(556.7)	0.351
Dietary pattern scores					
Vegetables-fruits	0.015	(1.002)	−0.187	(0.958)	**0.004**
Q1	651	(24.3)	76	(34.9)	**0.002**
Q2	677	(25.2)	49	(22.5)	
Q3	669	(24.9)	55	(25.2)	
Q4	687	(25.6)	38	(17.4)	
Snacks-drinks-milk products	0.022	(1.004)	−0.272	(0.915)	**<0.001**
Q1	646	(24.1)	81	(37.2)	**<0.001**
Q2	662	(24.7)	62	(28.4)	
Q3	684	(25.5)	43	(19.7)	
Q4	692	(25.8)	32	(14.7)	
Meat-fish	0.004	(0.996)	−0.045	(1.051)	0.487
Q1	669	(24.9)	56	(25.7)	0.441
Q2	665	(24.8)	61	(28.0)	
Q3	670	(25.0)	56	(25.7)	
Q4	680	(25.3)	45	(20.6)	
Female (%)	1075	(40.1)	87	(39.9)	0.967
Education level (%)					
Primary or below	1697	(63.2)	157	(72.0)	**0.014**
Secondary / Matriculation	636	(23.7)	45	(20.6)	
University or above	351	(13.1)	16	(7.3)	
Marital status (%)					
Married or living with a partner	2085	(77.7)	155	(71.1)	**0.004**
Widowed, separated or divorced	546	(20.3)	52	(23.9)	
Single	53	(2.0)	11	(5.0)	
Smoking status (%)					
Never smoke	1583	(59.0)	110	(50.5)	**0.003**
Ex-smoker	910	(33.9)	80	(36.7)	
Current smoker	191	(7.1)	28	(12.8)	
Alcohol use (%)					
Never	2203	(82.1)	181	(83.0)	0.191
Ex-drinker	55	(2.0)	8	(3.7)	
Current drinker	426	(15.9)	29	(13.3)	
Self-reported medical history (%)					
Diabetes mellitus	350	(13.0)	38	(17.4)	0.067
Hypertension	1118	(41.7)	100	(45.9)	0.225
Heart diseases or stroke	552	(20.6)	71	(32.6)	**<0.001**
IADLs					
No impairment	2141	(79.8)	138	(63.3)	**<0.001**
Some impairments	543	(20.2)	80	(36.7)	

[1]Differences between groups were assessed by independent *t* test or chi square test.

Table 4. Odds ratios (95% CI) for the cross-sectional association between dietary patterns and depressive symptoms (GDS> =8) at baseline (n = 2,902).

Dietary pattern	Case / Control	Crude			Model 1[2]			Model 2[3]			Model 3[4]		
		OR	(95% CI)	P_{trend}[1]	OR	(95% CI)	P_{trend}	OR	(95% CI)	P_{trend}	OR	(95% CI)	P_{trend}
Vegetables-fruits													
Q1	76/651	1		0.001	1		0.001	1		0.019	1		0.017
Q2	49/677	0.62	0.43–0.90		0.62	0.43–0.91		0.67	0.46–0.98		0.68	0.46–0.99	
Q3	55/669	0.70	0.49–1.01		0.71	0.49–1.02		0.81	0.56–1.18		0.83	0.57–1.20	
Q4	38/687	0.47	0.32–0.71		0.48	0.32–0.72		0.56	0.37–0.84		0.55	0.36–0.83	
Snacks- drinks-milk products													
Q1	81/646	1		<0.001	1		<0.001	1		<0.001	1		<0.001
Q2	62/662	0.75	0.53–1.06		0.75	0.53–1.06		0.76	0.53–1.09		0.77	0.54–1.10	
Q3	43/684	0.50	0.34–0.74		0.51	0.34–0.74		0.51	0.34–0.76		0.52	0.35–0.78	
Q4	32/692	0.37	0.24–0.56		0.37	0.24–0.57		0.40	0.25–0.62		0.41	0.26–0.65	
Meat-fish													
Q1	56/669	1		0.221	1		0.273	1		0.269	1		0.199
Q2	61/665	1.10	0.75–1.60		1.10	0.76–1.61		1.18	0.80–1.73		1.18	0.80–1.73	
Q3	56/670	1.00	0.68–1.47		1.01	0.69–1.49		1.08	0.73–1.61		1.06	0.71–1.58	
Q4	45/680	0.79	0.53–1.19		0.81	0.54–1.22		0.80	0.53–1.22		0.77	0.51–1.18	

[1]Test for trend was examined by entering dietary pattern score quartiles as a fixed factor and testing the contrast by using the polynomial option in all models.
[2]Model 1: adjusted for age, sex and daily energy intake.
[3]Model 2: further adjusted for BMI, PASE, number of IADLs, smoking status, alcohol use, education and marital status.
[4]Model 3: further adjusted for self-reported history of diabetes mellitus, hypertension, heart disease and stroke, and CSI-D score.

Table 5. Odds ratios (95% CI) for the longitudinal association between baseline dietary patterns and 4-year incidence of depressive symptoms (GDS$>$ = 8) (n = 2,211).

Dietary pattern	Case / Control	Crude			Model 1[2]			Model 2[3]			Model 3[4]		
		OR	(95% CI)	P_{trend}[1]	OR	(95% CI)	P_{trend}	OR	(95% CI)	P_{trend}	OR	(95% CI)	P_{trend}
Vegetables-fruits													
Q1	25/494	1		0.415	1		0.432	1		0.903	1		0.931
Q2	17/547	0.61	0.33–1.15		0.62	0.33–1.17		0.71	0.38–1.35		0.73	0.38–1.38	
Q3	18/534	0.67	0.36–1.24		0.66	0.36–1.24		0.77	0.41–1.45		0.80	0.42–1.50	
Q4	21/555	0.75	0.41–1.35		0.76	0.42–1.37		0.94	0.51–1.73		0.94	0.51–1.74	
Snacks- drinks-milk products													
Q1	24/494	1		0.430	1		0.569	1		0.845	1		0.824
Q2	13/514	0.52	0.26–1.03		0.54	0.27–1.07		0.61	0.31–1.21		0.62	0.31–1.24	
Q3	27/550	1.01	0.58–1.77		1.07	0.61–1.89		1.28	0.71–2.29		1.28	0.71–2.31	
Q4	17/572	0.61	0.33–1.15		0.65	0.34–1.24		0.84	0.43–1.65		0.85	0.43–1.68	
Meat-fish													
Q1	23/530	1		0.880	1		0.822	1		0.935	1		0.957
Q2	17/530	0.74	0.39–1.40		0.74	0.39–1.41		0.78	0.41–1.49		0.79	0.41–1.50	
Q3	16/533	0.69	0.36–1.32		0.71	0.37–1.36		0.74	0.38–1.44		0.75	0.39–1.45	
Q4	25/537	1.07	0.60–1.91		1.09	0.61–1.97		1.05	0.57–1.92		1.04	0.56–1.90	

[1]Test for trend was examined by entering dietary pattern score quartiles as a fixed factor and testing the contrast by using the polynomial option in all models.
[2]Model 1: adjusted for age, sex and daily energy intake at baseline.
[3]Model 2: further adjusted for BMI, PASE, number of IADLs, smoking status, alcohol use, education and marital status at baseline.
[4]Model 3: further adjusted for self-reported history of diabetes mellitus, hypertension, heart disease and stroke, and CSI-D score at baseline.

may have limited the power of the longitudinal analysis. Although we found significant associations between "vegetables-fruits" and "snacks-drinks-milk products" patterns and depressive symptoms in the cross-sectional analysis, the directionality of the associations was uncertain. The possibility of reverse causation may not be ruled out. People with major depression may change their eating behavior and food choices, either adopting an unhealthy diet (i.e. high-calorie foods) or reducing food intake [47,52], thus interpreting the relationship between diet and depression may be difficult in view of the bidirectional changes in diet as a consequence of mental health symptoms. We tried to conduct a sensitivity analysis excluding participants with extreme GDS (i.e. GDS≥11 (n = 56)) and the significant association between dietary patterns and depressive symptoms remained at baseline. These results possibly suggest that reverse causation seems an unlikely explanation for the significant findings in our cross-sectional analysis. Furthermore, we did not have dietary data at the 4-year follow-up whereas dietary patterns may have changed between baseline and follow-up. Moreover, although we controlled for various common factors and major chronic conditions in the analysis, residual potential confounding from some other factors related to the development of depression, such as family history of depression and recent life stress events might still be present. In addition, our sample as a whole was of a higher educational standard compared with the general Hong Kong population, and there were some differences in the baseline characteristics between those who included and those who excluded in the analysis, and between those who completed and those who discontinued the 4-year follow-up. Therefore, the results may not be generalized to the general population.

In conclusion, our cross-sectional analysis suggested significant associations between 'vegetables-fruits' dietary pattern and 'snacks-drinks-milk products' dietary pattern and the presence of depressive symptoms in the community-dwelling Chinese older people in Hong Kong. However, the longitudinal analyses did not support that dietary patterns are predictive of the occurrence of depressive symptoms.

Acknowledgments

We would like to give thanks for Ms Kay Yuen for coordination of this study.

Author Contributions

Conceived and designed the experiments: RC JW. Analyzed the data: RC DC JW. Contributed to the writing of the manuscript: RC DC JW

References

1. World Health Organization (2008) Global Burden of Disease: 2004 Update. Geneva: World Health Organization.
2. Hasin DS, Goodwin RD, Stinson FS, Grant BF (2005) Epidemiology of major depressive disorder: results from the National Epidemiologic Survey on Alcoholism and Related Conditions. Arch Gen Psychiatry 62: 1097–1106.
3. Blazer DG (2003) Depression in late life: review and commentary. J Gerontol A Biol Sci Med Sci 58: 249–265.
4. Fiske A, Wetherell JL, Gatz M (2009) Depression in older adults. Annu Rev Clin Psychol 5: 363–389.
5. Collins PY, Patel V, Joestl SS, March D, Insel TR, et al. (2011) Grand challenges in global mental health. Nature 475: 27–30.
6. Rogers PJ (2001) A healthy body, a healthy mind: long-term impact of diet on mood and cognitive function. Proc Nutr Soc 60: 135 143.
7. Stanger O, Fowler B, Piertzik K, Huemer M, Haschke-Becher E, et al. (2009) Homocysteine, folate and vitamin B12 in neuropsychiatric diseases: review and treatment recommendations. Expert Rev Neurother 9: 1393–1412.
8. Murakami K, Sasaki S (2010) Dietary intake and depressive symptoms: a systematic review of observational studies. Mol Nutr Food Res 54: 471–488.
9. Hu FB (2002) Dietary pattern analysis: a new direction in nutritional epidemiology. Curr Opin Lipidol 13: 3–9.
10. van Dam RM (2005) New approaches to the study of dietary patterns. Br J Nutr 93: 573–574.
11. Jacka FN, Pasco JA, Mykletun A, Williams LJ, Hodge AM, et al. (2010) Association of Western and traditional diets with depression and anxiety in women. Am J Psychiatry 167: 305–311.
12. Samieri C, Jutand MA, Feart C, Capuron L, Letenneur L, et al. (2008) Dietary patterns derived by hybrid clustering method in older people: association with cognition, mood, and self-rated health. J Am Diet Assoc 108: 1461–1471.
13. Crichton GE, Bryan J, Hodgson JM, Murphy KJ (2013) Mediterranean diet adherence and self-reported psychological functioning in an Australian sample. Appetite 70: 53–59.
14. Nanri A, Kimura Y, Matsushita Y, Ohta M, Sato M, et al. (2010) Dietary patterns and depressive symptoms among Japanese men and women. Eur J Clin Nutr 64: 832–839.
15. Sugawara N, Yasui-Furukori N, Tsuchimine S, Kaneda A, Tsuruga K, et al. (2012) No association between dietary patterns and depressive symptoms among a community-dwelling population in Japan. Ann Gen Psychiatry 11: 24 doi: 10.1186/1744-859X-11-24.
16. Suzuki T, Miyaki K, Tsutsum A, Hashimoto H, Kawakami N, et al. (2013) Japanese dietary pattern consistently relates to low depressive symptoms and it is modified by job strain and worksite supports. J Affect Disord 150: 490–498.
17. Sa' nchez-Villegas A, Delgado-Rodr'guez M, Alonso A, Schlatter J, Lahortiga F, et al. (2009) Association of the Mediterranean Dietary Pattern With the Incidence of Depression The Seguimiento Universidad de Navarra/University of Navarra Follow-up (SUN) Cohort. Arch Gen Psychiatry 66: 1090–1098.
18. Akbaraly TN, Brunner EJ, Ferrie JE, Marmot MG, Kivimaki M, et al. (2009) Dietary pattern and depressive symptoms in middle age. Br J Psychiatry 195: 408–413.
19. Le Port A, Gueguen A, Kesse-Guyot E, Melchior M, Lemogne C, et al. (2012) Association between dietary patterns and depressive symptoms over time: a 10-year follow-up study of the GAZEL cohort. PLOS ONE 7: e51593.
20. Chocano-Bedoya PO, O'Reilly EJ, Lucas M, Mirzaei F, Okereke OI, et al. (2013) Prospective study on long-term dietary patterns and incident depression in middle-aged and older women. Am J Clin Nutr 98: 813–820.
21. Lucas M, Chocano-Bedoya P, Shulze MB, Mirzaei F, O'Reilly EJ, et al. (2013) Inflammatory dietary pattern and risk of depression among women. Brain Behav Immun 36: 46–53.
22. Rienks R, Dobson AJ, Mishra GD (2013) Mediterranean dietary pattern and prevalence and incidence of depressive symptoms in mid-aged women: results from a large community-based prospective study. Eur J Clin Nutr 67: 75–82.
23. Hodge A, Almeida OP, English DR, Giles GG, Flicker L (2013) Patterns of dietary intake and psychological distress in older Australians: benefits not just from a Mediterranean diet. Int Psychogeriatr 25: 456–466.
24. Jacka FN, Cherbuin N, Anstey KJ, Butterworth P (2014) Dietary Patterns and Depressive Symptoms over Time: Examining the Relationships with Socioeconomic Position, Health Behaviours and Cardiovascular Risk. PLOS ONE 9: e87657.
25. Ruusunen A, Lehto SM, Mursu J, Tolmunen T, Tuomainen TP, et al. (2014) Dietary patterns are associated with the prevalence of elevated depressive symptoms and the risk of getting a hospital discharge diagnosis of depression in middle-aged or older Finnish men. J Affect Disord 159: 1–6.
26. Jacka FN, Kremer PJ, Berk M, de Silva-Sanigorski AM, Moodie M, et al. (2011) A prospective study of diet quality and mental health in adolescents. PLOS ONE 6: e24805.
27. Weng TT, Hao JH, Qian QW, Cao H, Fu JL, et al. (2011) Is there any relationship between dietary patterns and depression and anxiety in Chinese adolescents? Public Health Nutr 15: 673–682.
28. Tsai AC, Chang TL, Chi SH (2012) Frequent consumption of vegetables predicts lower risk of depression in older Taiwanese - results of a prospective population-based study. Public Health Nutr 15: 1087–1092.
29. Woo J, Lynn H, Lau WY, Leung J, Lau E, et al. (2006) Nutrient intake and psychological health in an elderly Chinese population. Int J Geriatr Psychiatry 21: 1036–1043.
30. Wong SY, Kwok T, Woo J, Lynn H, Griffith JF, et al. (2005) Bone mineral density and the risk of peripheral arterial disease in men and women: results from Mr. and Ms Os, Hong Kong. Osteoporos Int 16: 1933–1938.
31. Census and Statistics Department (2006) Hong Kong 2006 Population Bycensus Thematic Report: Older Persons. Hong Kong: Census and Statistics Department.
32. Prince M, Acosta D, Chiu H, Scazufca M, Varghese M, et al. (2003) Dementia diagnosis in developing countries: a cross-cultural validation study. Lancet 361: 909–917.
33. Washburn RA, Smith KW, Jette AM, Janney CA (1993) The Physical Activity Scale for the Elderly (PASE): development and evaluation. J Clin Epidemiol 46: 153–162.
34. Liu B, Woo J, Tang N, Ng K, Ip R, et al. (2001) Assessment of total expenditure in a Chinese population by a physical activity questionnaire: examination of validity. Int J Food Sci Nutr 52: 269–282.

35. Yesavage JA, Brink TL, Rose TL, Lum O, Huang V, et al. (1983) Development and validation of a geriatric depression screening scale. A preliminary report. J Psychiatr Res 17: 37–49.
36. Lee HB, Chiu HFK, Kwok WY, Leung CM, Kwong PK, et al. (1993) Chinese elderly and the GDS short form: a preliminary study. Clin Gerontol 14: 37–39.
37. Woo J, Leung SSF, Ho SC, Lam TH, Janus ED (1997) A food frequency questionnaire for use in the Chinese population in Hong Kong: Description and examination of validity. Nutr Res 17: 1633–1641.
38. Paul AA, Southgate DAT (1978) McCance & Widdowson's: The Composition of Foods. London: HMSO.
39. Yang Y, Wang G, Pan X (2002) China Food Composition 2002; Institute of Nutrition & Food Safety CC, editor. Peking: University Medical Press.
40. Chan R, Chan D, Woo J (2012) Associations between dietary patterns and demographics, lifestyle, anthropometry and blood pressure in Chinese community-dwelling older men and women. J Nutr Sci 1: e20 doi:10.1017/jns.2012.19
41. Reedy J, Wirfalt E, Flood A, Mitrou PN, Krebs-Smith SM, et al. (2010) Comparing 3 dietary pattern methods–cluster analysis, factor analysis, and index analysis–With colorectal cancer risk: The NIH-AARP Diet and Health Study. Am J Epidemiol 171: 479–487.
42. Field A (2005) Discovering Statistics Using SPSS; Wright DB, editor. London: Sage Publications.
43. Roman MW, Callen BL (2008) Screening instruments for older adult depressive disorders: updating the evidence-based toolbox. Issues Ment Health Nurs 29: 929–941.
44. Bodnar LM, Wisner KL (2005) Nutrition and depression: implications for improving mental health among childbearing-aged women. Biol Psychiatry 58: 679–685.
45. Bottiglieri T (2005) Homocysteine and folate metabolism in depression. Prog Neuro-Psychopharmacol Biol Psychiatry 29: 1103–1112.
46. Fava M, Mischoulon D (2009) Folate in depression: efficacy, safety, differences in formulations, and clinical issues. J Clin Psychiatry 70 Suppl 5: 12–17.
47. Jeffery RW, Linde JA, Simon GE, Ludman EJ, Rohde P, et al. (2009) Reported food choices in older women in relation to body mass index and depressive symptoms. Appetite 52: 238–240.
48. Crawford GB, Khedkar A, Flaws JA, Sorkin JD, Gallicchio L (2011) Depressive symptoms and self-reported fast-food intake in midlife women. Prev Med 52: 254–257.
49. Camfield DA, Owen L, Scholey AB, Pipingas A, Stough C (2011) Dairy constituents and neurocognitive health in ageing. Br J Nutr 106: 159–174.
50. Quirk SE, Williams;L.J.;, O'Neil A, Pasco JA, Jacka FN, et al. (2013) The association between diet quality, dietary patterns and depression in adults: a systematic review. BMC Psychiatry 175.
51. Sánchez-Villegas A, Martínez-González MA, Estruch R, Salas-Salvadó J, Corella D, et al. (2013) Mediterranean dietary pattern and depression: the PREDIMED randomized trial. BMC Medicine 11.
52. Lai JS, Hiles S, Bisquera A, Hure AJ, McEvoy M, et al. (2014) A systematic review and meta-analysis of dietary patterns and depression in community-dwelling adults. Am J Clin Nutr 99: 181–197.

24

Efficacy and Safety of Intravesical OnabotulinumtoxinA Injection on Elderly Patients with Chronic Central Nervous System Lesions and Overactive Bladder

Yuan-Hong Jiang[1], Chun-Hou Liao[2], Dong-Ling Tang[1], Hann-Chorng Kuo[1]*

1 Department of Urology, Buddhist Tzu Chi General Hospital and Tzu Chi University, Hualien, Taiwan, **2** Department of Urology, Cardinal Tien Hospital and School of Medicine, Fu-Jen Catholic University, New Taipei, Taiwan

Abstract

Purpose: Intravesical injection of onabotulinumtoxinA is an effective treatment for overactive bladder (OAB). Nonetheless, the treatment outcome is unclear in OAB patients with central nervous system (CNS) lesions. This study evaluated the efficacy and safety of intravesical onabotulinumtoxinA treatment in elderly patients with chronic cerebrovascular accidents (CVAs), Parkinson's disease (PD) and dementia.

Materials and Methods: Patients with CVA, PD, dementia, and OAB refractory to antimuscarinic therapy were consecutively enrolled in the study group. Age-matched OAB patients without CNS lesions were selected to serve as a control group. OnabotulinumtoxinA (100 U) was injected into the bladder suburothelium at 20 sites. The clinical effects, adverse events, and urodynamic parameters were assessed at baseline and 3 months post-treatment. The Kaplan-Meier method was used to compare long-term success rates between groups.

Results: A total of 40 patients with OAB due to CVA (23), PD (9), dementia (8) and 160 control patients were included in this retrospetive analysis. Improvement of urgency severity scale, increased bladder capacity and increased post-void residual volume were comparable between the groups at 3 months. Patients with CNS lesions did not experience increased risks of acute urinary retention and urinary tract infection; nonetheless, patients with CVA experienced a higher rate of straining to void. Long-term success rates did not differ between the patients with and without CNS lesions.

Conclusion: Intravesical injection of 100 U of onabotulinumtoxinA effectively decreased urgency symptoms in elderly OAB patients with CNS lesions. The adverse events were acceptable, and long-term effects were comparable to OAB patients in general. Nonetheless, the possibility of longstanding urinary retention and chronic catheterization need careful evaluation for this very vulnerable population before choosing intravesical onabotulinumtoxinA treatment.

Editor: Neal Shore, Carolina Urologic Research Center, United States of America

Funding: The authors have no support or funding to report.

Competing Interests: The authors have declared that no competing interests exist.

* Email: hck@tzuchi.com.tw

Introduction

OAB is highly prevalent in elderly patients and involves both peripheral and CNS factors [1]. The incidence of OAB increases with age, especially in patients with CNS disorders such as CVA and PD. White matter disease causing dementia increases significantly with age and can also cause OAB and urinary incontinence [2]. The reported incidence of urinary incontinence varied from 33% to 79% in patients with CVA [3], 33.1% with PD, and 50.9% with multiple sclerosis [4]. Most of the patients with CNS disorders and OAB had NDO.

The incidence of OAB increases with aging; thus, degeneration of the CNS in the elderly is proposed as one of the pathogenic factors of OAB [1]. In patients older than 60 years with irritative urinary symptoms, brain magnetic resonance imaging showed subclinical high-intensity ischemic changes in basal ganglia in 82.6% of elderly OAB patients. Thus, aging and CNS lesions play key roles in the pathogenesis of OAB among elderly patients [5]. Both storage and voiding symptoms occur in patients with CNS disorders, resulting in a complex combination of complaints [6]. The HR-QoL in patients with CNS lesions and OAB is worse than in patients with OAB in general [7].

Antimuscarinic agents are the predominant pharmacological treatment for patients with OAB [8]. Although antimuscarinic treatment has a high success rate, cognitive dysfunction during treatment with nonselective antimuscarinic agents for OAB is of growing concern [9]. In the recent decade, intravesical injection of BoNT-A emerged as an effective treatment for OAB among patients refractory or intolerable to antimuscarinic agents [10]. BoNT-A significantly improves OAB symptoms and urodynamic parameters in NDO and OAB. However, increased PVR volume and risk of UTI after BoNT-A treatment remain concerns among frail elderly patients [11].

Although intravesical BoNT-A injections for patients with NDO due to spinal cord injury or idiopathic OAB have been extensively investigated, data on BoNT-A treatment for patients with CNS lesion such as CVA, PD, and dementia are rare. Because CNS lesions usually occur in elderly patients and their bladder symptoms are more complicated to manage than those caused by OAB in general, intravesical BoNT-A treatment might not be as effective and safe as in other OAB patients. This study evaluated the efficacy and safety of intravesical onabotulinumtoxinA (100 U) treatment on patients with chronic CNS lesions and OAB due to CVA, PD, or dementia.

Methods

This study encompassed a retrospective analysis of therapeutic effects and adverse events in elderly patients with CNS lesions and OAB. Because this was a retrospective study, we could not enroll patients based on a power calculation. Patients with chronic CVA, PD, dementia, and OAB refractory to antimuscarinic therapy were consecutively enrolled in the study group from 2005 through 2012. These studies have been approved by the institutional review board of the Buddhist Tzu Chi General Hospital, No: 094-08, 095-73 and 095-10. Written informed consent was given by participants for their clinical records to be used in this study.

The patients with CNS lesion were diagnosed by neurologists and regularly treated at the hospital's neurology department. OAB patients without CNS lesions treated during the same period were selected as a control group. The OAB patients included in the study were older than 60 years of age and were selected from previous clinical trials at the hospital [12–15]. The institutional review board and ethics committee of the hospital approved the studies. All patients were informed about possible adverse events related to onabotulinumtoxinA injection and gave written, informed consent before treatment.

The inclusion criteria were OAB symptoms with or without urinary incontinence refractory to previous behavioral modification and antimuscarinic therapy for more than 3 months. Patients with CVA, PD, and dementia had to be ambulatory, able to communicate, and record a voiding diary. Exclusion criteria were inability to ambulate (bed-ridden or completely wheel chair bound), acute or chronic urinary tract infection, presence of bladder outlet obstruction, abnormal liver function, elevated serum creatinine, and PVR volume >150 ml at enrollment.

Patients received suburothelial injections of onabotulinumtoxinA (Allergan, Irvine, CA, USA) at 20 sites using a 23-gauge needle in a rigid cystoscopic injection instrument (22 Fr, Richard-Wolf, Knittlingen, Germany). One hundred units of onabotulinumtoxinA were reconstituted to 10 ml with normal saline. The injection sites were equally distributed on the lateral and posterior bladder walls, and 0.5 ml (5 U) was injected into the suburothelial space at each site, sparing the trigone. During the injections, the

Table 1. Changes of Voiding Diary and Urodynamic Variables after OnabotulinumtoxinA Treatment in Overactive Bladder Patients with Central Nervous System Lesion and Control Patients.

		CNS lesion	Control	P values[#]
		(n = 40)	(n = 160)	
USS	Baseline	3.72±0.67	3.68±0.64	0.777
	3 months	2.83±1.30	2.70±1.17	
	P =	0.003	<0.0001	
Urgency	Baseline	45.1±24.7	56.8±28.7	0.623
per 3 days	3 months	34.4±25.7	40.5±28.3	
	P =	0.071	0.138	
UUI/3 days	Baseline	12.4±12.7	19.3±18.5	0.963
	3 months	4.25±9.80	10.7±15.5	
	P =	0.010	0.035	
Cystometric	Baseline	220±119	248±119	0.067
Bladder	3 months	347±165	309±147	
Capacity(ml)	P =	0.001	<0.0001	
Pdet.Qmax	Baseline	26.5±16.0	26.8±13.7	0.996
(cmH$_2$O)	3 months	22.1±12.6	22.3±12.6	
	P =	0.123	<0.0001	
Qmax (ml/s)	Baseline	9.95±4.54	13.1±7.56	0.067
	3 months	11.3±6.57	11.4±6.14	
	P =	0.353	0.019	
PVR (ml)	Baseline	47.9±46.0	41.4±66.4	0.214
	3 months	157±130	120±116	
	P =	<0.0001	<0.0001	

[#]Comparison of the changes of variables from baseline to 3 months within each group.
CNS: central nervous system, OAB: overactive bladder, USS: urgency severity score, UUI: urgency urinary incontinence, Qmax: maximum flow rate, Pdet.Qmax: detrusor pressure at Qmax, PVR: post-void residual.

Table 2. Changes of Voiding Diary and Urodynamic Variables after OnabotulinumtoxinA Treatment in Overactive Bladder Patients with Cerebrovascular Disease, Parkinson's Disease, Dementia and Patients without Central Nervous System Lesion.

		N=	Baseline	3 months	p values[#]
USS	CVA	23	3.57±0.79	3.00±1.29	0.103
	PD	9	3.71±0.76	2.43±1.27	0.022
	Dementia	8	4.00±0.00	3.25±1.50	0.391
	Control	160	3.68±2.70	2.70±1.17	<0.0001
Urgency	CVA	23	36.8±24.0	28.5±27.1	0.047
Per 3 days	PD	9	56.0±26.4	43.0±16.3	0.329
	Dementia	8	41.3±23.3	30.5±37.5	0.513
	Control	160	56.8±28.7	40.5±28.3	0.138
UUI/3 days	CVA	23	13.5±12.5	5.67±1.21	0.050
	PD	9	10.8±16.8	9.67±15.0	0.749
	Dementia	8	13.3±7.85	1.50±3.00	0.087
	Control	160	19.3±18.5	10.7±15.5	0.035
Cystometric	CVA	23	198±108	358±162	0.002
Bladder	PD	9	266±121	283±181	0.780
Capacity(ml)	Dementia	8	202±97.8	448±89.0	0.001
	Control	160	248±119	309±147	<0.0001
Pdet.Qmax	CVA	23	31.0±21.8	27.3±18.2	0.334
(cmH$_2$O)	PD	9	26.3±13.6	21.1±7.34	0.409
	Dementia	8	18.0±2.0	13.7±1.53	0.006
	Control	160	26.8±13.7	22.3±12.6	<0.0001
Qmax	CVA	23	9.04±4.567	12.2±6.47	0.106
(ml/s)	PD	9	12.1±4.81	11.6±7.83	0.872
	Dementia	8	8.75±2.50	7.33±2.01	0.109
	Control	160	13.1±7.56	11.4±6.4	0.019
PVR	CVA	23	56.5±53.7	169±131	0.002
(ml)	PD	9	36.7±32.4	114±109	0.048
	Dementia	8	37.2±35.6	194±165	0.125
	Control	160	56.5±53.7	120±116	<0.0001

[#]Comparison of the changes of variables from baseline to 3 months within each group. CVA: cerebrovascular accident, PD: Parkinson's disease, USS: urgency severity score, UUI: urgency urinary incontinence, Qmax: maximum flow rate, Pdet.Qmax: detrusor pressure at Qmax, PVR: Post-void residual.

bladder volume was kept at 100–150 ml and injection into blood vessels was avoided.

All procedures were performed under intravenous general anesthesia in the operating room. Anticoagulant therapy was discontinued 1 week before onabotulinumtoxinA injection. A 14-Fr Foley indwelling catheter was inserted overnight, and the patients were discharged the next morning. Broad-spectrum prophylactic antibiotics were given postoperatively for 3 days. Patients who developed acute urinary retention or PVR volumes greater than 250 ml were advised to perform clean intermittent catheterization (CIC) or clean intermittent self-catheterization (CISC) until the PVR decreased to less than 200 ml.

All patients were closely monitored every month after onabotulinumtoxinA injection until the response to onabotulinumtoxinA had disappeared. Urgency episodes and UUI were verified using a 3-day voiding diary. A validated USS questionnaire was used to grade the severity of urgency, which was linguistically translated from the validated Patients Perception of Intensity of Urgency Scale [16]. The USS graded urgency as 0, 1, 2, 3, or 4 corresponding to no feeling of urgency, mild, moderate, severe feeling of urgency, and inability to hold urine, respectively

[17]. After each visit, all patients graded the treatment outcome of onabotulinumtoxinA injection based on changes to the USS. An improvement in USS by ≧1 was considered successful treatment. Any adverse event considered possibly related to the onabotulinumtoxinA treatment was recorded. These events included acute urinary retention, hematuria, general weakness, large PVR, straining to void, and UTI during the follow-up period.

Patients routinely underwent VUDS at baseline for diagnosis of DO and detection of BOO and 3 months after treatment. The parameters included CBC, Qmax, Pdet.Qmax, and PVR volume. VUDS was performed and terminology was defined according to the standards of the International Continence Society [18].

Parametric, continuous data are expressed as means and standard deviations while categorical data are expressed as numbers and percentages. Mean values of continuous variables were compared using the Mann-Whitney U-test, whereas categorical variables were compared using the Fisher exact test. Kaplan-Meier survival plots were constructed to analyze the cumulative success rates with time among groups. A p value<0.05 was considered statistically significant.

Table 3. Success Rates and Adverse Events among Overactive Bladder Patients with Cerebrovascular Disease, Parkinson's Disease, Dementia, and Patients without Central Nervous System Lesion.

	Age (years)	AUR	PVR >150 ml	Straining to void	Hematuria	UTI	General weakness
CVA (n = 23)	73.6±7.5	4 (17.4%)	12 (52.2%)	17 (73.9%)	2 (8.7%)	1 (4.3%)	1 (4.3%)
PD (n = 9)	73.6±11.2	1 (11.1%)	3 (33.3%)	1 (11.3%)	1 (11.1%)	2 (22.2%)	1 (11.1%)
Dementia (n = 8)	76.2±9.7	0	1 (12.5%)	2 (25.0%)	0	0	0
Control (n = 160)	74.6±7.5	16 (10%)	63 (39.3%)	81 (50.6%)	16 (10%)	22 (13.8%)	6 (3.8%)
P values	0.864	0.682	0.224	0.021	0.886	0.247	0.464

CVA: cerebrovascular accident, PD: Parkinson's disease, AUR: acute urinary retention, PVR: post void residual, UTI: urinary tract infection.

Results

This retrospective study included 40 patients with OAB due to CNS lesions (23 with CVA, 9 with PD, 8 with dementia) and 160 OAB patients without CNS lesions. The mean age of the patients with and without CNS lesions was 74.6±7.5 and 74.0±9.3 years, respectively (p = 0.661). The mean age was comparable among the three subgroups with CNS lesions. The mean duration of CNS lesions from diagnosis was 4.3±3.1 years.

The voiding diary, USS, and urodynamic parameters at baseline did not differ significantly between the patient groups with and without CNS lesions (Table 1). Patients with and without CNS lesions experienced significant improvements of USS and UUI episodes per 3 days 3 months after onabotulinumtoxinA treatment. Urodynamic parameters also showed significant increases of CBC and PVR in both groups with and without CNS lesions. The Pdet.Qmax and Qmax did not change in patients with CNS lesions, and there was no significant difference between the groups.

Table 2 lists the changes of voiding diary variables and urodynamic parameters after onabotulinumtoxinA treatment for each CNS lesion group and control group. Patients with PD and patients in the control group experienced significant improvement of USS. Urgency and UUI episodes also improved among CVA and control patients. CBC significantly increased in CVA, dementia, and control patients. Compared with baseline, PVR volume increased significantly 3 months after therapy in patients with CVA, PD, and the control group; however, the PVR change did not significantly different from the control group (p = 0.214).

Table 3 shows the incidences of adverse events in the CVA, PD, dementia, and control groups after onabotulinumtoxinA treatment. The incidence of straining to void was significantly greater in CVA subgroup. The other adverse events such as acute urinary retention, large PVR, and UTI did not significantly differ among the groups with and without CNS lesions. No adverse CNS event related to onabotulinumtoxinA injection occurred.

During the follow-up period, the therapeutic duration of onabotulinumtoxinA was similar among all subgroups with CNS lesions and the control group (Table 4). Figure 1 shows the cumulative success rates after onabotulinumtoxinA treatment between OAB patients with and without CNS lesions and among control OAB patients and subgroup patients with CNS lesions. The results show that the long-term success did not differ between patients with and without CNS lesions or among CNS lesion subgroups (all p>0.05).

Discussion

The results showed that elderly patients with OAB due to CNS lesions such as CVA, PD, or dementia refractory to antimuscarinic therapy can be effectively treated with intravesical injection of 100 U onabotulinumtoxinA. The adverse events and incidences of acute urinary retention and UTI were comparable to OAB patients in general.

Among elderly people with CNS lesions, OAB is common. In a community health survey, 31% of patients with CNS disease reported OAB symptoms, and the overall prevalence of neurogenic OAB was 0.6%. Patients with neurogenic OAB have poorer HR-QoL compared to patients with general OAB.[7] Among neurogenic OAB patients, CVA, PD, and multiple sclerosis are frequently encountered and cause NDO and UUI [1]. The pathogenesis of OAB in cerebral events involves not only sensory perception but also the impairment of detrusor contractility. In addition, patients with CVA or PD have impaired detrusor contractility or detrusor underactivity resulting in increased PVR

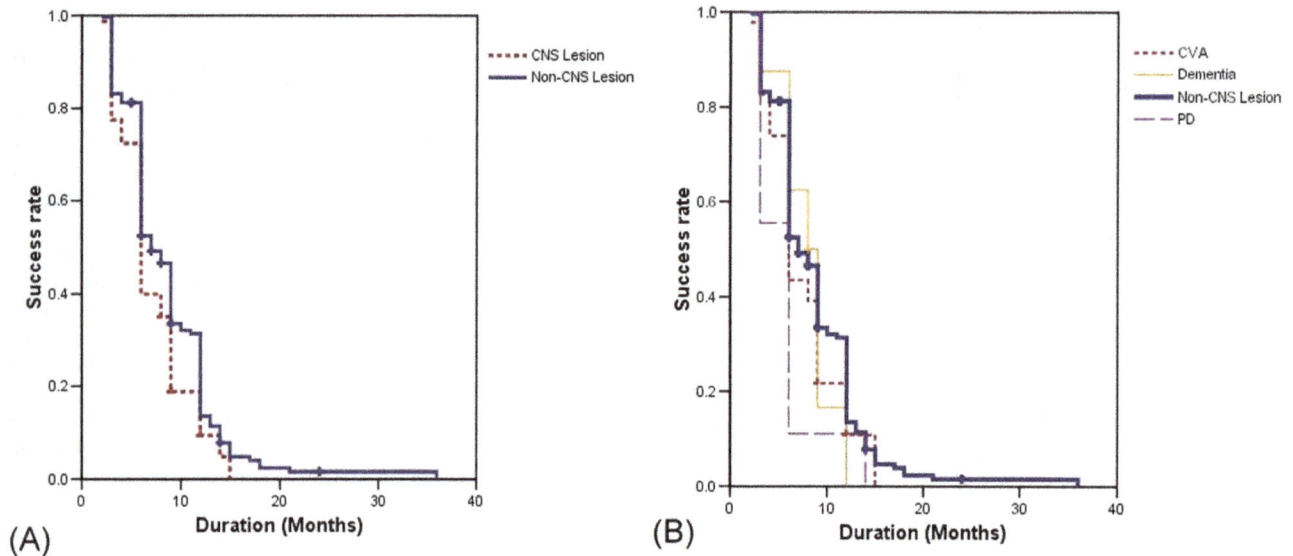

Figure 1. Kaplan-Meier survival curves for long-term success rates of patients with CNS lesions and the control group after intravesical onabotulinumtoxinA injection for OAB refractory to antimuscarinic therapy. (A) Success rates between OAB patients with and without CNS lesions. (B) Success rates among patients with different CNS lesions and the control group.

volumes [19,20]. Urethral sphincter dyssynergia, poor relaxation of the external urethral sphincter, and poor relaxation of the pelvic floor muscles are associated with DO in patients with CVA and PD [21]. Anticholinergic treatment of OAB among patients with CNS lesions could cause CNS adverse events and impaired bladder emptying.

Previous studies showed beneficial effects for 200-U onabotulinumtoxinA injections into the detrusor for patients with OAB due to PD and multiple system atrophy [22]. A recent study using 100 U onabotulinumtoxinA on patients with OAB due to PD showed similarly effective outcomes [23]. In addition, we previously reported suburothelial injections of 200 U onabotulinumtoxinA improved OAB symptoms and increased bladder volume in patients with CVA [24]. Nonetheless, PVR volume and voiding difficulty also increased after treatment. We found no clinical report of onabotulinumtoxinA effects among patients with dementia and OAB.

The pathogenesis of OAB and DO due to CNS lesions is not well known. Impaired sensory perception during bladder filling before reaching bladder capacity could play a key role in patients with OAB due to CNS lesions such as CVA, PD, and dementia.

Therefore, the guarding time for these patients to prevent urinary incontinence could be shorter than that for OAB patients in general. Intravesical onabotulinumtoxinA injections decrease detrusor contractility and also modulate afferent fibers in NDO [25]. A higher dose of onabotulinumtoxinA could impair detrusor contractility and sensory input too much, causing large PVR volumes, difficult urination, or overflow incontinence. Under these considerations, a small dose of BoNT-A such as 100 U of onabotulinumtoxinA could be an optimal dose for OAB due to CNS lesions.

Intravesical injection of 100 U of onabotulinumtoxinA effectively improved OAB symptoms and voiding diary and urodynamic parameters without increasing the risks of adverse events. The long-term therapeutic effects of onabotulinumtoxinA treatment of OAB patients with CNS lesions were similar to those of OAB patients in general. These results confirm that the intravesical injection of 100 U of onabotulinumtoxinA is an effective and safe treatment option for patients with OAB due to CVA, PD, and dementia. However, most of the patients with CNS lesions are vulnerable and usually cannot handle bladder management by themselves. The risk of UTI increases when

Table 4. The Long-term Therapeutic Duration of Overactive Bladder Patients with Cerebrovascular Disease, Parkinson's Disease, Dementia, and Patients without Central Nervous System Lesion.

Therapeutic duration				
	1–3 months	4–6 months	7–12 months	>12 months
CVA (n = 23)	4 (17.4%)	9 (39.1%)	9 (39.1%)	1 (4.3%)
PD (n = 9)	4 (44.4%)	4 (44.4%)	0	1 (11.1%)
Dementia (n = 8)	1 (12.5%)	2 (25.0%)	5 (62.5%)	0
Control (n = 160)	27 (16.9%)	53 (33.1%)	61 (38.1%)	19 (11.9%)
Total (n = 200)	3 (18.0%)	68 (34.0%)	75 (37.5%)	21 (10.5%)

CVA: cerebrovascular accident, PD: Parkinson's disease.

PVR increases after onabotulinumtoxinA injection, and the risk of CIC/CISC also increases [26,27]. The recovery duration from chronic urinary retention is also significantly increased in these frail elderly patients [11].

The patients enrolled in this study were patients with mild CVA, PD or dementia who were ambulatory, able to communicate, record a voiding diary and had PVR volume <150 ml. Patient selection in this vulnerable patient population is important because patients with CNS lesions and severe physical or mental impairment might have impaired bladder sensation after intravesical onabotulinumtoxinA injection and develop chronic urinary retention and recurrent UTI. When acute urinary retention or large PVR volume develops after onabotulinumtoxinA injection, a temporary indwelling Foley catheter is mandatory to prevent overdistention of the bladder. However, if patients wish to be completely dry and avoid an indwelling catheter, a care-giver should be instructed on CIC to empty the patient's bladder periodically. In patients who can accept and be instructed to perform CIC/CISC before onabotulinumtoxinA injection, the QoL and patient satisfaction are not affected by the need for CIC [28]. Nevertheless, the complications of UTI, possibility of chronic urinary retention, and its potential impact on health cost and burden on the caregiver still should be thoroughly discussed with patients' families for decision making [29]. All OAB patients with CVA, PD, or dementia should be informed of the possible adverse events and bladder management strategies before institution of onabotulinumtoxinA treatment.

The main limitations of the study were the small number of patients with CNS lesions and the lack of a randomized control group for comparison. In addition, only patients with mild physical impairment were studied, which limits the application of the results to all patients with CNS lesions and OAB. Nevertheless, because intravesical onabotulinumtoxinA injection ameliorated OAB symptoms without adverse CNS events due to anticholinergic effects, we recommend it as an alternative treatment for patients with refractory OAB due to CNS lesions.

Conclusion

The results confirmed that intravesical onabotulinumtoxinA 100 U injection effectively decreased urgency symptoms in patients with CVA, PD or dementia. The patients selected in this study had mild CNS lesions; adverse events were acceptable, and long-term effects were comparable to OAB patients in general. Nonetheless, the possibility of longstanding urinary retention and chronic catheterization need careful evaluation for this very vulnerable population before choosing intravesical onabotulinumtoxinA treatment.

Acknowledgments

This study was approved by the Research Ethics Committee of the hospital, TCGH IRB 094-08, 095-73 and 095-10.

Author Contributions

Conceived and designed the experiments: HCK. Performed the experiments: YHJ CHL DLT HCK. Analyzed the data: CHL DLT HCK. Contributed reagents/materials/analysis tools: HCK. Contributed to the writing of the manuscript: YHJ CHL HCK.

References

1. Andersson KE (2004) Mechanisms of disease: central nervous system involvement in overactive bladder syndrome. Nat Clin Pract Urol 1: 103–108.
2. Sakakibara R, Panicker J, Fowler CJ, Tateno F, Kishi M, et al. (2014) Is overactive bladder a brain disease? The pathophysiological role of cerebral white matter in the elderly. Int J Urol 21: 33–38.
3. McKenzie P, Badlani GH (2012) the incidence and etiology of overactive bladder in patients after cerebrovascular accident. Curr Urol Rep 13: 402–406.
4. Ruffion A, Castro-Diaz D, Patel H, Khalaf K, Onyenwenyi A, et al. (2013) Systematic review of the epidemiology of urinary incontinence and detrusor overactivity among patients with neurogenic overactive bladder. Neuroepidemiology 41: 146–155.
5. Kitada S, Ikei Y, Hasui Y, Nishi S, Yamaguchi T, et al. (1992) Bladder function in elderly men with subclinical brain magnetic resonance imaging lesions. J Urol 147: 1507–1509.
6. Winge K, Fowler CJ (2006) Bladder dysfunction in Parkinsonism: mechanisms, prevalence, symptoms, and management. Mov Disord 21: 737–745.
7. Tapia CI, Khalaf K, Berenson K, Globe D, Chancellor M, et al. (2013) Health-related quality of life and economic impact of urinary incontinence due to detrusor overactivity associated with a neurologic condition: a systematic review. Health Qual Life Outcomes 2013 Jan 31; 11: 13. doi:10.1186/1477-7525-11-13.
8. Gormley EA, Lightner DJ, Burgio KL, Chai TC, Clemens JQ, et al. (2012) Diagnosis and treatment of overactive bladder (non-neurogenic) in adults: AUA/SUFU guideline. J Urol 188: 2455–2463.
9. Kay GG, Abou-Donia MB, Messer WS Jr, Murphy DG, Tsao JW, et al. (2005) Antimuscarinic drugs for overactive bladder and their potential effects on cognitive function in older patients. J Am Geriatr Soc 53: 2195–2201.
10. Chapple C, Sievert KD, MacDiarmid S, Khullar V, Radziszewski P, et al. (2013) OnabotulinumtoxinA 100 U significantly improves all idiopathic overactive bladder symptoms and quality of life in patients with overactive bladder and urinary incontinence: a randomised, double-blind, placebo-controlled trial. Eur Urol 64: 249–256.
11. Liao CH, Kuo HC (2013) Increased risk of large post-void residual urine and decreased long-term success rate after intravesical onabotulinumtoxinA injection for refractory idiopathic detrusor overactivity. J Urol 189: 1804–1810.
12. Liu HT, Chancellor MB, Kuo HC (2009) Urinary nerve growth factor levels are elevated in patients with detrusor overactivity and decreased in responders to detrusor botulinum toxin-A injection. Eur Urol 56: 700–706.
13. Kuo HC (2006) Will suburothelial injection of small dose of botulinum A toxin have similar therapeutic effects and less adverse events for refractory detrusor overactivity? Urology 68: 993–997.
14. Kuo HC (2007) Comparison of effectiveness of detrusor, suburothelial and bladder base injections of botulinum toxin a for idiopathic detrusor overactivity. J Urol 178: 1359–1363.
15. Kuo HC (2011) Bladder base/trigone injection is safe and as effective as bladder body injection of onabotulinumtoxinA for idiopathic detrusor overactivity refractory to antimuscarinics. Neurourol Urodyn 30: 1242–1248.
16. Cartwright R, Srikrishna S, Cardozo L, Robinson D (2011) Validity and reliability of the patient's perception of intensity of urgency scale in overactive bladder. BJU Int 107: 1612–1617.
17. Ke QS, Kuo HC (2010) Strong correlation between the overactive bladder symptom score and urgency severity score in assessment of patients with overactive bladder syndrome. Tzu Chi Med J 22: 82–86.
18. Haylen BT, de Ridder D, Freeman RM, Swift SE, Berghmans B, et al. (2010) An International Urogynecological Association (IUGA)/International Continence Society (ICS) joint report on the terminology for female pelvic floor dysfunction. Neurourol Urodynam 29: 4–20.
19. Natsume O (2008) Detrusor contractility and overactive bladder in patients with cerebrovascular accident. Int J Urol 15: 505–510.
20. Terayama K, Sakakibara R, Ogawa A, Haruta H, Akiba T, et al. (2012) Weak detrusor contractility correlates with motor disorders in Parkinson's disease. Mov Disord 27: 1775–1780.
21. Meng NH, Lo SF, Chou LW, Yang PY, Chang CH, et al. (2010) Incomplete bladder emptying in patients with stroke: is detrusor external sphincter dyssynergia a potential cause? Arch Phys Med Rehabil 91: 1105–1109.
22. Giannantoni A, Rossi A, Mearini E, Del Zingaro M, Porena M, et al. (2009) Botulinum toxin A for overactive bladder and detrusor muscle overactivity in patients with Parkinson's disease and multiple system atrophy. J Urol 182: 1453–1457.
23. Anderson RU, Orenberg EK, Glowe P (2014) OnabotulinumtoxinA Office Treatment for Neurogenic Bladder Incontinence in Parkinson's Disease. Urology 83: 22–27.
24. Kuo HC (2006) Therapeutic effects of suburothelial injection of botulinum a toxin for neurogenic detrusor overactivity due to chronic cerebrovascular accident and spinal cord lesions. Urology 67: 232–236.
25. Conte A, Giannantoni A, Proietti S, Giovannozzi S, Fabbrini G, et al. (2012) Botulinum toxin A modulates afferent fibers in neurogenic detrusor overactivity. Eur J Neurol 19: 725–732.
26. Dmochowski R, Chapple C, Nitti VW, Chancellor M, Everaert K, et al. (2010) Efficacy and safety of onabotulinumtoxinA for idiopathic overactive bladder: a double-blind, placebo controlled, randomized, dose ranging trial. J Urol 184: 2416–2422.

27. Mangera A, Apostolidis A, Andersson KE, Dasgupta P, Giannantoni A, et al. (2014) An updated systematic review and statistical comparison of standardised mean outcomes for the use of botulinum toxin in the management of lower urinary tract disorders. Eur Urol 65: 981–990.

28. Schurch B, Carda S (2014) OnabotulinumtoxinA and multiple sclerosis. Ann Phys Rehabil Med. 2014 Jun 5. pii: S1877-0657(14)01723-0. doi:10.1016/j.rehab.2014.05.004. [Epub ahead of print].

29. Apostolidis A, Dasgupta P, Denys P, Elneil S, Fowler CJ, et al. (2009) Recommendations on the use of botulinum toxin in the treatment of lower urinary tract disorders and pelvic floor dysfunctions: a European consensus report. Eur Urol 55: 100–119.

Permissions

The contributors of this book come from diverse backgrounds, making this book a truly international effort. This book will bring forth new frontiers with its revolutionizing research information and detailed analysis of the nascent developments around the world.

We would like to thank all the contributing authors for lending their expertise to make the book truly unique. They have played a crucial role in the development of this book. Without their invaluable contributions this book wouldn't have been possible. They have made vital efforts to compile up to date information on the varied aspects of this subject to make this book a valuable addition to the collection of many professionals and students.

This book was conceptualized with the vision of imparting up-to-date information and advanced data in this field. To ensure the same, a matchless editorial board was set up. Every individual on the board went through rigorous rounds of assessment to prove their worth. After which they invested a large part of their time researching and compiling the most relevant data for our readers.

The editorial board has been involved in producing this book since its inception. They have spent rigorous hours researching and exploring the diverse topics which have resulted in the successful publishing of this book. They have passed on their knowledge of decades through this book. To expedite this challenging task, the publisher supported the team at every step. A small team of assistant editors was also appointed to further simplify the editing procedure and attain best results for the readers.

Apart from the editorial board, the designing team has also invested a significant amount of their time in understanding the subject and creating the most relevant covers. They scrutinized every image to scout for the most suitable representation of the subject and create an appropriate cover for the book.

The publishing team has been an ardent support to the editorial, designing and production team. Their endless efforts to recruit the best for this project, has resulted in the accomplishment of this book. They are a veteran in the field of academics and their pool of knowledge is as vast as their experience in printing. Their expertise and guidance has proved useful at every step. Their uncompromising quality standards have made this book an exceptional effort. Their encouragement from time to time has been an inspiration for everyone.

The publisher and the editorial board hope that this book will prove to be a valuable piece of knowledge for researchers, students, practitioners and scholars across the globe.

List of Contributors

Holger Schulz
Institute of Epidemiology I, Helmholtz Zentrum München, German Research Center for Environmental Health, Neuherberg, Germany

Sandra Ortlieb
Institute of Epidemiology I, Helmholtz Zentrum München, German Research Center for Environmental Health, Neuherberg, Germany
Institute of Medical Statistics and Epidemiology, Technische Universita"t Mu"nchen, Munich, Germany

Lukas Gorzelniak and Klaus A. Kuhn
Institute of Medical Statistics and Epidemiology, Technische Universität München, Munich, Germany

Dennis Nowak
Institute and Outpatient Clinic for Occupational, Social and Environmental Medicine, Ludwig Maximilians-Universität, Munich, Germany
Comprehensive Pneumology Center Munich (CPC-M), Member of the German Center for Lung Research, Munich, Germany

Ralf Strobl and Eva Grill
Institute for Medical Information Processing, Biometrics and Epidemiology, Ludwig-Maximilians-Universität München, Munich, Germany
German Center for Vertigo and Balance Disorders, Ludwig-Maximilians-Universität München, Munich, Germany

Barbara Thorand and Annette Peters
Institute of Epidemiology II, Helmholtz Zentrum München, German Research Center for Environmental Health, Neuherberg, Germany

Stefan Karrasch
Institute of Epidemiology I, Helmholtz Zentrum München, German Research Center for Environmental Health, Neuherberg, Germany
Institute and Outpatient Clinic for Occupational, Social and Environmental Medicine, Ludwig Maximilians-Universität, Munich, Germany
Institute of General Practice, University Hospital Klinikum rechts der Isar, Technische Universität München, Munich, Germany

Alexander Horsch
Institute of Medical Statistics and Epidemiology, Technische Universität München, Munich, Germany
Department of Computer Science, University of Tromsø, Tromsø, Norway
Department of Clinical Medicine, University of Tromsø, Tromsø, Norway

Josef Yayan
Department of Internal Medicine, Division of Pulmonary, Allergy, and Sleep Medicine, Saarland University Medical Center, Homburg/Saar, Germany

Cyrille P. Launay and Anastasiia Kabeshova
Department of Neuroscience, Division of Geriatric Medicine, UPRES EA 4638, UNAM, Angers University Hospital, Angers, France

Laure de Decker
Department of Geriatrics, EA 1156–12, Nantes University Hospital, Nantes, France

Cédric Annweiler
Department of Neuroscience, Division of Geriatric Medicine, UPRES EA 4638, UNAM, Angers University Hospital, Angers, France
Robarts Research Institute, Schulich School of Medicine and Dentistry, the University of Western Ontario, London, Ontario, Canada

Olivier Beauchet
Department of Neuroscience, Division of Geriatric Medicine, UPRES EA 4638, UNAM, Angers University
Hospital, Angers, France
Biomathics, Paris, France

Pei-Ying Wu, Shan-Ping Yang, Yu-Zhen Luo and Jun-Yu Zhang
Center of Infection Control, National Taiwan University Hospital, Taipei, Taiwan

Mao-Yuan Chen, Szu-Min Hsieh, Hsin-Yun Sun and Wen-Chun Liu
Department of Internal Medicine, National Taiwan University Hospital and National Taiwan University College of Medicine, Taipei, Taiwan

Mao-Song Tsai
Department of Internal Medicine, Far Eastern Memorial Hospital, New Taipei City, Taiwan

Kuan-Yeh Lee
Department of Internal Medicine, National Taiwan University Hospital Hsin-Chu Branch, Hsin-Chu, Taiwan

Wang-Huei Sheng
Center of Infection Control, National Taiwan University Hospital, Taipei, Taiwan
Department of Internal Medicine, National Taiwan University Hospital and National
Taiwan University College of Medicine, Taipei, Taiwan

Chien-Ching Hung
Department of Internal Medicine, National Taiwan University Hospital and National
Taiwan University College of Medicine, Taipei, Taiwan
Department of Medical Research, China Medical University Hospital, Taichung, Taiwan
China Medical University, Taichung, Taiwan

Daniele Volpe and Maria Giulia Giantin
Department of Physical Medicine & Rehabilitation, S. Raffaele Arcangelo Fatebenefratelli Hospital, Venice, Italy

Alfonso Fasano
Morton and Gloria Shulman Movement Disorders Clinic and the Edmond J. Safra Program in Parkinson's Disease, Toronto Western Hospital and Division of Neurology, University of Toronto, Toronto, Ontario, Canada

L. Eduardo CofréLizama, Mirjam Pijnappels, Gert H. Faber and Jaap H. van Dieën
MOVE Research Institute Amsterdam, Faculty of Human Movement Sciences, VU University Amsterdam, Amsterdam, The Netherlands

Peter N. Reeves
College of Osteopathic Medicine, Michigan State University, East Lansing, Michigan, United States of America

Sabine M. Verschueren
Department of Rehabilitation Sciences, Faculty of Kinesiology and Rehabilitation Sciences, Katholieke Universiteit Leuven, Leuven, Belgium

Makoto Yamaguchi, Shinichi Akiyama, Sawako Kato, Takayuki Katsuno, Tomoki Kosugi, Waichi Sato, Naotake Tsuboi, Yoshinari Yasuda, Masashi Mizuno, Yasuhiko Ito, Seiichi Matsuo and Shoichi Maruyama
Department of Nephrology, Nagoya University Graduate School of Medicine, Nagoya, Japan

Masahiko Ando
Center for Advanced Medicine and Clinical Research, Nagoya University Hospital, Nagoya, Japan

Ryohei Yamamoto
Department of Geriatric Medicine and Nephrology, Osaka University Graduate School of Medicine, Suita, Japan

Antonio Nouvenne, Andrea Ticinesi, Erminia Ridolo, Loris Borghi and Tiziana Meschi
Internal Medicine and Critical Subacute Care Unit, Parma University Hospital, Parma, Italy
Department of Clinical and Experimental Medicine, University of Parma, Parma, Italy

Fulvio Lauretani
Geriatrics Unit, Parma University Hospital, Parma, Italy

Marcello Maggio
Department of Clinical and Experimental Medicine, University of Parma, Parma, Italy

Giuseppe Lippi
Laboratory of Clinical Chemistry and Hematology, Parma University Hospital, Parma, Italy

Loredana Guida and Ilaria Morelli
Internal Medicine and Critical Subacute Care Unit, Parma University Hospital, Parma, Italy

Melissa C. Kilby
Department of Kinesiology, The Pennsylvania State University, University Park, Pennsylvania, United States of America

Semyon M. Slobounov and Karl M. Newel
Department of Kinesiology, The Pennsylvania State University, University Park, Pennsylvania, United States of America
Center for Sport Concussion Research and Services, The Pennsylvania State University, University Park, Pennsylvania, United States of America

Achille E. Tchalla
Harvard Medical School, Boston, Massachusetts, United States of America
Division of Gerontology, Beth Israel Deaconess Medical Center, Boston, Massachusetts, United States of America
Institute for Aging Research, Hebrew SeniorLife, Boston, Massachusetts, United States of America
Department of Geriatric Medicine, University Hospital Center of Limoges, University of Limoges; EA 6310 HAVAE (Disability, Activity, Aging, Autonomy and Environment), Limoges, France

Alyssa B. Dufour, Thomas G. Travison, Brad Manor and Lewis A. Lipsitz
Harvard Medical School, Boston, Massachusetts, United States of America
Division of Gerontology, Beth Israel Deaconess Medical Center, Boston, Massachusetts, United States of America
Institute for Aging Research, Hebrew SeniorLife, Boston, Massachusetts, United States of America

Ikechukwu Iloputaife and Daniel Habtemariam
Institute for Aging Research, Hebrew SeniorLife, Boston, Massachusetts, United States of America

Michaela Dewar
Department of Psychology, School of Life Sciences, Heriot-Watt University, Edinburgh, United Kingdom Human Cognitive Neuroscience, Department of Psychology University of Edinburgh, United Kingdom
Centre for Cognitive Ageing and Cognitive Epidemiology, Psychology, University of Edinburgh, Edinburgh, United Kingdom

Jessica Alber
Human Cognitive Neuroscience, Department of Psychology, University of Edinburgh, United Kingdom

Nelson Cowan
Human Cognitive Neuroscience, Department of Psychology, University of Edinburgh, United Kingdom
Department of Psychology, University of Missouri, Columbia, Missouri, United States of America

Sergio Della Sala
Human Cognitive Neuroscience, Department of Psychology, University of Edinburgh, United Kingdom

Centre for Cognitive Ageing and Cognitive Epidemiology, Psychology, University of Edinburgh, Edinburgh, United Kingdom

Peng Zhang, Mian Xi, Lei Zhao, Qiao-Qiao Li, Li-Ru He, Shi-Liang Liu and Meng- Zhong Liu
Sun Yat-sen University Cancer Center, State Key Laboratory of Oncology in South China, Collaborative Innovation Center for Cancer Medicine, Department of Radiation Oncology, Cancer Center, Sun Yat-sen University, Guangzhou, People's Republic of China

Jing-Xian Shen
Sun Yat-sen University Cancer Center, State Key Laboratory of Oncology in South China, Collaborative Innovation Center for Cancer Medicine, Imaging Diagnosis and Interventional Center, Cancer Center, Sun Yat-sen University, Guangzhou, People's Republic of China

Aarón Salinas-Rodríguez, Betty Manrique-Espinoza,Karla Moreno-Tamayo and Martha María Téllez-Rojo Solís
Center for Evaluation Research and Surveys, National Institute of Public Health, Cuernavaca, Mexico

Ma. Del Pilar Torres-Pereda
Center for Health Systems Research, National Institute of Public Health, Cuernavaca, Mexico

Britta Müller and Peter Kropp
Institute of Medical Psychology and Medical Sociology, Medical Faculty, University of Rostock, Rostock, Germany

Christoph A. Nienaber
Medical Center Rostock, Department of Cardiology and Angiology, Rostock University Hospital, University of Rostock, Rostock, Germany

Olaf Reis
Clinic for Child and Adolescent Psychiatry, Rostock University Hospital, University of Rostock, Rostock, Germany

Wolfgang Meyer
Queen Mary University of London, Barts and the London School of Medicine and Dentistry, London, United Kingdom

Oliver Reich and Roland Rapold
Department of Health Sciences, Helsana Group, Zurich, Switzerland

Thomas Rosemann and Oliver Senn
Institute of General Practice and Health Services Research, University Hospital, Zurich, Switzerland

Eva Blozik
Department of Primary Medical Care, University Medical Center Hamburg-Eppendorf, Hamburg, Germany

Enrique Rey, Marta Barcelo, Angel Alvarez-Sanchez and Manuel Diaz-Rubio
Division of Digestive Diseases, Hospital Clinico San Carlos, Universidad Complutense, Instituto de Investigacion Sanitaria San Carlos (IdISSC), Madrid, Spain

Maria Jose Jiménez Cebrián
Centro Valdeluz, Madrid, Spain
Spanish Society of Nursing Homes Physicians (Sociedad Espan~ola de Medicos de Residencias – SEMER), Madrid, Spain

Alberto Lopez Rocha
Spanish Society of Nursing Homes Physicians (Sociedad Española de Medicos de Residencias – SEMER), Madrid, Spain

Marion J. Torres
Univ. Bordeaux, ISPED, Centre INSERM U897-Epidé´miologie-Biostatistique, F-33000, Bordeaux, France
INSERM, ISPED, Centre INSERM U897-Epidé´miologie- Biostatistique, F-33000, Bordeaux, France
Nutricia Advanced Medical Nutrition, Danone Research, Saint-Ouen, France

Béatrice Dorigny
Nutricia Advanced Medical Nutrition, Danone Research, Saint-Ouen, France

Mirjam Kuhn
Nutricia Research, Advanced Medical Nutrition, Utrecht, Netherlands

Claudine Berr
INSERM, U1061, Neuropsychiatrie: recherche épidémiologique et clinique, UniversitéMontpellier I, Hôpital La Colombiére, F-34093, Montpellier, France

Pascale Barberger-Gateau and Luc Letenneur
Univ. Bordeaux, ISPED, Centre INSERM U897-Epidémiologie-Biostatistique, F-33000, Bordeaux, France
INSERM, ISPED, Centre INSERM U897-Epidémiologie-Biostatistique, F-33000, Bordeaux, France

Chih-Kuang Liang and Yu-Te Lin
Center for Geriatrics and Gerontology, Kaohsiung Veterans General Hospital, Kaohsiung, Taiwan
Division of Neurology, Department of Medicine, Kaohsiung Veterans General Hospital Kaohsiung, Taiwan
Aging and Health Research Center, National Yang Ming University, Taipei, Taiwan

Chin-Liang Chu
Center for Geriatrics and Gerontology, Kaohsiung Veterans General Hospital, Kaohsiung, Taiwan
Aging and Health Research Center, National Yang Ming University, Taipei, Taiwan
Department of Psychiatry, Kaohsiung Veterans General Hospital, Kaohsiung, Taiwan

Ming-Yueh Chou
Center for Geriatrics and Gerontology, Kaohsiung Veterans General Hospital, Kaohsiung, Taiwan
Aging and Health Research Center, National Yang Ming University, Taipei, Taiwan
Department of Family Medicine, Kaohsiung Veterans General Hospital, Kaohsiung, Taiwan

Ti Lu
Department of Psychiatry, Kaohsiung Veterans General Hospital, Kaohsiung, Taiwan

Chien-Jen Hsu
Department of Orthopaedics, Kaohsiung Veterans General Hospital, Kaohsiung, Taiwan

Liang-Kung Chen
Aging and Health Research Center, National Yang Ming University, Taipei, Taiwan
Center for Geriatrics and Gerontology, Taipei Veterans General Hospital, Taipei, Taiwan

Cynthia Chen, Bee Choo Tai, Angela CheongNgan and Phoon Fong
Saw Swee Hock School of Public Health, National University of Singapore, National University Health System, Singapore, Singapore

Isaac Sia
College of Public Health and Health Professions, University of Florida, Gainesville, Florida, United States of America

Hon-ming Ma
Departments of Medicine and Therapeutics, Prince of Wales Hospital, The Chinese University of Hong Kong, Hong Kong SAR, China

Shi YuJulia Tan
Yong Loo Lin School of Medicine, National University of Singapore, National University Health System, Singapore, Singapore

Kin Ming Chan
Medical Services, Ang Mo Kio Thye Hua Kwan Hospital, Singapore, Singapore

Boon Yeow Tan
Medical Services, St Luke's Hospital, Singapore, Singapore

Edward Menon
Medical Services, St Andrew's Community Hospital, Singapore, Singapore

Chye Hua Ee and Kok Keng Lee
Bright Vision Hospital, Singapore, Singapore

Yee Sien Ng
Department of Rehabilitation Medicine, Singapore General Hospital, Singapore, Singapore

Yik Ying Teo
Saw Swee Hock School of Public Health, National University of Singapore, National University Health System, Singapore, Singapore
Genome Institute of Singapore, Agency for Science, Technology, and Research, Singapore, Singapore
Graduate School for Integrative Science and Engineering, National University of Singapore, Singapore, Singapore
Department of Statistics and Applied Probability, National University of Singapore, Singapore, Singapore

Stefan Ma and Derrick Heng
Ministry of Health, Singapore, Singapore

Gerald Choon-Huat Koh
Saw Swee Hock School of Public Health, National University of Singapore, National University Health System, Singapore,Singapore

Yong Loo Lin School of Medicine, National University of Singapore, National University Health System, Singapore, Singapore

Yingyan Ma, Haiyun Liu, Lin Bai, Xun Xu and Xi Zhang
Department of Ophthalmology, Shanghai First People's Hospital, Shanghai Jiao Tong University, Shanghai, China

Xiaohua Ying and Xiaocheng Xu
School of Public Health, Fudan University, Shanghai, China

Haidong Zou
Department of Ophthalmology, Shanghai First People's Hospital, Shanghai Jiao Tong University, Shanghai, China
Shanghai Eye Disease Prevention & Treatment Center, Shanghai, China

Dzenita Smailhodzic, Carel B. Hoyng, B. Jeroen Klevering, Freekje van Asten." Johannes P. H. van de Ven, Ramon A. C. van Huet and Yara T. E. Lechanteur
Department of Ophthalmology, Radboud university medical center, Nijmegen, the Netherlands

Anna M. Blom and Frida C. Mohlin
Section of Medical Protein Chemistry, Department of Laboratory Medicine Malmo, Lund University, Malmo, Sweden

Anneke I. den Hollander1
Department of Ophthalmology, Radboud university medical center, Nijmegen, the Netherlands
Department of Human Genetics, Radboud university medical center, Nijmegen, the Netherlands

Joannes M. M. Groenewoud and Gert Jan van der Wilt
Department for Health Evidence, Radboud university medical center, Nijmegen, the Netherlands

Yuan Tian and Tos T. J. M. Berendschot
University Eye Clinic Maastricht, Maastricht, the Netherlands

Sascha Fauser
Department of Ophthalmology, University of Cologne, Cologne, Germany

Chris de Bruijn
Innomedics, Düsseldorf, Germany

Mohamed R. Daha
Department of Nephrology, Leiden University Medical Center, Leiden, the Netherlands

Wen-Ying Ting and Ming-Che Lee
Department of Chest Medicine, Taipei Veterans General Hospital, Taipei, Taiwan, R.O.C.

Shiang-Fen Huang
Division of Infectious Disease, Department of Internal Medicine, Taipei Veterans General Hospital, Taipei, Taiwan, R.O.C.
School of Medicine, National Yang-Ming University, Taipei, Taiwan, R.O.C.

Yung-Yang Lin
Institute of Clinical Medicine and Institute of Brain Science, National Yang-Ming University, Taipei, Taiwan, R.O.C.
Laboratory of Neurophysiology and Department of Neurology, Taipei Veterans General Hospital, Taipei, Taiwan, R.O.C.

Yu-Chin Lee and Wei-Juin Su
Department of Chest Medicine, Taipei Veterans General Hospital, Taipei, Taiwan, R.O.C.
School of Medicine, National Yang-Ming University, Taipei, Taiwan, R.O.C.

Jia-Yih Feng
Department of Chest Medicine, Taipei Veterans General Hospital, Taipei, Taiwan, R.O.C.
Institute of Clinical Medicine, School of Medicine, National Yang-Ming University, Taipei, Taiwan, R.O.C.

Ruth Chan and Jean Woo
Department of Medicine and Therapeutics, The Chinese University of Hong Kong, Shatin, Hong Kong

Dicken Chan
The Jockey Club School of Public Health and Primary Care, The Chinese University of Hong Kong, Shatin, Hong Kong

Yuan-Hong Jiang, Dong-Ling Tang and Hann-Chorng Kuo
Department of Urology, Buddhist Tzu Chi General Hospital and Tzu Chi University, Hualien, Taiwan

Chun-Hou Liao
Department of Urology, Cardinal Tien Hospital and School of Medicine, Fu-Jen Catholic University, New Taipei, Taiwan

Index

www.ingramcontent.com/pod-product-compliance
Lightning Source LLC
Chambersburg PA
CBHW061245190326
41458CB00011B/3589